Oxford Textbook of

Axial Spondyloarthritis

Titles in the Oxford Textbooks in Rheumatology series

Oxford Textbook of Vasculitis 3e
Edited by Gene V. Ball, Barri J. Fessler, and S. Louis Bridges, Jr.

Oxford Textbook of Clinical and Biochemical Disorders of the Skeleton
By Roger Smith and Paul Wordsworth

Oxford Textbook of Axial Spondyloarthritis
Edited by Robert D. Inman and Joachim Sieper

Oxford Textbook of Osteoarthritis and Crystal Arthropathy 3e (*forthcoming*)
Edited by Michael Doherty, Nigel Arden, Hans Bijlsma, David Hunter, and Nicola Dalbeth

Oxford Textbook of Psoriatic Arthritis (*forthcoming*)
Edited by Oliver Fitzgerald and Dafna Gladman

Oxford Textbook of

Axial Spondyloarthritis

Titles in the Oxford Textbooks in Rheumatology series

Oxford Textbook of Vasculitis 3e
Edited by Gene V. Ball, Barri J. Fessler, and S. Louis Bridges, Jr.

Oxford Textbook of Clinical and Biochemical Disorders of the Skeleton
By Roger Smith and Paul Wordsworth

Oxford Textbook of Axial Spondyloarthritis
Edited by Robert D. Inman and Joachim Sieper

Oxford Textbook of Osteoarthritis and Crystal Arthropathy 3e (*forthcoming*)
Edited by Michael Doherty, Nigel Arden, Hans Bijlsma, David Hunter, and Nicola Dalbeth

Oxford Textbook of Psoriatic Arthritis (*forthcoming*)
Edited by Oliver Fitzgerald and Dafna Gladman

Oxford Textbook of
Axial Spondyloarthritis

Edited by

Robert D. Inman

Director Spondylitis Program,
University Health Network,
Professor of Medicine and Immunology,
University of Toronto
Toronto, Canada

Joachim Sieper

Medical Department I, Rheumatology,
Charite University Hospital, Campus Benjamin Franklin
Berlin, Germany

OXFORD
UNIVERSITY PRESS

OXFORD
UNIVERSITY PRESS

Great Clarendon Street, Oxford, OX2 6DP,
United Kingdom

Oxford University Press is a department of the University of Oxford.
It furthers the University's objective of excellence in research, scholarship,
and education by publishing worldwide. Oxford is a registered trade mark of
Oxford University Press in the UK and in certain other countries

First Edition published in 2016
Impression: 1

Published in the United States of America by Oxford University Press
198 Madison Avenue, New York, NY 10016, United States of America

British Library Cataloguing in Publication Data
Data available

Library of Congress Control Number: 2016937493

ISBN 978–0–19–873444–4

We are pleased to dedicate this book to all those around the world living with axial spondyloarthritis, whom it is a privilege to care for, and from whom the clinicians and researchers contributing to this text continue to draw inspiration.

We also take the opportunity to dedicate this work to our wives Straughn and Inge, for their love, patience, and support throughout our careers.

Rob Inman
Joachim Sieper

Preface

It is particularly timely that a multidisciplinary and multinational team of experts come together for a major textbook on axial spondyloarthritis (axSpA).

The conceptual framework of the disease itself has evolved beyond ankylosing spondylitis (AS) to encompass a broader concept of axial inflammation. AS was originally anchored in the demonstration of damage in the sacroiliac joints on pelvic X-rays, but that always left excluded those patients with inflammatory back pain who had not developed radiographic sacroiliitis. The advent of magnetic resonance imaging and the utility of a combination of clinical and laboratory parameters have contributed substantially to the clinical recognition of this non-radiographic form of axSpA. Earlier recognition has opened the door to earlier intervention.

The understanding of the biologic basis of axSpA has also seen significant advances in recent years. While the familial nature of axSpA was recognized for centuries, the discovery of the HLA-B27 relationship in 1973 coincided with the advent of a revolution in genetics with the development of new techniques in molecular biology. The era of genome-wide association studies has laid the groundwork for the discovery of over 40 additional genes, beyond HLA-B27, which confer susceptibility to axSpA. Concurrently, techniques applied to defining the immune response have seen dramatic advances in immunophenotyping human diseases. Microarray analysis of gene expression and flow cytometry with the capacity to stain for a wide array of surface proteins have led to an appreciation of new cytokines which contribute to the inflammation of axSpA. Subsets of immune cells of unanticipated diversity—innate lymphoid cells, mucosa-associated invariant T cells, Th17 cell subsets—have been discovered with these newer techniques, and are now shining new light on the pathogenesis of axSpA.

However, it is the rapidity of the translation of these immunological insights into therapeutics that has constituted a sea change in this disease. From therapeutic options limited to non-steroidal anti-inflammatory drugs (NSAIDs) and analgesics just 20 years ago, there is now a range of monoclonal antibodies targeting a rapidly expanding list of proinflammatory cytokines which includes TNF, IL-17, and IL-23. It is increasingly realistic to achieve symptomatic control of the disease and its progression through the timely introduction of biologic therapies. Above all, this has provided hope to patients around the world for whom the diagnosis used to mean an inexorable course of chronic pain and increasing disability. This has been achieved through the partnerships reflected in the breadth of expertise among the authors of this text—genetics, molecular biology, immunology, epidemiology, and clinics—on the part of researchers and clinicians. Furthermore, perhaps most critically has been the active involvement of patients themselves in this journey of discovery. It is they who ultimately will be the beneficiaries of the new knowledge described in this book.

Contents

List of contributors *xi*

Symbols and abbreviations *xiii*

1 **Spondyloarthritis in antiquity and in history** *1*
Bruce Rothschild and Ernst Feldtkeller

2 **Epidemiology of axial spondyloarthritis** *13*
Lianne Gensler, Michael Weisman, and Liron Caplan

3 **Diagnosis and classification of axial spondyloarthritis** *19*
Floris van Gaalen, Désirée van der Heijde, and Maxime Dougados

4 **Diagnosis, classification, and management of peripheral spondyloarthritis** *29*
Martin Rudwaleit and Atul Deodhar

5 **Genetics of spondyloarthritis** *37*
Matthew A. Brown and John Reveille

6 **Immune mechanisms: HLA-B27** *45*
Robert A. Colbert and Paul Bowness

7 **Immune mechanisms: innate immunity** *53*
Troy Noordenbos and Dominique Baeten

8 **Immune mechanisms: adaptive immunity** *63*
Maxime Breban and Hill Gaston

9 **Infection and spondyloarthritis** *71*
Marjatta Leirisalo-Repo and John D. Carter

10 **Pathology: bone** *81*
Rik J. Lories and Georg Schett

11 **Clinical features** *91*
Muhammad Asim Khan

12 **Clinical outcomes** *101*
Astrid van Tubergen and Robert Landewé

13 **Imaging: sacroiliac joints** *111*
Walter P. Maksymowych and Robert G.W. Lambert

14 **Imaging: spine** *123*
Xenofon Baraliakos and Kay-Geert A. Hermann

15 **Juvenile-onset spondyloarthritis** *133*
Ruben Burgos-Vargas and Shirley M.L. Tse

16 **Extra-articular manifestations: uveitis** *145*
James T. Rosenbaum

17 **Extra-articular manifestations: inflammatory bowel disease** *151*
Dirk Elewaut, Heleen Cypers, Matthew L. Stoll, and Charles O. Elson

18 **Extra-articular manifestations: psoriasis** *167*
Wolf-Henning Boehncke and Dafna D. Gladman

19 **Non-pharmacological management in axial spondyloarthritis** *175*
Laura Passalent and Salih Ozgocmen

20 **Treatment: NSAIDs** *189*
Jonathan Chan and Nigil Haroon

21 **Treatment: DMARDs** *199*
Denis Poddubnyy and Hildrun Haibel

22 **Treatment: biologics** *203*
Juergen Braun and Irene E. van der Horst-Bruinsma

23 **Treatment: spinal surgery** *213*
Heinrich Boehm and Y. Raja Rampersaud

24 **Patient registries** *229*
Elisabeth Lie, Tore Kristian Kvien, and Mikkel Østergaard

25 **Cost-of-illness and economic evaluations in axial spondyloarthritis** *239*
Annelies Boonen

26 **Physical functioning and work ability** *251*
Michael M. Ward

27 **Patient support and advocacy** *259*
Seoirse Smith and Laurie M. Savage

28 **Axial spondyloarthritis in Asia** *267*
Huji Xu, Feng Huang, Chan-Bum Choi, and Tae-Hwan Kim

29 **Axial spondyloarthritis in Latin America** *277*
Percival Sampaio-Barros and Rafael Valle-Oñate

30 **Axial spondyloarthritis in India** *285*
Anand Malaviya and Ashok Kumar

Index *299*

List of contributors

Dominique Baeten, Department of Clinical Immunology and Rheumatology, Academic Medical Center/University of Amsterdam, Amsterdam, The Netherlands

Xenofon Baraliakos, Rheumazentrum Ruhrgebiet, Ruhr-University Bochum, Herne, Germany

Heinrich Boehm, Klinik fuer Wirbelsaeulenchirurgie, Zentralklinik Bad Berka, Germany

Wolf-Henning Boehncke, Division of Dermatology and Venerology, Geneva University Hospital, Geneva, Switzerland, and Department of Pathology and Immunology, University of Geneva

Annelies Boonen, Department of Internal Medicine, Division of Rheumatology, Maastricht University Medical Center, The Netherlands, and Caphri Research School, Maastricht University, Maastricht, The Netherlands

Paul Bowness, Professor of Experimental Rheumatology, Nuffield Department of Orthopaedics, Rheumatology and Musculoskeletal Sciences, University of Oxford, Oxford, UK

Juergen Braun, Rheumazentrum Ruhrgebiet, Herne, Ruhr-University Bochum, Herne, Germany

Maxime Breban, Department of Rheumatology, Ambroise Paré Hospital, Boulogne-Billancourt, France, and Chronic Inflammation and Immune System Research Unit, NSERM UMR1173, University of Versailles-Saint-Quentin, Saint-Quentin-en-Yvelines, France

Matthew A. Brown, Institute of Health and Biomedical Innovation, Queensland University of Technology, Translational Research Institute, Brisbane, Australia

Ruben Burgos-Vargas, Department of Rheumatology, Hospital General de Mexico, Mexico City, Mexico

Liron Caplan, Department of Veterans Affairs and University of Colorado School of Medicine, Denver, Colorado, USA

John D. Carter, Department of Internal Medicine, Division of Rheumatology, University of South Florida College of Medicine, Tampa, Florida, USA

Jonathan Chan, Department of Internal Medicine, Division of Rheumatology, University of British Columbia, Vancouver, Canada

Chan-Bum Choi, Hanyang University Hospital for Rheumatic Diseases, Seoul, South Korea

Robert A. Colbert, Pediatric Translational Research Branch, National Institute of Arthritis, Musculoskeletal and Skin Diseases, National Institutes of Health, Bethesda, Maryland, USA

Heleen Cypers, Department of Rheumatology, Ghent University Hospital, Ghent, Belgium, and Unit for Molecular Immunology and Inflammation, VIB Inflammation Research Center, Ghent University, Belgium

Atul Deodhar, Division of Arthritis and Rheumatic Diseases OP-09, Oregon Health and Science University, Portland, Oregon, USA

Maxime Dougados, Professor of Rheumatology, René Descartes University and Hôpital Cochin, Paris, France

Dirk Elewaut, Department of Rheumatology, Ghent University Hospital, Ghent, Belgium, and Unit for Molecular Immunology and Inflammation, VIB Inflammation Research Center, Ghent University, Belgium

Charles O. Elson, Department of Medicine, University of Alabama at Birmingham, Birmingham, Alabama, USA

Ernst Feldtkeller, Deutsche Vereinigung Morbus Bechterew, Munich, Germany

Floris van Gaalen, Department of Rheumatology, Leiden University Medical Center, Leiden, The Netherlands

Hill Gaston, Department of Medicine, University of Cambridge, UK

Lianne Gensler, Director, Ankylosing Spondylitis Clinic, UCSF Medical Center, San Francisco, California, USA

Dafna D. Gladman, Psoriatic Arthritis Program, Toronto Western Hospital, Canada

Hildrun Haibel, Rheumatology, Medical Department I, Charité Universitätsmedizin Berlin, Germany

Nigil Haroon, University Health Network, University of Toronto, Toronto, Ontario, Canada

Désirée van der Heijde, Department of Rheumatology, Leiden University Medical Center, Leiden, The Netherlands

Kay-Geert A. Hermann, Department of Radiology, Charité–University Medicine Berlin, Berlin, Germany

Irene E. van der Horst-Bruinsma, Department of Rheumatology, VU University Medical Centre, Amsterdam, The Netherlands

Feng Huang, Department of Rheumatology, Chinese PLA General Hospital, Beijing, China

Muhammad Asim Khan, Case Western Reserve University, Cleveland, Ohio, USA

Tae-Hwan Kim, Hanyang University Hospital for Rheumatic Diseases, Seoul, Republic of Korea

Ashok Kumar, Director and Head, Department of Rheumatology, FORTIS Hospital, Vasant Kunj, New Delhi, India

Tore Kristian Kvien, Department of Rheumatology, Diakonhjemmet Hospital, Oslo, Norway

Robert G.W. Lambert, Department of Radiology and Diagnostic Imaging, University of Alberta, Edmonton, Alberta, Canada

Robert Landewé, Department of Clinical Immunology and Rheumatology, Academic Medical Center/University of Amsterdam, The Netherlands, and Atrium Medical Center, Heerlen, The Netherlands

Marjatta Leirisalo-Repo, Professor, Helsinki University Central Hospital, Department of Medicine, Division of Rheumatology, Helsinki, Finland

Elisabeth Lie, Department of Rheumatology, Diakonhjemmet Hospital, Oslo, Norway

Rik J. Lories, Division of Rheumatology, University Hospitals Leuven, Leuven, Belgium

Walter P. Maksymowych, Department of Medicine, University of Alberta, Edmonton, Alberta, Canada

Anand Malaviya, Department of Rheumatology, ISIC Superspeciality Hospital, Vasant Kunj, New Delhi, India

Troy Noordenbos, Department of Clinical Immunology and Rheumatology, Academic Medical Center/University of Amsterdam, Amsterdam, The Netherlands

Mikkel Østergaard, Copenhagen Center for Arthritis Research, Center for Rheumatology and Spine Diseases, Rigshospitalet, Glostrup, and Department of Clinical Medicine, University of Copenhagen, Copenhagen, Denmark

Salih Ozgocmen, Department of Physical Medicine and Rehabilitation, Division of Rheumatology, Erciyes University, Faculty of Medicine, Kayseri, Turkey

Laura Passalent, Physiotherapist Practitioner, Toronto Western Hospital, University Health Network, Toronto, Ontario, Canada

Denis Poddubnyy, Rheumatology, Medical Department I, Charité Universitätsmedizin Berlin, Berlin, Germany

Y. Raja Rampersaud, Division of Orthopaedic Surgery, Arthritis Program, Toronto Western Hospital, University Health Network, Toronto, Ontario, Canada

John Reveille, University of Texas Health Science Center at Houston, Texas, USA, and MD Anderson Cancer Center, Houston, Texas, USA

James T. Rosenbaum, Casey Eye Institute, Oregon Health & Sciences University, and Legacy Devers Eye Institute, Portland, Oregon, USA

Bruce Rothschild, Professor of Medicine, Northeast Ohio Medical University, Rootstown, Ohio, USA; and Research Associate, Carnegie Museum (ICST), Pittsburgh, Pennsylvania, USA

Martin Rudwaleit, Klinikum Bielefeld, Charité University Medicine, Berlin, Germany, and Ghent University, Belgium

Percival Sampaio-Barros, Division of Rheumatology, University of São Paulo, São Paulo, Brazil

Laurie M. Savage, Spondylitis Association of America, Sherman Oaks, California, USA

Georg Schett, Department of Internal Medicine 3, University of Erlangen-Nuremberg, Erlangen, Germany

Seoirse Smith, Ankylosing Spondylitis International Federation, Dublin, Ireland, and Ankylosing Spondylitis Association of Ireland, Dublin, Ireland

Matthew L. Stoll, Department of Pediatric Rheumatology, University of Alabama at Birmingham, Birmingham, Alabama, USA

Shirley M.L. Tse, Division of Rheumatology, Department of Pediatrics, The Hospital for Sick Children, University of Toronto, Toronto, Ontario, Canada

Astrid van Tubergen, Department of Medicine, Division of Rheumatology, Maastricht University Medical Center, Maastricht, The Netherlands

Rafael Valle-Oñate, Rheumatology and Clinical Immunology Service, Military Hospital/Salud Reinun, Bogota, Colombia

Michael M. Ward, Intramural Research Program, National Institute of Arthritis and Musculoskeletal and Skin Diseases, National Institutes of Health, Bethesda, Maryland, USA

Michael Weisman, Director, Rheumatology, Cedars-Sinai Medical Center, Los Angeles, California, USA

Huji Xu, Chairman of Department of Internal Medicine, Head and Chief, Division of Rheumatology and Immunology, Changzheng Hospital, Second Military Medical University, Shanghai, China

Symbols and abbreviations

5-ASA	5-aminosalicylic acid
6-MWT	6-minute walking test
AAA	atlantoaxial ankylosis
AAS	atlantoaxial subluxation
AAU	acute anterior uveitis
ACEi	angiotensin-converting enzyme inhibitor
ACR	American College of Rheumatology
ACSM	American College of Sports Medicine
AGORA	Platform of Organizations of People with Rheumatic Diseases in Southern Europe
ALS	amyotrophic lateral sclerosis
AMI	acute myocardial infarction
ANA	antinuclear antibody
AP	anteroposterior
APC	antigen-presenting cell
APS1	autoimmune polyendocrine syndrome-1
ARA	American Rheumatism Association
ARAD	Australian Rheumatology Association Database
ARB	angiotensin II receptor antagonist
ARTIS	Antirheumatic Therapies in Sweden
AS	ankylosing spondylitis
ASA	Ankylosing Spondylitis Association
ASAS	Assessment of SpondyloArthritis international Society
ASAS HI	Assessment of SpondyloArthritis international Society Health Index
ASAS-PR	ASAS partial remission
ASCEND	A Study of Cardiovascular Events in Diabetes
ASDAS	Ankylosing Spondylitis Disease Activity Score
ASIF	Ankylosing Spondylitis International Federation
ASPECT	adenovirus-mediated gene therapy with sitimagene ceradenovec followed by intravenous ganciclovir for patients with operable high-grade glioma
ASQoL	Ankylosing Spondylitis Quality of Life Questionnaire
aTNF	tumour-necrosis-factor antagonists
axSpA	axial spondyloarthritis
BAFF	B-cell activation factor
BASDAI	Bath Ankylosing Spondylitis Disease Activity Index
BASFI	Bath Ankylosing Spondylitis Functional Index
BASMI	Bath Ankylosing Spondylitis Metrology Index
BASRI	Bath Ankylosing Spondylitis Radiographic Index
BCR	B cell receptor
BEI	Berlin Enthesitis Index
κ2m	beta 2-microglobulin
BID	twice a day
BIOBADASER	Base de Datos de Productos Biológicos de la Sociedad Española de Reumatología
BiP	binding immunoglobulin protein
BMD	bone mineral density
BME	bone marrow oedema
BMP	bone morphogenetic protein
BP	years before present
BSRBR	British Society for Rheumatology Biologics Registry
CAM	complementary and alternative medicine
CARD9	caspase recruitment domain-containing protein 9
CASPAR	Classification of Psoriatic Arthritis
CCP	cyclic citrullinated peptide
CCR	Canadian C-spine Rule
CD	Crohn's disease
CDAI	Crohn's Disease Activity Index
CDC	Centers for Disease Control and Prevention
CES	cauda equina syndrome
CEUS	contrast-enhanced ultrasound
CF	cystic fibrosis
CHEERS	Consolidated Health Economic Evaluation Reporting Standards
CHOP	C/EBP homologous protein
CIA	collagen-induced arthritis
CiReA	Chlamydia-induced ReA
CLASS	Celecoxib Long-term Arthritis Safety Study
CME	continuing medical education
CNV	copy number variant
COI	cost-of-illness
COPCORD	Community Orientated Program for the Control of Rheumatic Diseases
COX	cyclooxygenase
CPPD	calcium pyrophosphate deposition disease
CR	conventional X-ray
CRP	C-reactive protein

CS	corticosteroids
CT	computed tomography
CTLA	cytotoxic T lymphocyte antigen
CTLSO	cervical or thoracic-lumbar-sacral orthosis
CVD	cardiovascular disease
Cys	cysteine
Cys67	cysteine residue at position 67
DANBIO	Danish Registry for Biologic Therapies in Rheumatology
DC	dendritic cell
DC-ART	disease-controlling antirheumatic treatment
DES	discrete event simulation
DESIR	Devenir des Spondyloarthropathies Indifférenciées Récentes
DFI	Dougados Functional Index
DIP	distal interphalangeal
DISH	diffuse idiopathic skeletal hyperostosis
DISH	diffuse idiopathic skeletal hyperostosis
DITRA	deficiency of interleukin thirty-six receptor antagonist
DLQI	Dermatology Life Quality Index
DLS	dorsal lordosating spondylodesis
DMARD	disease-modifying antirheumatic drug
DPYD	deoxypyridinoline
DVMB	Deutsche Vereinigung Morbus Bechterew
DZ	dizygotic
EAE	experimental autoimmune encephalomyelitis
EAM	extra-articular manifestation
EASi-QoL	Evaluation of Ankylosing Spondylitis Quality of Life
EC	European Community
EDASMI	Edmonton Ankylosing Spondylitis Metrology Index
EEN	exclusive enteral nutrition
EFCCA	European Federation of Crohn's and Ulcerative Colitis Associations
EHR	electronic health record
ELISA	enzyme-linked immunosorbent assay
EM	electron microscope
EMA	European Medicines Agency
EMT	emergency medical technician
ENRADAS	Effects of Non-Steroidal Anti-Inflammatory Drugs on Radiographic Damage in Ankylosing Spondylitis
EQ-5D	European Quality of Life 5 Dimensions Questionnaire
ER	endoplasmic reticulum
ERA	enthesitis-related arthritis
ERAD	endoplasmic reticulum-associated degradation
ERAP	endoplasmic reticulum aminopeptidase
ERASURE	Efficacy of Response and Safety of Two Fixed Secukinumab Regimens in Psoriasis
ES	effect sizes
ESR	erythrocyte sedimentation rate
ESSG	European Spondylarthropathy Study Group
ESTHER	Evidence-based Stimulation Trial with Human rFSH in Europe and Rest of World
eSUN	Spondylitis Update Newsletter
ETN	etanercept
EULAR	European League Against Rheumatism
FABERE	flexion, abduction, external rotation, and extension
FC	flow cytometry
FDA	US Food and Drug Administration
FGF	fibroblast growth factor
FHC	free heavy chains
FIXTURE	Full Year Investigative Examination of Secukinumab versus Etanercept Using Two Dosing Regimens to Determine Efficacy in Psoriasis
FMF	Familial Mediterranean Fever
FMT	faecal microbial transplantation
FY	fiscal year
GC	glucocorticoid
Gd	gadolinium
GDP	gross domestic product
GE	gradient echo
GESPIC	German Spondyloarthritis Inception Cohort
GHI	Global Hunger Index
GI	gastrointestinal
GINA	Genetic Information Non-Discrimination Act
Glu	glutamic acid
GP	general practitioner
GPR	global posture re-education
GRAPPA	Group for Research and Assessment of Psoriasis and Psoriatic Arthritis
GRP78	glucose-regulated protein 78 kDa
GWAS	genome-wide association studies
H2RA	high-dose histamine 2 receptor antagonist
HAQ	Health Assessment Questionnaire
HBV	hepatitis B virus
HCA	human capital productivity cost
HIRA	Health Insurance Review and Assessment Service
HLA-B27	human leukocyte antigen B27
HNF4A	hepatocyte nuclear factor 4 alpha
HR	hazard ratio
HRCT	high-resolution computed tomography
HRQoL	Health-Related Quality of Life
HS	hidradenitis suppurativa
HUNT	Nord-Trøndelag Health Study
hκ2m	human beta 2-microglobulin
IBD	inflammatory bowel disease
IBP	inflammatory back pain
ICD	International Classification of Disease
iCER	incremental cost-effectiveness ratio
ICF	International Classification of Functioning, Disability, and Health
ICOS	inducible co-stimulatory molecule
ICOSLG	inducible T-cell co-stimulator ligand
iCUR	incremental cost-utility ratio
IFN	interferon
IFPA	International Federation of Psoriasis Associations
Ig	immunoglobulin
IgG1κ	human immunoglobulin G1κ
IGRA	interferon-gamma release assay
IHD	ischaemic heart disease

IHH	Indian hedgehog
IHR	internal rotation of the hip
IL	interleukin
IL-23R	interleukin-23 receptor
ILAR	International League of Associations for Rheumatology
ILC	innate lymphoid cell
IMD	intermalleolar distance
IMID	immune-mediated inflammatory disease
IMS-ELISA	immunomagnetic separation and enzyme-linked immunosorbent assay
INFAST	Infliximab for Treatment of Axial Spondyloarthritis
iNKT	innate natural killer T
INSPIRE	International Spondyloarthritis Inter-Observer Reliability Exercise
IP	interphalangeal
IPTW	inverse probability of treatment weighting
IRA	Indian Rheumatology Association
ISG	Indian Society of Gastroenterology
JAK	janus kinase
JIA	juvenile idiopathic arthritis
JoSpA	juvenile-onset spondyloarthritis
KIR	killer immunoglobulin receptor
Kp	*Klebsiella pneumoniae*
LBP	lipopolysaccharide binding protein
LCE	late cornified envelope
LDQ	Leeds Disability Questionnaire
LEI	Leeds Enthesitis Index
LFN	leflunomide
LILRB4	leukocyte immunoglobulin-like receptor, subfamily B, member 4
LMP2	low molecular weight protein 2
LPS	lipopolysaccharide
LR	likelihood ratio
LTBI	latent tuberculosis infection
MACE	major adverse cardiac events
MADCAM	mucosal addressin cell adhesion molecule
MAIT	mucosal-associated invariant T
MASES	Maastricht Ankylosing Spondylitis Enthesitis Score
MCID	minimal clinically important difference
MCP-1	monocyte chemoattractant protein-1
MCS	Mental Component Score
M-CSF	macrophage colony stimulating factor
MDP	muramyl dipeptide
MEI	Mander Enthesitis Index
MHC	major histocompatibility complex
MIC	macrophage inhibitory cytokine
MICA	major histocompatibility complex class I chain-related gene A
MID	minimal important difference
miDVO-R	minimally invasive dorso-ventral osteotomy and reconstruction
MMP	matrix metalloproteinase
mNY	modified New York
MP	methylprednisolone
MPR	medical possession rate
MRI	magnetic resonance imaging

MRP	myeloid-related protein
MS	multiple sclerosis
mSASSS	modified Stoke Ankylosing Spondylitis Spinal Score
MTP	metatarsophalangeal
MTX	methotrexate
MyD88	myeloid differentiation factor
MZ	monozygotic
NAPSI	Nail Psoriasis Severity Index
NASC	North American Spondylitis Consortium
NASS	National Ankylosing Spondylitis Society
NFκB	nuclear factor κB
NHANE	National Health and Nutrition Examination Survey
NHIS	National Health Interview Survey
NIAMS	National Institute of Arthritis and Musculoskeletal and Skin Diseases
NIH	National Institutes of Health
NK	natural killer
NOD	nucleotide oligomerization domain
NOR-DMARD	Norwegian Disease-Modifying Antirheumatic Drug Register
nr-axSpA	non-radiographic axial spondyloarthritis
NRS	numerical rating scale
NSAID	non-steroidal anti-inflammatory drug
NSAR	non-steroidal antirheumatic
NTM	non-tuberculous mycobacteria
OASIS	Outcome in Ankylosing Spondylitis International Study
OCI	osteitis condensans ilii
OMERACT	Outcome Measures in Rheumatology Clinical Trials
Omp	outer membrane protein
OPG	osteoprotegerin
OR	odds ratio
ORMDL3	orosomucoid-like 3
OSKAR	Observation Study of Spondyloarthropathy Registry
OVMB	Österreichische Vereinigung Morbus Bechterew
OWD	occiput-to-wall distance
P	position
PA	postero-anterior
pANCA	peripheral antineutrophil cytoplasmic antibodies
PARE	People with Arthritis and Rheumatism
PASI	Psoriasis Area and Severity Index
PCR	polymerase chain reaction
PCS	Physical Component Score
PEERS	People Educated and Empowered to Rise above Spondylitis
PET	positron emission tomography
PGA	Physician Global Assessment
PGE2	prostaglandin E2
PIP	proximal interphalangeal
PIR	paired immunoglobulin receptor
PPI	proton pump inhibitor
PPM1A	protein phosphatase magnesium-dependent 1A
PROMIS	Patient-Reported Outcome Measurement Information System

PRR	pattern recognition receptor
PsA	psoriatic arthritis
PSO	pedicle subtraction osteotomy
PSOAS	Prospective Study of Outcomes in Ankylosing Spondylitis
PSORS	psoriasis susceptibility locus
PSpARC40	peripheral spondyloarthritis response criterion 40
PTGER	prostaglandin E receptor
PTGS	prostaglandin endoperoxide synthase
PTHrP	parathyroid hormone-related protein
PULSAR	Program to Understand the Longterm Outcomes in Spondyloarthritis
PY	person years
PYD	pyridinoline
QALY	quality-adjusted life years
QID	four times a day
RA	rheumatoid arthritis
RANKL	receptor activator of nuclear factor κB ligand
RASSS	Radiographic Ankylosing Spondylitis Spinal Score
r-axSpA	radiographic axial spondyloarthritis
RBE	Registro Brasileiro de Espondiloartrites
RDCI	Rheumatic Diseases Comorbidity Index
ReA	reactive arthritis
REGISPONSER	Registro Español de Espondiloartritis de la Sociedad Española de Reumatologia
RESPONDIA	Registro Ibero-Americano de Espondiloartrites
RF	rheumatoid factor
ROB-FIN	Register of Biologic Treatment in Finland
ROR-γt	receptor orphan receptor γt
RR	relative risk
RT	real-time
RUNX	runt-related transcription factor
SAA	Spondylitis Association of America
SAPHO	synovitis, acne, pustulosis, hyperostosis, and osteitis
SCI	Science Citation Index
SCQM	Swiss Clinical Quality Management
SD	standard deviation
SDD	smallest detectable difference
sDMARD	synthetic disease-modifying antirheumatic drug
SE	spin echo
SEC	secukinumab
SF-36	36-item Short-Form Health Survey
SFB	segmented filamentous bacteria
SFI	San Francisco Enthesitis Index
SI	sacroiliac
SIR	standardized incidence ratio
SIRAS	Scotland Registry for Ankylosing Spondylitis
SLE	systemic lupus erythematosus
SMARD	symptom-modifying antirheumatic drug
SNP	single nucleotide polymorphism
SpA	spondyloarthritis
SPACE	Spondyloarthritis Caught Early
SPARCC	Spondyloarthritis Research Consortium of Canada
SPARTAN	Spondyloarthritis Research and Treatment Network
SPF	specific pathogen-free
SPO	Smith-Petersen osteotomy
SSA	seronegative spondarthritis
SSATG	South Swedish Arthritis Treatment Group
SSS	Sacroiliac Joint Structural Score
SSZ	sulfasalazine
STAT3	signal transducer and activator of transcription 3
STIR	short tau inversion recovery
sTNF	soluble tumour necrosis factor
STURE	Stockholm TNF Uppfölgnings Registry
SUN	Standardization of Uveitis Nomenclature
SWIFT	Spondylitis Web Info for Teens
T1FS	T1 fat saturated
T1W	T1-weighted
T2FS	T2 fat saturated
T2W	T2-weighted
TAP	transporter associated with antigen processing
TASC	The Australo-Anglo-American Spondylitis Consortium
TB	tuberculosis
Tc1	type 1 cytotoxic T
TCM	traditional Chinese medicine
TCR	T cell receptor
TENS	transcutaneous electrical nerve stimulation
TGF-β1	transforming growth factor-beta 1
TICOPA	Tight Control of Psoriatic Arthritis
TIRM	turbo inversion recovery magnitude
TLR	Toll-like receptor
TLSO	thoracic-lumbar-sacral orthosis
tmTNF	transmembrane tumour necrosis factor
TNF	tumour necrosis factor
TNFi	tumour necrosis factor inhibitor
TNFRSF1A	tumour necrosis factor receptor superfamily member 1A
TRAP	tartrate-resistant acid phosphatase
TRAPS	tumour necrosis factor-receptor-associated periodic syndrome
Treg	regulatory T
TWD	tragus-to-wall distance
TWEAK	tumour necrosis factor-like weak inducer of apoptosis
UC	ulcerative colitis
UPR	unfolded protein response
US	ultrasound
uSpA	undifferentiated spondyloarthritis
UST	ustekinumab
VAS	visual analogue scale
VCAM	vascular cell adhesion molecule
WALS	Workplace Activity Limitations Scale
WHO	World Health Organization
WLQ-25	Work Limitations Questionnaire
WPAI	Work Productivity and Activity Impairment
WPS-RA	Rheumatoid Arthritis Specific Work Productivity Survey
XBP-1	X-box binding protein 1

CHAPTER 1

Spondyloarthritis in antiquity and in history

Bruce Rothschild and Ernst Feldtkeller

Spinal ankylosis in palaeontological fossils

Past evaluation had difficulty determining whether ankylosed vertebrae were caused by inflammation, degeneration, or trauma. We therefore limit discussion to those cases/series wherein diagnosis is verified with current criteria.

One of the earliest reviews of this topic was written by Zorab (1), citing isolated cases in cave bear, sheep, Egyptian oxen, and sacred monkeys, *Bos indicus* from India, the monk seal *Monachus monachus*, a late-seventeenth-century church burial, and in mummies from the Roman period (30 BC), in neolithic Sweden, and in the Medici family. This chapter expands on his insightful commentary.

Spondyloarthropathy, with 1–8% prevalence in ancient human populations, is found as early as the Permian period (270–225 million years ago) (2). It is certainly the oldest non-infectious skeletal disease. Rheumatoid arthritis (RA) does not appear in the skeletal record until the Holocene period (6500 years ago) (3). The earliest case of gout was apparently in the Cretaceous period (135–65 million years ago), in *Tyrannosaurus rex* (4). Infection of bone (osteomyelitis) or of joints (septic arthritis) is poorly represented in the palaeontological record.

The differential diagnosis of axial spondyloarthropathy (axSpA) includes such entities as diffuse idiopathic skeletal hyperostosis (DISH), hypervitaminosis A, fluorosis, infectious spondylitis, fusions related to healing of traumatic damage, and congenital disease (5, 6).

The issue is even more complicated as calcium pyrophosphate deposition disease (CPPD) is thought to produce calcification of the anulus fibrosus (7–13). It is unclear whether that is an intrinsic characteristic of CPPD, or the co-occurrence with spondyloarthropathy. Study of the Komodo dragon (which has clear and separate evidence of both diseases) suggests the latter, as CPPD complicates 50% of cases of spondyloarthropathy in *Varanus komodiensis* and does not occur in its absence (2). Distinguishing direct vertebral infection in skeletons from spondyloarthropathy is predicated on observation of infection-related resorptive damage distinctive (5).

Osteoarthritis is exceptionally rare in nature, so the chance of finding a primary case is remote, perhaps explaining its absence in the early vertebrate palaeontological record.

The contemporary zoological record

Systematic survey of mammalian families led to recognition that spondyloarthropathy was essentially pan-mammalian (4, 6, 14–26). Frequencies of 25% in bears (independent of species), 35% in rhinoceros, 6% in lamas, 5% in lions, 5–10% in marsupials, and 6% specifically in koala have been reported (Table 1.1).

Given the transmammalian nature of spondyloarthropathy, it seemed appropriate to explore its occurrence in other classes of animals. Examination of over 50,000 birds confirmed that class not to be susceptible (27), but examination of reptiles revealed a different picture (28). Spondyloarthropathy was extremely rare, except in two families, crocodylidae and varanidae. It is present in a species-specific manner, affecting 2–20% of members of the genus *Varanus* (28). The Komodo dragon *Varanus komodoiensis, Varanus salvadorii*, and *Varanus gouldii* were especially susceptible.

The fossil record

The phylogenetic distribution and frequency of spondyloarthropathy in contemporary animals suggested that this disease has a long history worthy of investigation in the fossil record (2, 14, 18–21, 23, 24, 26, 29). Isolated reports illustrated occurrence of spondyloarthropathy in the saber-toothed tiger *Smilodon*, the mammoth *Mammutus* (23, 29), and even in the ground sloths *Mylodon* and *Eremotherium* and armadillo-like *Glyptodon* (30). Spondyloarthropathy may even be responsible for the Höhlengicht (cave gout) designation that the eminent pathologist Rudolf Virchow used to describe afflicted cave-dwelling animals (31).

Systematic evaluation of the prevalence of disease as a population phenomenon in the fossil record is limited by the numerical representation of families (e.g. mammalian) and extinction events. Tracing the antiquity of spondyloarthropathy in the Tertiary–Quaternary record, now referred to as the Cenozoic, examines the correlation with the rise of mammals after the demise of the dinosaurs. Spondyloarthropathy was quite prevalent in mammals in the oldest Cenozoic times, the Paleocene and Eocene (38–65 years before present (YBP)). Twenty-five percent of Uintatheriidae (order Dinocerata), 12.5% of Coryphodontidae (order Pantodonta), and 13% of Brontotheridae were affected (32). It was even present (7%) in the cloven-hoofed, horse-like Chalicotheriidae in the Oligocene. Failure of these families to survive those epochs (their extinction) precludes assessment of disease time-variation. Subsequent analysis of the population prevalence of disease in slightly more recent evolutionary lines revealed geometric increase over time for primates (e.g. 4–30% for baboons), horses (1% in the Miocene to 7% today), and rhinoceros (Oligocene at 9%; Miocene 15%; Pleistocene 20%; today 35%) (15, 26). Curiously, the prevalence in some groups (elephants) did not change. Mammoths were equally

Table 1.1 Prevalence of spondyloarthropathy in mammals

Affected animals	Prevalence (%)
Ape	17–28
Old World monkey	3–20
New World monkey (in affected species)	1–4
Elephant	5–8
Horse/ass	8/21
Rhinoceros	35
Cow	27
Hog	5–25 (7 in domestic)
Goat	4–29, especially markhor
Bison	7 American; 19 European
Lama	6
Hippopotamus	10–20
Dog-like canids (in affected species)	1–40
Fox	0 (except Fennec fox 18)
Hyaena	17
Bears	25
Large/small cats	1–4/0–25
Racoon	2
Rabbit	0
Porcupine	2 American; 11 European
Dolphin	7–15
Anteater	20
Duckbill platypus	6
Opossum	1
Kangaroo	5–10
Koala	6

affected as elephants today, although the mastodons were apparently spared (23).

Recognition of spondyloarthropathy as transmammalian led to the natural question as to how long this condition has been present. Examination of the fossil record allowed its recognition, but addressing the epidemiology of its occurrence and prevalence through time was more complex. The fossil record is somewhat compromised by the limited number of investigators able to find, extract, and identify fossils, and the incomplete nature of many of the discovered skeletons. It is often difficult to locate sufficient numbers of animals of a given species, or even genus, to allow recognition of evolution of the disease over time. By 'evolution' as used here, we mean change in population prevalence over time. The character of disease and its skeletal distribution actually are little changed over time or across phylogeny. Examination of the disease in a gorilla sample revealed an identical skeletal distribution of disease, frequency of peripheral joint fusion, and pattern of disease to that noted in affected humans. The search was most productive in the odd-toed perissodactyls, horses and rhinoceros. The prevalence in the Oligocene was 1% and 5% in horses and rhinoceros, respectively. It increased geometrically over time to the current levels of 8% and 35% (26).

Serendipitous observations in the sauropod *Camarasaurus* led to recognition of its occurrence in dinosaurs (33). Previous studies had identified DISH in this group—actually with quite high prevalence in some genera (25–50%), suggesting that it might represent a sexual ontological phenomenon in that group (34). This contrasted with the zygapophyseal joint erosions in the other sauropod with spondyloarthropathy (33). The findings were clearly distinguishable from DISH and their polyostotic character precluded the diagnosis of infectious arthropathy. Availability of sufficient dinosaur skeletons for epidemiological analysis has been even more complex than that for mammals. While the latter could be established by examination of the collections of 20 or 30 museums, dinosaur skeletons are more scattered over the world. Thus, study at present is limited to reporting distribution among dinosaur families. The latter include the Ceratopsia (horned dinosaurs such as Triceratops), orinthomimids, and possibly even *Tyrannosaurus rex* (4, 35).

Perhaps some readers are surprised that an apparently relatively low-frequency population phenomenon such as spondyloarthropathy has been recognized in dinosaurs. Perhaps the scrutiny the group receives is a factor, but the much smaller denominator for earlier organisms (low number of skeletons of most dinosaurs and early archosaurs) makes observation of that disease more impressive.

Dinosaurs were not the only ancient reptiles in which spondyloarthropathy has been recognized. Similar to contemporary crocodilians, characteristics clearly documenting the disease have been reported in Cenozoic crocodiles *Tomistoma dowsoni* and *Leidyosuchus formidabilis* (36, 37). Witzmann et al. (38) reported occurrence in the Late Triassic (220 million years ago) in the phytosaur '*Angistorhinopsis ruetimeyeri*'. Dinosaurs were not the only reptiles of the Mesozoic period. Marine reptiles were also present and at least one family was affected (28).

Since spondyloarthropathy was clearly present in dinosaurs, the next question was: how early is the disease identifiable? Thus, study of the Permian fossil record has been pursued, revealing the presence of spondyloarthropathy in the sail-backed reptile *Dimetrodon* and the less commonly known ancient reptiles *Diadectes* and *Ctenorhachis*. These pre-date recognition of the disease in an early Triassic reptile (Fig. 1.1) (39).

Human spondyloarthritis in archaeological excavations

Isolated reports compatible with our diagnostic of spondyloarthritis (SpA) are well represented in the human skeletal disease literature (1, 40–45). This contrasts with more informative population studies which are rare (42). The prevalence of SpA in ancient human populations clearly has a sanitation signature (46), identifying faecal–oral contamination opportunities.

The first clinical description of SpA in North America was by Jayson (47). New World penetrance of the disease, however, antedated this observation by many millennia (48, 49). Spondyloarthritis has extensive representation in the human skeletal record of North America, but South America is less well studied. Arriaza (50) reported 7% prevalence in 4000 YBP Chile. The oldest North American case is dated at 5000–8000 YBP (51). The 4.6% prevalence in the Late Archaic, Frontenac Island site is statistically

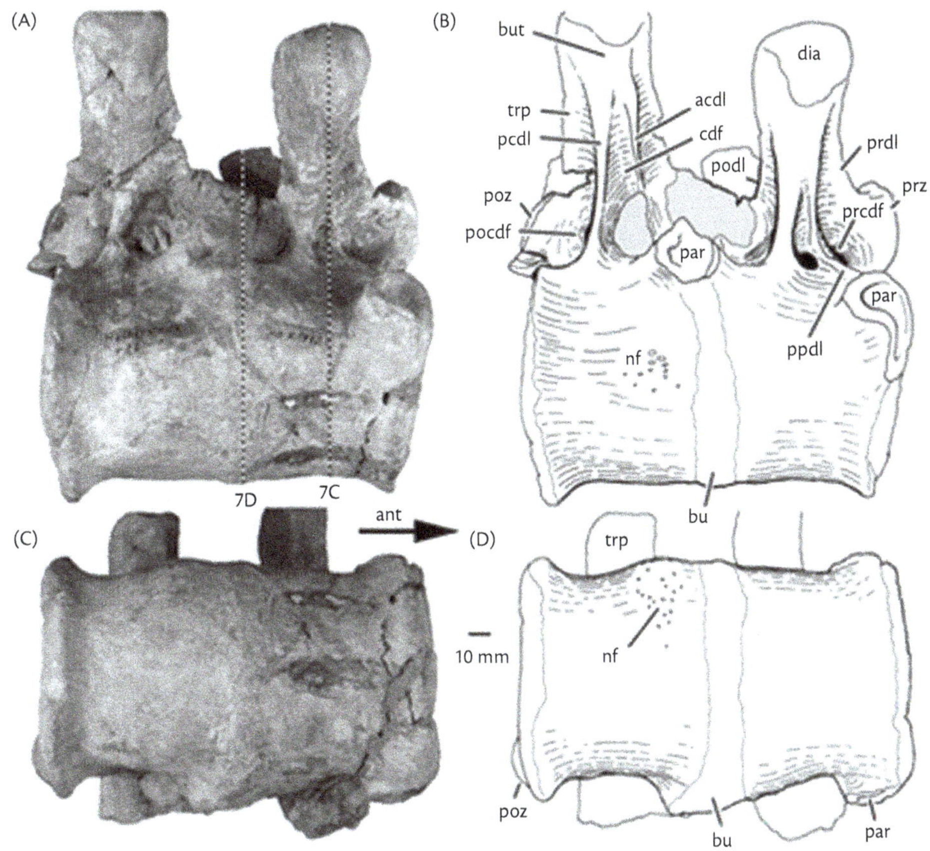

Fig. 1.1 (See colour plate section). Fused thoracic segment of *Phytosauria indet* from the Late Triassic of Halberstadt. (A, B) Right lateral view; (C, D) ventral view. Witzmann F, Schwarz-Wings D, Hampe O, Fritsch G, Asbach P 2014: Evidence of Spondyloarthropathy in the Spine of a Phytosaur (Reptilia: Archosauriformes) from the Late Triassic of Halberstadt, Germany. Plos One 9:e85511.

indistinguishable (Chi square = 0.09) from the 5.4% found in the early-twentieth-century New York Highland Park site. Noting the latter's problematic sanitation (52, 53) and infectious diarrhoea initiation of at least some forms of SpA (5), the prevalence of SpA in such populations may be explained. This perspective is confirmed by study of eastern and western gorilla and chimpanzee. The geographically disparate gorillas and chimpanzee subspecies had indistinguishable spondyloarthropathy prevalence, but presented with different patterns of disease (16, 17). The latter pauci and polyarticular patterns correlated with specific infectious agents known to cause the disease. The prevalence (49) of SpA in skeletal populations dated from 4700 to 400 YBP (Table 1.2) and ranged from 0.7% to 5.1% (49), independent of genetic relationships, time (Chi square = 2.30, NS), and geography (Fisher's exact test $p = 0.066$).

Old World spondyloarthritis

Well documented (1, 54–57), mostly European reports of SpA appear to represent isolated cases, with accurate prevalence information unavailable to date. It is difficult to assess literature reports of SpA. Some have suggested the presence of ankylosing spondylitis (AS) in pharaohs of the eighteenth and nineteenth dynasties of Old Egypt: Amenhotep (Amenophis) II, Ramses II ('the Great', Fig. 1.2), and his son Merenptah (58, 59). Chhem et al. (60) as well as Saleem and Hawass (61), who took computer tomographs of the royal mummies, suggested that Rameses II and other pharaohs actually had

Table 1.2 Prevalence of SpA in North American archaeological excavations

Provenance (BP)	Site	Prevalence (%)
<3000	Frontenac Island, New York	4.6
	Ala-307, California	0.7
	Sci-1, California	1.5
2000	Klunk Mound, Illinois	1.8
	CCo-295, California	1.3
	Kodiak Island, Alaska	0.8
>1000	4 Counties, Wisconsin	0.7
	Madisonville, Ohio	4.0
	Dickson Mound, Illinois	4.1
	Pueblo Bonito, New Mexico	3.0
	Pueblo San Cristobal, New Mexico	2.2
>500	Hardin Village, Kentucky	0.9
	Kuaua Mound, New Mexico	1.5
	Pottery Mound, New Mexico	5.1
500	Amelia Island, Florida	2.5
	Yokem Mound, Illinois	2.3

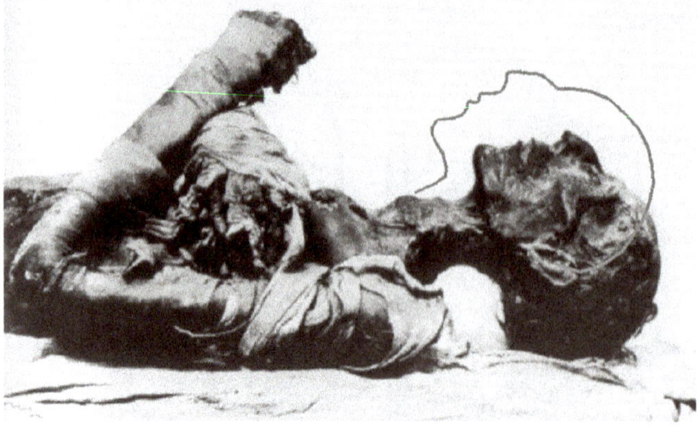

Fig. 1.2 The mummy of Ramses II 'The Great' in his sarcophagus. Additionally drawn is the head position that would result if his post-mortem fracture were rearranged correctly.
Balout L, Roubet C, Desroches-Noblecourt C 1985: La Momie de Ramsès II. Paris, Éditions Recherche sur les Civilisations.

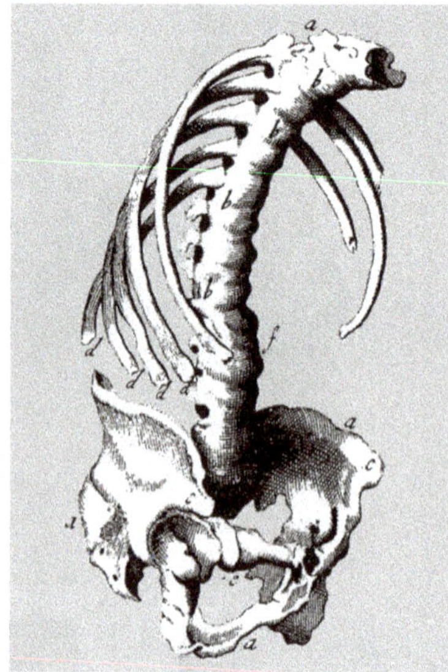

Fig. 1.3 The skeletal remains described by Bernard Connor in 1695.

DISH and concluded that AS may be—similar to RA—a relatively new disease. While the diagnosis of AS is generally ruled out when sacroiliac (SI) joints are pristine, other forms of SpA often spare those joints (46, 49). DISH actually has a history almost as long as that of spondylitis, both having been noted in early mammals and in dinosaurs (62, 63). Thus the diagnosis in pharaohs appears dependent upon one's perspective of the character of these entities.

Another famous example is the Coptic Saint Apa Bane living in the fourth century in a monastery of Middle Egypt. He slept standing, leaned upon a wall erected for him in his cell. After his death his tomb was the destination of many pilgrims. Excavations in 1992 revealed an active AS as a possible contributor to this ascetic behaviour (64).

The historical literature is even more difficult to assess, given changes in language and interpretations of the times. It is actually the correspondence between physicians that would have to be reviewed in the original language that would permit the necessary insights, and that is beyond the scope of the present discussion. Thus the suggestion that the Medici family was afflicted by SpA (65) adds to their mystique, but provides little in the way of new understanding of life and health of the times.

Two-thousand-year-old skeletons from Ein Gedi, Israel (66, 67) suggest long-standing presence in the Near East. Indeed, Ruffer (43, 55) reported the disease in 2980–2900 BCE III Dynasty Nefermaat at Meydum, and Frohlich et al. (68) reported occurrence in a third-millennium BC Hamad Town burial mound.

SpA has a long presence in northeast Africa, originally recognized by Ruffer and Rietti (69) to date back at least 3000 years. González et al. (70) reported a case of AS in Canary Island guanches (aborigines). Subsequent evaluation revealed prevalence of SpA in the Nile River west bank Semna South Meriotic Nubian site (2000–1600 YBP) at 4%, compared to 6% in the 4500-YBP northern Mali Hassi el Abiod sites and 10% of Egyptians in the Elessa/van Luschan collections of the American Museum of Natural History (63, 71).

Predecessors of spondyloarthritis research in the seventeenth to nineteenth centuries

A description of the history of AS research has been given by Buess and Koelbing (72) and—partially based on this description—by Bywaters (73). In the following, we rely essentially on these excellent descriptions, which will not be cited again.

Probably the first to describe the skeletal remains of a human with AS was Bernard Connor (1666–1698), born in Ireland. Together with other students studying anatomy in France, he came across a most unusual skeleton found in a graveyard in which the ilium and sacrum and the 15 lowest vertebrae and adjoining ribs formed one continuous bone (Fig. 1.3). The group decided that Connor should publish this extraordinary finding. Connor fully realized the importance of his discovery and reported it in three languages: in French in a letter to Sir William de Waldegrave published in 1693 (74), in Latin published in Oxford in 1695 (75), and in English in his thesis published by the Royal Society in 1695 (76). He concluded from the unification of the ribs with the spine that this deformation must have been developed already before the individual began to breathe (i.e. before birth), because a fracture never heals if it is not immobilized.

Several similar descriptions followed in the next centuries. In contrast to Connor's finding which was certainly a case of AS, diagnoses from today's perspective are often not possible. Before the ankylosis could be defined as the result of a specific disease and not as just a curiosity, a systematic comparison of many similar cases was necessary. An opportunity for such a comparison were scientific collections of pathologic-anatomic findings like that collected by John Hunter (1728–1793) in London which is today the pride of the Royal College of Surgeons of England (77), and that collected by Eduard Sandifort (1742–1814) in Leiden (78). Examples of AS can be found in both collections and in the publications by their collectors (77, 78).

In the nineteenth century, physicians tried to differentiate several diseases leading to ankylosis of the spine and to detect and treat the process in living patients. One of them was Carl Wenzel (1769–1827) in Frankfurt am Main, who published in his great monography of 1824 (79) the results of his careful studies concerning spinal diseases. He does not differentiate between inflammatory and degenerative diseases but concludes—in contrast to his contemporaries—that the cause of the ankylosis is not the result

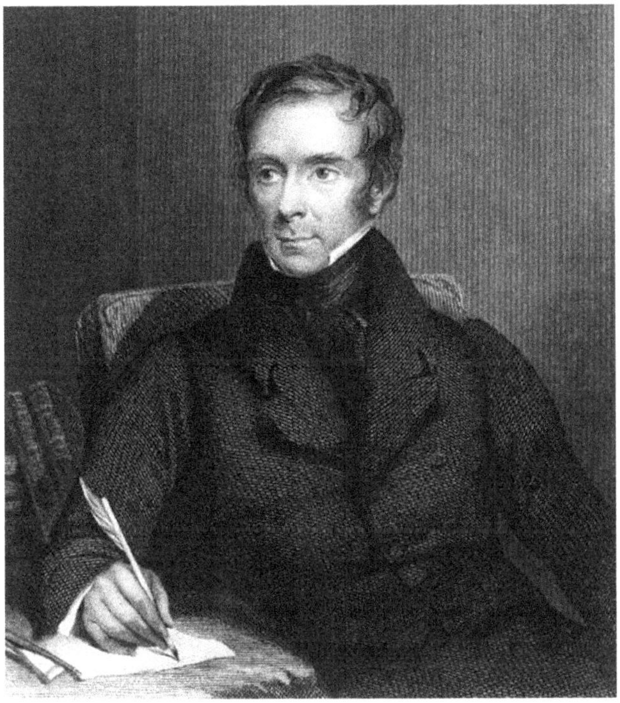

Fig. 1.4 Sir Benjamin Collins Brodie (1783–1862), surgeon in London.

of a disease in the spinal cord but a kind of hyperalimentation of bones, possibly as reaction to an inflammatory lesion of the bone.

The first clinical description of the typical presentation of AS was by Benjamin Collins Brodie (1783–1862, Fig. 1.4), a surgeon in London. In 1850, he described a patient who obviously suffered from AS with back pain and involvement of the legs (80). The disease was complicated by occasional eye inflammations of unknown nature. Brodie sees the origins of the disease as being long-lasting chronic inflammation. He reported that in patients whom he observed, the disease lasted several years and ended with complete immobility of a large part of the spine.

Charles Hilton Fagge (1838–1883), a physician at Guy's Hospital in London, was the first doctor of medicine (in contrast to surgeons) who described this nearly unknown disease in 1877 (81). Also he was the first to describe the clinical as well as the anatomical aspects of the disease and distinguished it from osteoarthritis, which was well known at the time. He left it to the future to give this new disease a name.

Meanwhile, sufficient interest in this disease had built up to allow Adolf Strümpell (1853–1925, Fig. 1.5), an internist in Leipzig, to mention the disease in his textbook of 1884 (82, 83). He cites two patients with complete ankylosis of the spine and hip joints. He was also the first to include in his textbook a photograph of a person living with AS (Fig. 1.6).

The next name is not mentioned because of essential contributions to SpA research but because in central, northern, and eastern Europe the disease is erroneously named after him: Wladimir Michailowitsch Bechterew (1857–1927). He insisted on a neurological emphasis which has since been invalidated. As Buess and Koelbing (72) succinctly put it in the French edition of their booklet: 'Bechterew sowed confusion and reaped glory'. In 1893, Bechterew (84) described five cases observed by him with a disease

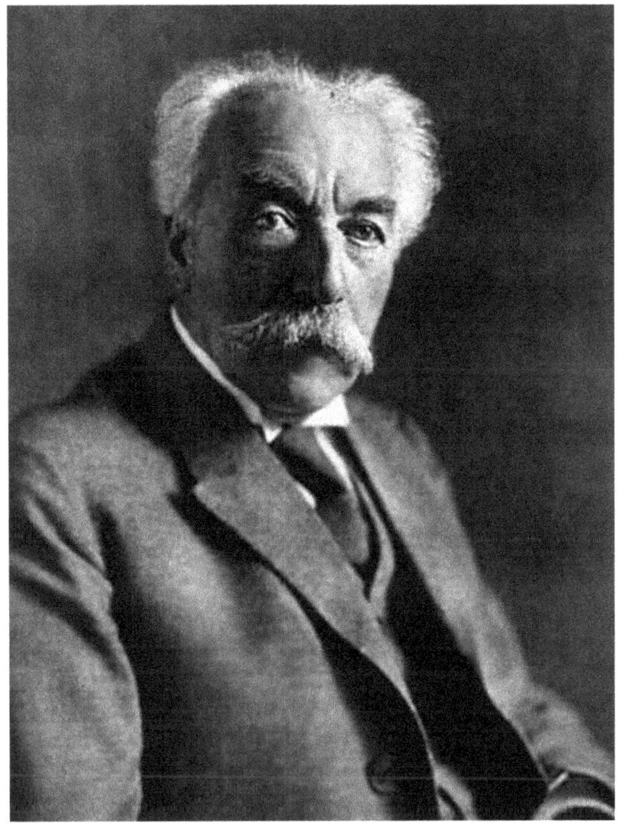

Fig. 1.5 Adolf Strümpell (1853–1925), professor of internal medicine in Leipzig.

for which he had not found any description in the neuropathologic literature, with one of them indeed suffering apparently from AS; for the two mentally ill patients, the true diagnosis remains unclear for us; the two elderly ladies, however, certainly did not have AS, but either spondylosis in connection with familiar Scheuermann's disease (85) or senile kyphosis (86, 87). For Bechterew, however, there was no doubt that all five had the same disease.

The circumstances of Bechterew's tragic death in 1927 were revealed under the *perestroika* in 1988: as Keitel (88) reports, citing Russian authors, Bechterew was asked by Stalin's treating physician, the neuropathologist professor Kramer, to visit Stalin who suffered from muscle atrophy in his left hand. During his participation at a congress in Moscow, Bechterew spent 3 hours with his difficult patient. After leaving Stalin, he mentioned his psychological impression of having talked to a paranoid patient. There followed a theatre visit and an invitation by the theatre director to a small meal. On his way back to the hotel, he complained of stomach problems and had to vomit. After medical treatment on the next day with injections by two physicians (possibly collaborating with the secret police, the GPU), Bechterew died of 'heart failure'. It is widely held that Stalin ordered his death to avoid Bechterew's diagnosis becoming known to others. The height of hypocrisy was that in 1952, still during Stalin's life, a special postage stamp (Fig. 1.7) was issued in the Soviet Union on the occasion of the 25th anniversary of the death of this famous physician.

It is Pierre Marie (1853–1940, Fig. 1.8) who is now agreed generally to have given in 1898 the most detailed and characteristic clinical description of the disease (89) which was then acknowledged

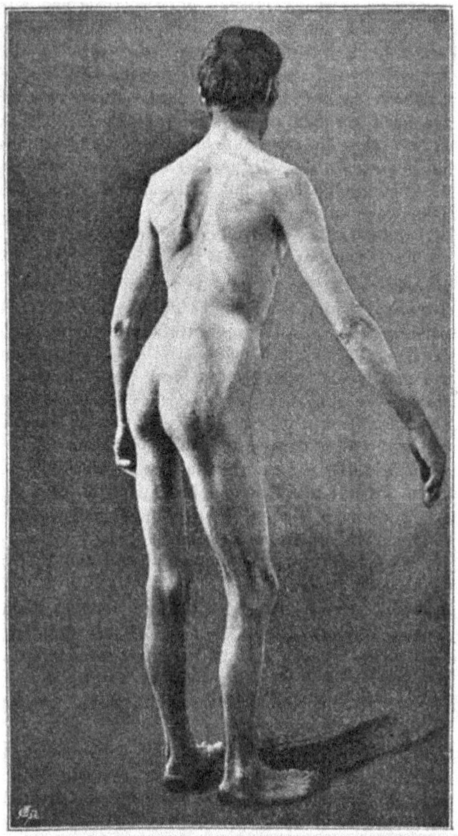

Fig. 1.6 The first published photograph of a patient with AS, published by Adolf Strümpell in 1897.

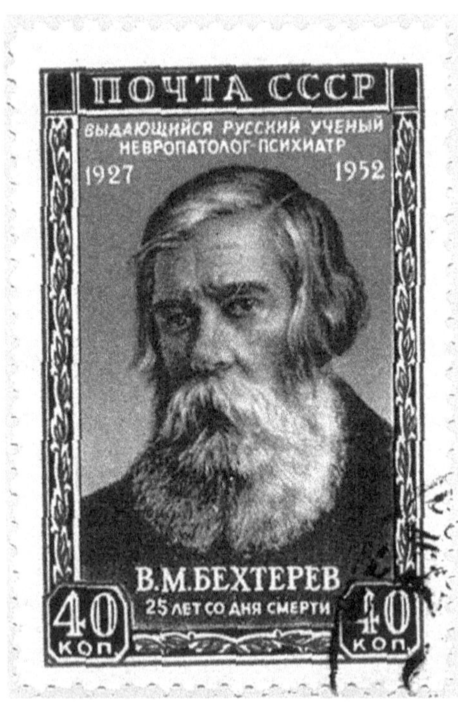

Fig. 1.7 Wladimir Michailowitsch Bechterew (1857–1927), professor of neurology and psychiatry in St Petersburg, appeared on a stamp in 1952, marking the 25th anniversary of his death.

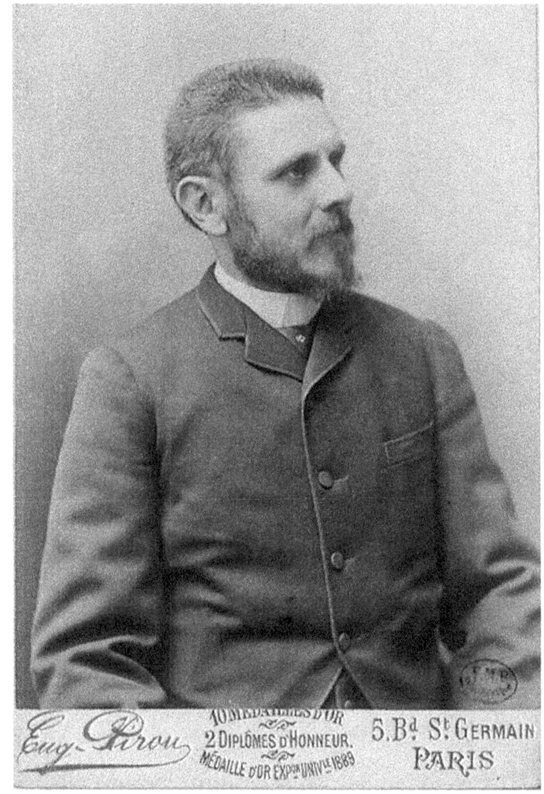

Fig. 1.8 Pierre Marie (1853–1940), professor of neurology in Paris.

as a separate disease. With his photographs (Fig. 1.9) published in 1906 (90), he characterized the variability of the kyphosis of the ankylosed spine. Marie called the disease 'spondylose rhizomélique', involving the joints at the roots (ριζα) of the limbs. He also reported the onset in early adult age with pain in the low back, with palpable bony growth (syndesmophytosis), ankylosis of the hip joints, dorsal kyphosis, limitation of chest expansion, and a development of stiffness from the lower to the upper parts of the spine. A description of his life and work was published by Michel Benoist in 1995 (91).

After dealing with the works of Strümpell and Marie, Bechterew distinguished in his autobiography (92) between a 'Morbus Bechterew' (with spinal stiffness and pronounced nervous symptoms) and a 'Morbus Strümpell–Bechterew–Marie' (with real ankylosis of the spine) (88). In simplification of this differentiation, a 'Bechterew type' of the disease (without peripheral joint involvement) was distinguished in the early twentieth century from a 'Marie–Strümpell type' (with peripheral joint involvement). Yet Fraenkel in 1903/04 (93) and Schlayer in 1906 (94) mentioned that this differentiation is not justified because there are no different processes leading to these forms of the disease and patients may change from one to the other form during their life.

Was it the authority of Bechterew that made the term 'Morbus Bechterew' or 'Bechterew's disease' for AS so popular in central, northern, and eastern Europe, as Buess and Koelbing (72) assume? Or was it the differentiation from the 'Marie–Strümpell type' of AS which made the term 'Morbus Bechterew' for the Bechterew type and finally for all types of AS so popular? Today the term Morbus Bechterew is better known than AS in central, northern, and eastern Europe, at least to patients, and this is why also the patient

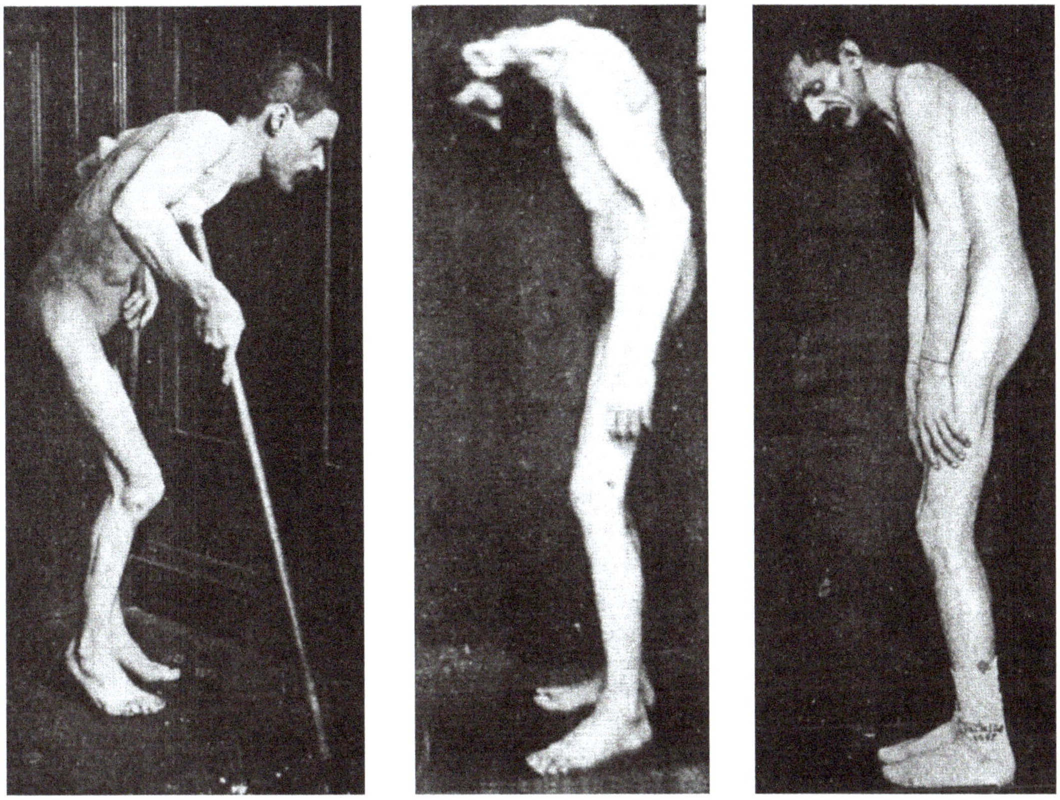

Fig. 1.9 Variability in the shape of the ankylosed spine in photographs published by Pierre Marie and André Léri in 1906.

organizations in these countries adopted this wrong appellation as the name of their associations.

Progress in spondyloarthritis diagnostics in the twentieth century

Diagnosis of the disease that is today called AS was essentially facilitated after the detection of X-rays in 1895 by Wilhem Röntgen (1845–1923, Nobel Prize 1901).

Eugen Fraenkel (1853–1925), a pathologist in Hamburg, investigated intensively the pathologic and radiological differential diagnosis of degenerative and inflammatory spine affections (93). He observed that inflammatory spine disease commonly affects, in its early stages, also the joints between the processus articulares, and he introduced in his publication of 1903/04 on this disease the term arthritis chronica ankylopoetica.

After several anatomic samples of spines showing AS were X-rayed by others, C.R. Schlayer in 1906 (94) was the first to present the spine with AS in X-rays of living patients (Fig. 1.10). The diagnosis based on X-rays of the spine was, however, only possible in advanced disease, as it may take several years until spinal changes in X-rays are visible. Schlayer uses the term spondylarthritis ankylopoetica, which was the name of the disease in Europe still in 1959 when the author of this chapter (EF) received this diagnosis.

Walter Geilinger (95) provided in 1917 one of the first clear radiographic descriptions of the typical syndesmophytes that led to spinal fusion in AS (96). Walter Krebs (97) noticed in 1930 the precocity and relative specificity of SI joint lesions. The diagnosis of AS could now be made before the development of spinal ankylosis.

The first description of cardiac involvement in AS was given by A.O. Fischer and O. Vontz in 1931 (98), who reported valvular heart diseases in 11% of patients with AS. T.B. Mallory in 1936 was the first to describe aortitis in patients with AS (99). The association of

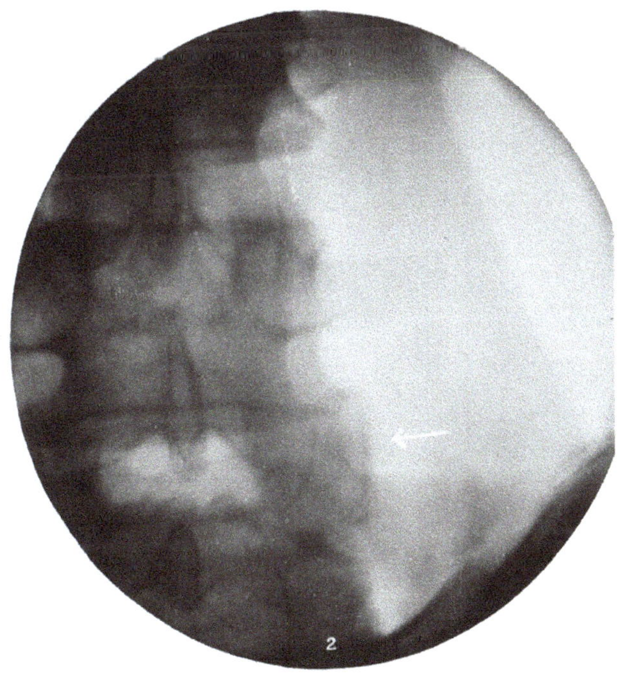

Fig. 1.10 One of the first X-rays of a living patient with AS, published by Schlayer in 1906.

conduction disturbances and AS was described for the first time in 1966 by Weed et al. (100).

The association of iritis and AS had already been mentioned by Bechterew in 1893 (84), but iritis as a manifestation of AS was first suggested independently by the German opthalmologists E. Kunz and E. Kraupa in 1933 as mentioned by Benedek in his historical introduction (101). Jacques Forestier and P. Robert emphasized in 1934 the distinction between syndesmophytes and osteophytes (73,102).

Particularly in the USA, the disease was inappropriately also known as 'rheumatoid spondylitis' during the first half of the twentieth century, because of the false belief that it was a variant of RA. A number of factors led to final abandonment of this term, for instance the widespread acceptance of the relevance of the rheumatoid factor test for RA and the persistent seronegativity of patients with AS. It was only in 1963 that the American Rheumatism Association officially adopted the term AS. In Europe, on the other hand, the term AS and its variants 'spondylitis ankylosans' and 'spondylarthritis ankylopoetica' have been in wide use for more than 100 years. The development of the Rome criteria (103) ended the use of 'rheumatoid spondylitis' as a descriptive term, even by its most diehard supporters (96,104).

E. Bowie and G. Glasgow (105) were the first to describe the cauda equina syndrome as an infrequent complication of longstanding AS. The typical radiologic feature is lumbar dural ectasia. Slow insidious progression of the symptoms eventually results in severe pain, muscle wasting, sensory loss in the lower spinal nerve root territories, and sphincter dysfunction (106).

The knowledge that AS is a familial disease and shows marked racial differences was an important factor leading to the application of new tissue antigen techniques (originally based on transplantation needs) to the rheumatic diseases. The resultant major breakthrough of HLA-B27 being associated with the spondyloarthritides in 1973 by Lee Schlosstein et al. (107) and independently by Derek Brewerton et al. (108) led in turn to further important discoveries in the HLA range in other diseases, and to an expansion of the SpA concept (73).

In 1974, Moll et al. (109) introduced the concept of 'seronegative spondyloarthropathy' on the basis of overlapping clinical and radiologic features within a number of different diseases (104). Although this concept has meanwhile been modified (e.g. Behçet's disease has been excluded), the concept is now generally accepted and is the basis of the classification criteria by Amor et al. (110) and by the European Spondylarthropathy Study Group (ESSG) (111).

Spondyloarthritis therapy in antiquity and history

In antiquity and until the Middle Ages, diseases were treated not only with medications and physical therapy but also by declarations of magical enchantments in the presence of the patient (112). Some remedies and magical texts against muscular complaints, rheumatic troubles, and stiffness in general were excavated in 1896 from the tomb of a magician and medical practitioner of the twelfth dynasty of Ancient Egypt (about 1900 BC), detected in the area of the Ramesseum temple near Luxor (Figs 1.11 and 1.12) (113). We can

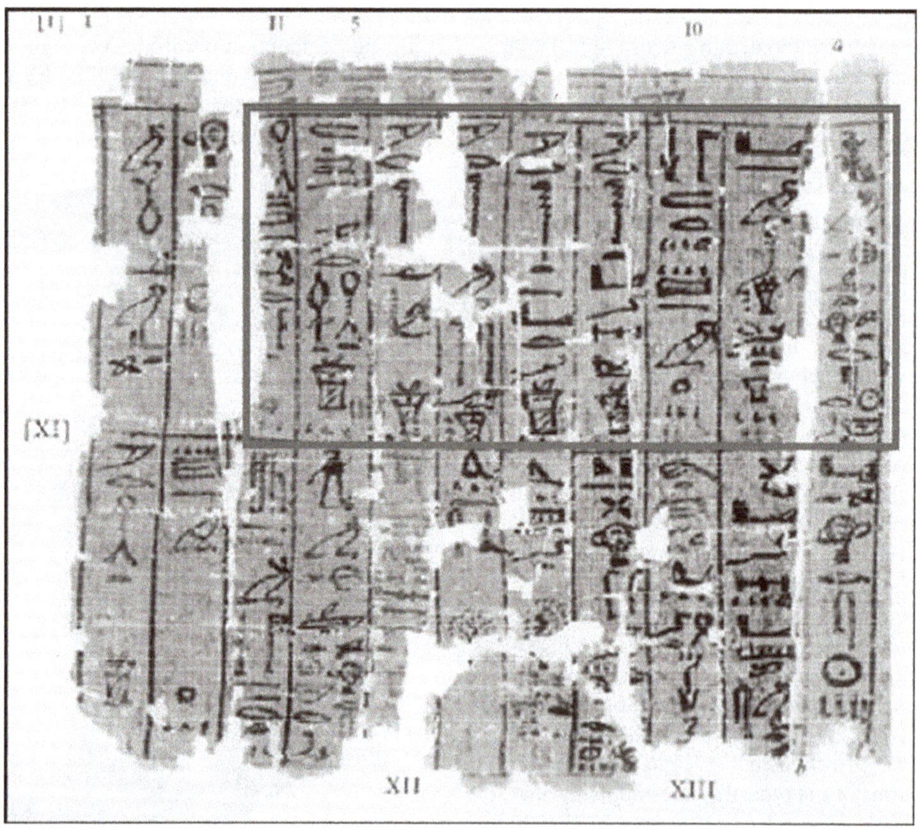

Fig. 1.11 Part of the papyrus 'Ramesseum V' circa 1900 BC (113) with (in the rectangle): 'Remedy for easing everything which is stiff: natron, beans, white oil, hippopotamus oil, crocodile oil, silurus-fish oil, mullet oil, incense, sweet myrrh, honey, to be cooked together, bandage with it every day until he is comfortable'.
Barns JWB (Hg.) 1956: Five Ramesseum Papyri. Oxford University Press, Oxford.

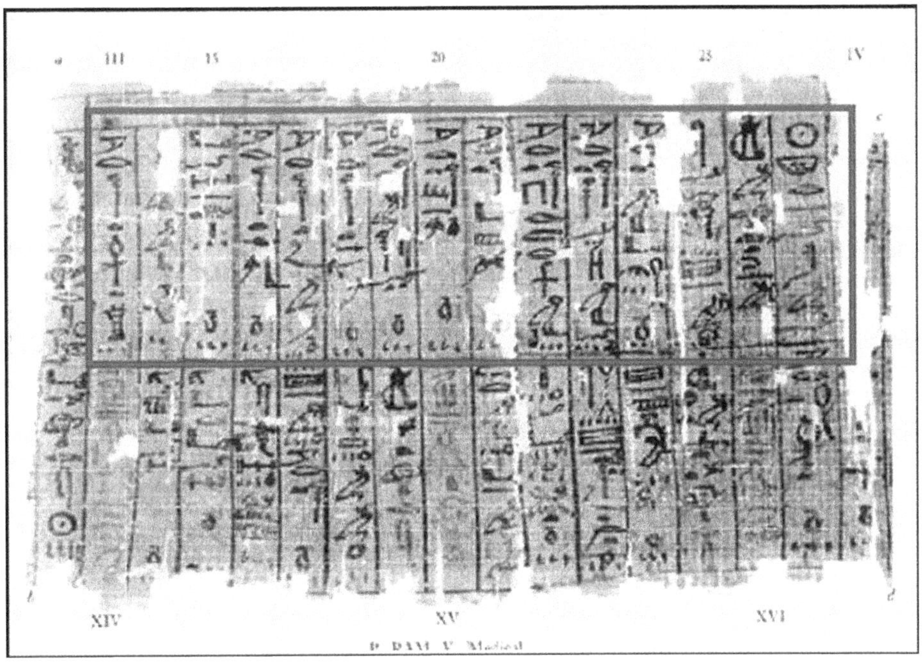

Fig. 1.12 Another part of the papyrus 'Ramesseum V' (Gardiner 1955) with (in the rectangle): 'To ease what is stiff and straighten what is warped: white oil, moringa, fat of centipede, hippopotamus oil, lion oil, donkey oil, crocodile oil, mouse oil, lizard oil, snake oil, ... to be cooked together, anoint with it every day until he is comfortable'. Barns JWB (Hg.) 1956: Five Ramesseum Papyri. Oxford University Press, Oxford.

only assume that pharaoh Ramses the Great (twentieth dynasty) with his AS (see section 'Old World spondyloarthritis') was also treated with a similar mixture and corresponding magical incantations.

The Hippocratic School understood all diseases—including spinal deformities—as the consequence of disturbed balance between the humours, and proposed cupping, bleeding, and purging to restore this balance, even up until the seventeenth century. Besides this humoral therapy, the Hippocratic School applied mechanical forces in the hope of correcting spinal deformities regarded as luxations (Fig. 1.13). An example of the Hippocratic luxation table may be found in the Wellcome Historical Medical Museum in London (72).

A principle to apply no pressure but only tension led Francis Glisson (1597–1677) to recommend in 1650 the extension device (traction slings) named after him (72), which is still available today.

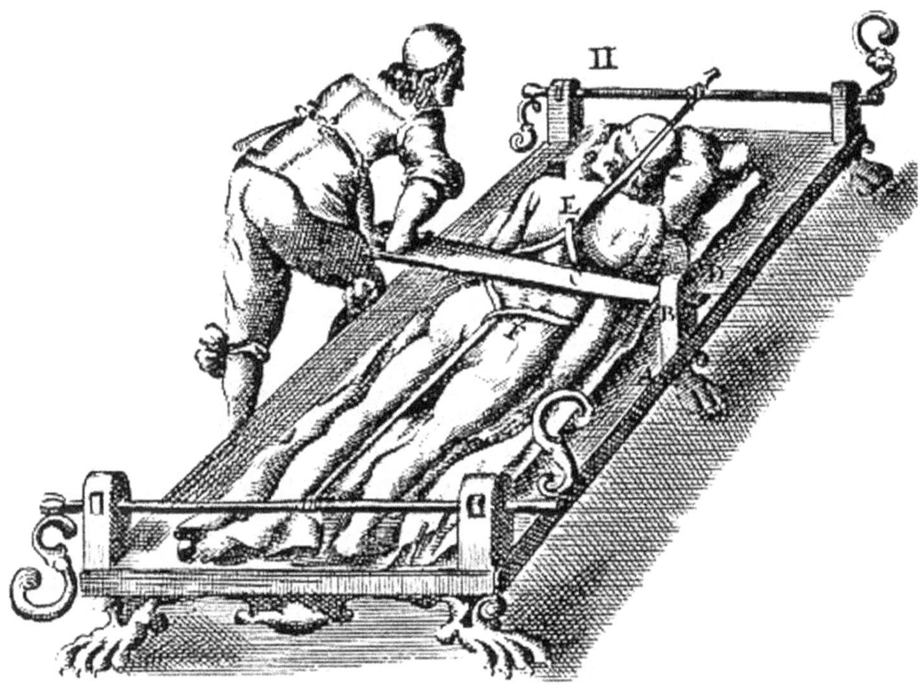

Fig. 1.13 Use of the Hippocratic luxation table in a baroque illustration contained in the 6th Latin edition of Armamentarium Chirurgiae Io. Sculteti, Amsterdam, 1672.

Carl Wenzel (79) discussed in his book of 1824 the use of mechanical equipment and stated that mechanical forces can never cure the reaction to inflammatory lesions of the bone. He proposed to educate patients to avoid long-during flexion of the spine, to avoid inappropriate clothing, and to lie flat on a firm surface. He recommended strategies to strengthen the muscles of the back and blister plasters as stimuli against the inflammation.

Bechterew in 1897 recommended treatment with warm baths, stretching of the spine, derivatives, massage, and potentially the intake of iodine (114). Hot-water spas were visited by patients in Roman antiquity. Some of them with healthy mineral waters attracted especially patients with rheumatic diseases. First notice of the use of the thermal spring water in Bad Gastein (Austria) for medical treatment goes back to the year 1350. After Antoine Henri Becquerel (1852–1908, Nobel Prize 1903) detected radioactivity in 1896, Karl Aschoff (1867–1945, a pharmacist in Bad Kreuznach, Germany) detected in 1904 that the therapeutic effect of spas like Bad Kreuznach and Bad Gastein is due to the radioactive noble gas radon dissolved in the water. Radon containing water and radon gas in former mining galleries are today successfully used in many spas for the therapy of rheumatic diseases including AS. Injury by radioactivity in this concentration has not been observed in any case (115).

Soon after the separation of the radioactive isotope radium-224 in 1902, there was great interest in its potential therapeutic use. A. Bickel in 1913 was the first to report the treatment of AS with this new radionuclide (116). The subsequently recognized leukaemia risk curtailed this approach to use only in the most severe cases. Radium-224 (also called Thorium-X) injections were successfully applied in several countries, including Germany until 1990 when the production of radium-224 for injection purposes was discontinued due to technical and commercial reasons (117).

In 1926, Kohler (118) was the first to employ X-rays for AS therapy. It was not until 1955 that Court-Brown and Abbatt (119) drew attention to the high incidence of leukaemia in people who had received high doses of radiation for AS (72).

About 100 years ago, the importance of regular physiotherapy for patients with AS was not generally recognized. Patients were often immobilized by a plaster mold, corset, or by bed rest to release them from pain, with the result that they became quickly ankylosed. In the course of the twentieth century the therapy saw a radical development: dynamic-active movement therapy became increasingly preferred, initiated by Walter Krebs in 1934 who recommended spa courses with balneotherapy, systematic motion exercises, heat applications, and massage, besides treatment with aminophenazon, a pain killer which was brought to the market as Pyramidon® in 1897 (120, 121).

Bywaters (73) commented on this development: 'Today's more active treatment is based on the fact that ultimate function depends on maintenance of good posture and actively maintained movement during the inflammatory period. Yesterday's dependence on drugs is now seen to be illusory, although they still have a useful symptomatic function to serve. The failures of earlier times visible on the streets today were due to the lack of education both of patient and doctor, and often a failure to recognise and diagnose the disease and its insidious nature.'

References

1. Zorab PA. The historical and prehistorical background of ankylosing spondylitis. Proc R Soc Med 1961;54:415–20.
2. Rothschild BM, Schultz HP, Pellegrini R. Herpetological Osteopathology. New York, Springer, 2012.
3. Rothschild BM, Woods RJ, Ortel W. Rheumatoid arthritis in the buff: erosive arthritis in representative defleshed bones. Am J Phys Anthropol 1990;82:441–9.
4. Rothschild BM, Tanke D, Carpenter K. Gout in Tyrannosaurus rex and other tyrannosaurids. Nature 1997;387:357.
5. Resnick D. Diagnosis of Bone and Joint Disorders. Philadelphia, Saunders, 2002.
6. Rothschild BM, Woods RJ. Spondyloarthropathy: erosive arthritis in representative defleshed bones. Am J Phys Anthropol 1991;85:125–34.
7. Doherty M, Dieppe P, Watt I. Low incidence of calcium pyrophosphate dihydrate crystal deposition in rheumatoid arthritis, with modification of radiographic features in coexistant disease. Arthritis Rheum 1984;27:1002–9.
8. Martel W, McCarter DK, Solsky MA, et al. Further observations on the arthropathy of calcium pyrophosphate crystal deposition disease. Radiology 1981;141:1–15.
9. McCarty DJ. Diagnostic mimicry in arthritis patterns of joint involvement associated with calcium pyrophosphate dihydrate crystal deposits. Bull Rheum Dis 1975;25:804–9.
10. Menkes CJ, Decraemere W, Postel M, Forest M. Chondrocalcinosis and rapid destruction of the hip. J Rheumatol 1985;12:130–3.
11. Reginato A, Valanzuela F, Martinez Passano G, Sergo Daza K. Polyarticular and familial chondrocalcinosis. Arthritis Rheum 1970;13:197–213.
12. Resnick D, Shapiro RF, Wiesner KB. Diffuse idiopathic skeletal hyperostosis (DISH) (ankylosing hyperostosis of Forestier and Rotes-Querol). Semin Arthritis Rheum 1978;7:153–87.
13. Zitnan D, Sitaj S. Chondrocalcinosis articularis. Acta Rheumatol Baln Pistiniana 1966;2:1–77.
14. Rothschild BM, Rothschild C. No laughing matter: spondyloarthropathy in Hyaenidae. J Zoo Wildlife Med 1994;25:259–63.
15. Rothschild BM, Rothschild C. Trans-mammalian pandemic of inflammatory arthritis (spondyloarthropathy variety): persistence since the Pleistocene. Paleontol Soc Publ 1996;8:330.
16. Rothschild BM, Rühli FJ. Comparison of arthritis characteristics in lowland Gorilla gorilla and mountain Gorilla beringei. Am J Primatol 2005;66:205–18.
17. Rothschild BM, Rühli FJ. Etiology of reactive arthritis in Pan paniscus, Pan troglodytes troglodytes and Pan schweinfurthii. Am J Primatol 2005;66:219–31.
18. Rothschild BM, Woods RJ. Spondyloarthropathy in gorillas. Semin Arthritis Rheum 1989;18:267–76.
19. Rothschild BM, Woods RJ. Osteoarthritis, calcium pyrophosphate deposition disease, and osseous infection in Old World primates. Am J Phys Anthropol 1992;87:341–7.
20. Rothschild BM, Woods RJ. Erosive arthritis and spondyloarthropathy in Old World primates. Am J Phys Anthropol 1992;88:389–400.
21. Rothschild BM, Woods RJ. Arthritis in New World monkeys: osteoarthritis, calcium pyrophosphate deposition disease and spondyloarthropathy. Int J Primatol 1993;14:61–78.
22. Rothschild BM, Wang X-M, Cifelli R. Spondyloarthropathy in Ursidae: a sexually transmitted disease? National Geographic Research and Exploration 1993;9:382–4.
23. Rothschild BM, Wang X-M, Shoshani J. Spondyloarthropathy in proboscideans. J Zoo Wildlife Med 1994;25:360–6.
24. Rothschild BM, Rothschild C, Woods RJ. Inflammatory arthritis in large cats: an expanded spectrum of spondyloarthropathy. J Zoo Wildlife Med 1998;29:279–84.
25. Rothschild BM, Rothschild C, Woods RJ. Inflammatory arthritis in canids: spondyloarthropathy. J Zoo Wildl Med 2001;32:58–64.
26. Rothschild BM, Prothero DR, Rothschild C. Origins of spondyloarthropathy in Perissodactyla. Clin Exp Rheumatol 2001;19:628–32.
27. Rothschild BM, Panza RK. Epidemiologic assessment of trauma-independent skeletal pathology in non-passerine birds from museum collections. Avian Pathol 2005;34:212–19.

28. Rothschild BM. Scientifically rigorous reptile and amphibian osseous pathology: lessons for forensic herpetology from comparative and paleo-pathology. Appl Herpetol 2008;10:39–116.
29. Bjorkengren AG, Sartoris DJ, Shermis S, Resnick D. Patterns of paravertebral ossification in the prehistoric saber-toothed cat. Am J Roentgenol 1987;148:779–82.
30. Estudos FJ. Multidisciplinares. In: Goncalves de Araujo AJ, Ferreira LF (eds) Non-human Vertebrate Paleopathology. Brazil, Panorama, 1988, pp. 213–34.
31. Dubos R. Man Adapting. New Haven, Yale University Press, 1965.
32. Rothschild BM, Sebes JI, Rothschild C. Antiquity of arthritis spondyloarthropathy identified in the Paleocene of North America. Clin Exp Rheumatol 1998;16:573–5.
33. Rothschild BM. Origin of spondyloarthropathy in the Jurassic. Lancet 2002;360:1454.
34. Rothschild BM, Berman D. Fusion of caudal vertebrae in late Jurassic sauropods. J Vert Paleontol 1991;11:29–36.
35. Bell PR, Rothschild BM, Tanke DH. First report of gout in an ornithomimid (Dinosauria: Theropoda) from the horseshoe Canyon Formation, Alberta. New Mexico Mus Natl Hist Bull 2011;53:166–8.
36. Ruffer MA. A pathological specimen dating from the lower Miocene period. (Extrait de Contributions à l'étude des Vertébrés miocène de l'Egypte.) Cairo Survey Depart 1917:1–7.
37. Sawyer GT, Erickson BR. Paleopathology of the Paleocene crocodile *Leidyosuchus (=Borealosuchus) formidabilis*. Sci Mus Minnesota St Paul Monog 1998;4:1–38.
38. Witzmann F, Schwarz-Wings D, Hampe O, Fritsch G, Asbach P. Evidence of spondyloarthropathy in the spine of a phytosaur (Reptilia: Archosauriformes) from the Late Triassic of Halberstadt, Germany. PLoS One 2014;9:e85511.
39. Cisneros JC, Cabral UG, de Beer F, Damiani R, Fortier DC. Spondarthritis in the Triassic. PLoS One 2010;5:e13425.
40. Anderson B. Did Benvenuto Cellini (1500–1571) have Reiter's disease? Sex Transm Dis 1989;32:47–8.
41. Hrdlička A, Merbs CF, Tyson RA, Dyer Alcauskas ES. Catalogue of the Hrdlička Paleopathology Collection. San Diego, Diego Museum of Man, 1980.
42. Rothschild BM, Rothschild C. Evolution of osseous/radiologic signs of tuberculosis. In: Palfi G, Dutour O, Deak J, Hutas I (eds) Tuberculosis Past and Present. Budapest, Golden Book Publisher, Tuberculosis Foundation, 1999, pp. 293–8.
43. Ruffer MA. Studies in the paleopathology of Egypt. Chicago, University of Chicago Press, 1921, pp. 187–9.
44. Smith GE, Jones FW. The Archaeological Survey of Nubia: Report for 1907–1908. Volume II: Report on the Human Remains. Cairo, National Printing Department, 1910.
45. Suzuki T. Paleopathological and paleoepidemiological investigation of human skeletal remains of early Hawaiians from Mokapu Site, Oahu Island, Hawaii. Japan Rev 1993;4:83–128.
46. Rothschild BM, Rothschild C. 19th century spondyloarthropathy independent of socioeconomic status: lack of skeletal collection bias. J Rheumatol 1992;20:314–19.
47. Jayson MI. Leonard Trask—the wonderful invalid. The first American description of ankylosing spondylitis. Arthritis Rheum 2003;48:612–13.
48. Kidd KE. Note on the palaeopathology of Ontario. Am J Phys Anthropol 1954;12:610–15.
49. Rothschild BM, Woods RJ. Character of pre-Columbian North American spondyloarthropathy. J Rheumatol 1992;19:1229–35.
50. Arriaza BT. Seronegative spondyloarthropathies and diffuse idiopathic skeletal hyperostosis in ancient northern Chile. Am J Phys Anthropol 1993;91:263–378.
51. Neumann HW. A preliminary sruvey of the paleopathology of an archaic American Indian population. Bull Tulane Univ Med Fac 1966;25:195–206.
52. Lamphear KM. Health and Mortality in a Nineteenth Century Poorhouse Skeletal Sample. Ann Arbor, Michigan, University Microfilms, 1988.
53. McKelvey B. Rochester, The Water-Power City, 1812–1854. Cambridge, Harvard University Press, 1945.
54. Bourke JB. A review of the paleopathology of arthritic diseases in antiquity. In: Brothwell D, Sandison AT (eds) Diseases in Antiquity: A Survey of the Diseases, Injuries and Surgery of Early Populations. Springfield, IL, Charles C. Thomas, 1967, pp. 352–70.
55. Ruffer A. Arthritis deformans and spondylitis in ancient Egypt. J Pathol Bacteriol 1919;22:152–96.
56. Tamás H, Erzsébet F, Sándor É. Articular abnormalities of skeletal remains from the Zsámbék-Premontre archeological site. Osteologiai Közlemények 2006;19–24.
57. Thould AK, Thould BT. Arthritis in Roman Britain. Brit Med J 1983;287:1909–11.
58. Harris JE, Wente EF (eds). An X-Ray Atlas of the Royal Mummies. Chicago, University of Chicago Press, 1980.
59. Massare C. Anatomo-radiologie et vérité historique a propos du bilan xéroradiographique de Ramsès II. Brux Méd 1979;59:163–70.
60. Chhem RK, Schmit P, Fauré C. Did Ramesses II really have ankylosing spondylitis? A reappraisal. Can Assoc Radiol J 2004;55:211–17.
61. Saleem SN, Hawass Z. Ankylosing spondylitis or diffuse idiopathic skeletal hyperostosis in Royal Egyptian mummies of the 18th–20th dynasties? Computed tomography and archaeology studies. Arthritis Rheumatol 2014;66:3311–16.
62. Rothschild BM. Diffuse idiopathic skeletal hyperostosis as reflected in the paleontologic record: dinosaurs and early mammals. Semin Arthritis Rheum 1987;17:119–25.
63. Rothschild BM, Martin LD. Skeletal Impact of Disease. Albuquerque, New Mexico Museum of Natural History and Science, 2006.
64. Buschhausen H. Das Mönchswesen in Abu Fano. In: Falck v. M, Lichtwark F (eds) Ägypten, Schätze aus dem Wüstensand. Wiesbaden, Dr Ludwig Richter, 1996, pp. 59–68.
65. Weisz GM, Matucci-Cerinic M, Albury WR, Lippi D. The Medici syndrome: a medico-historical puzzle. Int J Rheumatic Dis 2010;13:125–31.
66. Bloom RA, Smith P. On the antiquity of the seronegative spondyloarthropathies: evidence from ancient Judea. Skeletal Radiol 1992;24:111–14.
67. Rothschild BM, Rothschild C. Inflammatory arthritis in the first century Negev. Prog Rheum 1992;5:112–15.
68. Frohlich B, Ortner DJ, Al-Khalifa H. Human disease in the Ancient Middle East. J Bahrain Hist Archaeol Soc 1987/1988;14:61–73.
69. Ruffer MA, Rietti A. On osseous lesions in Ancient Egyptians. J Pathol Bacteriol 1912;16:439–40.
70. González T, Garcia C, Rodriguez C, González-Antón R. Ankylosing spondylitis in aborigines (guanches) of the Canary Islands. Arthritis Rheum 1990;33:1294–5.
71. Rothschild BM, Arriaza B, Woods RJ, Dutour O. Spondyloarthropathy identified as the etiology of Nubian erosive arthritis. Am J Phys Anthropol 1999;109:259–67.
72. Buess H, Koelbing HM. Kurze Geschichte der ankylosierenden Spondylitis und Spondylose. Acta Rhumatol 1964;22.
73. Bywaters EGL. Historical introduction. In: Moll JMH (ed) Ankylosing Spondylitis. Edinburgh, Churchill Livingstone, 1980, pp. 1–15.
74. Connor B. Lettre écrite à Monsieur le chevalier Guillaume de Waldegrave, premier médecin de sa Majesté Britannique. Paris, 1693.
75. Connor B. An extract of a letter to Sir Charles Walgrave, published in French at Paris, giving an account of an extraordinary human skeleton whose vertebrae of the back, the ribs, and several bones down to the os sacrum, were all firmly united into one solid bone, without jointing or cartilage. Philos Trans R Soc 1695;19:21.
76. Connor B, Cole B, Clements H. Dissertationes Medico-Physicae: De Stupendo Ossium Coalitu. Oxford, Sheldonian Theatre, 1695.
77. Hunter J. The Works of John Hunter, posthumously edited by JF Palmer, 4 volumes and atlas. London, Longman, 1835.
78. Sandifort E. Museum Anatomicum Academiae Lugduno-Batavae, Vols 1 and 2. Leiden, University of Leiden, 1793.

79. Wenzel C. Über die Krankheiten am Rückgrathe. Bamberg, Wesché, 1824.
80. Brodie BC. Pathological and surgical observations on the diseases of the joints, 5th edition with alterations and additions. London, Longman, Brown, Green and Longmans, 1850.
81. Fagge Ch H. A case of simple synostosis of the ribs to the vertebrae, and of the arches and the articular processes of the vertebrae themselves, and also of one hip joint. Trans Pathological Soc London 1877;28:201.
82. Strümpell A. Lehrbuch der Speziellen Pathologie und Therapie der inneren Krankheiten, Vol. 2. Leipzig, Vogel, 1884.
83. Strümpell A. Bemerkung über die chronische ankylosierende Entzündung der Wirbelsäule und der Hüftgelenke. Dtsch Z Nervenheilk 1897;11:338.
84. Bechterew WM. Steifigkeit der Wirbelsäule und ihre Verkrümmung als besondere Erkrankungsform. Neurologisches Zentralblatt 1893;12:426–34.
85. Ott VR, Wurm H. Spondylitis Ankylopoetika (Morbus Strümpell–Marie–Bechterew), 2nd edn. Darmstadt, Steinkopf, 1957.
86. Knaggs RL. Spondylitis deformans. Br J Surg 1924/1925;12:524.
87. Collins DH. The Pathology of Articular and Spinal Diseases. London, Arnold, 1949.
88. Keitel W. Ein Opfer Stalins? Wladimir Michailowitsch Bechterew (1857–1927). Z Rheumatol 2002;61:201–6.
89. Marie P. Sur la spondylose rhizomélique. Rev Méd 1898;18:285–315.
90. Marie P, Léri A. La spondylose rhizomélique. Nouvelle Iconogr Salpêtrière, Clin Maladies Syst Nerveux 1906;19:32.
91. Benoist M. Historical perspective: Pierre Marie, pioneer investigator in ankylosing spondylitis. Spine 1995;20:849–52.
92. Bechterew WM. Autobiography. In: Grote LR (ed) Die Medizin der Gegenwart in Selbstdarstellungen, vol. 6. Meiner, Leipzig, 1927.
93. Fraenkel E. Über chronische ankylosierende Wirbelsäulenversteifung. Fortschr Geb Röntgenstr 1903/1904;7:62.
94. Schlayer CR. Über chronische Wirbelsäulenversteifung. Fortschr Geb Röntgenstr 1906;10:261.
95. Geilinger W. Ankylosierende Spondylitis. Stuttgart, Union Deutsche Verlagsges, 1917.
96. Khan MA. Clinical features of ankylosing spondylitis. In: Hochberg MC, Silman AJ, Smolen JS, Weinblatt ME, Weisman MH (eds) Rheumatology, 3rd edn. London, Mosby, 2003, pp. 1161–81.
97. Krebs W. Zur Frage der sogenannten rheumatischen Erkrankungen der Wirbelsäule. Dtsch Med Wochenschr 1930;56:220–2, 270–2.
98. Fischer AO, Vontz O. Klinik der spondylarthritis ankylopoetica. In: Mikulicz von J, Naunyn B (eds) Mitteilungen aus den Grenzgebieten der Medizin und Chirurgie. Jena, Gustav Fischer, 1931;42:586–95.
99. Mallory TB. Case records of the Massachusetts General Hospital. New Engl J Med 1936;214:690–8.
100. Weed CL, Kulander PG, Massarella JA, Decker JL. Heart block in ankylosing spondylitis. Arch Internal Med 1966;117:800–6.
101. Benedek TG. History of the rheumatic diseases. In: Klippel JH (ed) Primer on the Rheumatic Diseases, 11th edn. Atlanta, Arthritis Foundation, 1997, pp. 1–5.
102. Forestier J, Robert P. Ostéophytes et syndesmophytes. Gazette Méd Fr (Radiol Suppl) 1934;192.
103. Kellgren JH, Jeffrey MR, Ball J (eds). The epidemiology of chronic rheumatism, Vol. I. Oxford, Blackwell Scientific Publications, 1963, pp. 326–7.
104. Russell AS. Ankylosing spondylitis: history. In: Hochberg MC, Silman AJ, Smolen JS, Weinblatt ME, Weisman MH (eds) Rheumatology, 3rd edn. London, Mosby, 2003, pp. 1145–7.
105. Bowie E, Glasgow G. Cauda equina lesions associated with ankylosing spondylitis: report of three cases. Br Med J 1961;2:24–7.
106. Cornec D, Devauchelle Pensec V, Joulin SJ, Saraux A. Dramatic efficacy of infliximab in cauda equina syndrome complicating ankylosing spondylitis. Arthritis Rheum 2009;60:1657–60.
107. Schlosstein L, Terasaki PI, Bluestone R, Pearson CM. High association of an HL-A antigen, W27, with ankylosing spondylitis. New Engl J Med 1973;288:704–6.
108. Brewerton DA, Hart FD, Nicholls A, Caffrey M, James DCO, Sturrock RD. Ankylosing spondylitis and HL-A 27. Lancet 1973;1:904–7.
109. Moll J, Haslock I, MacRae IF, Wright V. Association between ankylosing spondylitis, psoriatic arthritis, Reiter's disease, the intestinal arthropathies, and Behçet's syndrome. Medicine 1974;53:343–64.
110. Amor B, Dougados M, Mijiyawa M. Critères de classification des spondylarthropathies. Rev Rhumatisme 1990;57:85–9.
111. Dougados M, van der Linden S, Juhlin R, et al. The European Spondylarthropathy Study Group preliminary criteria for the classification of spondylarthropathy. Arthritis Rheum 1991;34:1218–27.
112. Schmitz R. Geschichte der Pharmazie, Vol. 1: Von den Anfängen bis zum Ausgang des Mittelalters. Eschborn, Govi, 1998.
113. Gardiner A. The Ramesseum papyri. Oxford, Oxford University Press, 1955.
114. Bechterew WM. Von der Verwachsung oder Steifigkeit der Wirbelsäule. Dtsch Z Nervenheilk 1897;11:327–37.
115. Jöckel H. Praktische Erfahrungen mit der Radontherapie. In: Pratzel G, Deetjen P (eds) Radon in der Kurortmedizin. Geretsried, I.S.M.H., 1997, pp. 84–91.
116. Bickel A. Weitere Beiträge zur ThX-Therapie bei Anämie, Leukämie und rheumatischen Erkrankungen. Berl Klin Wochenschrift 1913;50:346–8.
117. Wick RR, Gössner W. History and current uses of 224Ra in ankylosing spondylitis and other diseases. Environ Int 1993;19:467–73.
118. Kohler A. Über die Röntgenbehandlung der Arthritis deformans und der Spondylitis deformans. Klin Wochenschr 1926;5:204.
119. Court-Brown WM, Abbatt JD. The incidence of leukaemia in ankylosing spondylitis with X-ray treatment. Lancet 1955;1:1283.
120. Krebs W. Das Röntgenbild des Beckens bei der Bechterewschen Krankheit. Fortschr Geb Röntgenstr 1934;50:537–42.
121. Krebs W, Vontz O. Entstehung und Verlauf der Spondylitis ankylopoetica (Bechterew). Dtsch Med Wochenschr 1934;60:100–2.

CHAPTER 2

Epidemiology of axial spondyloarthritis

Lianne Gensler, Michael Weisman, and Liron Caplan

Axial spondyloarthritis (axSpA) is an inflammatory arthritis of the sacroiliiac joints and spine. The prototype is ankylosing spondylitis (AS), the radiographic form of the disease; however, more recently, an earlier or less differentiated form has been described termed non-radiographic axial spondyloarthritis (nr-axSpA). Extra-articular manifestations (EAMs) commonly include anterior uveitis, inflammatory bowel disease (IBD), and psoriasis. There is a strong association with the HLA-B27 allele and the prevalence of the disease tends to follow the frequency of this gene. Epidemiologic studies in axSpA are relevant in the population studied and therefore have limited external validity. This chapter describes the epidemiology of axSpA.

How to assess epidemiology in chronic disease

In order to define the epidemiology of disease, it is necessary to have a clear and stable definition of the disease. The incidence and prevalence must also be truthfully captured in the populations studied. The study population should be generalizable and reflect the population that surrounds it. Disease incidence is typically defined as the proportion of newly developed cases divided by the number of individuals at risk for the same outcome during a specified time interval. Disease prevalence measures the frequency of an existing outcome, particularly important in chronic diseases such as axSpA. Prevalence can be determined in a cross-sectional manner, at one point in time, and is termed point prevalence, or in a given period, when it is termed period prevalence. In chronic disease, finding the 'incident' time point can be difficult to pin-point, as described in the section 'Limitations of epidemiologic studies in axial spondyloarthritis', below. Furthermore, those in the healthcare system, who are more likely to identify the more severe end of the disease spectrum, may bias the prevalence. Population-based registries and longitudinal electronic health record systems have the potential to address some of these issues surrounding incidence, especially with lead-time data when healthy people enter the population studied and then develop disease.

Limitations of epidemiologic studies in axial spondyloarthritis

A number of methodological and scientific issues complicate efforts to characterize axSpA in epidemiologic terms. First and foremost, the various criteria used to define disease over the past few decades identify overlapping, but inconsistent populations. The Rome (1), New York (2), and modified New York (mNY) criteria (3) identify patients with well-established AS by requiring abnormalities on plain radiographs. The ESSG, Amor (4), and the clinical arm of the Assessment of SpondyloArthritis international Society (ASAS) classification criteria (5), by contrast, do not require abnormalities on imaging (Table 2.1). A number of these criteria do not require inflammatory back pain. As a consequence, the relatively insensitive Rome, New York, and mNY criteria identify only a subset of patients with axSpA, resulting in lower prevalence estimates than those of more recent classification systems.

Second, these criteria rely on radiographs, which take years to display clear evidence of bony damage and therefore cannot precisely distinguish a specific year of disease onset. This imprecision would be anticipated to produce unstable annual incidence estimates. The prolonged interval between symptom onset and disease diagnosis substantiate these concerns (6, 7). Another limitation is that imaging data might not be available as this is expensive to perform, particularly on a population level, and thus limits the utility of classifying populations accordingly.

Third, figures based on administrative data contain a number of shortcomings. These primarily result from the lack of a specific coding for the concept of axSpA. International Classification of Disease, 9th Clinical Modification (ICD-9-CM) edition contain codes for AS (720.0), sacroiliitis (720.2), spinal enthesopathy (720.1), and other inflammatory spondylopathy (720.8 and 720.9)—codes that remain largely unaltered in the 10th Clinical Modification (ICD-10-CM). Not surprisingly, these codes likely reflect the same issues plaguing the classification criteria described above, including insensitivity and misclassification due to a reliance on imaging. While the planned 11th edition of ICD codes should incorporate axial (as well as peripheral) SpA, its release is not scheduled prior to 2017, with adoption likely to occur years later. Codes for disease associated with axial involvement (psoriatic arthritis (PsA), ICD-9-CM 696.0, and enteropathic-associated arthritis, ICD-9-CM 713.1) also do not discriminate between axial and peripheral involvement, thereby limiting their utility due to similar problems with misclassification.

Another limitation with using administrative data is that it requires that patients be identified and diagnosed with the disease. Because of the significant delay to diagnosis and the tendency to attempt self-management, which often occurs in patients with

Table 2.1 Criteria for axSpA

	Rome (1961)	New York (1966)	mNY (1984)	Amor (1990)	ESSG (1991)	ASAS, MRI arm (2009)	ASAS, clinical arm
Requires radiographic changes§	No	Yes	Yes	No	No	No	No
Includes radiographic changes§	Yes	Yes	Yes	Yes	Yes	Yes	No
Includes MRI sacroiliitis	No	No	No	No	No	Yes	No
Requires back pain	No	No	No	No	Yes*	Yes	Yes
Includes HLA-B27	No	No	No	Yes	No	Yes	Yes
Includes uveitis	Yes	No	No	Yes	No	Yes	Yes
Includes psoriasis	No	No	No	Yes	Yes	Yes	Yes
Includes IBD	No	No	No	Yes	Yes	Yes	Yes
Includes metrology	No	Yes	Yes	No	No	No	No
Includes Achilles tendonitis	No	No	No	Yes	Yes	Yes	Yes
Includes family history	No	No	No	Yes	Yes	Yes	Yes
Includes raised CRP	No	No	No	No	No	Yes	Yes

CRP, C-reactive protein.

§Grade 2 bilateral or grade 3 or 4 unilateral.

*For axSpA.

axSpA, the prevalence estimates may underrepresent the overall frequency of axSpA by neglecting more subtle presentations and will be biased by a relative overrepresentation of the most severe cases. The inverse may also be true, when patients are misdiagnosed with axSpA in the setting of a potential mimic. However, based on the significant number of undiagnosed patients with axSpA in the primary care setting, the former is likely to be more problematic (8).

Finally, the use of the HLA-B27 allele for diagnostic and classification purposes presents a number of challenges. These difficulties arise from the apparent changing prevalence of HLA-B27 by age (9) and variations in the association of HLA-B27 subtypes with disease susceptibility and protection (10). Major differences in the prevalence of HLA-B27 between ethnic groups and minor variations in the commercially available assays (11) may also have implications for determining the incidence and prevalence of disease. Not all prevalence studies collect the HLA-B27-status, making this aspect of classification difficult to use uniformly and difficult to analyse across heterogeneous studies.

Assessment of prevalence of inflammatory back pain

Inflammatory back pain (IBP) is the hallmark feature of axSpA. A number of criteria have been developed to classify patients with IBP (12–14). The criteria alone are not a perfect test and the sensitivity and specificity of this feature is only 80% and 72%, respectively (14). When this type of back pain was assessed in the US population, it was found that prevalence was between 5% and 6%, depending on the criteria used (15). It was also noted that amongst those with any chronic axial pain (lasting at least 3 months), one-third had IBP. When evaluated by race/ethnicity, non-Hispanic whites were more likely to have IBP compared to non-Hispanic blacks. In the UK, the prevalence of IBP was determined in a primary care population using three of the published IBP criteria (16). In this population of 17 177 patients in Norfolk, patients with at least one visit for back pain were assessed for IBP by survey. Based on three published criteria, the prevalence of IBP ranged between 7.7% and 15.4%. It was not different between genders or age groups. Hamilton and colleagues extrapolated these data to the practice population and determined that the prevalence of IBP in the primary care population between the ages of 18 and 80 years old was between 1.7% and 3.4%, depending on the criteria set used.

Assessment of HLA-B27 in different populations

The prevalence of axSpA, and especially the radiographic form AS, follows the frequency of HLA-B27 in a given population (Fig. 2.1). This general rule holds, though there are some subtypes (HLA-B27*09 in Sardinians and HLA-B27*06 in South Asians) that are not strongly associated with disease susceptibility (17–19).

It is also interesting to note that within populations, certain HLA-B27 serotypes are greater risk alleles. For example, on mainland China, HLA-B27*04 is a greater risk allele than HLA-B27*05 (the most common allele found in Caucasian AS patients) (20). In the northern hemisphere, there appears to be a gradient from north to south and west to east (21). The highest HLA-B27 prevalence is in the indigenous Northern Americans, the Inuit and Yupik, ranging between 25% and 50%. In Northern Eurasia, the prevalence ranges between 10% and 16% in countries like Iceland, Norway, and Sweden (22). In the UK, the prevalence is 9.5% (23), whereas the prevalence in South East Asia approaches 12% compared to 2–6% on the mainland of China (24). Because disease prevalence so closely follows the allele prevalence in a given population, understanding the population prevalence of HLA-B27 will allow extrapolated rough estimates of disease prevalence. It is very helpful to determine the true allele prevalence in the population. For the first time this was assessed in the US population using the National

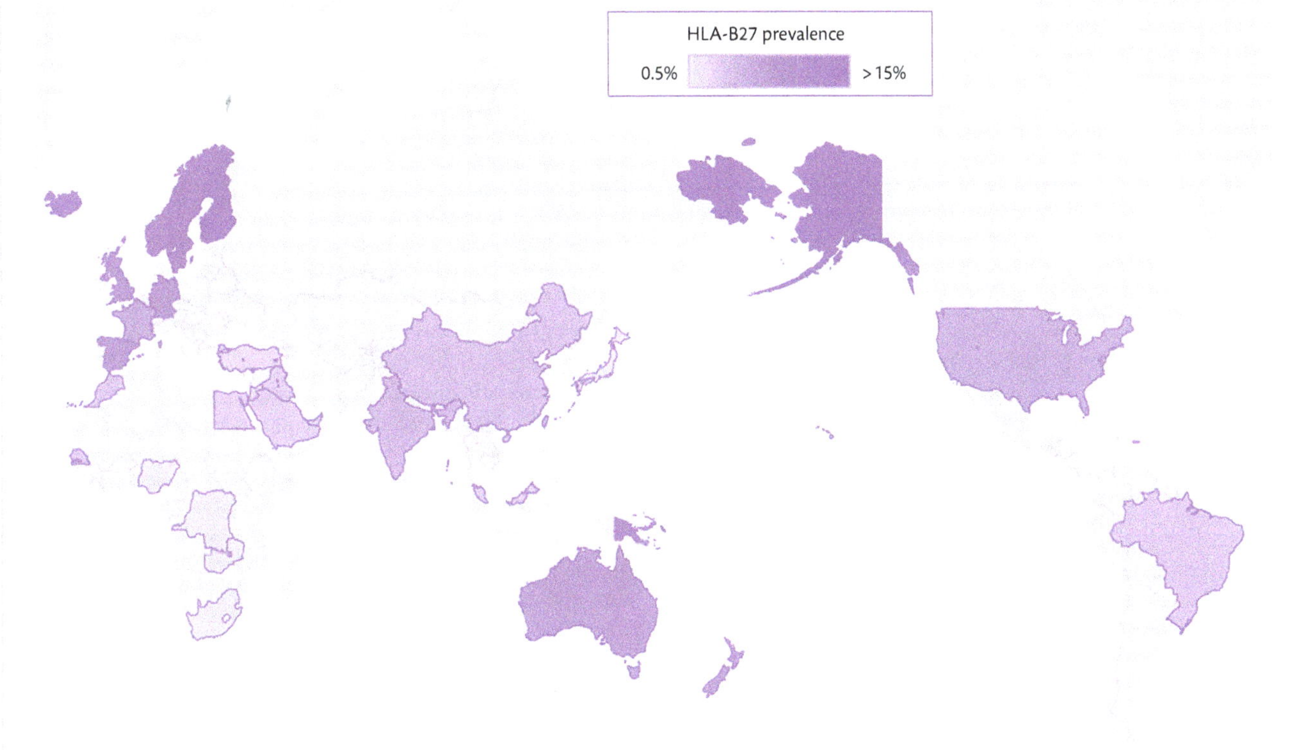

Fig. 2.1 Map of HLA-B27 prevalence. Global prevalence of HLA-B27 is ascertained where there are available population data. Most countries have no data available in control populations and therefore are not shown as shaded (48).
Gonzalez-Galarza, F.F., Takeshita, L.Y.C., Santos, E.J.M., Kempson, F., Maia, M.H.T., Silva, A.L.S.D., Silva, A.L.T.E., et al. (2015). Allele frequency net 2015 update: new features for HLA epitopes, KIR and disease and HLA adverse drug reaction associations. Nucleic Acids Research, 43/D1: D784–8. Oxford University Press. DOI: 10.1093/nar/gku1166.

Health and Nutrition Examination Survey (2009–2010 cycle) (9). There was a 6.1% (95% CI 4.6–8.2) age adjusted prevalence in the overall population. When evaluated by race/ethnicity, the prevalence was 7.5% (95% CI 5.3–10.4) among non-Hispanic whites and 3.5% (95% CI 2.5–4.8) amongst all other US races/ethnicities combined.

Incidence and prevalence of axial spondyloarthritis

The prevalence of axSpA is difficult to determine from administrative data. This is because there is no ICD-9-CM or 10-CM code for axSpA. There is a plan for ICD-11-CM to include the more updated categories of SpA, including both axial and peripheral disease, but this is several years away. Therefore, in order to understand prevalence using administrative data, investigators must rely on the current codes for AS (720.0), sacroiliitis (720.2), spinal enthesopathy (720.1), and other inflammatory spondyloarthropathy (720.8 and 720.9).

Another limitation in interpreting the current definitions is that in order to get the tumour necrosis factor inhibitors (TNFi) approved for the axial form of disease in the USA, the code for AS (720.0) needs to be used at this time, which further confuses the true prevalence of disease using administrative data. Though several studies have assessed the prevalence of axSpA and AS in various cohort settings, fewer studies have been generalizable to the population that surrounds it. It is difficult to compare non-population-based studies; therefore the data below are limited to those that are most representative of the surrounding population.

In 1979, the prevalence of AS was determined to be 129 per 100 000 in Caucasians living in Rochester, Minnesota (25). In 2008, the National Arthritis Data workgroup published data on the prevalence of arthritis in the USA, using the National Health Interview Survey (NHIS) (26). The investigators determined that 0.6–2.4 million adults (346–1310 per 100 000 adults ≥ 25 years and older) were affected by SpA, but they could not estimate the prevalence of AS based on available data. Most recently, using the National Health and Nutrition Examination Survey (NHANEs) 2009–2010 cycle, the prevalence of SpA (and mostly axial disease) using the ESSG and Amor criteria was determined (27). The Amor criteria revealed a prevalence estimate of 0.9% (95% CI 0.7–1.1) and the ESSG criteria a prevalence estimate of 1.4% (95% CI 1.0–1.9). Not all criteria were collected and no radiographic data were available, so that these estimates are likely an underrepresentation of the true prevalence. In the state of Alaska, the ESSG and Amor criteria were assessed in all native residents of the two study regions (28). There was an overall prevalence of SpA of 2.5%, though many of these patients were classified as 'undifferentiated SpA', and may have been considered nr-axSpA using today's classification criteria.

In Canada, Haroon et al. used the provincial health administrative database of Ontario to determine the age- and sex-standardized incidence and prevalence of AS between 1995 and 2010 (29). The authors found that the prevalence in Ontario had almost tripled over the prior two decades (from 79/100 000 in 1995 to 213/100 000 in 2010).

They also noted that the proportion of new diagnoses in women was increasing, though the standardized incidence rates were stable over the same period (between 14 and 16 per 100 000). In Canada, the ICD-9 code 720 reflects both radiographic disease (AS) and non-radiographic disease (nr-axSpA). Because the terminology for nr-AxSpA was only defined towards the end of this study period, and with no other way to code these patients, the prevalence and gender effects may partially, but not completely, be explained this way. Not well reflected in the Canadian data is the high prevalence of AS among the Haida and Bella Coola Native Americans off the coast of British Columbia. In these groups, the prevalence of HLA-B27 is 50% and 25%, respectively, and the associated prevalence of AS with radiographic sacroiliitis was found to be 10% and 2%, respectively (30).

In northern Norway, Bakland et al. established the incidence and prevalence of AS between 1960 and 1993 by a cohort design, as the university hospital was the only rheumatology centre serving the region (31). They used the date of onset of clinical disease in patients with AS to define the incidence rates. For the purpose of defining primary AS, they excluded patients who had EAMs, including psoriasis and IBD. This exclusion likely underestimated the findings, but resulted in a very high HLA-B27 frequency of 93%. The annual incidence of primary AS was 7.26, while estimated point prevalence rose from 0.036% in 1970, to 0.10% in 1980, and to 0.21% in 1990, with a period prevalence of 0.26% suggesting stable disease incidence over the study period. In another Norwegian population-based study, investigators used the Nord-Trøndelag Health Study (HUNT) over two study periods to determine incident AS (32). They found 107 incident cases of AS (of 35 385 participants). This resulted in an incident rate of 16.6–27 per 100 000, depending on case definition used. These are higher than previously reported incidence rates, and it was thought that, because the diagnosis was self-reported, people with non-radiographic disease were being included. The authors also found that current smoking was significantly associated with the development of the disease.

Exarchou et al. used the Swedish National Patient Register to identify the prevalence of clinically diagnosed AS (33). The investigators found 11 030 AS cases, with a stricter definition in 8538 living cases between 16 and 64 years old. This resulted in a point prevalence in 2009 of 0.18%. Northern Sweden had a higher prevalence than southern Sweden and men had a significantly higher prevalence than woman (0.23% vs 0.14%). They used ICD coding to identify cases, and required that patients have a diagnosis from a rheumatologist or internist, to improve specificity, such that more severe disease was likely selected for. This may have also led to the lower prevalence and differences between the genders.

In the Chukotka settlements of Russia, the prevalence of SpA was ascertained by interview and medical examination in 355 of the 498 residents (34). The authors found a prevalence of AS in 1.1% of the population, though 2.5% had SpA, suggesting that the spectrum of axSpA prevalence falls between these two numbers.

In a Japanese nationwide survey, cases of SpA were ascertained and recruited from hospital and clinic records (35). Based on this study, it was estimated that the prevalence of AS (and probably axSpA) was 0.0065%, based on Amor and ESSG criteria. This was based on the assumption that 1/10 of the population was surveyed. There were several limitations of this study, including the selection of predominantly university clinics and hospitals, the response rate of these locations, and the requirement for cases to have been seen and diagnosed in this setting. However, the low prevalence of HLA-B27 in the Japanese population would be expected to associate with this low prevalence of disease.

In Marche, Italy, a survey was administered to a gender and age stratified population with a response rate of only 58%, suggesting at least some selection bias (36). The positive responders were then assessed and diagnosed by a rheumatologist, with an AS prevalence of 0.37% in this single region of Italy.

The Community Orientated Program for the Control of Rheumatic Diseases (COPCORD) protocol, primarily an International League of Associations for Rheumatology (ILAR) and World Health Organization (WHO) collaboration, has produced several studies attempting to determine the prevalence of various rheumatic diseases (37). Limitations of some of these studies include the non-random selection of locations studied and the selection bias associated with response. Other prevalence studies have been performed in specific cohorts, such as university employees (38) and employees of the French national gas and electricity company (39). These studies are not discussed in this chapter, as they have limited external validity.

A meta-analysis of the global prevalence of AS (using the New York or mNY criteria) was performed (40). The authors reported, based on 36 eligible studies, that the AS prevalence was 238 per 100 000 in Europe, 167 per 100 00 in Asia, 319 per 100 000 in North America, 102 per 100,000 in Latin America, and 74 per 100 000 in Africa (Table 2.2).

Axial spondyloarthritis in chronic back pain populations

Underwood and Dawes surveyed 313 back pain sufferers in the primary care setting (41). They noted that 15% of patients had IBP, and two patients were found to have radiographic AS, where another 18 (39%) had other features of SpA, suggesting that 5% of patients may have undiagnosed disease, possibly including the spectrum of nr-axSpA. Bakland et al. studied 807 participants from a Norwegian population survey who reported back pain lasting more than 4 weeks (42). The participants were invited to come in for a clinical, laboratory, and imaging evaluation. They found that 8.4% met the ASAS criteria for axSpA. The mNY criteria were met in 2.4%, while 6% fulfilled the clinical arm only. They also found that 20% of participants with clinical SpA progressed to radiographic disease after a median of 8 years. A Dutch study determined the prevalence of axSpA in the primary care setting in undiagnosed patients by recruiting patients with chronic back pain between the ages of 20 and 45 years for further evaluation (8). The investigators found that 24% of the 364 patients they evaluated met the ASAS criteria for axSpA, and 7% of patients met the mNY criteria. These results should be interpreted with caution, as the prevalence of HLA-B27 in the cases was only 20%, which is unexpected for axSpA; however, it does suggest an underdiagnosis of axSpA in younger patients in primary care clinics, despite the recorded history of chronic back pain.

Gender differences in axial spondyloarthritis

It is widely accepted that patients with the radiographic form of the disease, AS, have a slightly higher male predominance. A global

Table 2.2 Global prevalence of axSpA based on published studies

Country	Prevalence (%)	Study design	Study size	Definition/criterion used	Limitations
Canada (29)	0.21	Retrospective study of Ontario provincial health administrative database	6930 cases per 8 720 499 population (1995) to 24 976 cases per 11 016 692 population (2010)	At least two physician service claims with ICD-9 code 720 or ICD-10 M45 by a rheumatologist or one similar code associated with procedure or discharge	Retrospective, diagnosis with ICD coding—includes both radiographic and non-radiographic disease; single province in Canada
China (including Taiwan) (45)	0.2–0.54	Pooled analysis of survey data	120 451	New York or mNY criteria	Most studies performed in Han Chinese
Finland (46)	0.15	Population-based	8000	Required patients to be receiving speciality medication	Age > 30 years old
Italy (36)	0.37	Random questionnaires to age/gender stratified population in Marche seen in 16 GP settings, followed by rheumatology evaluation	2155	Physician diagnosis	58% response rate (selection bias)
Japan (47)	0.0065	Nationwide survey of hospitals and clinics	~ 1/10 Japanese population recruited with 426 and 638 cases across two surveys	Amor and ESSG criteria	Required cases with hospital records; selection bias
Northern Norway (31)	0.21 (1990)	Population-based	534 cases of ~ 217 000 population	mNY criteria, excluding cases with EAMs	Cases required rheumatology diagnosis of AS
Russia (Chukotka) (34)	1.1	Chukotka settlement	355 assessed of 498 population	mNY criteria	71% response
Sweden (33)	0.18 (2009)	Population-based using National Patient Register	8538–11 030 cases	ICD-9 diagnosis	ICD coding requiring clinical diagnosis, which may include AS and nr-axSpA
USA (27)	0.9–1.4	Population based	43–70 cases per 5103 population	Amor and ESSG	Not all criterion collected

meta-analysis, performed by continent, reported a European and Asian mean male:female ratio of 3.8:1 and 2.3:1, respectively (40). The authors limited study selection to those where New York or mNY criteria were met, and the clinical diagnosis was made by a rheumatologist, in addition to population-based studies. The ASAS classification criteria have enabled the assessment of those with the disease, but without radiographic damage (nr-axSpA). These studies suggest there is a more balanced gender distribution in the overall spectrum, with more women than men in the nr-axSpA group (43, 44). Men have more radiographic damage and a higher burden of inflammation, so that the detection of women in the non-radiographic form of the disease is important and may reflect the broader radiographic spectrum of disease.

Conclusion

The prevalence of axSpA follows the prevalence of HLA-B27, though this is especially true for the radiographic form of the disease, AS. As criteria evolve, these rates will change, and likely reflect the change in criteria, not a change in the disease prevalence. Estimating period prevalence that crosses the boundaries of several published criteria makes assessment of epidemiology complex and difficult to interpret. Finally, currently available ICD coding does not adequately cover the spectrum of disease, making administrative data difficult to use for epidemiologic purposes. Advances have been made with the development of the ASAS classification criteria with the ability to include magnetic resonance imaging (MRI) findings. However, MRI needs to be easily accessible or HLA-B27 prevalence needs to perform well in the population it is being tested.

References

1. Bennett PH, Wood PHN (eds). Population Studies of the Rheumatic Diseases. Amsterdam, Excerpta Medica Foundation. International Congress Series No. 148, 1963, p. 456.
2. Kellgren JH, Jeffrey MR, Ball J. The Epidemiology of Chronic Rheumatism, Vol. 1. Oxford, Blackwell Scientific Publications, 1963.
3. van der Linden S, Valkenburg HA, Cats A. Evaluation of diagnostic criteria for ankylosing spondylitis. A proposal for modification of the New York criteria. Arthritis Rheum 1984;27(4):361–8.
4. Amor B, Dougados M, Mijiyawa M. [Criteria of the classification of spondyloarthropathies.] Rev Rhum Mal Osteoartic 1990;57(2):85–9.
5. Rudwaleit M, van der Heijde D, Landewe R, et al. The development of Assessment of SpondyloArthritis international Society classification criteria for axial spondyloarthritis (part II): validation and final selection. Ann Rheum Dis 2009;68(6):777–83.
6. Feldtkeller E, Khan MA, Heijde DVD, van der Linden S, Braun J. Age at disease onset and diagnosis delay in HLA-B27 negative vs. positive patients with ankylosing spondylitis. Rheumatol Int 2003;23(2):61–6.

7. Ozgocmen S, Ardicoglu O, Kamanli A, et al. Pattern of disease onset, diagnostic delay, and clinical features in juvenile onset and adult onset ankylosing spondylitis. J Rheum 2009;36(12):2830–3.
8. van Hoeven L, Luime J, Han H, Vergouwe Y, Weel A. Identifying axial spondyloarthritis in Dutch primary care patients, ages 20–45 years, with chronic low back pain. Arthritis Care Res 2014;66(3):446–53.
9. Reveille JD, Hirsch R, Dillon CF, Carroll MD, Weisman MH. The prevalence of HLA-B27 in the US: data from the US National Health and Nutrition Examination Survey. Arthritis Rheum 2012;64(5):1407–11.
10. Reveille JD. An update on the contribution of the MHC to AS susceptibility. Clin Rheumatol 2014;33(6):749–57.
11. Seipp MT, Erali M, Wies RL, Wittwer C. HLA-B27 typing: evaluation of an allele-specific PCR melting assay and two flow cytometric antigen assays. Cytometry B Clin Cytom 2005;63(1):10–15.
12. Calin A, Porta J, Fries JF, Schurman DJ. Clinical history as a screening test for ankylosing spondylitis. JAMA 1977; 237(24):2613–14.
13. Rudwaleit M, Metter A, Listing J, Sieper J, Braun J. Inflammatory back pain in ankylosing spondylitis: a reassessment of the clinical history for application as classification and diagnostic criteria. Arthritis Rheum 2006;54(2):569–78.
14. Sieper J, van der Heijde D, Landewe R, et al. New criteria for inflammatory back pain in patients with chronic back pain: a real patient exercise by experts from the Assessment of SpondyloArthritis international Society (ASAS). Ann Rheum Dis 2009;68(6):784–8.
15. Weisman MH, Witter JP, Reveille JD. The prevalence of inflammatory back pain: population-based estimates from the US National Health and Nutrition Examination Survey, 2009–10. Ann Rheum Dis 2013;72(3):369–73.
16. Hamilton L, Macgregor A, Warmington V, Pinch E, Gaffney K. The prevalence of inflammatory back pain in a UK primary care population. Rheumatology 2013;53(1):161–4.
17. Lopez-Larrea C, Sujirachato K, Mehra NK, et al. HLA-B27 subtypes in Asian patients with ankylosing spondylitis. Evidence for new associations. Tissue Antigens 1995;45(3):169–76.
18. Nasution AR, Mardjuadi A, Kunmartini S, et al. HLA-B27 subtypes positively and negatively associated with spondyloarthropathy. J Rheum 1997;24(6):1111–14.
19. Paladini F, Taccari E, Fiorillo MT, et al. Distribution of HLA-B27 subtypes in Sardinia and continental Italy and their association with spondylarthropathies. Arthritis Rheum 2005;52(10):3319–21.
20. Liu Y, Jiang L, Cai Q, et al. Predominant association of HLA-B*2704 with ankylosing spondylitis in Chinese Han patients. Tissue Antigens 2009;75(1):61–4.
21. Mathieu A, Cauli A, Fiorillo MT, Sorrentino R. HLA-B27 and ankylosing spondylitis geographic distribution as the result of a genetic selection induced by malaria endemic? A review supporting the hypothesis. Autoimmunity Rev 2008;7(5):398–403.
22. Khan MA. HLA-B27 and its subtypes in world populations. Editorial review. Curr Opin Rheum 1995;7(4):263.
23. Brown MA, Pile KD, Kennedy LG, et al. HLA class I associations of ankylosing spondylitis in the white populations in the United Kingdom. Ann Rheum Dis 1996;55(4):268–70.
24. Khan MA. HLA-B27 and its subtypes in world populations. Curr Opin Rheum 1995;7(4):263–9.
25. Carter ET, McKenna CH, Brian DD, Kurland LT. Epidemiology of ankylosing spondylitis in Rochester, Minnesota, 1935–1973. Arthritis Rheum 1979;22(4):365–70.
26. Helmick CG, Felson DT, Lawrence RC, et al. Estimates of the prevalence of arthritis and other rheumatic conditions in the United States: Part I. Arthritis Rheum 2007;58(1):15–25.
27. Reveille JD, Witter JP, Weisman MH. Prevalence of axial spondylarthritis in the United States: estimates from a cross-sectional survey. Arthritis Care Res 2012;64(6):905–10.
28. Boyer GS, Templin DW, Cornoni-Huntley JC, et al. Prevalence of spondyloarthropathies in Alaskan Eskimos. J Rheum 1994;21(12):2292–7.
29. Haroon N, Paterson JM, Li P, Haroon N. Increasing proportion of female patients with ankylosing spondylitis: a population-based study of trends in the incidence and prevalence of AS. BMJ Open 2014;4(12):1–7.
30. Gofton JP, Chalmers A, Price GE, Reeve CE. HL-A27 and ankylosing spondylitis in B.C. Indians. J Rheum 1984;11(5):572–3.
31. Bakland G, Nossent HC, Gran JT. Incidence and prevalence of ankylosing spondylitis in northern Norway. Arthritis Rheum 2005;53(6):850–5.
32. Videm V, Cortes A, Thomas R, Brown MA. Current smoking is associated with incident ankylosing spondylitis—the HUNT population-based Norwegian health study. J Rheum 2014;41(10):2041–8.
33. Exarchou S, Lindström U, Askling J, et al. The prevalence of clinically diagnosed ankylosing spondylitis and its clinical manifestations: a nationwide register study. Arthritis Res Ther 2015;17:118.
34. Alexeeva L, Krylov M, Vturin V, Mylov N, Erdesz S, Benevolenskaya L. Prevalence of spondyloarthropathies and HLA-B27 in the native population of Chukotka, Russia. J Rheum 1994;21(12):2298–300.
35. Hukuda S, Minami M, Saito T, et al. Spondyloarthropathies in Japan: nationwide questionnaire survey performed by the Japan Ankylosing Spondylitis Society. J Rheum 2000;28(3):554–9.
36. Salaffi F, De Angelis R, Grassi W. Prevalence of musculoskeletal conditions in an Italian population sample: results of a regional community-based study. I. The MAPPING study. Clin Exp Rheum 2005;23(6):819–28.
37. Goycochea-Robles M-V, Sanin LH, Moreno-Montoya J, et al. Validity of the COPCORD Core Questionnaire as a classification tool for rheumatic diseases. J Rheum 2011;86(38):31–5.
38. Onen F, Solmaz D, Cetin P, et al. Prevalence of inflammatory back pain and axial spondyloarthritis among university employees in Izmir, Turkey. J Rheum 2015;1–6.
39. Costantino F, Talpin A, Said-Nahal R, et al. Prevalence of spondyloarthritis in reference to HLA-B27 in the French population: results of the GAZEL cohort. Ann Rheum Dis 2013;74:689–93.
40. Dean LE, Jones GT, MacDonald AG, Downham C, Sturrock RD, Macfarlane GJ. Global prevalence of ankylosing spondylitis. Rheumatology 2014; 53(4):650–7.
41. Underwood MR, Dawes P. Inflammatory back pain in primary care. Br J Rheum 1995;34:1074–7.
42. Bakland G, Alsing R, Singh K, Nossent JC. Assessment of SpondyloArthritis International Society criteria for axial spondyloarthritis in chronic back pain patients with a high prevalence of HLA-B27. Arthritis Care Res 2013;65(3):448–53.
43. Boonen A, Sieper J, van der Heijde D, et al. The burden of non-radiographic axial spondyloarthritis. Semin Arthritis Rheum 2015;44(5):556–62.
44. Wallis D, Haroon N, Ayearst R, Carty A, Inman RD. Ankylosing spondylitis and nonradiographic axial spondyloarthritis: part of a common spectrum or distinct diseases? J Rheum 2013;40(12):2038–41.
45. Zeng QY, Chen R, Darmawan J, et al. Rheumatic diseases in China. Arthritis Res Ther 2008;10(1):R17.
46. Kaipiainen-Seppanen O, Aho K, Heliovaara M. Incidence and prevalence of ankylosing spondylitis in Finland. J Rheum 1997;24(3):496–9.
47. Hukuda S, Minami M, Saito T, et al. Spondyloarthropathies in Japan: nationwide questionnaire survey performed by the Japan Ankylosing Spondylitis Society. J Rheum 2001;28(3):554–9.
48. Gonzalez-Galarza FF, Takeshita LYC, Santos EJM, et al. Allele frequency net 2015 update: new features for HLA epitopes, KIR and disease and HLA adverse drug reaction associations. Nucleic Acids Res 2015;43:D784–8.

CHAPTER 3

Diagnosis and classification of axial spondyloarthritis

Floris van Gaalen, Désirée van der Heijde, and Maxime Dougados

Introduction to diagnosis and classification

AxSpA is a potentially disabling chronic inflammatory disease affecting the spine and the SI joints. Lead symptoms of the disease are chronic back pain and stiffness.

The disease is called radiographic axSpA (r-axSpA) or AS when on plain radiographs bone changes consistent with sacroiliitis are present. When no evidence of sacroiliitis is seen on radiographs the disease is called nr-axSpA. In such cases, the diagnosis is made based on evidence of active inflammation of the SI joints on MRI and clinical and laboratory features, or a combination of clinical and laboratory features only.

Apart from affecting the spine and SI joints, axSpA may involve peripheral joints (e.g. knee and ankle) and entheses (insertion of ligaments or tendons at the bone), and can be associated with EAMs such as uveitis, psoriasis, and IBD.

In this chapter, diagnosis and classification of axSpA are discussed, including the use of MRI in detecting sacroiliitis and the difference between clinical diagnosis and disease classification.

Nomenclatures and stages of disease

SpA describes a group of interrelated diseases, including AS, PsA, arthritis with IBD, and reactive arthritis (ReA). The clinical presentation can be very heterogeneous, but patients with SpA can be distinguished according to their presentation as predominantly axial or predominantly peripheral SpA. SpA is called peripheral SpA when symptoms of peripheral arthritis, dactylitis, and/or enthesitis dominate the clinical presentation. Peripheral SpA is discussed in detail in Chapter 4. SpA with predominant involvement of the vertebral column and the SI joints is called axSpA. The most well-known form of axSpA is AS.

The term ankylosing spondylitis is derived from the Greek root *ankylosis* meaning stiffening of a joint, and *spondylos* which refers to a vertebra. AS thus refers to an inflammatory disorder associated with fibrous or bony bridging of joints in the spine, including the bridging of one or more intervertebral discs. Other terms used historically for AS include Bechterew's disease and Marie-Strümpell disease (1).

Diagnosis and classification of AS relies on the presence of a combination of clinical symptoms plus unequivocal radiographic sacroiliitis on radiographs of at least grade 2 bilaterally or grade 3 unilaterally (2) (Table 3.1).

Table 3.1 Grading of radiographic sacroiliitis

Grade 0 Normal
Grade 1 Suspicious changes
Grade 2 Minimal abnormality—small localized areas with erosion or sclerosis, without alteration in the joint width
Grade 3 Unequivocal abnormality—moderate or advanced sacroiliitis with one or more of the following: erosions, evidence of sclerosis, widening, narrowing, or partial ankylosis
Grade 4 Severe abnormality—total ankylosis

Source: Data from Bennett PH, Wood, PH (eds) Population studies in the rheumatic disease. Amsterdam. Excerpta Medica Foundation International Congress Series 148, 1966;456–457.

Examples of radiographic sacroiliitis are given in Fig. 3.1. However, radiographs of the SI joint are often normal when first symptoms of axSpA appear and it usually takes several years for definite radiographic sacroiliitis to evolve. As a result, the diagnosis of AS is commonly delayed by 8–11 years after the onset of symptoms (3–5). Inflammation in SI joints can in most cases be shown by MRI before the occurrence of structural damage, and MRI inflammation has also been shown to be predictive for developing sacroiliitis on radiographs later on (6). Rudwaleit and colleagues proposed that the presence and absence of radiographic sacroiliitis in patients with SpA represent different stages of a single disease continuum and, thereby, the same disease entity (7).

The term axSpA was introduced as the umbrella term for the two stages of disease. R-axSpA indicates the presence of sacroiliitis on radiographs and nr-axSpA refers to patients with SpA that have no sacroiliitis on radiographs but may have signs of active sacroiliitis on MRI (Fig. 3.2).

R-axSpA and nr-axSpA are increasingly considered together, although some uncertainty remains regarding whether these categories represent distinct but overlapping disorders or simply different points in the severity or chronology of illness along a single spectrum (8, 9).

Evaluation of suspected axial spondyloarthritis

AxSpA, including r-axSpA and nr-axSpA, should be considered in men and women with chronic back pain with an onset before the

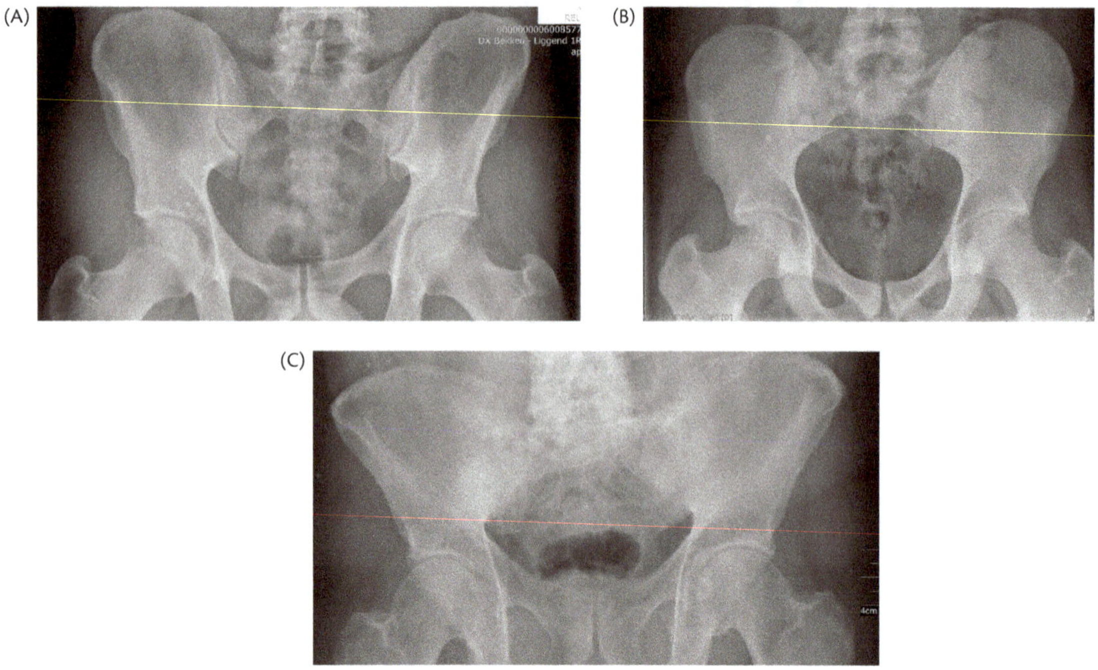

Fig. 3.1 Signs of sacroiliitis on radiographs. The panels show three different patients with different grades of sacroiliitis. Upper panel (A): No abnormalities on the SI joints. Grade zero ('normal') bilaterally. Middle panel (B): Bilateral grade 2 sacroiliitis with irregularity of the articular surface of the SI joint bilaterally due to erosions with sclerotic changes on the iliac side of the SI joint. Lower panel (C): Bilateral grade 4 sacroiliitis with fusion of the SI joints.

age of 45 years. A history of chronic low back pain that has been almost continuous for 3 months or more is present in most patients with axSpA and should prompt further evaluation to establish whether other features of SpA are present and, if so, whether they are sufficient to establish a diagnosis of axSpA.

Patients suspected of axSpA should undergo a thorough medical history, physical examination, and selected laboratory testing. Early referral to a rheumatologist based upon a limited set of symptoms and findings may facilitate diagnosis and institution of effective treatment (10). For example, a study in 16 countries found that axSpA could be diagnosed after referral to a rheumatologist in about 35% of patients in a primary care setting with chronic back pain for more than 3 months who were positive for HLA-B27, inflammatory back pain, (IBP) or sacroiliitis on imaging (11). Referral strategies using other sets of referral parameters have also been shown to be effective (12). ASAS recommendations for referral were published recently in April 2015 (13).

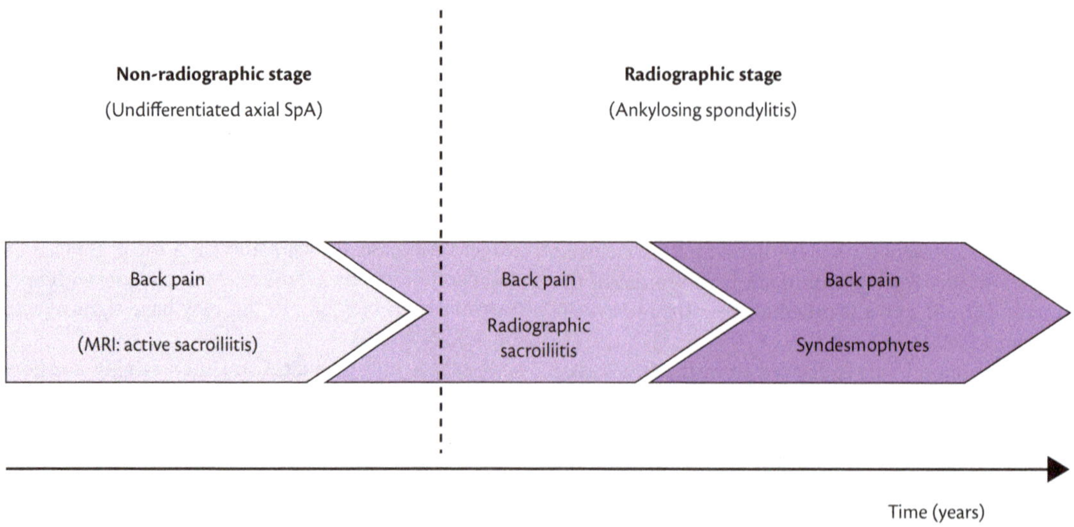

Fig. 3.2 Radiographic and non-radiographic stages in axSpA.Unifying concept of axSpA as proposed by Rudwaleit et al. (7), showing schematically the transition from early to late axSpA. AxSpA often starts without sacroiliitis detectable by conventional radiography, but, with time (often several years), sacroiliitis and possibly syndesmophytes (bony growth in the ligaments of the spine) may become detectable by conventional radiography. Back pain as the leading symptom may be present throughout the disease course. During the early disease stage, MRI may detect acute inflammatory lesions in the absence of radiographic sacroiliitis. Vertical dotted line indicates the distinction between nr-axSpA and r-axSpA also known as ankylosing spondylitis.

Patient history

IBP: chronic back pain is the leading symptom in patients with axSpA. In order to clinically differentiate back pain caused by inflammation of the SI joints and lower spine from other causes, attempts have been made to describe and to define clinical criteria for this specific kind of back pain, which has been termed IBP. Over the years, several attempts have been made to capture IBP in criteria sets, generally based on expert opinion, comparing AS patients with patients with mechanical back pain.

The 2009 ASAS experts IBP criteria were developed based on the opinion of 13 SpA experts investigating 20 patients with back pain, which were labelled as IBP or not by the experts. The criteria are met if four out of five of the following features are present:

- Onset of back pain before the age of 40 years
- Insidious onset of back pain
- Improvement of back pain with exercise
- No improvement of back pain with rest
- Pain at night (with improvement upon getting up)

These criteria were validated against expert judgement on the presence or absence of IBP in an international cohort of 648 patients with suspected SpA. The sensitivity of the ASAS experts IBP criteria was 79.6% and the specificity was 72.4%. For comparison, the previously published IBP criteria by Calin and the Berlin IBP criteria had a sensitivity and specificity of 89.9 and 52.5 and 70.0 and 81.4, respectively, in the same cohort (14). It is important to emphasize that IBP is a possible symptom of axSpA but is not present in all patients with SpA, and IBP can be present in patients without SpA. Nevertheless, IBP is suggestive for SpA and has also been successfully used as a screening parameter for axSpA in young patients with chronic low back pain seen by primary care physicians or orthopaedists (15).

Alternating buttock pain: pain alternating between the right and left gluteal regions is thought to be suggestive of axSpA.

Good response to non-steroidal anti-inflammatory drugs (*NSAIDs*): although patients with back pain of many causes may improve when treated with anti-inflammatory doses of an NSAID, marked improvement in pain within 24–48 hours supports the diagnosis of axSpA.

A history of anterior uveitis, IBD, or psoriasis: this needs to have been diagnosed by a physician and preferably an expert for this manifestation, e.g. an ophthalmologist in cases of uveitis.

A previous or current diagnosis of arthritis, dactylitis, or enthesitis: preferably made by a rheumatologist.

A family history of SpA: presence in first-degree or second-degree relatives of any of the following—AS, psoriasis, uveitis, ReA, or IBD—increases the risk for axSpA in a patient. First-degree relatives are parents, siblings, and offspring. Second-degree relatives are grandparents, grandchildren, uncles, aunts, nephews, nieces, and half-siblings.

Physical examination

All patients suspected of axSpA should undergo a thorough physical examination. Due to possible multiorgan involvement, physical examination of spine, peripheral joints, skin, nails, and eyes may provide important clues to the diagnosis of axSpA (Fig. 3.3). Other findings may help identify or exclude alternative diagnoses or comorbidities and establish a baseline measurement for ongoing clinical assessment of the patient.

The following features when present are thought to be suggestive of axSpA:

- Impairment of spinal mobility: impairment of spinal mobility is an important clinical sign of axSpA and is one of the central

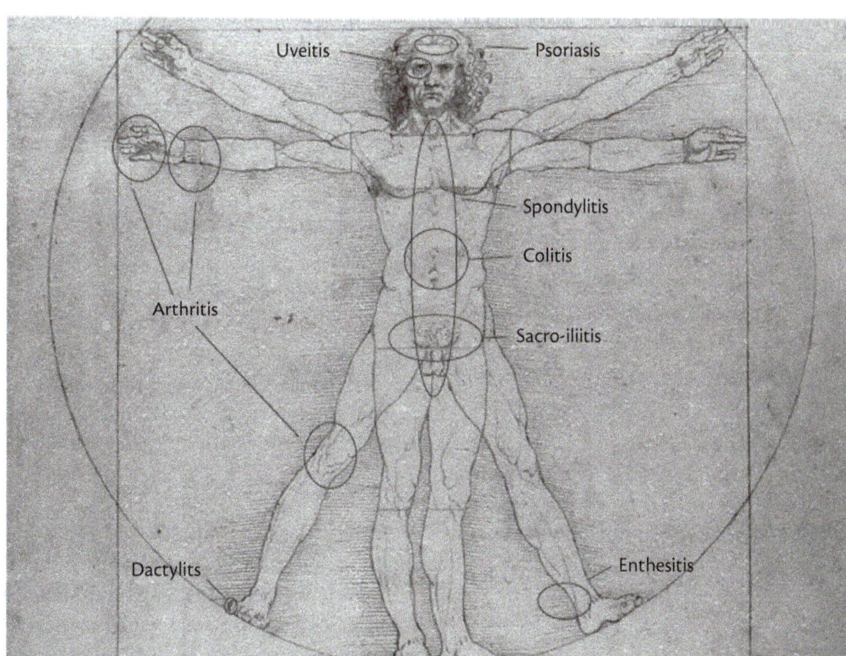

Fig. 3.3 (See colour plate section). Multiorgan involvement in SpA indicated on Leonardo da Vinci's Vitruvian Man.

outcomes in treatment studies in axSpA. However, it is not part of the new ASAS classification criteria and not part of the proposed diagnosed algorithm for axSpA because spinal mobility is often not or only slightly restricted early in the course of the disease and may not differentiate well from other diseases, such as degenerative spine disease. Spinal mobility measures recommended by ASAS are chest expansion, modified Schober test, occiput-to-wall distance, cervical rotation, and either lateral spinal flexion test or Bath Ankylosing Spondylitis Metrology Index (BASMI) (see (16) for reference including descriptions on how to perform these measures). An early clinical sign is disappearance of the lumbar lordosis.

- Recent data from a long-term study of AS patients showed that lateral spinal flexion and lumbar flexion as measured by the modified Schober test are most frequently impaired, followed by involvement of the thoracic and cervical spine. These data suggested that in clinical practice the lateral spinal flexion test and modified Schober test suffice to screen for impairment in spinal mobility (17). In case any of these two tests are impaired, a full examination of all the above-mentioned spinal mobility tests is warranted. To aid clinicians in identifying impairments in spinal mobility, age-specific reference intervals for spinal mobility in non-disease controls are available (18).
- Arthritis: in patients with arthralgia, the peripheral joints, including the hands, wrists, elbows, shoulders, hips, knees, ankles, and feet, should be examined to determine the number of swollen and/or tender joints, as well as those with deformities and/or loss of range of motion. An asymmetric oligoarthritis, predominantly involving the lower limbs, is the most typical pattern for peripheral arthritis in SpA.
- Dactylitis: dactylitis is a diffuse swelling of the digits of toes or fingers, also termed 'sausage digit'. A past history of a swollen finger or toe should prompt a physical examination, since after an inflammatory episode of dactylitis, the affected toe or finger may remain swollen to a varying degree. Dactylitis in SpA often coexists with psoriasis.
- Heel enthesitis: enthesitis is an inflammation at sites where tendons or ligaments insert into the bone. Although any enthesis can be affected in axSpA, the site where physical examination can most reliably identify enthesitis is the heel. At the heels, tenderness and swelling at the insertions of the plantar fascii and Achilles tendon into the calcaneus should be investigated.
- Eyes: patients with symptoms or signs suggestive of (unilateral) anterior uveitis, such as eye pain, visual disturbance, or redness, should be referred for evaluation and treatment by an expert in uveitis, normally an ophthalmologist, and require examination using a slit lamp to confirm the diagnosis.
- Skin and nails: skin and nails should be examined for evidence of psoriasis. Since psoriasis may be mild, a systematic evaluation of the most frequently affected areas (including nails, scalp, and elbows but also navel and gluteal fold) is recommended.

Laboratory testing

Acute phase reactants

Acute phase reactants, including the erythrocyte sedimentation rate (ESR) and CRP, should be measured in patients suspected of axSpA. If only one test can be done, CRP is the preferred test. Elevated CRP levels are observed in about 40% of patients with axSpA (19). Thus a normal CRP does not exclude axSpA. In patients with established axSpA, CRP levels are used in composite measures to assess disease activity (20).

HLA-B27 testing

HLA-B27 is the most important genetic risk factor for axSpA and remains one of the strongest genetic associations with any common human disease. About 80% of Caucasoid AS patients are positive for HLA-B27, compared to only 8–10% of the population. Nonetheless, only a minority (about 5%) of B27-positive individuals develop AS. Thus a positive test for HLA-B27 alone is not diagnostic for disease. The frequency of HLA-B27 in nr-axSpA has been reported to be about 60–85% (8, 21, 22).

Imaging

Radiography of sacroiliac joints

Radiography of SI joints and spine has been used since the 1930s for diagnosis and staging of patients with AS (23). In contrast to MRI, radiographs can only detect chronic bony changes (damage), which are the consequence of inflammation and not inflammation itself. Nevertheless, in patients suspected of axSpA, a plain film radiograph of the pelvis should be considered to evaluate the SI joints (24). A standard anteroposterior (AP) view of the pelvis has the advantage of including the hips, which are relatively frequently affected in axSpA. Presence of abnormalities of the SI joint on radiographs, including sclerosis, erosions, changes in joint width, or ankylosis, strongly supports the diagnosis of AS. Each SI joint on radiography can be graded from 0 (normal) to 4 (total ankylosis) based upon the degree of abnormalities (Table 3.1). A patient is regarded as positive for radiographic sacroiliitis if the score is greater than or equal to grade 2 bilaterally or if the score is greater than or equal to grade 3 unilaterally.

Reading radiographs of the SI joints is considered difficult. Interobserver and intra-observer variations are substantial particularly in grade 1 and 2 abnormalities (25). Unfortunately, training in reading radiography does not reduce intra-observer variation. As a result, sacroiliitis on radiographs is not seldom missed or incorrectly diagnosed (26).

Radiography of the spine

Radiographs of the spine are generally not required for a diagnosis of axSpA, but AP and lateral views should be performed in patients diagnosed with axSpA for assessment of the severity of disease, with a focus on the presence of syndesmophytes. Syndesmophytes are rare in the absence of radiographic sacroiliitis, but in certain cases when interpretation of the changes in the SI joints is difficult, presence of syndesmophytes helps make a diagnosis of axSpA.

MRI of the sacroiliac joints

In patients with clear signs of sacroiliitis on radiographs, additional imaging, such as MRI, is not necessary for diagnosis. However, radiography is often inadequate to detect early disease, as patients may have symptoms for several years before abnormalities can be seen on radiographs (27). Studies have shown that MRI can detect inflammation in the SI joints of patients at a high risk of having AS years before these joints develop sacroiliitis on radiographs (6).

So, MRI of the SI joint, unlike plain radiographs, can reveal inflammatory changes before structural abnormalities are present.

Recommended sequences to detect inflammatory lesions on MRI of the SI joints are short tau inversion recovery (STIR) and T1 fat-saturated after gadolinium used in conjunction with T1-weighted (T1W) sequence. While the STIR sequence shows active inflammation as increased signal intensity due to the presence of increased amounts of free water, T1 plus gadolinium depicts areas of increased vascularization due to increased diffusion of gadolinium into the interstitial space. However, gadolinium administration is contraindicated in patients with renal disease and increases costs of performing MRI. More importantly, however, in clinical practice, T1/gadolinium has not been shown to provide additional value over STIR in clinical practice (28, 29).

The ASAS/Outcome Measures in Rheumatology Clinical Trials (OMERACT) MRI working group has published a consensus among experts on what defines active sacroiliitis on MRI of the SI joints (30). According to the definition, active inflammatory lesions should appear on STIR sequences as bone marrow oedema (BME), highly suggestive of SpA, and must be clearly present and located in typical anatomical areas (subchondral or periarticular bone marrow of the SI joints). The lesions are hyperintense ('white') on STIR and hypointense 'dark' signal on T1W images. A positive MRI should show at least two BME lesions on the same slice, or one lesion on at least two consecutive slices (Fig. 3.4).

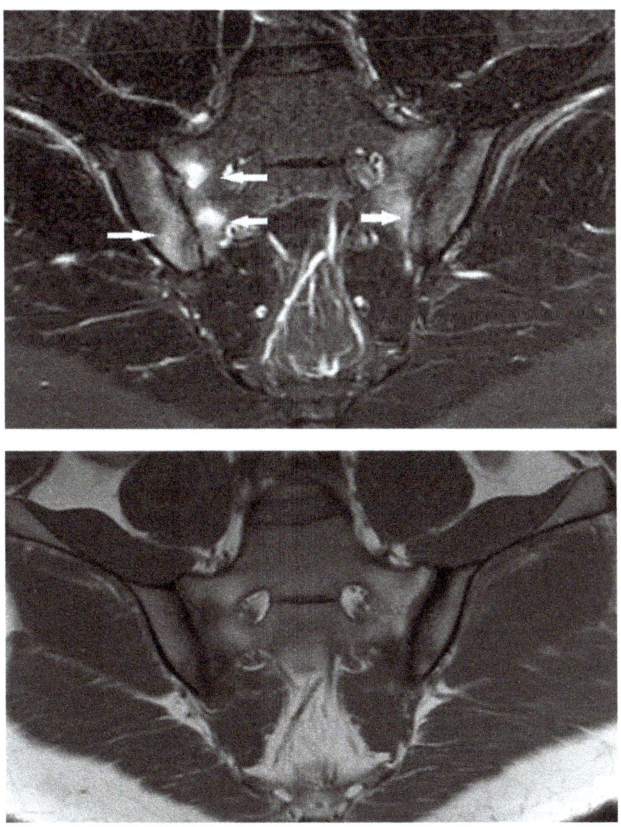

Fig. 3.4 MRI of a patient with active sacroiliitis. Upper panel shows STIR sequence and lower panel T1 sequence. Bright white areas in STIR are areas of BME (arrows). On T1 sequences, areas of BME are dark. Given that on this one MRI slice at least two areas of BME highly suggestive of axSpA are seen, the MRI is positive for sacroiliitis according to the ASAS/OMERACT definition.

In order to use this definition, several technical requirements must be met: besides using the previously mentioned MRI sequences, a slice thickness of 3 or 4 mm is needed, and the SI joints are to be imaged using a semicoronal orientation along the long axis of the sacral bone (see Chapter 13 for more details).

A positive MRI by itself or with chronic back pain alone is not diagnostic of axSpA. Presence of BME on MRI has been observed in about 10% of controls either with chronic back pain without SpA or even in individuals without back pain (31, 32).

Besides BME, which is thought to reflect active inflammation in patients with SpA, MRI of the SI joints may show structural changes due to previous inflammation, including fat deposition, sclerosis, erosions, and bony ankylosis in the T1 sequence. Incorporation of structural changes into the definition of a positive sacroiliac MRI for SpA has been advocated (33), as this could improve the diagnostic value of MRI, but a generally accepted definition of what constitutes structural changes consistent with SpA has yet to be decided (for more details see Chapter 13).

MRI of the spine

Abnormalities of the spine on MRI are not used in the routine diagnosis of axSpA. However, detection of inflammatory or structural lesions in the spine might improve the diagnostic utility of MRI scanning in axSpA. A consensus-based definition of a positive spinal MRI for inflammatory lesions (spondylitis) and structural changes (fat deposition) has been published (34), and spinal inflammation detected in the absence of inflammation in the SI joints has been observed in SpA patients (35). More research is needed, but in certain cases MRI of the spine could be considered in patients with a very high level of suspicion for nr-axSpA that have a normal radiograph and MRI of the SI joints (for more details see Chapter 13).

Classification of axial spondyloarthritis

Classification criteria are usually developed for the identification of patients for inclusion in clinical trials. Although classification criteria are not for diagnosis in clinical practice, the value of classification criteria lies in their ability to identify typical cases of a particular disease using a standardized and often abbreviated form of the diagnostic process. Items in classification criteria reflect the essential features of a disease and thereby are an *aide-mémoire* to the key points used in making a clinical diagnosis.

Since the introduction of radiography in medicine, sacroiliitis on radiographs has been considered the hallmark of AS (23). As a result, sacroiliitis on radiographs has been given a very prominent place in classification criteria (36, 37) since the 1960s where sacroiliitis on radiographs had to be present to fulfil the classification criteria.

The last set of classification criteria to exclusively focus on AS, the mNY criteria published in 1984, classifies patients as having definite AS if the radiologic criterion of radiographic sacroiliitis is met and one clinical criterion is present. Clinical criteria in the mNY criteria are a history of chronic low back pain and stiffness which improves with exercise but is not relieved by rest, limitation in the lumbar spine on physical examination, or limitation of chest expansion on physical examination (see Table 3.2 for details).

Since publication, the mNY criteria have been the most widely used criteria for classification of AS, and most likely also for

Table 3.2 mNY criteria for AS

1. Clinical criteria
a) Low back pain and stiffness for more than 3 months which improves with exercise but is not relieved by rest
b) Limitation of motion of the lumbar spine in both the sagittal and frontal planes
c) Limitation of chest expansion relative to normal values corrected for age and sex
2. Radiologic criterion
Sacroiliitis grade ≥ 2 bilaterally or sacroiliitis grade 3–4 unilaterally

Definite AS if the radiologic criterion is associated with at least one clinical criterion.

Source: Data from van der Linden S, Valkenburg HA, Cats A. Evaluation of diagnostic criteria for ankylosing spondylitis. A proposal for modification of the New York criteria. Arthritis Rheum 1984 Apr; 27(4):361–8.

diagnosis of AS. The Amor criteria from 1990 (38) and ESSG preliminary classification criteria published in 1991 (39) also allow classification of AS patients, but both were developed to be able to classify the entire group of SpA, which includes SpA with axial manifestations but also SpA with exclusively peripheral disease.

In the Amor criteria, points are given for the presence of disease features, with six points needed for classification of SpA. In patients with AS, radiographic sacroiliitis gives three points, so it needs to be present together with one or more of nine clinical items (each 1 or 2 points), HLA-B27 positivity (2 points), positive family history (2 points), or a good response to NSAIDs (2 points) (38). In the ESSG criteria, to classify AS, the presence of sacroiliitis on radiographs is usually combined with IBP. However, the ESSG criteria are also met when IBP is present in combination with any one of the following features: a positive family history of SpA, psoriasis, IBD, alternating buttock pain, enthesopathy, or onset of (peripheral) arthritis 1 month after an episode of urethritis, cervicitis, or acute diarrhoea within 1 month before onset of (peripheral) arthritis (39).

The mNY criteria have been widely accepted and perform well in established AS; they do not perform well in early disease where radiographic sacroiliitis may not yet be present. So while the mNY criteria lack sensitivity in early AS, the ESSG criteria may lack specificity because, in addition to IBP, only one further clinical parameter such as psoriasis needs to be present to classify a patient as SpA. It has been argued that this combination of clinical features is not sufficient in classifying patients with early AS (40, 41). The Amor criteria may provide a better specificity than the ESSG criteria because to reach the 6-point cut-off, at least three SpA parameters are needed in order to fulfil the criteria.

A few years after publication of the ESSG and Amor criteria, MRI emerged as a diagnostic tool to visualize acute inflammation in the SI joints. Subsequently, a prospective study showed that in a cohort of 25 HLA-B27-positive patients with IBP, signs of active inflammation on MRI preceded development of sacroiliitis on radiographs after 3 years with a positive predictive value of 60% (6). Several years later, another prospective study showed that in IBP patients with a symptom duration of less than 2 years, inflammatory lesion in the SI joint on MRI predicted development of radiographic sacroiliitis at 7 years of follow-up. The effect was most pronounced in HLA-B27-positive patients with a lot of inflammation on MRI at baseline (42). Together, these studies supported the predictive validity of MRI as an imaging instrument in early axSpA, and in particular for detecting patients with nr-axSpA.

The mNY criteria were never intended to classify patients with nr-axSpA and are exclusively for r-axSpA. Although the ESSG and Amor criteria were intended for the entire spectrum of SpA, including nr-axSpA, they had been developed before MRI techniques detecting SI joint inflammation were available.

ASAS classification criteria for axial spondyloarthritis

In 2009, ASAS developed criteria for the classification of axSpA that are applicable to both r-axSpA and nr-axSpA. A specific aim was to develop SpA criteria for application in early disease and thereby facilitate conduct of clinical trials and observational studies in early axSpA.

A two-step process was followed to create the new classification criteria. First, candidate classification criteria were constructed following assessment of 71 patients with chronic back pain of unknown origin suspected of having axSpA, with the majority of patients (69 out of 71) without radiographic sacroiliitis. Clinical data, laboratory tests, and imaging results were presented on paper to 20 SpA experts from around the world. Experts were asked to classify patients as axSpA or no axSpA and provide their level of confidence for each assessment. From these assessments, candidate criteria were constructed. As it was felt that the new criteria should include the possibility to classify axSpA solely on the basis of clinical criteria, the two candidate criteria sets both consisted of two parts. In both candidate sets, patients could be classified as axSpA if sacroiliitis was present on imaging (either MRI or radiography of SI joints) and one additional criterion was present. In addition, in candidate set 1, a patient could be classified as axSpA if three SpA features other than imaging were present, and in candidate set 2, a patient could also be classified as axSpA if IBP was present together with two other (non-imaging) SpA features (43).

In the second phase, the two sets of candidate criteria for classification of axSpA were validated and refined. For that purpose, a validation cohort of consecutively referred patients suspected of having axSpA was created. In total, 25 centres of ASAS members from 16 countries provided clinical, laboratory, and imaging data from 649 patients. In the cohort, 391 patients had axSpA (60.2%) and 258 did not (39.8%), as diagnosed by the local rheumatologist. This diagnosis of the rheumatologist served as the external standard in creation of the classification criteria. In addition to testing the prespecified candidate criteria and comparing performance against the ESSG and Amor criteria, both the original criteria and versions including MRI in addition to radiographs were investigated.

Overall, both candidate sets performed equally well in the validation cohort, and in a modified version of the Amor criteria where MRI had been added candidates performed similarly. The ESSG criteria, however, with or without the addition of MRI, performed less well. When the specificity of the candidate criteria set 1 was analysed separately for its 'imaging arm' (sacroiliitis on radiographs or MRI plus one or more SpA feature) and for its 'clinical arm' (three or more SpA features), the specificity of the imaging arm was excellent at 97.3%, but that of the clinical arm was only 76.7%. To refine the clinical arm, several alternatives were made. One alternative for the clinical arm of the criteria set was the presence of HLA-B27 plus two or more other SpA features in order to classify a patient as having axSpA. This alternative was shown to have a better specificity (83.3–84.9%).

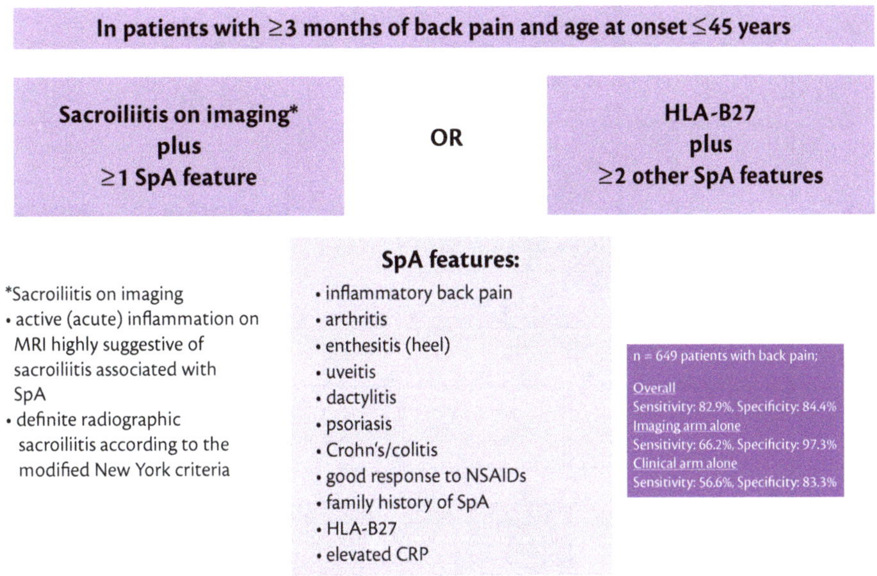

Fig. 3.5 ASAS classification criteria for axSpA.
Reproduced from Ann Rheum Dis, Rudwaleit M et al., 68, 777–783s, 2009 with permission from BMJ Publishing Group Ltd.

Finally, all ASAS members were allowed to vote which set of candidate criteria would be the final set: besides candidate criteria sets 1 and 2, and a modified version of the ESSG and Amor criteria, two alternatives were presented. The majority of ASAS members voted for the criteria set with HLA-B27 plus two or more other SpA features as the clinical arm (19) (Fig. 3.5).

Similar to the candidate criteria sets, the final ASAS classification criteria consist of two parts. According to the imaging arm, a patient with chronic back pain with an onset before the age of 45 is classified as axSpA if sacroiliitis is unequivocally present on radiographs or MRI (as subchondral bone marrow oedema) of the SI and at least one other SpA feature is present. According to the clinical arm, patients with chronic back pain with an onset before the age of 45 are classified as axSpA if they test positive for HLA-B27 and at least two other features are present. In the validation cohort, the criteria had a sensitivity of 82.9% and a specificity of 84.4%, with the diagnosis of the rheumatologist as the reference.

Although these ASAS criteria are to be used primarily as classification criteria, the ASAS criteria might perform well as diagnostic criteria if used by rheumatologists in situations where prevalence of SpA is high (e.g. in the validation cohort where prevalence of SpA was 60%). How the ASAS criteria perform in clinics with a low prevalence of SpA, such as in primary care, is not known, but it is likely that many patients will be classified who do not have the diagnosis. Therefore it is not recommended to use these classification criteria for diagnostic purposes in primary care.

The ASAS classification criteria have clearly met the goal of enabling clinical trials in early axSpA. Since publication, the classification criteria have been studied in early disease cohorts, and many clinical trials using the ASAS classification criteria have been performed (e.g. 44–48). Another example for the general acceptance of these criteria is that at the time of writing this chapter over 20 active clinical trials and studies using the ASAS classification criteria were listed in the ClinicalTrials.gov online database (https://clinicaltrials.gov/).

Making a diagnosis of axial spondyloarthritis

Classification criteria are developed to provide a clear 'yes' or 'no' answer, usually to decide whether a patient would be suitable for inclusion in a clinical trial, and are applied after the rheumatologist has made the diagnosis. In clinical practice, a more flexible approach is necessary, although the same parameters are used for classification and diagnostic purposes (7). AxSpA is a heterogeneous disorder for which no single specific distinguishing feature is available (49). Therefore a diagnosis is always based on the presence of more than one feature suggestive of the disease.

In diagnosis, negative findings are taken into account, while this is not the case if classification criteria are applied. For example, if radiographs and MRI of the SI joints and the spine are available but do not show any evidence of inflammation or structural damage typical for SpA, this can then be taken as a strong argument against the diagnosis, even if the clinical arm of the classification criteria would be fulfilled (50). Furthermore, in a diagnostic procedure using differential diagnosis, other causes for a patient's symptoms are investigated and other causes for SpA-associated features (e.g. arthritis due to gout, elevated CRP due to a recent infection, subchondral bone marrow oedema on MRI due to mechanical stress) are considered. A recent publication by Braun and colleagues, reporting on a selection of patient cases with an incorrect diagnosis of axSpA referred to a tertiary centre outpatient clinic, provides excellent insights into possible errors made in the diagnosis of axSpA (50).

A helpful tool in the early diagnosis of axSpA is the 2013 ASAS modified Berlin diagnostic algorithm (Fig. 3.6). The algorithm was developed to provide cost-effective guidance for rheumatologists to assess whether an individual patient referred for evaluation could be diagnosed as having axSpA. The algorithm was validated in SPondyloarthritis Caught Early (SPACE) (22) and the ASAS cohort.

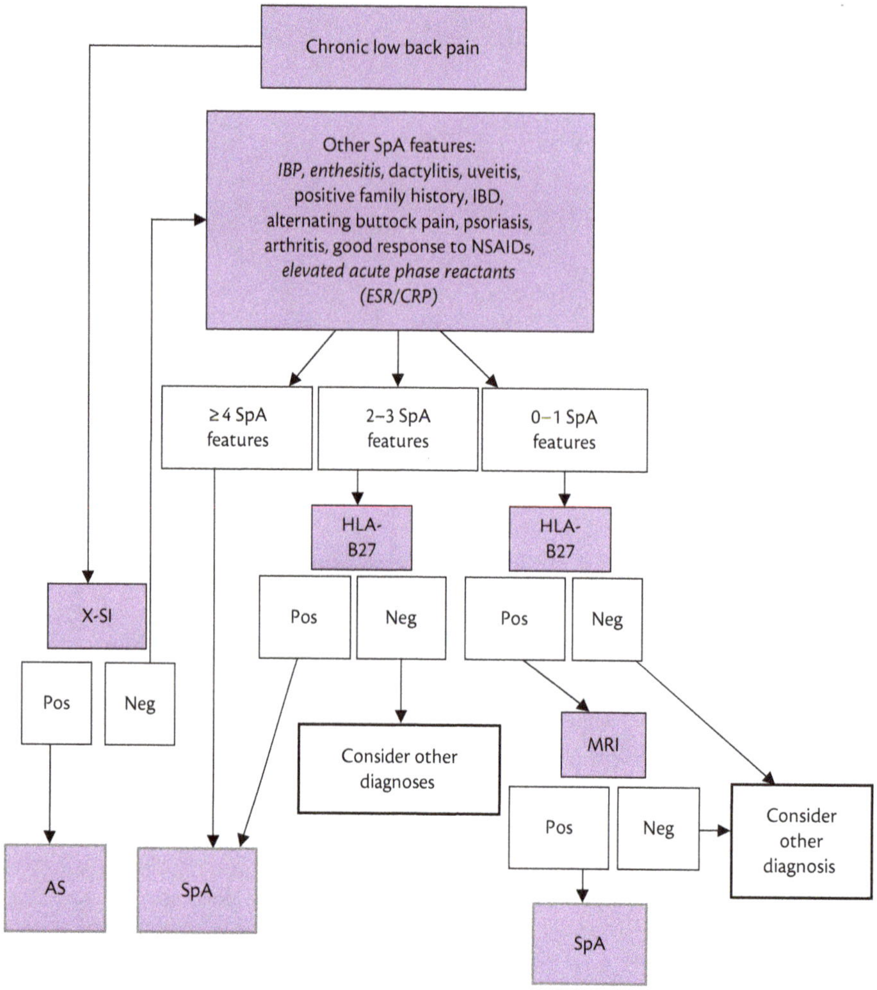

Fig. 3.6 ASAS modification of the Berlin algorithm for diagnosing axSpA.
Reproduced from Ann Rheum Dis, van den Berg et al., 72, 1646–53, 2013 with permission from BMJ Publishing Group Ltd.

Here we present the application of this algorithm using the results of the Leiden SPACE cohort. This cohort consisted of young adults with chronic back pain referred to a rheumatologist. Patients had had back pain for longer than 3 months but less than 2 years. In the SPACE cohort, for research purposes all diagnostic testing thought to be relevant for SpA is done in all patients, including HLA-B27 testing and an MRI of the SI joints. Thirty-eight percent of patients from the SPACE cohort used in the algorithm evaluation had been classified as axSpA.

After going through the steps, for each box the algorithm gives a yes or no answer on whether a patient probably has axSpA (Fig. 3.6). Applying this algorithm to a patient with chronic back pain of at least 3 months' duration with an onset before age 45, as a first step a radiograph of the pelvis is made. If a patient has clear sacroiliitis (at least grade 2 bilaterally or grade 3 unilaterally) the algorithm states that the patient has r-axSpA or AS. In the SPACE cohort, with a low number of AS patients, 11 out of 12 (92%) AS patients could be classified according to the ASAS criteria.

If the radiograph of the pelvis shows no convincing sacroiliitis, additional tests may be ordered based on the number of SpA features a patient has according to history, physical examination, and testing for acute phase reactants. When a patient has less than four SpA features, the algorithm advises HLA-B27 testing. In patients with no or only one SpA feature that are HLA-B27 negative, the algorithm advises to consider another diagnosis. In the SPACE cohort, the yield of MRI SI if performed as the next step was very low. After performing MRI SI in HLA-B27-negative patients with maximally one SpA feature, only 2.3% was classified as axSpA. In patients with no or one SpA feature who are HLA-B27 positive, MRI SI provides an answer if patients have SpA or not. In SpA patients with two or three features testing positive for HLA-B27, the algorithm states that all have SpA, and indeed all patients in the SPACE cohort in this category were classified as axSpA. In SpA patients with two or three features testing negative for HLA-B27, the algorithm states that patients do not have axSpA. However, in the SPACE cohort, 16% of these patients had a positive MRI and could be classified as axSpA. In patients in this category, an MRI of the SI joints may be considered in particular if a patient has SpA features that have a strong association with the disease (Fig. 3.6: SpA features in bold). If a patient has four or more features (without HLA-B27 and MRI results available), the algorithm indicates that a patient has SpA. In the SPACE cohort, after making an MRI of the SI joints and/or HLA-B27 testing, 70% of patients could be classified as axSpA, but 30% not.

The modified algorithm has both a sensitivity and specificity of about 80% for axSpA in patients with back pain for more than 3 months but less than 2 years with an onset of pain before the age of 45. Thus it provides only a general guideline for the diagnosis of individual cases, and it might be necessary in some patients to have all clinical, laboratory, and imaging results available before making a final diagnosis.

In some patients, diagnostic uncertainty remains, despites extensive testing. In such patients, a 'wait-and-see' policy regarding the diagnosis and symptomatic treatment with regular follow-up assessments will often be the most appropriate approach. Selected patients may benefit from additional imaging studies, such as patients with normal SI joint imaging on plain radiography and MRI, but prominent spinal pain and other features of SpA, for whom evidence of spondylitis shown on imaging of the spine may support a diagnosis of axSpA, rather than another cause of back pain. Similarly, ultrasonography has been used by some experts to document the presence of enthesitis when there is uncertainty regarding whether enthesitis is present (51). An initially negative MRI of the SI joints may become positive if repeated after 1 year, particularly in male patients who are HLA-B27 positive (52).

Conclusion

AxSpA is the umbrella term for SpA patients with predominant involvement of the axial skeleton. AxSpA is composed of r-axSpA or AS typically with radiographic sacroiliitis on plain radiography, and nr-axSpA, without plain radiographic changes of sacroiliitis.

AxSpA can generally be diagnosed based upon the recognition of a pattern of clinical, laboratory, and imaging findings characteristic of axSpA, including chronic back pain, sacroiliitis on imaging, and the presence of HLA-B27 and other features; the likelihood of the diagnosis varies depending upon the specific findings that are present. There is no single historical feature or diagnostic study with sufficient specificity to make the diagnosis without the presence of additional abnormalities, nor are there widely accepted and well-established diagnostic criteria or checklists on which to base the diagnosis.

In 2009, ASAS developed classification criteria for axSpA, which have been successfully used in clinical trials and cohort studies. SpA features in the ASAS classification criteria are the cornerstone for diagnosis of axSpA, and an ASAS-endorsed diagnostic algorithm is available to provide cost-effective guidance for rheumatologists to assess whether an individual patient could be diagnosed as having axSpA.

References

1. Calabro JJ, Maltz BA. Ankylosing spondylitis. N Engl J Med 1970;282(11):606–10.
2. van der Linden S, Valkenburg HA, Cats A. Evaluation of diagnostic criteria for ankylosing spondylitis. A proposal for modification of the New York criteria. Arthritis Rheum 1984;27(4):361–8.
3. Khan MA. Ankylosing spondylitis: introductory comments on its diagnosis and treatment. Ann Rheum Dis 2002;61(Suppl 3):iii3–7.
4. Mau W, Zeidler H, Mau R, et al. Clinical features and prognosis of patients with possible ankylosing spondylitis. Results of a 10-year followup. J Rheumatol 1988;15(7):1109–14.
5. Feldtkeller E, Khan MA, van der Heijde D, van der Linden S, Braun J. Age at disease onset and diagnosis delay in HLA-B27 negative vs. positive patients with ankylosing spondylitis. Rheumatol Int 2003;23(2):61–6.
6. Oostveen J, Prevo R, den BJ, van de Laar M. Early detection of sacroiliitis on magnetic resonance imaging and subsequent development of sacroiliitis on plain radiography. A prospective, longitudinal study. J Rheumatol 1999;26(9):1953–8.
7. Rudwaleit M, Khan MA, Sieper J. The challenge of diagnosis and classification in early ankylosing spondylitis: do we need new criteria? Arthritis Rheum 2005;52(4):1000–8.
8. Kiltz U, Baraliakos X, Karakostas P, et al. Do patients with non-radiographic axial spondylarthritis differ from patients with ankylosing spondylitis? Arthritis Care Res (Hoboken) 2012;64(9):1415–22.
9. Deodhar A, Reveille JD, Van Den Bosch F, et al. The concept of axial spondyloarthritis: joint statement of the spondyloarthritis research and treatment network and the Assessment of SpondyloArthritis international Society in response to the US Food and Drug Administration's comments and concerns. Arthritis Rheumatol 2014;66(10):2649–56.
10. Rudwaleit M, Sieper J. Referral strategies for early diagnosis of axial spondyloarthritis. Nat Rev Rheumatol 2012;8(5):262–8.
11. Sieper J, Srinivasan S, Zamani O, et al. Comparison of two referral strategies for diagnosis of axial spondyloarthritis: the Recognising and Diagnosing Ankylosing Spondylitis Reliably (RADAR) study. Ann Rheum Dis 2013;72(10):1621–7.
12. Braun A, Gnann H, Saracbasi E, et al. Optimizing the identification of patients with axial spondyloarthritis in primary care—the case for a two-step strategy combining the most relevant clinical items with HLA B27. Rheumatology (Oxford) 2013;52(8):1418–24.
13. Poddubnyy D, van Tubergen A, Landewe R, Sieper J, van der Heijde DA. Development of an ASAS-endorsed recommendation for the early referral of patients with a suspicion of axial spondyloarthritis. Ann Rheum Dis 23 Apr 2015; doi: 10.1136/annrheumdis-2014-207151.
14. Sieper J, van der Heijde D, Landewe R, et al. New criteria for inflammatory back pain in patients with chronic back pain: a real patient exercise by experts from the Assessment of SpondyloArthritis international Society (ASAS). Ann Rheum Dis 2009;68(6):784–8.
15. Brandt HC, Spiller I, Song IH, Vahldiek JL, Rudwaleit M, Sieper J. Performance of referral recommendations in patients with chronic back pain and suspected axial spondyloarthritis. Ann Rheum Dis 2007;66(11):1479–84.
16. Sieper J, Rudwaleit M, Baraliakos X, et al. The Assessment of SpondyloArthritis international Society (ASAS) handbook: a guide to assess spondyloarthritis. Ann Rheum Dis 2009;68(Suppl 2):ii1–44.
17. Ramiro S, Landewé R, van der Heijde D, et al. A spinal mobility gets impaired in a fixed order in patients with ankylosing spondylitis: 12-year OASIS results. Arthritis Rheum 2013;65(Suppl 10):1525.
18. Ramiro S, van Tubergen A, Stolwijk C, van der Heijde D, Royston P, Landewe R. Reference intervals of spinal mobility measures in normal individuals: the mobility study. Ann Rheum Dis 2015;74(6):1218–24.
19. Rudwaleit M, van der Heijde D, Landewe R, et al. The development of Assessment of SpondyloArthritis international Society classification criteria for axial spondyloarthritis (part II): validation and final selection. Ann Rheum Dis 2009;68(6):777–83.
20. van der Heijde D, Lie E, Kvien TK, et al. ASDAS, a highly discriminatory ASAS-endorsed disease activity score in patients with ankylosing spondylitis. Ann Rheum Dis 2009;68(12):1811–18.
21. Robinson PC, Brown MA. The genetics of ankylosing spondylitis and axial spondyloarthritis. Rheum Dis Clin N Am 2012;38(3):539–53.
22. van den Berg R, de Hooge M, van Gaalen F, Reijnierse M, Huizinga T, van der Heijde D. Percentage of patients with spondyloarthritis in patients referred because of chronic back pain and performance of classification criteria: experience from the Spondyloarthritis Caught Early (SPACE) cohort. Rheumatology (Oxford) 2013;52(8):1492–9.
23. Forestier J. The importance of sacro-iliac changes in the early diagnosis of ankylosing spondylarthritis 1: Marie–Strumpell–Bechterew disease. Radiology 1939;33(3):389–402.
24. Mandl P, Navarro-Compan V, Terslev L, et al. EULAR recommendations for the use of imaging in the diagnosis and management of spondyloarthritis in clinical practice. Ann Rheum Dis 2015;74(7):1327–39.

25. van Tubergen A, Heuft-Dorenbosch L, Schulpen G, et al. Radiographic assessment of sacroiliitis by radiologists and rheumatologists: does training improve quality? Ann Rheum Dis 2003;62(6):519–25.
26. van den Berg R, Lenczner G, Feydy A, et al. Agreement between clinical practice and trained central reading in reading of sacroiliac joints on plain pelvic radiographs. Results from the DESIR cohort. Arthritis Rheumatol 2014;66(9):2403–11.
27. Feldtkeller E, Bruckel J, Khan MA. Scientific contributions of ankylosing spondylitis patient advocacy groups. Curr Opin Rheumatol 2000;12(4):239–47.
28. de Hooge M, van den Berg R, Navarro-Compan V, et al. Magnetic resonance imaging of the sacroiliac joints in the early detection of spondyloarthritis: no added value of gadolinium compared with short tau inversion recovery sequence. Rheumatology (Oxford) 2013;52(7):1220–4.
29. van Onna M, van Tubergen A, van der Heijde D, Jurik AG, Landewe R. Gadolinium contrast-enhanced MRI sequence does not have an incremental value in the assessment of sacroiliitis in patients with early inflammatory back pain by using MRI in combination with pelvic radiographs: a 2-year follow-up study. Clin Exp Rheumatol 2014;32(2):225–30.
30. Rudwaleit M, Jurik AG, Hermann KGA, et al. Defining active sacroiliitis on magnetic resonance imaging (MRI) for classification of axial spondyloarthritis: a consensual approach by the ASAS/OMERACT MRI group. Annal Rheum Dis 2009;68(10):1520–7.
31. Weber U, Pedersen SJ, Ostergaard M, Rufibach K, Lambert RG, Maksymowych WP. Can erosions on MRI of the sacroiliac joints be reliably detected in patients with ankylosing spondylitis?—A cross-sectional study. Arthritis Res Ther 2012;14(3):R124.
32. Weber U, Zubler V, Pedersen SJ, et al. Development and validation of a magnetic resonance imaging reference criterion for defining a positive sacroiliac joint magnetic resonance imaging finding in spondyloarthritis. Arthritis Care Res (Hoboken) 2013;65(6):977–85.
33. Weber U, Lambert RGW, Pedersen SJ, Hodler J, Ostergaard M, Maksymowych WP. Assessment of structural lesions in sacroiliac joints enhances diagnostic utility of magnetic resonance imaging in early spondylarthritis. Arthritis Care Res 2010;62(12):1763–71.
34. Hermann KG, Baraliakos X, van der Heijde DM, et al. Descriptions of spinal MRI lesions and definition of a positive MRI of the spine in axial spondyloarthritis: a consensual approach by the ASAS/OMERACT MRI study group. Ann Rheum Dis 2012;71(8):1278–88.
35. van der Heijde D, Sieper J, Maksymowych WP, et al. Spinal inflammation in the absence of sacroiliac joint inflammation on MRI in patients with active non-radiographic axial spondyloarthritis. Arthritis Rheum 2014;66(3):667–73.
36. Moll JM, Wright V. New York clinical criteria for ankylosing spondylitis. A statistical evaluation. Ann Rheum Dis 1973;32(4):354–63.
37. Gofton JP, Lawrence JS, Bennett PH, Burch TA. Sacro-ilitis in eight populations. Ann Rheum Dis 1966;25(6):528–33.
38. Amor B, Dougados M, Mijiyawa M. Criteria of the classification of spondylarthropathies. Rev Rhum Mal Osteoartic 1990;57(2):85–9.
39. Dougados M, van der Linden S, Juhlin R, et al. The European Spondylarthropathy Study Group preliminary criteria for the classification of spondylarthropathy. Arthritis Rheum 1991;34(10):1218–27.
40. Rudwaleit M, Khan MA, Sieper J. The challenge of diagnosis and classification in early ankylosing spondylitis: do we need new criteria? Arthritis Rheum 2005;52(4):1000–8.
41. Collantes E, Veroz R, Escudero A, et al. Can some cases of 'possible' spondyloarthropathy be classified as 'definite' or 'undifferentiated' spondyloarthropathy? Value of criteria for spondyloarthropathies. Spanish Spondyloarthropathy Study Group. Joint Bone Spine 2000;67(6):516–20.
42. Bennett AN, McGonagle D, O'Connor P, et al. Severity of baseline magnetic resonance imaging-evident sacroiliitis and HLA-B27 status in early inflammatory back pain predict radiographically evident ankylosing spondylitis at eight years. Arthritis Rheum 2008;58(11):3413–18.
43. Rudwaleit M, Landewe R, van der Heijde D, et al. The development of Assessment of SpondyloArthritis international Society classification criteria for axial spondyloarthritis (part I): classification of paper patients by expert opinion including uncertainty appraisal. Ann Rheum Dis 2009;68(6):770–6.
44. Dougados M, van der Heijde D, Sieper J, et al. Symptomatic efficacy of etanercept and its effects on objective signs of inflammation in early nonradiographic axial spondyloarthritis: a multicenter, randomized, double-blind, placebo-controlled trial. Arthritis Rheumatol 2014;66(8):2091–102.
45. Sieper J, Lenaerts J, Wollenhaupt J, et al. Efficacy and safety of infliximab plus naproxen versus naproxen alone in patients with early, active axial spondyloarthritis: results from the double-blind, placebo-controlled INFAST study, part 1. Ann Rheum Dis 2014;73(1):101–7.
46. van den Berg R, de Hooge M, van Gaalen F, Reijnierse M, Huizinga T, van der Heijde D. Percentage of patients with spondyloarthritis in patients referred because of chronic back pain and performance of classification criteria: experience from the Spondyloarthritis Caught Early (SPACE) cohort. Rheumatology (Oxford) 2013;52(8):1492–9.
47. Dougados M, d'Agostino MA, Benessiano J, et al. The DESIR cohort: a 10-year follow-up of early inflammatory back pain in France: study design and baseline characteristics of the 708 recruited patients. Joint Bone Spine 2011;78(6):598–603.
48. Aydin SZ, Maksymowych WP, Bennett AN, McGonagle D, Emery P, Marzo-Ortega H. Validation of the ASAS criteria and definition of a positive MRI of the sacroiliac joint in an inception cohort of axial spondyloarthritis followed up for 8 years. Ann Rheum Dis 2012;71(1):56–60.
49. van Tubergen A, Weber U. Diagnosis and classification in spondyloarthritis: identifying a chameleon. Nat Rev Rheumatol 2012;8(5):253–61.
50. Braun J, Baraliakos X, Kiltz U, Heldmann F, Sieper J. Classification and diagnosis of axial spondyloarthritis—what is the clinically relevant difference? J Rheumatol 2015;42(1):31–8.
51. Eder L, Barzilai M, Peled N, Gladman DD, Zisman D. The use of ultrasound for the assessment of enthesitis in patients with spondyloarthritis. Clin Radiol 2013;68(3):219–23.
52. van Onna M, Jurik AG, van der Heijde D, van Tubegren A, Heuft-Dorenbosch L, Landewe R. HLA-B27 and gender independently determine the likelihood of a positive MRI of the sacroiliac joints in patients with early inflammatory back pain: a 2-year MRI follow-up study. Ann Rheum Dis 2011;70(11):1981–5.

CHAPTER 4

Diagnosis, classification, and management of peripheral spondyloarthritis

Martin Rudwaleit and Atul Deodhar

Introduction to diagnosis, classification, and management of peripheral spondyloarthritis

Some would argue that the term 'peripheral spondyloarthritis' is an oxymoron since 'spondyloarthritis' would indicate that spine ('spondylo') involvement is mandatory in this disease process. However, ever since the inflammatory rheumatic diseases affecting the spine were first differentiated from RA by Moll and Wright in 1974, it is well known that these conditions frequently involve the peripheral skeleton along with the spine, and sometimes the peripheral musculoskeletal symptoms are clinically more predominant and more troublesome to the patient than the spinal involvement (1). Hence 'peripheral spondyloarthritis' is a group of conditions that falls under the larger umbrella term of 'spondyloarthritis', with principal involvement of peripheral joints, enthesis, and tendons more so than the involvement of spine and axial skeleton (2).

The clinical features of peripheral SpA typically include an asymmetric, mono-, or oligoarticular (less than five joints), inflammatory arthritis that involves the lower limbs more than the upper limbs, seronegativity for rheumatoid factor, absence of nodules (to differentiate these conditions from RA), and various combinations of clinical features that include enthesitis, tendonitis, dactylitis, uveitis, IBD, and psoriasis. There may be preceding infection with specific bacteria (i.e. *Salmonella, Shigella, Yersinia, Campylobacter*, and *Chlamydia*) in some patients. Family history of similar arthritides and presence of the HLA-B27 gene would also be consistent with this diagnosis. These patients may also develop IBP and subsequent sacroiliitis, though at presentation the predominant feature would be involvement of the non-axial skeleton, hence they would be considered to have peripheral SpA rather than axSpA.

While Moll and Wright included Behçet's syndrome and Whipple's disease in the original group, these conditions are no longer considered to belong to the SpA spectrum. More recently, acne-associated arthritis, synovitis, acne, pustulosis, hyperostosis, and osteitis (SAPHO) syndrome, and arthritis associated with hidradenitis suppurativa (HS) are also considered under the term peripheral SpA by various authors (3–5). Juvenile idiopathic arthritis (JIA) has a subset that presents with uveitis and asymmetric peripheral inflammatory arthritis that too could be included under this umbrella. The full spectrum of peripheral SpA is shown in Table 4.1.

Table 4.1 Spectrum of peripheral SpA

Peripheral SpA conditions	Other predominant clinical features
Conditions commonly included under 'peripheral SpA'	
PsA	Psoriasis and nail involvement, usually preceding arthritis
IBD-associated arthritis	CD or UC
ReA	Urethritis, history of preceding infection with *Salmonella, Shigella, Yersinia, Campylobacter*, and *Chlamydia*, mucosal ulcers, keratoderma blennorrhagicum
Undifferentiated peripheral SpA	Enthesitis, dactylitis, family history of SpA, HLA-B27, uveitis, and not fitting into any of the other conditions mentioned above
Conditions with no clear consensus for inclusion under 'peripheral SpA'	
SAPHO syndrome	Synovitis, acne, pustulosis, hyperostosis, osteitis, typical involvement of anterior chest wall joints
Acne-associated arthritis	Acne conglobata, peripheral arthritis
HS-associated arthritis	HS, peripheral arthritis, occasionally sacroiliitis
JIA-associated uveitis	Uveitis, asymmetric inflammatory arthritis typically involving lower limbs (knee)

To lump or to split?

While the conditions described under peripheral SpA share many common clinical features, as described in the Introduction, they also differ from each other in several ways. These diseases vary in prognosis, outcomes, response to therapies, and even choice of therapies. For example, reactive arthritis (ReA) has a high spontaneous remission rate that is not seen in PsA (6), and post-*Chlamydia* ReA may respond to long-term antibiotics while other peripheral SpA conditions will not (7). Most conditions under peripheral SpA have association with HLA-B27, but the proportion varies widely between 70% in white Caucasian patients with ReA to no association seen in peripheral enteropathic arthritis (8). The functional, imaging, and outcome measures validated in PsA patients have not been tested in other peripheral SpA conditions, and we do not know if they will work as well in non-psoriatic peripheral SpA. Because of these differences, some would prefer to study these conditions separately (the 'splitters'). Others would concentrate on the commonalities and lump them together under one umbrella term (the 'lumpers') (9). Arguments have been made in favour of 'splitters' as noted in the Introduction, but there are distinct advantages of considering these conditions under one umbrella. Familial clustering is a feature of these conditions; hence lumping and considering them together is likely to help with early diagnosis in family members. Also, it is less likely that large-scale clinical trials will ever be conducted on conditions such as ReA, SAPHO, or enteropathic arthritis. On the other hand, the divergences of these conditions regarding genetic background, the natural course, and outcome make lumping these questionable. A single clinical trial of a therapeutic agent conducted on 'peripheral SpA' without psoriasis was a big effort and may get approval to use that drug on all entities under 'peripheral SpA' (10).

Epidemiology

PsA, a major member of peripheral SpA, has been described separately and will not be discussed in detail here. There are no national-level studies on the prevalence of 'peripheral SpA' as a general term, since the terminology is relatively new (11). Some studies have combined ReA, enteropathic arthritis, and undifferentiated SpA to get an idea of the prevalence of peripheral SpA in the community. A cross-sectional study conducted in an adult population in Marche, a region located in central Italy, found that 0.42% of the population was found to have PsA, and an additional 0.09% of the population had either ReA or arthritis associated with IBD or undifferentiated SpA (12).

Several studies have looked at targeted populations, to assess the prevalence of (such as in patients with known IBD) or incidence of (such as after an outbreak of gastroenteritis due to salmonella) peripheral SpA.

In a population-based study conducted on culture-confirmed infection with bacterial enteric pathogens (*Salmonella*, *Shigella*, *Yersinia*, *Campylobacter*, and *E. coli* O157) in Oregon, USA, the incidence of ReA was found to be between 0.6 and 3.1 cases per 100 000 (13). This incidence of ReA found in the general population with background infections with enteropathic organisms is much lower than the incidence seen after an acute outbreak of similar infections. For example, after a large outbreak of *Campylobacter jejuni* infection in Finland, the frequency of ReA was 2.6% (14), whereas another food-borne infection with *Yersinia pseudotuberculosis* serotype O:3 also in Finland led to 14% of patients developing ReA (15). In a Canadian outbreak of food-borne gastroenteritis caused by *Salmonella typhimurium*, 7.6% of patients developed ReA (16).

Inflammatory arthritis is the most common extra-intestinal manifestation in patients with IBD (17, 18). The frequency of inflammatory arthritis appears to be similar in both Crohn's disease (CD) and ulcerative colitis (UC) (18). In a study conducted in Turkish patients with established diagnosis of IBD attending a tertiary clinic, 29% were found to have peripheral SpA and almost half of these patients were not diagnosed before this study was conducted (19). In IBD patients attending the rheumatology and gastroenterology clinics of Kuwait University Hospital, 31.5% were found to have peripheral SpA (20). In a study conducted on the Puerto Rican population with IBD, 42% had spondyloarthropathy (16% had axSpA and 26% had peripheral SpA) (17). Overall, the prevalence of peripheral SpA in carefully examined IBD patients appears to be close to 30% (21) (see Table 4.2).

Similar studies to find the prevalence of peripheral SpA have been conducted on HS patients. In a systematic investigation on all patients with HS referred to three dermatology university hospital centres, the crude prevalence of SpA was 3.7% according to the ESSG criteria (3).

Varying presentations of peripheral SpA (with IBD, food poisoning, psoriasis, uveitis, etc.) indicate how this diagnosis can be missed in clinics such as gastroenterology, ophthalmology, dermatology, and infectious diseases, unless the specialist specifically asks about musculoskeletal symptoms.

Diagnosis of peripheral spondyloarthritis

Peripheral SpA is a clinical diagnosis based on 'pattern recognition' and usually does not need many confirmatory investigations. The patient—typically a young adult in his or her 20s to 40s—would present with a subacute onset of inflammatory arthritis that involves less than five joints ('oligoarthritis', but occasionally a monoarthritis) in an asymmetric manner (Fig. 4.1). Lower extremity large joints (for example a knee) would be commonly involved. A targeted enquiry may reveal history of tendonitis, enthesitis, or dactylitis. There may be personal or family history of psoriasis, IBD, uveitis, or IBP. The clinical examination would confirm the inflammatory nature of the arthritis (synovitis, joint warmth, effusion, etc.), and may also reveal evidence of enthesitis in other areas (Achilles tendon, patellar, and quadriceps tendon insertion would be typical), dactylitis, or psoriasis. This type of presentation would be sufficient to make the diagnosis of peripheral SpA. Further investigations that would aid with this diagnosis would include a negative rheumatoid factor and a negative cyclic citrullinated peptide (CCP), high inflammatory markers such as sedimentation rate and CRP (seen in about 30% of cases), and positive HLA-B27 gene (between 30% and 50% of cases, depending upon the underlying condition). If a joint has effusion, examination of the synovial fluid will show 'inflammatory' characteristics (white cell counts of more than 2000/CC).

Several other diagnoses may mimic peripheral SpA. A common differential diagnosis would be a fibromyalgia patient with several tender points that could be mistaken for 'enthesitis'. It is therefore important to actively search for evidence of inflammation by history and by examination (e.g. swollen joint with effusion, dactylitis, uveitis); or look for tenderness and swelling of entheses that are generally not involved in fibromyalgia (e.g. plantar fascia insertion on calcaneum, Achilles tendon, patellar tendon insertion on lower pole of patella or tibia). A peripheral SpA patient presenting with monoarthritis needs to undergo investigation to rule out crystal-induced arthritis or septic arthritis. Lyme arthritis is another condition to be excluded in patients with knee arthritis.

Table 4.2 Epidemiology of IBD-associated arthritis. (Adapted from Salvarani 2009 (18).)

Author	Year	Country	Patients	AS (%)	SI (%)	Peripheral arthritis (%)	Enthesopathy (%)	Overall (%)
Scarpa (43)	1992	Italy	79 (UC)	25.3	43	18.9	–	62
Veloso (44)	1996	Portugal	792	3.0	–	16.2	–	–
Orchard (45)	1998	Great Britain	1459	1.0	–	7.4	–	21.4
Suh (46)	1998	Korea	129	1.6	6.2	15.5	–	17.1
De Vlam (47)	2000	Netherlands	103 (CD)	3.8	21.8		7	39
Queiro (48)	2000	Spain	62 (UC)	3.2	24.2	30.6	–	–
Salvarani (49)	2001	Italy, Netherlands	160	2.6	3.6	10.6	10	33.1
Christodoulou (50)	2002	Greece	252	–	5.9	2.8	–	17.0
Palm (51)	2002	Norway	406	2.4	2.0	17	26	32.5
Turkcapar (52)	2006	Turkey	162	9.9	45.7	14.8	50.0	–
Peeters (53)	2008	Belgium	251 (CD)	6	27	29	–	–
Rodriguez (17)	2008	Puerto Rico	100	2.6	13	5	–	–
Lanna (54)	2008	Brazil	130	6.2	9.2	25.4	5.4	31.5
Beslek (19)	2009	Turkey	122	8.2				28.7
Resende (55)	2013	Brazil	1472	2.5		0.7 (peripheral arthritis), 3.2 (enteroarthritis)		
Al-Jarrallah (20)	2013	Kuwait	130	8.5	3.1	31.5	5.4	34.6

Source: Salvarani C, Fries W. Clinical features and epidemiology of spondyloarthritides associated with inflammatory bowel disease. World J Gastroenterol. 2009;15(20):2449–55.

'Oligo' or 'mono' arthritis without a clear diagnosis ('undifferentiated arthritis') can be seen in 50% of patients presenting in 'early arthritis' (disease duration less than 1 year) clinics (22). Apart from a thorough history and physical examination, as well as extensive work-up, it is very important to follow these patients for over 1 year to determine if they indeed develop 'peripheral SpA'. Sieper et al. applied the Bayes' theorem to calculate the post-test probability of such patients having ReA (23). By their calculations, if a patient presents with asymmetric mono-/oligoarticular arthritis predominantly of the lower extremities, and other diagnoses (gout, osteoarthritis, trauma) have been excluded, the probability of ReA is 40%. If there is evidence of a genitourinary or gastrointestinal (GI) infection with an organism associated with ReA, the probability of ReA increases to 90%. *Chlamydia* detected in the urine without history of *Chlamydia* infection makes the probability of ReA 60%, and stool culture positive for bacteria associated with ReA makes the probability 70%.

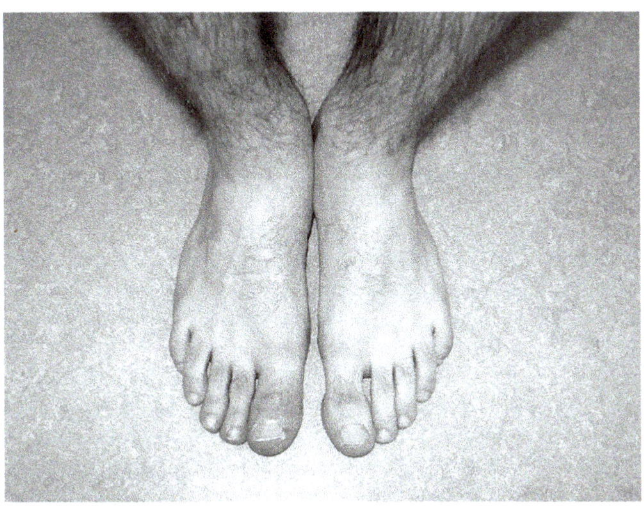

Fig. 4.1 (See colour plate section). A 25-year-old man, HLA-B27 positive, presenting with arthritis of the right toe and right ankle. This pattern of arthritis is typical of SpA. Courtesy of M. Rudwaleit.

With the new terminology dividing 'spondyloarthritis' into two broad groups, namely 'peripheral' and 'axial', the old term 'undifferentiated spondyloarthritis' needs to be retired. If patients have clinical features of SpA, depending upon their major musculoskeletal manifestation, they can be classified as either 'axial' or 'peripheral' SpA, without using the term 'undifferentiated'.

The long-term outcome of peripheral SpA depends upon the subtype, as well as on the therapy used. Observational studies on SpA have included patients with different entry criteria, and hence it can be difficult to draw clear conclusions about spontaneous or drug-induced remissions (6). ReA has high rates of spontaneous remission (50–60% by 2.5 years), but PsA and IBD-associated arthritis are unlikely to remit spontaneously (6). One drug study on peripheral SpA has reported drug-induced remission rates (after 12 weeks of treatment with adalimumab) of 42%, compared to 0% in the placebo group (24).

Pathology and histopathology of peripheral spondyloarthritis

Enthesitis, dactylitis, and peripheral oligoarthritis are the key clinical features of peripheral SpA. It is particularly dactylitis and enthesitis that, if present, help the clinician to distinguish SpA from other types of arthritides. However, enthesitis is more common by far than dactylitis. Earlier investigations suggested a role of MR imaging in distinguishing RA from SpA by the greater presence of bone 'oedema', reflecting enthesitis in affected joints in SpA, as compared to RA and more pronounced synovitis in RA (25). However, this differentiating imaging feature could not be confirmed in a recent study in which a comparable degree of bone oedema on MRI, enthesitis, and synovitis in RA and SpA was demonstrated (26).

Synovial tissue from inflamed joints obtained by mini-arthroscopy revealed inflammatory cellular infiltrates that include infiltrating CD3+ T cells, CD22+ B cells, and macrophages. The degree of synovitis and particularly the number of CD68+ macrophages in the synovial lining and sublining was not a differentiating feature between SpA and RA patients in previous studies (26, 27). However, the number of CD163+ macrophages was about two-fold higher in SpA synovitis as compared to RA synovitis and was related to inflammatory disease activity in SpA (26). CD163 is a marker of alternative activation (M2) and associates with the cytokines IL-4, IL-13, and IL-10. The concentration of these cytokines in synovial fluid, however, was not different between RA and SpA, whereas lymphocyte activation was impaired (28, 29). Of importance, when comparing PsA and non-psoriatic SpA, no great differences in the composition of the inflammatory cell infiltrations were found, suggesting that PsA is clearly related to the spectrum of SpA (27). Upon effective treatment with TNFi, a dramatic reduction of the infiltration of synovial tissue with inflammatory cells (T cells and macrophages) but not of B cells and plasma cells can be observed in SpA. The implications of the latter are as yet unknown (30).

Animal models of peripheral SpA further contribute to our understanding of the pathophysiology of SpA. A recent mouse model identified entheseal resident T cells with a specific phenotype (ROR-γt+CD3+CD4−CD8−) that upon stimulation by overexpression of IL-23 become activated, produce IL-17 and IL-22, and are involved in the induction of enthesitis and entheseal new bone formation with resemblance to the human disease (31). Another animal model elegantly demonstrated the importance of biomechanical stress for the induction of enthesitis and new bone formation (32).

Table 4.3 Amor and ESSG criteria

Amor criteria for SpA	ESSG criteria for SpA
A. *Past or current clinical manifestations*	*Inflammatory back pain OR synovitis*
1. Back pain at night and/or back stiffness in the morning (1 point)	◆ asymmetric or
2. Asymmetric oligoarthritis (2 points)	◆ predominantly lower limb
3. Gluteal pain without other details (1 point) or alternating gluteal pain (2 points)	*AND* one or more of the following:
4. Sausage-like digit or toe (2 points)	◆ positive family history
5. Heel pain or other enthesopathy (2 points)	◆ psoriasis ◆ IBD
6. Iritis (2 points)	◆ urethritis, cervicitis, or acute diarrhoea within 1 month before arthritis
7. Non-gonococcal urethritis within 1 month before the onset of arthritis (1 point)	◆ buttock pain alternating between right and left gluteal areas
8. Diarrhoea within 1 month before the onset of arthritis (1 point)	◆ enthesopathy
9. Past or current psoriasis and/or balanitis and/or IBD (2 points)	◆ SI (X-rays)
B. *Roentgenographic changes*	
10. Sacroiliitis grade 2 or more if bilateral, grade 3 or more if unilateral (3 points)	
C. *Predisposing genetic factors*	
11. Presence of HLA-B27 antigen and/or positive family history for AS, Reiter's syndrome, psoriasis, uveitis, or chronic bowel disease (2 points)	
D. *Responsiveness to treatment*	
12. Improvement within 48 hours after initiation of an NSAID and/or recurrence within 48 hours after discontinuation of an NSAID (2 points)	

Definite SpA if ≥ 6 points, probable SpA if 5 points

Classification of peripheral spondyloarthritis

The Amor and ESSG criteria (Table 4.3) were both the first generation of criteria that encompassed the entire spectrum of SpA, including PsA, arthritis associated with IBD, AS, and ReA (33, 34). In addition, these criteria enabled researchers for the first time to classify a patient with peripheral arthritis as SpA in the absence of psoriasis, IBD, a preceding infection, and X-ray sacroiliitis. At that time, the term 'undifferentiated SpA' emerged as a consequence for the classification of this group of patients that did not qualify for one of the specified SpA subtypes. Thus the term 'undifferentiated SpA' was applied to both patients with predominant axSpA, yet not exhibiting typical X-ray sacroiliitis, and patients with predominant peripheral SpA, yet not qualifying for ReA, PsA, or IBD arthritis.

When attempts were undertaken to diagnose AS earlier, and along these efforts the concept of axSpA and peripheral SpA evolved as an alternative to the concept of specific SpA subgroups, criteria for predominant peripheral SpA were revisited and new criteria elaborated and validated. This most recent set of classification criteria for peripheral SpA developed by ASAS (Table 4.4) encompasses all manifestations and features of SpA (11). The entry manifestation in these criteria is either peripheral arthritis of the SpA pattern (oligoarticular, usually lower limb, asymmetric) or peripheral enthesitis or dactylitis. In addition, psoriasis, IBD, uveitis, HLA-B27, preceding infection, or sacroiliitis must be present, or at least two of peripheral arthritis, enthesitis, dactylitis, previous IBP, or family history.

In contrast to the ESSG criteria, the new ASAS criteria allow the classification of a patient with peripheral enthesitis or dactylitis but without peripheral arthritis. In contrast to the Amor criteria with a requirement of 6 points for fulfilment, the ASAS peripheral SpA criteria are less strict, and allow also the classification of patients who would score according to the Amor criteria 3 to 4 points only. Thus the sensitivity of the ASAS criteria (77.8%) is higher compared to the ESSG criteria (62.5%) and much higher compared to the Amor criteria (39.8%), at a reasonable specificity (82.2%). The higher sensitivity allows the classification of patients for clinical trials with early SpA and of patients with 'pauci-symptomatic' peripheral SpA,

Table 4.4 ASAS criteria for peripheral SpA (11)

Arthritis or enthesitis or dactylitis	
Plus ≥ one of:	*Plus ≥ two of the remaining:*
◆ Psoriasis	◆ Arthritis
◆ IBD	◆ Enthesitis
◆ Preceding infection	◆ Dactylitis
◆ HLA-B27	◆ IBP in the past
◆ Uveitis	◆ Positive family history for SpA
◆ Sacroiliitis on imaging (radiographs or MRI)	

Peripheral arthritis: usually predominantly lower limb and/or asymmetric arthritis; enthesitis: clinically assessed; dactylitis: clinically assessed.

Source: Rudwaleit M, van der Heijde D, Landewe R, Akkoc N, Brandt J, Chou CT, et al. The Assessment of SpondyloArthritis International Society classification criteria for peripheral spondyloarthritis and for spondyloarthritis in general. Ann Rheum Dis. 2011;70(1):25–31.

Table 4.5 Current treatment options and their efficacy for peripheral SpA according to clinical manifestations

	Synovitis	**Enthesitis**	**Dactylitis**
NSAIDs	+	(+)	+
Local steroid injections	+++	+ (difficult to perform at some sites)	+
Low-dose prednisolone (≤7.5 mg per day)	−/+	?	?
SSZ	+++	−	?
MTX	++	−	?
LFN	++	−	?
TNFi	+++	+++	+++

The grading of efficacy reflects both available evidence from the literature and the clinical experience of the authors.

in other words the classification of peripheral SpA patients who have not yet experienced the full set of clinical manifestations that can occur with SpA. The criteria have been applied for the first time in a large placebo-controlled trial with adalimumab in peripheral SpA (see 'Therapy of peripheral spondyloarthritis') (35). As is the case for the ASAS axSpA criteria, the ASAS criteria for peripheral SpA are not intended to be applied as diagnostic criteria since an exclusion of other conditions is not required.

Therapy of peripheral spondyloarthritis

NSAIDs are often used in alleviating symptoms of enthesitis, dactylitis, and peripheral synovitis. While NSAIDs are particularly effective for the treatment of IBP in SpA with predominant axial involvement (sacroiliitis, spondylitis), their effectiveness for peripheral disease is less well studied. In addition, local steroid injections are effective for synovitis (intra-articular injections) and for some enthesitic sites such as plantar fascia enthesitis. Yet injecting the entheseal bone insertion site is often a painful procedure. Low-dose systemic steroid therapy does not have an established role in peripheral SpA. Clinical experience suggests that low dose steroids are more effective in RA than in SpA, yet clinical trials are lacking (Table 4.5).

Among the synthetic disease-modifying antirheumatic drugs (sDMARDs), sulfasalazine (SSZ) is the preferred sDMARD to be used in peripheral synovitis since it is the best-studied drug in peripheral SpA (36). SSZ is also recommended by the ASAS/European League Against Rheumatism (EULAR) for the management of AS if peripheral synovitis is a dominating feature (37). Usual doses of SSZ are 2 g per day, with occasional increases to 3 g per day if needed. If SSZ does not provide sufficient efficacy, other sDMARDs such as methotrexate (MTX) and leflunomide (LFN) can be tried. Yet evidence from controlled clinical trials demonstrating the efficacy of these drugs in peripheral SpA is lacking. Data from uncontrolled studies in AS as well as clinical experience suggest, however, that these drugs may be effective in peripheral synovitis in SpA.

The efficacy of sDMARDs on enthesitis has not been well studied either. Even less data are available for dactylitis. Yet clinical experience suggests that none of the sDMARDs is particularly effective. In contrast, clinical experience and data from trials of AS and PsA patients treated with TNFi strongly point to a role of TNFi in the treatment of enthesitis and dactylitis (38). While both enthesitis and dactylitis were always a secondary outcome parameter at best in all clinical AS trials, a single controlled study focused on enthesitis as the primary outcome. In this trial, 24 patients with MRI-proven enthesitis of the heel were treated with either etanercept (ETN) or placebo for 12 weeks. ETN-treated patients had a significantly better clinical improvement and a tendency for greater improvement on MRI as well compared to placebo treatment (39).

The TNFi adalimumab has been studied in a smaller (n = 40) and a larger (n = 165, ABILITY2) placebo-controlled trial in peripheral non-psoriatic SpA. In both trials, adalimumab led to a significant clinical improvement (24, 35). In the second trial, a new response index, peripheral SpA response criterion 40 (PSpARC40), has been applied as the primary outcome after 12 weeks. This response criterion was defined as ≥40% improvement from baseline (≥20-mm absolute improvement on a visual analogue scale) in patients' global assessments of disease activity and pain, and ≥40% improvement in at least one of the following features: swollen joint and tender joint counts, total enthesitis count, or dactylitis count. After 12 weeks, PSpARC40 was obtained by 39% of patients treated with adalimumab and 20% treated with placebo (35). In this study, enthesitis, which was assessed by various assessment instruments, also improved to a greater degree with adalimumab compared to placebo, as did dactylitis. Thus TNFi are effective treatment options not only for axSpA but also for synovitis, enthesitis, and dactylitis in peripheral SpA. Other promising drugs are targeting IL-17, for example secukinumab, which has been shown to be effective in AS and in PsA in phase 3 trials (40).

Treatment of reactive arthritis

The principles of the treatment of ReA are not different from peripheral SpA without evidence of a preceding infection of the genitourinary tract by *Chlamydia* or of the GI tract by *Salmonella, Shigella, Yersinia*, or *Campylobacter*. ReA has a high tendency for spontaneous remission after several weeks to 6 months in many patients, although manifestations of SpA may recur later again. The therapeutic role of antibiotics has been studied in several earlier and recent studies with no proven benefit in acute ReA (41, 42).

A single placebo-controlled trial in patients with chronic (disease duration 10–14 years), *Chlamydia*-proven ReA (as evidenced by polymerase chain reaction (PCR) demonstration of *Chlamydia* in either peripheral blood or synovium) showed a clear benefit for a 6 months' combination treatment (either doxycycline plus rifampin or azithromycin plus rifampin, n = 27) compared to placebo (n = 12) (7). Although the study results were highly intriguing, they have yet to be confirmed in another trial. Accordingly and considering the potential risks and side-effects of long-term antibiotic therapy, to date, most rheumatologists do not give long-term combination antibiotics to their patients with chronic ReA, and rather use local treatment, DMARDs, or TNFi.

References

1. Moll JM, Haslock I, Macrae IF, Wright V. Associations between ankylosing spondylitis, psoriatic arthritis, Reiter's disease, the intestinal arthropathies, and Behçet's syndrome. Medicine (Baltimore) 1974;53(5):343–64.
2. Garg N, van den Bosch F, Deodhar A. The concept of spondyloarthritis: where are we now? Best Pract Res Clin Rheumatol 2014;28(5):663–72.
3. Richette P, Molto A, Viguier M, et al. Hidradenitis suppurativa associated with spondyloarthritis—results from a multicenter national prospective study. J Rheumatol 2014;41(3):490–4.
4. Magrey M, Khan MA. New insights into synovitis, acne, pustulosis, hyperostosis, and osteitis (SAPHO) syndrome. Curr Rheumatol Rep 2009;11(5):329–33.
5. Lim DT, James NM, Hassan S, Khan MA. Spondyloarthritis associated with acne conglobata, hidradenitis suppurativa and dissecting cellulitis of the scalp: a review with illustrative cases. Curr Rheumatol Rep 2013;15(8):346.
6. Poddubnyy D, Gensler LS. Spontaneous, drug-induced, and drug-free remission in peripheral and axial spondyloarthritis. Best Pract Res Clin Rheumatol 2014;28(5):807–18.
7. Carter JD, Espinoza LR, Inman RD, et al. Combination antibiotics as a treatment for chronic *Chlamydia*-induced reactive arthritis: a double-blind, placebo-controlled, prospective trial. Arthritis Rheum 2010;62(5):1298–307.
8. Reveille JD. The genetic basis of spondyloarthritis. Ann Rheum Dis 2011;70(Suppl 1):i44–50.
9. Nash P, Mease PJ, Braun J, van der Heijde D. Seronegative spondyloarthropathies: to lump or split? Ann Rheum Dis 2005;64(Suppl 2):ii9–13.
10. Mease P, Sieper J, Van den Bosch F, Rahman P, Karunaratne PM, Pangan AL. Randomized controlled trial of adalimumab in patients with nonpsoriatic peripheral spondyloarthritis. Arthritis Rheumatol 2015;67(4):914–23.
11. Rudwaleit M, van der Heijde D, Landewe R, et al. The Assessment of SpondyloArthritis international Society classification criteria for peripheral spondyloarthritis and for spondyloarthritis in general. Ann Rheum Dis 2011;70(1):25–31.
12. De Angelis R, Salaffi F, Grassi W. Prevalence of spondyloarthropathies in an Italian population sample: a regional community-based study. Scand J Rheumatol 2007;36(1):14–21.
13. Townes JM, Deodhar AA, Laine ES, et al. Reactive arthritis following culture-confirmed infections with bacterial enteric pathogens in Minnesota and Oregon: a population-based study. Ann Rheum Dis 2008;67(12):1689–96.
14. Hannu T, Kauppi M, Tuomala M, Laaksonen I, Klemets P, Kuusi M. Reactive arthritis following an outbreak of *Campylobacter jejuni* infection. J Rheumatol 2004;31(3):528–30.
15. Hannu T, Mattila L, Nuorti JP, et al. Reactive arthritis after an outbreak of *Yersinia pseudotuberculosis* serotype O:3 infection. Ann Rheum Dis 2003;62(9):866–9.
16. Inman RD, Johnston ME, Hodge M, Falk J, Helewa A. Postdysenteric reactive arthritis. A clinical and immunogenetic study following an outbreak of salmonellosis. Arthritis Rheum 1988;31(11):1377–83.
17. Rodriguez VE, Costas PJ, Vazquez M, et al. Prevalence of spondyloarthropathy in Puerto Rican patients with inflammatory bowel disease. Ethn Dis 2008;18(2 Suppl 2):S2-225-9.
18. Salvarani C, Fries W. Clinical features and epidemiology of spondyloarthritides associated with inflammatory bowel disease. World J Gastroenterol 2009;15(20):2449–55.
19. Beslek A, Onen F, Birlik M, et al. Prevalence of spondyloarthritis in Turkish patients with inflammatory bowel disease. Rheumatol Int 2009;29(8):955–7.
20. Al-Jarallah K, Shehab D, Al-Azmi W, Al-Fadli A. Rheumatic complications of inflammatory bowel disease among Arabs: a hospital-based study in Kuwait. Int J Rheum Dis 2013;16(2):134–8.
21. Olivieri I, Cantini F, Castiglione F, et al. Italian Expert Panel on the management of patients with coexisting spondyloarthritis and inflammatory bowel disease. Autoimmun Rev 2014;13(8):822–30.
22. Hulsemann JL, Zeidler H. Undifferentiated arthritis in an early synovitis out-patient clinic. Clin Exp Rheumatol 1995;13(1):37–43.
23. Sieper J, Rudwaleit M, Braun J, van der Heijde D. Diagnosing reactive arthritis: role of clinical setting in the value of serologic and microbiologic assays. Arthritis Rheum 2002;46(2):319–27.
24. Paramarta JE, De Rycke L, Heijda TF, et al. Efficacy and safety of adalimumab for the treatment of peripheral arthritis in spondyloarthritis patients without ankylosing spondylitis or psoriatic arthritis. Ann Rheum Dis 2013;72(11):1793–9.
25. McGonagle D, Gibbon W, Emery P. Classification of inflammatory arthritis by enthesitis. Lancet 1998;352(9134):1137–40.
26. Paramarta JE, van der Leij C, Gofita I, et al. Peripheral joint inflammation in early onset spondyloarthritis is not specifically related to enthesitis. Ann Rheum Dis 2014;73(4):735–40.
27. Kruithof E, Baeten D, De Rycke L, et al. Synovial histopathology of psoriatic arthritis, both oligo- and polyarticular, resembles spondyloarthropathy more than it does rheumatoid arthritis. Arthritis Res Ther 2005;7(3):R569–80.
28. Vandooren B, Noordenbos T, Ambarus C, et al. Absence of a classically activated macrophage cytokine signature in peripheral spondylarthritis, including psoriatic arthritis. Arthritis Rheum 2009;60(4):966–75.
29. Baeten D, Moller HJ, Delanghe J, Veys EM, Moestrup SK, De Keyser F. Association of CD163+ macrophages and local production of soluble CD163 with decreased lymphocyte activation in spondylarthropathy synovitis. Arthritis Rheum 2004;50(5):1611–23.
30. Kruithof E, Baeten D, Van den Bosch F, Mielants H, Veys EM, De Keyser F. Histological evidence that infliximab treatment leads to downregulation of inflammation and tissue remodelling of the synovial membrane in spondyloarthropathy. Ann Rheum Dis 2005;64(4):529–36.
31. Sherlock JP, Joyce-Shaikh B, Turner SP, et al. IL-23 induces spondyloarthropathy by acting on ROR-γt+ CD3+CD4–CD8– entheseal resident T cells. Nat Med 2012;18(7):1069–76.
32. Jacques P, Lambrecht S, Verheugen E, et al. Proof of concept: enthesitis and new bone formation in spondyloarthritis are driven by mechanical strain and stromal cells. Ann Rheum Dis 2014;73(2):437–45.
33. Amor B, Dougados M, Mijiyawa M. [Criteria of the classification of spondylarthropathies.] Rev Rhum Mal Osteoartic 1990;57(2):85–9.
34. Dougados M, van der Linden S, Juhlin R, et al. The European Spondylarthropathy Study Group preliminary criteria for the classification of spondylarthropathy. Arthritis Rheum 1991;34(10):1218–27.
35. Mease P, Sieper J, Van den Bosch F, Rahman P, Karunaratne PM, Pangan AL. Randomized controlled trial of adalimumab in patients with non-psoriatic peripheral spondyloarthritis. Arthritis Rheumatol 2015;67(4):914–23.
36. Clegg DO, Reda DJ, Abdellatif M. Comparison of sulfasalazine and placebo for the treatment of axial and peripheral articular manifestations of the seronegative spondylarthropathies: a

Department of Veterans Affairs cooperative study. Arthritis Rheum 1999;42(11):2325–9.
37. Braun J, van den Berg R, Baraliakos X, et al. 2010 update of the ASAS/EULAR recommendations for the management of ankylosing spondylitis. Ann Rheum Dis 2011;70(6):896–904.
38. Baraliakos X, van den Berg R, Braun J, van der Heijde D. Update of the literature review on treatment with biologics as a basis for the first update of the ASAS/EULAR management recommendations of ankylosing spondylitis. Rheumatology (Oxford) 2012;51(8):1378–87.
39. Dougados M, Combe B, Braun J, et al. A randomised, multicentre, double-blind, placebo-controlled trial of etanercept in adults with refractory heel enthesitis in spondyloarthritis: the HEEL trial. Ann Rheum Dis 2010;69(8):1430–5.
40. McInnes IB, Mease PJ, Kirkham B, et al. Secukinumab, a human anti-interleukin-17A monoclonal antibody, in patients with psoriatic arthritis (FUTURE 2): a randomised, double-blind, placebo-controlled, phase 3 trial. Lancet 2015;386(9999):1137–46.
41. Kuuliala A, Julkunen H, Paimela L, et al. Double-blind, randomized, placebo-controlled study of three-month treatment with the combination of ofloxacin and roxithromycin in recent-onset reactive arthritis. Rheumatol Int 2013;33(11):2723–9.
42. Barber CE, Kim J, Inman RD, Esdaile JM, James MT. Antibiotics for treatment of reactive arthritis: a systematic review and metaanalysis. J Rheumatol 2013;40(6):916–28.
43. Scarpa R, del Puente A, D'Arienzo A, et al. The arthritis of ulcerative colitis: clinical and genetic aspects. J Rheumatol 1992;19(3):373–7.
44. Veloso FT, Carvalho J, Magro F. Immune-related systemic manifestations of inflammatory bowel disease. A prospective study of 792 patients. J Clin Gastroenterol 1996;23(1):29–34.
45. Orchard TR, Wordsworth BP, Jewell DP. Peripheral arthropathies in inflammatory bowel disease: their articular distribution and natural history. Gut 1998;42(3):387–91.
46. Suh CH, Lee CH, Lee J, et al. Arthritic manifestations of inflammatory bowel disease. J Korean Med Sci 1998;13(1):39–43.
47. de Vlam K, Mielants H, Cuvelier C, De Keyser F, Veys EM, De Vos M. Spondyloarthropathy is underestimated in inflammatory bowel disease: prevalence and HLA association. J Rheumatol 2000;27(12):2860–5.
48. Queiro R, Maiz O, Intxausti J, et al. Subclinical sacroiliitis in inflammatory bowel disease: a clinical and follow-up study. Clin Rheumatol 2000;19(6):445–9.
49. Salvarani C, Vlachonikolis IG, van der Heijde DM, et al. Musculoskeletal manifestations in a population-based cohort of inflammatory bowel disease patients. Scand J Gastroenterol 2001;36(12):1307–13.
50. Christodoulou DK, Katsanos KH, Kitsanou M, Stergiopoulou C, Hatzis J, Tsianos EV. Frequency of extraintestinal manifestations in patients with inflammatory bowel disease in northwest Greece and review of the literature. Dig Liver Dis 2002;34(11):781–6.
51. Palm O, Moum B, Jahnsen J, Gran JT. The prevalence and incidence of peripheral arthritis in patients with inflammatory bowel disease, a prospective population-based study (the IBSEN study). Rheumatology (Oxford) 2001;40(11):1256–61.
52. Turkcapar N, Toruner M, Soykan I, et al. The prevalence of extraintestinal manifestations and HLA association in patients with inflammatory bowel disease. Rheumatol Int 2006;26(7):663–8.
53. Peeters H, Vander Cruyssen B, Mielants H, et al. Clinical and genetic factors associated with sacroiliitis in Crohn's disease. J Gastroenterol Hepatol 2008;23(1):132–7.
54. Lanna CC, Ferrari Mde L, Rocha SL, Nascimento E, de Carvalho MA, da Cunha AS. A cross-sectional study of 130 Brazilian patients with Crohn's disease and ulcerative colitis: analysis of articular and ophthalmologic manifestations. Clin Rheumatol 2008;27(4):503–9.
55. Resende GG, Lanna CC, Bortoluzzo AB, et al. Enteropathic arthritis in Brazil: data from the Brazilian Registry of Spondyloarthritis. Rev Bras Reumatol 2013;53(6):452–9.

CHAPTER 5

Genetics of spondyloarthritis

Matthew A. Brown and John Reveille

Introduction to the genetics of spondyloarthritis

In addition to sharing clinical, histopathological, and immunological features, SpA encompasses a group of diseases that are genetically linked through shared associations with *HLA-B27*, as well as other genes of the *IL23R* and aminopeptidase groups. Great progress has been made since the development of the genome-wide association study approach, with better dissection of the HLA-associations of this group of diseases, as well as the discovery of multiple genetic loci found outside of the major histocompatibility complex (MHC) in AS in particular. These genetic data shed light on the related pathogenesis of AS and PsA, IBD-related arthritis, and ReA. Genetic associations also strengthen the suggestive data that Behçet's disease and Familial Mediterranean Fever (FMF) are also related to the more classical forms of SpA.

Genetic epidemiology of spondyloarthropathies

In developed countries, SpAs are very common, with an estimated 7 million Americans suffering from this group of diseases (1), compared with 1.3 million suffering from RA (1). The prevalence of AS varies in proportion to the prevalence of HLA-B27 in the population. In populations of European descent, where roughly 8% of health individuals carry HLA-B27, AS has a prevalence of around 0.5%. HLA-B27 is rare amongst people of African-American descent and in Australian Aboriginals, largely explaining the rarity of AS in these groups (2, 3). Psoriasis is even more common than SpA, with a prevalence of 2–3% in people of white European ancestry, with the disease being less common in people of Asian and African ancestry (4, 5). Whether this difference in population frequency also has genetic explanations is unclear.

HLA-B27 carriers have an age of onset typically approximately 5 years younger than HLA-B27-negative cases (6) and have a demonstrable higher frequency of acute anterior uveitis (AAU) (8). AS has a moderate male predominance (approximately 2–3:1), whereas IBD-related arthritis has a more balanced gender distribution. Psoriatic SpA also has a strong male predominance, whereas psoriasis and peripheral PsA have equal or female-predominant gender distributions. These gender differences are likely to have genetic explanations, but these have yet to be resolved.

AS runs very strongly in families, the risk of developing AS in siblings or children of AS patients being about 12% (Table 5.1). As is typical of polygenic diseases, the likelihood of recurrent disease in more distant relatives is much lower (≤1%) (7). Twin studies indicate that the risk of developing AS is primarily genetic, with

Table 5.1 Risk of AS in relatives of cases (7)

	HLA-B27 status unknown	HLA-B27 positive	HLA-B27 negative
Identical twin	60%	60%	–
Parent/sibling/child	10%	15%	0%
Grandparent	1%	5%	0%

heritability in excess of 90%, suggesting that the environmental triggers for the disease are ubiquitous (8, 9). Twin and family studies also indicate that the severity of AS is highly heritable, with the heritability of radiographic severity measures being 62% (10), with family studies indicating significant heritability of disease activity and severity measures such as the Bath Ankylosing Spondylitis Disease Activity Index (BASDAI) and Bath Ankylosing Spondylitis Functional Index (BASFI), as well as age of symptom onset (11, 12).

Psoriasis is also known to be highly heritable; the concordance rate in monozygotic (MZ) twins is significantly higher than in dizygotic (DZ) twins (35–72% vs 12–23%), indicating greater sharing of risk factors, most probably genetic (estimated heritability 66–80%) (13, 14). PsA also runs strongly in families; siblings of a first-degree relative with PsA are 12–49 times more likely to develop the condition themselves than relatives of individuals without PsA, though only four times more frequently than in spouse controls, suggesting that there is a significant environmental component to PsA risk (15, 16). A strong environmental influence is also suggested by the finding in twin studies of similar concordance rates for PsA between identical (MZ) and non-identical (DZ) twin pairs (17). Concordance of the pattern of PsA within families does not appear to be strong, suggesting that in psoriasis there is an underlying predisposition for synovitis/enthesitis rather than for a specific disease pattern (15).

The major histocompatibility complex and spondyloarthritis

The classical MHC lies between HLA-F and HLA-DP, covering 3.6 megabases. Within this locus, 224 known genes are encoded, most of which have immunological functions. The locus is characterized by extreme and complex patterns of linkage disequilibrium that extend more than 10 megabases either side of the MHC. This extreme linkage disequilibrium is presumed to persist because of survival advantage related to combinations of alleles at different loci on preserved haplotypes. Within the MHC, the HLA alleles are characterized by extreme allelic heterogeneity, which is thought to provide a survival advantage due to the increased likelihood of heterozygosity increasing the range of antigens that can be presented. All the SpAs show association with HLA alleles, and for most there is evidence that other MHC genetic variants are involved, though this has been complex to tease out because of the complex genetic architecture of the locus.

The association of HLA-B27 with AS, first reported in the early 1970s, is amongst the strongest associations of any HLA allele with a common human disease. There are now at least 141 known subtypes of HLA-B27 (http://www.ebi.ac.uk/ipd/imgt/hla/allele.html) which are thought to have evolved from the common ancestor HLA-B27 allele, *HLA-B*2705*. Most subtypes are very rare, and, in most populations worldwide, variation within HLA-B27 makes no difference to the likelihood of these individuals developing the condition. In white European populations, the two most common subtypes, *HLA-B*2702* and *B*2705*, are equally disease-associated (18). Two other subtypes, *HLA-B*2706* which is found in Asians (19) and *HLA-B*2709* which is found in Sardinians (20), appear to be protective or neutrally associated with disease.

As mentioned in the Introduction, HLA-B27 is rare in most African populations, where the development of seronegative arthritis such as AS appears more closely related to HIV infection than genetic risk factors, although weaker associations with *HLA-B*2705* and *B*1403* have been noted (20). In Scandinavian countries and amongst the Inuit, HLA-B27 has a much higher prevalence (10–37%), suggesting that either HLA-B27 provides a survival advantage (perhaps through protection against an infectious disease) or that the high prevalence is due to a founder effect or genetic drift (21, 22). In the broader North American population, a decreasing prevalence of HLA-B27 has been demonstrated in older adults (23), suggesting that HLA-B27 may actually reduce survival, possibly due to associations with increased risk of cardiovascular disease (23).

It is now established that HLA-B27 homozygotes have increased risk of AS, with homozygotes having roughly double the risk of heterozygotes (6, 24, 25). Whether this influences clinical manifestations of the disease is unclear. HLA-B27-negative cases are more likely to have concomitant IBD and psoriasis and less uveitis, but otherwise show similar radiographic severity and clinical manifestations (6, 26).

The strength of the association of HLA-B27 with ReA is considerably lower than with primary AS, with most series reporting B27-carriage rates of 20–60%. Even in case series with axial involvement, the prevalence of HLA-B27 varies substantially (27). Because HLA-B27 is mandatory for the clinical but not imaging arm of the ASAS classification criteria (28), the HLA-B27 prevalence varies in part according to the balance of cases meeting the clinical or imaging arms of the criteria (27–29).

Psoriasis is associated with HLA-Cw6 rather than HLA-B27, but in patients with psoriatic SpA there is a strong association with HLA-B27. Suggestive evidence that other MHC genes may be involved (30) has recently been confirmed in a large HLA imputation study. This demonstrated significant association with HLA-A, -B, and -DQA1 alleles (31). No association with MICA alleles was demonstrated, refuting the long-standing suggestion that MICA alleles were psoriasis-associated (32). This study also showed that PsA was more strongly associated with HLA-B27 than psoriatic skin disease. No distinction was drawn between axial and peripheral PsA, so this may simply represent the known association of AS complicating psoriasis with HLA-B27.

There has been considerable research into the influence of MHC genes and HLA alleles other than HLA-B27 with AS. The association of HLA-B60 with AS is well established, having first been reported by Robinson et al. in 1989 (33), and subsequently confirmed in white Europeans (18) and in east Asians (34). HLA-B60 is split into two DNA sequence-defined alleles, HLA-B*40:01 and -B*40:02, both of which are associated with AS (odds ratio (OR) 1.22 and 1.59, respectively) (35). Risk associations have also been demonstrated with HLA-B*51:01, HLA-B*47:01, HLA-B*13:02, and protective associations with HLA-B*07:02 and HLA-B*57:01 (35). These differential associations are fully statistically explained by the amino acid found at position 97 in the HLA-B protein, suggesting that this is a critical residue in the mechanism by which HLA-B contributes to AS.

The finding of association with HLA-B*51 is of particular interest as this allele is also the major HLA risk allele for Behçet's disease (36), which is clinically associated with sacroiliitis, with AS complicating 5% of Behçet's disease cases (37).

Non-MHC genetic associations of spondyloarthropathies

Aminopeptidases and spondyloarthritis

The M1-aminopeptidases are a family of metalloproteinases with diverse physiological roles. Genetic associations with three genes from the family, *ERAP1*, *ERAP2*, and *NPEPPS* (puromycin-sensitive aminopeptidase), have been identified in genome-wide association studies (GWAS) performed in AS (25, 38), and have also been associated with other SpAs. Of great significance, endoplasmic reticulum aminopeptidase 1 (ERAP1) has been shown to interact with key disease-associated HLA-alleles in AS, psoriasis, and Behçet's disease (see Table 5.2), which has implications for the mechanism by which these HLA alleles operate to cause AS.

ERAP1 encodes an aminopeptidase which is expressed in the endoplasmic reticulum (ER), and which is involved in preparing peptides for MHC class I presentation to immune effector cells. Its association with AS is restricted to *HLA-B27*-positive cases, the first confirmed human example of gene–gene interaction in any common human disease (39). Additionally, ERAP1 is associated in HLA-B*4001-positive AS, but not in HLA-B27- and HLA-B40-negative AS, indicating that there is gene–gene interaction with HLA-B40 and *ERAP1* as well (35). *ERAP1* has also recently been shown to be associated with psoriasis, and in this condition the association is restricted to *HLA-Cw6*-positive cases (40). *ERAP1* is also associated with Behçet's disease, and the association is restricted to HLA-B51 carriers (41), HLA-B51 being the major allelic risk factor for Behçet's disease. The direction of association of *ERAP1* alleles with Behçet's disease is the opposite to that observed with AS and psoriasis.

Whilst it is possible that each of these HLA class I alleles operate through different mechanisms in the respective disease involved, the common association and interaction with *ERAP1* suggests a similar underlying mechanism. ERAP1 acts as a 'molecular ruler', cleaving peptides down to the optimal nine amino acid length for presentation by HLA class I proteins (42). Protective *ERAP1* variants prevent conformational changes in ERAP1 which are thought to be required for peptide cleavage, and thus cause reduced function (41) and changes in the amount and sequence of peptide presented in the ER to HLA class I molecules (43, 44). The restriction

Table 5.2 Genetic associations achieving genome-wide significance in AS

Gene	Locus	SNP	Putative function	Key reference
IL23R	1p31	rs11209026	Activation/differentiation of IL-23R-expressing cells	(38)
		rs12141575		
RUNX3	1p36	rs6600247	Reduction in CD8 lymphocyte counts	(39)
IL6R	1q21	rs4129267	Th17 lymphocyte differentiation, multiple other immunological effects	(60)
FCGR2A	1q32	rs1801274	Unknown	(25)
		rs2039415		
GPR25-KIF21B	1q32	rs41299637	Unknown. ?Bacterial sensing	(61)
HHAT	1q32	rs12758027	Unknown	(25)
2p15	2p15	rs6759298	Unknown	(60)
IL1R2-R1	2q11	rs4851529	Influence on IL-1 cytokine response	(25)
		rs2192752		
UBE2E3	2q31	rs12615545	Ubiquination	(25)
GPR35	2q37	rs4676410	Receptor for 2-acyl lysophosphatidic acid, ?role in bacterial sensing	(25)
EOMES	3p24	rs13093489	T-lymphocyte differentiation	(25)
ANTXR2	4q21	rs12504282	Unknown	(60, 62)
PTGER4	5p13	rs12186979	Induction of IL23 expression, in turn driving activation/ differentiation of IL-23R-expressing cells; bone anabolism	(39)
IL7R	5p13	rs11742270	T-lymphocyte differentiation	(25)
ERAP1	5q15	rs30187	Peptide trimming prior to HLA class I presentation	(38)
		rs1065407		
ERAP2	5q15	rs2910686	Peptide trimming prior to HLA class I presentation	(25)
IL12B	5q33	rs6871626	Activation/differentiation of IL-23R-expressing cells	(61)
		rs6556416		
*HLA-A*0201*	6p21.3	rs2975033	Presentation of peptides to T cells	(25)
HLA-B	6p21.3	rs116488202*	Presentation of peptides to T cells, or misfolding leading to ER stress reaction, or homodimers formation leading to NK cell activation	(63–65)
*HLA-DRB1*0103*	6p21.3	rs17885388	Presentation of peptides to T cells	
HLA-DPB1	6p21.3	rs1126513	Presentation of peptides to T cells	
BACH2	6q15	rs17765610	B-cell differentiation	(25)
		rs639575		
GPR37	7q31	rs2402752	?Bacterial sensing	(25)
CARD9	9q34	rs1128905	Th17 activation after β-glucan exposure	(39)
ZMIZ1	10q22	rs1250550	T-lymphocyte differentiation	(25)
NKX2-3	10q24	rs11190133	T-lymphocyte differentiation	(25)
TNFR1/LTBR	12p13	rs1860545	TNF signalling	(39)
		rs7954567		
SH2B3	12q24	rs11065898	TCR signalling	(25)
GPR65	14q31	rs11624293	Receptor for glycosphingolipids, ?role in bacterial sensing	(25)
IL27	16p11	rs75301646	Th17/Th1 lymphocyte differentiation balance	(25)
		rs35448675		

(continued)

Table 5.2 Continued

Gene	Locus	SNP	Putative function	Key reference
NOS2	17q11	rs2531875	Nitric oxide synthesis	(25)
		rs2297518		
NPEPPS	17q21	rs9901869	Peptide trimming prior to HLA class I presentation	(25)
TBX21	17q21	rs11657479	Innate lymphoid cell differentiation	(39)
TYK2	19p13	rs35164067	Signalling from cytokine receptors, including IL-23R	(25)
		rs6511701		
21q22	21q22	rs2836883	Unknown	(60)
ICOSLG	21q22	rs7282490	T-lymphocyte differentiation	(25)
UBE2L3	22q11	rs2283790	Ubiquination	(25)

of the association of *ERAP1* with HLA-B27- and HLA-B40-positive AS indicates that HLA-B27 and HLA-B40 must operate in AS by a mechanism involving ERAP1, most likely by aberrant peptide handling.

ERAP2 is associated with AS (25, 45), psoriasis, and IBD, with the same alleles being associated in the same direction. ERAP2 also acts as an n-terminal aminopeptidase, although its peptide specificity is less well established. It has also been suggested that ERAP2 may form heterodimers with ERAP1, with the combined protein having different peptide cleavage properties than either ERAP1 or ERAP2 in isolation (46, 47). The protective *ERAP2* alleles all lie on a haplotype that carries the SNP rs2248374, which leads to nonsense-mediated decay of ERAP2 transcripts and absence of ERAP2 protein (48). Thus, as with *ERAP1*, loss-of-function variants of *ERAP2* lead to disease protection. The association of *ERAP2* with AS was initially only discovered having controlled either for the association of *ERAP1* or HLA-B27 (25); due to the strong interaction between these alleles, controlling for one is equivalent in AS cases to controlling for the other. Recently, further statistical analysis demonstrates that the *ERAP2* associations hold true for both HLA-B27-positive and -negative AS, in contrast to *ERAP1* where the association is restricted to HLA-B27-positive or HLA-B40-positive cases (45).

Whilst it is clear that the ERAP1 and ERAP2 protective variants for AS, psoriasis, and IBD are loss-of-function variants, it is possible that these lead to either reduced destruction of antigenic peptide (and thus increased cellular immunity) or reduced formation of antigenic peptide (and thus reduced cellular immunity) (49). Inhibition of aminopeptidases in cell lines has been shown to increase antigen presentation and cytotoxic T-cell responses (50). The effects of ERAP1 genetic variation on antigen processing are still being investigated, but it is clear that these are significantly affected by the antigen amino-acid sequence, with X-Pro bonds being resistant to ERAP1-mediated cleavage. This may explain how the same *ERAP1* variants have opposite directions of association in combination with different HLA alleles in different diseases (Table 5.3).

NPEPPS is expressed primarily in the cytosol and is thought to cleave peptides downstream of the proteasome but upstream of ERAP1 and ERAP2. Its structure has yet to be resolved and it is not known how the AS-associated genetic variants affect its function. A further closely related aminopeptidase, *LN-PEP* or *IRAP*, is encoded next to ERAP1 and ERAP2 at chromosome 5q15. Whilst it has not yet been shown to be associated with any disease, this is difficult to exclude given the complex linkage disequilibrium patterns at this site and interaction with HLA class I alleles. Association with IRAP would be of particular interest, as it is expressed in endosomes and involved in cleavage of internalized proteins, enabling their presentation by HLA class I proteins ('cross-presentation') (51).

The interleukin-23 (IL-23) pathway and spondyloarthropathies

IL23R encodes the receptor for the cytokine IL-23, which is involved in activation of a range of proinflammatory cells including Th17 lymphocytes, gamma-delta cells, mast cells, and others. Association with *IL23R* was first reported in 2007, and since then at least two common variants associated with SNPs have been demonstrated

Table 5.3 Genetic associations of aminopeptidases with immune-mediated diseases

Gene	SNP	Disease	Interacting HLA-allele	Reference
ERAP1	rs30187	AS	HLA-B27	(38)
	rs30187	AS	HLA-B40	(35)
	rs10050860	AS	?	(39)
	rs27524/ rs30187	Psoriasis	HLA-Cw6	(40)
	rs17482078	Behçet's disease	HLA-B*51	(41)
	rs30187	Enthesitis-related subtype, JIA	?	(66)
ERAP2	rs2248374	AS	–	(25, 45)
	rs2910686	Psoriasis	–	(67)
	rs2549794	IBD	–	(68)
	rs7705093	Birdshot retinopathy	?	(69)
LNPEP-ERAP2	rs27290	JIA	–	(66)
NPEPPS	rs9901869	AS	–	(25)

(39), as well as suggestive associations with rare variants (52). The major associated SNP in white Europeans, rs11209026, is not polymorphic in east Asians, where another variant, rs76418789, is the main associated variant (52). This variant is found in white Europeans but at much lower frequency, and is thus not easy to distinguish from the dominant common variant associations. The rs11209026 risk allele has been shown to be a gain-of-function variant (53).

Stimulated by the discovery of the association of *IL23R* with AS, trials of IL-17 blockade have been initiated in AS, and in a phase 2 study strong beneficial effects similar to those observed with TNF-antagonist medications have been reported (54).

Other genetic associations with AS with effects on the IL-23 pathway include *CARD9, EOMES, ICOSLG, IL1R1, IL1R2, IL6R, IL7R, IL12B, IL27, PTGER4, RUNX3, TBX21, TYK2*, and *ZMIZ1* (25). Whilst these genes all have influences on the IL-23 pathway, they also affect other pathways, and so it is not possible to be certain at this point whether their primary influence is directly through IL-23 or downstream to it. However, the large number of genes that influence this pathway strongly supports the hypothesis that this pathway is central to the pathogenesis of AS.

PTGER4 is of particular interest as it forms part of the mechanostat, linking physical stress at entheses with induction of IL-23 production and anabolic bone formation signals, thus identifying a mechanism by which inflammation may lead to bone formation in AS. The role of prostaglandins in the pathogenesis of the osteoproliferative process in AS was further supported by the finding of suggestive association of variants of PTGS1 (encoding cyclo-oxygenase 1) with cross-sectional severity of spinal radiographic change (55).

CARD9 encodes a protein involved in signalling between the innate immunity receptor dectin-1 and the nucleus, leading to IL-23 production. This is of particular interest given the recent demonstration in the Skg mouse model that dectin-1 stimulation by the fungal cell wall component beta-glucan induces SpA, episodic unilateral uveitis, and colitis resembling Crohn's disease (56). This shows a mechanism by which SpA can develop in the absence of HLA-B27 through innate immune pathways.

Particularly strong overlap has been noted between associations of IBD and AS with a 52-fold enrichment of IBD genetic loci, with nearly all shared loci being concordant (either increasing or decreasing risk in both diseases) and mostly with the same SNPs involved. Although overall there is marked overlap, some major differences exist (57). For example, the major AS allele, HLA-B27, is not associated with IBD, and the IBD loci *CARD15/NOD2* and *ATG16L1* show no association with AS to date. This suggests that these loci are particularly important in driving the phenotype which results in individuals that otherwise have similar underlying genetic predisposition.

GWAS have recently identified several genetic associations with psoriasis (see Table 5.4), many of which overlap with both AS and IBD, and genes involved in the IL-23R pathway are over-represented in psoriasis associations, and include *IL23R, IL12B,*

Table 5.4 Genetic associations achieving genome-wide significance in psoriasis and PsA

Gene	Locus	SNP	Putative function	Key reference
IL23R	1p31	rs11209026	Activation/differentiation of IL-23R-expressing cells	(70–73)
IL28RA	1p36	rs4649203	Along with IL-10RB forms receptor for IL-28A, -B, and -29	(40)
RUNX3	1p36	rs4649038	Control of CD8 and Th1 lymphocyte differentiation	(74)
Intergenic	1q31	rs10789285	Unknown	(75)
DENND1B	1q31	rs2477077	Clathrin-mediated endocytosis of proteins	(76)
SLC45A1/TNFRSF9	1p36	rs11121129	Unknown	(67)
LCE3D	1q21	rs4085613	Skin development	(77)
B3GNT2	2p15	rs10865331	Lymphocyte activation	(67)
REL	2p16	rs702873	Control of cytokine secretion including TNF	(40)
IFIH1	2q24	rs17716942	Innate viral recognition	(40)
PLCL2	3p24	rs4685408	Involved in thymic development	(75)
Intergenic	3p24	rs6809854	Unknown	(40)
NFκBIZ	3q12	rs4685408	IL-17 signalling via TRAF3IP2	(75)
CARD6	5p13	rs114934997	Receptor signalling/activation of NFκB	(75)
ERAP1	5q15	rs27524	Peptide trimming prior to HLA class I presentation	(40)
ERAP2	5q15		Peptide trimming prior to HLA class I presentation	
IL13/IL4	5q31	rs20541	IL-13 inhibits proinflammatory cytokine secretion including IFNγ	(78)
IL12B	5q33	rs3213094	T-lymphocyte differentiation/activation	(71–73)
TNIP1	5q33	rs1024995	Interacts with TNFAIP3	(78)
HLA	6p21		Antigen presentation	

(continued)

Table 5.4 Continued

Gene	Locus	SNP	Putative function	Key reference
EXOC2/IRF4	6p25	rs9504361	IRF4 is involved in T-lymphocyte differentiation	(67)
TRAF3IP2	6q21	rs240993	IL-17 receptor signalling	(40, 79)
		rs458017		(40)
TNFAIP3	6q23		TNF signalling control	(78)
TAGAP	6q25	rs2451258	RhoGTPAse-activating protein involved in T-cell activation	(67)
ELMO1	7p14	rs2700987	TLR-mediated interferon production by plasmacytoid dendritic cells	(67)
8DDX58	9p21	rs11795343	Antiviral receptor	(67)
KLF4	9p31	rs10979182	Transcription factor involved in skin barrier function and macrophage activating pathways	(67)
CAMK2G	10q22	rs2675662	Unknown	(75)
ZC3H12C	11q22	rs4561177	Unknown	(67)
ETS1	11q24	rs3802826	T-lymphocyte differentiation/activation	(67)
IL23A/STAT2	12q13	rs2066808	Activation/differentiation of IL-23R-expressing cells	(78)
GJB2	13q12	rs3751385	Encodes connexion-26 gap junction channel, mechanism unknown	(80)
NFκBIA	14q13	rs8016947	Control of cytokine secretion including TNF	(40, 81)
AKAP3	15q25	rs35343117	Unknown	(75)
FBXL19	16p11	rs10782001	Ubiquination, including of IL-1RL1	(81)
SOCS1	16p13	rs367569	Suppressor of cytokine signalling involved in TYK2-mediated and IFNγ signalling	(67)
NOS2	17q11	rs4795067	Produces nitric oxide which itself has diverse functions	(81)
STAT3	17q21	rs963986	Signalling from cytokine receptors including IL-23R. *PTRF/STAT5* nearby	(67)
CARD14	17q25	rs11652075	NFκB activation	(67)
STARD6,POLI, MBD2	18q21	rs545979	Unknown	(67)
ILF3,CARM1	19p13	rs892085	ILF3 coregulates IL-2 transcription	(67)
TYK2	19p13	rs12720356	Signalling from cytokine receptors including IL-23R	(40)
		rs280519		(40)
ZNF816A	19q13	rs9304742	Unknown	(80)
ZNF313/RNF114	20q13	rs495337	T-cell activation	(82)
UBE2L3	22q11	rs4821124	Ubiquination, target unknown	(67)

TYK2, and *IL23A*. These findings have been important in stimulating clinical trials in psoriasis of cytokine-inhibition therapy targeting this pathway, with clear beneficial effects. For example, ustekinumab, an antibody treatment targeting IL-12p40, is now a licensed treatment for psoriasis in many countries, and is effective for both psoriatic skin and joint disease (58). Anti-IL-17A antibody treatment has also been shown to be effective for both psoriasis and PsA (59).

Several genes that can broadly be said to act through nuclear factor κB1 (NFκB1) show association with psoriasis, something that is more a feature of seropositive diseases such as RA, perhaps explaining the clinical overlap of PsA with RA. These include *NFκB1A*, *REL*, *TRAF3IP2*, and *TNIP1*.

A surprise finding from genetic studies has been the association of genes involved in interferon signalling pathways and psoriasis. *IL28RA* encodes a type III interferon receptor subunit. *IFIH1* encodes an innate immunity receptor, stimulation of which by microbes leads to a type I interferon response. *TYK2* encodes a tyrosine kinase involved in signalling from various cytokine receptors including IL-23R and interferon receptors. This suggests that interferon signalling induced by microbial infection may be important in psoriasis pathogenesis.

Conclusion

There is extensive sharing of genetic risk factors across SpA, suggesting that a significant proportion of their shared clinical features relates to similar immunogenetic mechanisms. The findings of genetic studies have greatly advanced our understanding of the pathogenesis of these diseases and have led to new effective therapies for them. Only a minority of the genes involved have thus far been discovered, and further research is required both to identify a higher proportion of the genes involved and to determine the causal mechanisms underlying the known genetic associations.

References

1. Helmick CG, Felson DT, Lawrence RC, et al. Estimates of the prevalence of arthritis and other rheumatic conditions in the United States: Part I. Arthritis Rheum 2008;58(1):15–25.
2. Khan MA, Kushner I, Braun WE. Letter: low incidence of HLA-B27 in American blacks with spondyloarthropathies. Lancet 1976;1(7957):483.
3. Brown MA, Jepson A, Young A, Whittle HC, Greenwood BM, Wordsworth BP. Ankylosing spondylitis in West Africans—evidence for a non-HLA-B27 protective effect. Ann Rheum Dis 1997;56(1):68–70.
4. Gelfand JM, Stern RS, Nijsten T, et al. The prevalence of psoriasis in African Americans: results from a population-based study. J Am Acad Dermatol 2005;52(1):23–6.
5. Yip SY. The prevalence of psoriasis in the Mongoloid race. J Am Acad Dermatol 1984;10(6):965–8.
6. Jaakkola E, Herzberg I, Laiho K, et al. Finnish HLA studies confirm the increased risk conferred by HLA-B27 homozygosity in ankylosing spondylitis. Ann Rheum Dis 2006;65(6):775–80.
7. Brown MA, Laval SH, Brophy S, Calin A. Recurrence risk modelling of the genetic susceptibility to ankylosing spondylitis. Ann Rheum Dis 2000;59(11):883–6.
8. Brown MA, Kennedy LG, MacGregor AJ, et al. Susceptibility to ankylosing spondylitis in twins: the role of genes, HLA, and the environment. Arthritis Rheum 1997;40(10):1823–8.
9. Pedersen OB, Svendsen AJ, Ejstrup L, Skytthe A, Harris JR, Junker P. Ankylosing spondylitis in Danish and Norwegian twins: occurrence and the relative importance of genetic vs. environmental effectors in disease causation. Scand J Rheumatol 2008;37(2):120–6.
10. Brophy S, Hickey S, Menon A, et al. Concordance of disease severity among family members with ankylosing spondylitis? J Rheumatol 2004;31(9):1775–8.
11. Brown MA, Brophy S, Bradbury L, et al. Identification of major loci controlling clinical manifestations of ankylosing spondylitis. Arthritis Rheum 2003;48(8):2234–9.
12. Hamersma J, Cardon LR, Bradbury L, et al. Is disease severity in ankylosing spondylitis genetically determined? Arthritis Rheum 2001;44(6):1396–400.
13. Grjibovski AM, Olsen AO, Magnus P, Harris JR. Psoriasis in Norwegian twins: contribution of genetic and environmental effects. J Eur Acad Dermatol Venereol 2007;21(10):1337–43.
14. Duffy DL, Spelman LS, Martin NG. Psoriasis in Australian twins. J Am Acad Dermatol 1993;29(3):428–34.
15. Myers A, Kay LJ, Lynch SA, Walker DJ. Recurrence risk for psoriasis and psoriatic arthritis within sibships. Rheumatology (Oxford) 2005;44(6):773–6.
16. Moll JM, Wright V. Familial occurrence of psoriatic arthritis. Ann Rheum Dis 1973;32(3):181–201.
17. Pedersen OB, Svendsen AJ, Ejstrup L, Skytthe A, Junker P. On the heritability of psoriatic arthritis. Disease concordance among monozygotic and dizygotic twins. Ann Rheum Dis 2008;67(10):1417–21.
18. Brown MA, Pile KD, Kennedy LG, et al. HLA class I associations of ankylosing spondylitis in the white population in the United Kingdom. Ann Rheum Dis 1996;55(4):268–70.
19. Lopez-Larrea C, Sujirachato K, Mehra NK, et al. HLA-B27 subtypes in Asian patients with ankylosing spondylitis. Evidence for new associations. Tissue Antigens 1995;45(3):169–76.
20. D'Amato M, Fiorillo MT, Galeazzi M, Martinetti M, Amoroso A, Sorrentino R. Frequency of the new HLA-B*2709 allele in ankylosing spondylitis patients and healthy individuals. Dis Markers 1995;12(3):215–17.
21. Oen K, Postl B, Chalmers IM, et al. Rheumatic diseases in an Inuit population. Arthritis Rheum 1986;29(1):65–74.
22. Boyer GS, Templin DW, Cornoni-Huntley JC, et al. Prevalence of spondyloarthropathies in Alaskan Eskimos. J Rheumatol 1994;21(12):2292–7.
23. Walsh JA, Zhou X, Clegg DO, Teng C, Cannon GW, Sauer B. Mortality in American Veterans with the HLA-B27 gene. J Rheumatol 2015;42(4):638–44.
24. Khan M, Kushner I, Braun W, Zachary A, Steinberg A. HLA-B27 homozygosity in ankylosing spondylitis: relationship to risk and severity. Tissue Antigens 1978;11:434–8.
25. International Genetics of Ankylosing Spondylitis Consortium, Cortes A, Hadler J, et al. Identification of multiple risk variants for ankylosing spondylitis through high-density genotyping of immune-related loci. Nat Genet 2013;45(7):730–8.
26. Cortes A, Maksymowych WP, Wordsworth BP, et al. Association study of genes related to bone formation and resorption and the extent of radiographic change in ankylosing spondylitis. Ann Rheum Dis 2015;74(7):1387–93.
27. Robinson PC, Wordsworth BP, Reveille JD, Brown MA. Axial spondyloarthritis: a new disease entity, not necessarily early ankylosing spondylitis. Ann Rheum Dis 2013;72(2):162–4.
28. Zeidler H, Amor B. The Assessment in Spondyloarthritis international Society (ASAS) classification criteria for peripheral spondyloarthritis and for spondyloarthritis in general: the spondyloarthritis concept in progress. Ann Rheum Dis 2011;70(1):1–3.
29. Akkoc N, Khan MA. Looking into the new ASAS classification criteria for axial spondyloarthritis through the other side of the glass. Curr Rheumatol Rep 2015;17(6):515.
30. Knight J, Spain SL, Capon F, et al. Conditional analysis identifies three novel major histocompatibility complex loci associated with psoriasis. Hum Molec Genet 2012;21(23):5185–92.
31. Okada Y, Han B, Tsoi LC, et al. Fine mapping major histocompatibility complex associations in psoriasis and its clinical subtypes. Am J Hum Genet 2014;95(2):162–72.
32. Gonzalez S, Martinez-Borra J, Torre-Alonso JC, et al. The MICA-A9 triplet repeat polymorphism in the transmembrane region confers additional susceptibility to the development of psoriatic arthritis and is independent of the association of Cw*0602 in psoriasis. Arthritis Rheum 1999;42(5):1010–16.
33. Robinson WP, van der Linden SM, Khan MA, et al. HLA-Bw60 increases susceptibility to ankylosing spondylitis in HLA-B27+ patients. Arthritis Rheum 1989;32(9):1135–41.
34. Wei JC, Tsai WC, Lin HS, Tsai CY, Chou CT. HLA-B60 and B61 are strongly associated with ankylosing spondylitis in HLA-B27-negative Taiwan Chinese patients. Rheumatology (Oxford) 2004;43(7):839–42.
35. Cortes A, Pulit SL, Leo PJ, et al. Major histocompatibility complex associations of ankylosing spondylitis are complex and involve further epistasis with ERAP1. Nat Commun 2015;6:7146.
36. Meguro A, Inoko H, Ota M, et al. Genetics of Behçet disease inside and outside the MHC. Ann Rheum Dis 2010;69(4):747–54.
37. Ait Badi MA, Zyani M, Kaddouri S, Niamane R, Hda A, Algayres JP. [Skeletal manifestations in Behçet's disease. A report of 79 cases.] Rev Med Interne 2008;29(4):277–82.
38. Burton PR, Clayton DG, Cardon LR, et al. Association scan of 14,500 nonsynonymous SNPs in four diseases identifies autoimmunity variants. Nat Genet 2007;39(11):1329–37.
39. Evans DM, Spencer CC, Pointon JJ, et al. Interaction between ERAP1 and HLA-B27 in ankylosing spondylitis implicates peptide handling in the mechanism for HLA-B27 in disease susceptibility. Nat Genet 2011;43(8):761–7.
40. Strange A, Capon F, Spencer CC, et al. A genome-wide association study identifies new psoriasis susceptibility loci and an interaction between HLA-C and ERAP1. Nat Genet 2010;42(11):985–90.
41. Kirino Y, Bertsias G, Ishigatsubo Y, et al. Genome-wide association analysis identifies new susceptibility loci for Behçet's disease and epistasis between HLA-B*51 and ERAP1. Nat Genet 2013;45(2):202–7.
42. Chang SC, Momburg F, Bhutani N, Goldberg AL. The ER aminopeptidase, ERAP1, trims precursors to lengths of MHC class I peptides by a 'molecular ruler' mechanism. Proc Natl Acad Sci USA 2005;102(47):17107–12.

43. Alvarez-Navarro C, Martin-Esteban A, Barnea E, Admon A, Lopez de Castro JA. ERAP1 polymorphism relevant to inflammatory disease shapes the peptidome of the birdshot chorioretinopathy-associated HLA-A*29:02 antigen. Mol Cell Proteomics 2015;14(7):1770–80.
44. Sanz-Bravo A, Campos J, Mazariegos MS, Lopez de Castro JA. Dominant role of the ERAP1 polymorphism R528K in shaping the HLA-B27 peptidome through differential processing determined by multiple peptide residues. Arthritis Rheumatol 2015;67(3):692–701.
45. Robinson PC, Costello ME, Leo P, et al. ERAP2 is associated with ankylosing spondylitis in HLA-B27-positive and HLA-B27-negative patients. Ann Rheum Dis 2015;74(8):1627–9.
46. Saveanu L, Carroll O, Lindo V, et al. Concerted peptide trimming by human ERAP1 and ERAP2 aminopeptidase complexes in the endoplasmic reticulum. Nat Immunol 2005;6(7):689–97.
47. Evnouchidou I, Weimershaus M, Saveanu L, van Endert P. ERAP1-ERAP2 dimerization increases peptide-trimming efficiency. J Immunol 2014;193(2):901–8.
48. Andres AM, Dennis MY, Kretzschmar WW, et al. Balancing selection maintains a form of ERAP2 that undergoes nonsense-mediated decay and affects antigen presentation. PLoS Genet 2010;6(10):e1001157.
49. Evnouchidou I, Papakyriakou A, Stratikos E. A new role for Zn(II) aminopeptidases: antigenic peptide generation and destruction. Curr Pharm Des 2009;15(31):3656–70.
50. Zervoudi E, Saridakis E, Birtley JR, et al. Rationally designed inhibitor targeting antigen-trimming aminopeptidases enhances antigen presentation and cytotoxic T-cell responses. Proc Natl Acad Sci USA 2013;110(49):19890–5.
51. Saveanu L, Carroll O, Weimershaus M, et al. IRAP identifies an endosomal compartment required for MHC class I cross-presentation. Science 2009;325(5937):213–17.
52. Davidson SI, Jiang L, Cortes A, et al. Brief report: high-throughput sequencing of IL23R reveals a low-frequency, nonsynonymous single-nucleotide polymorphism that is associated with ankylosing spondylitis in a Han Chinese population. Arthritis Rheum 2013;65(7):1747–52.
53. Di Meglio P, Di Cesare A, Laggner U, et al. The IL23R R381Q gene variant protects against immune-mediated diseases by impairing IL-23-induced Th17 effector response in humans. PloS One 2011;6(2):e17160.
54. Baeten D, Baraliakos X, Braun J, et al. Anti-interleukin-17A monoclonal antibody secukinumab in treatment of ankylosing spondylitis: a randomised, double-blind, placebo-controlled trial. Lancet 2013;382(9906):1705–13.
55. Cortes A, Maksymowych WP, Wordsworth BP, et al. Association study of genes related to bone formation and resorption and the extent of radiographic change in ankylosing spondylitis. Ann Rheum Dis 2015;74(7):1387–93.
56. Ruutu M, Thomas G, Steck R, et al. β-glucan triggers spondyloarthropathy and Crohn's-like ileitis in SKG mice. Arthritis Rheum 2012;64(7):2211–22.
57. Parkes M, Cortes A, van Heel DA, Brown MA. Genetic insights into common pathways and complex relationships among immune-mediated diseases. Nat Rev Genet 2013;14(9):661–73.
58. Gottlieb A, Menter A, Mendelsohn A, et al. Ustekinumab, a human interleukin 12/23 monoclonal antibody, for psoriatic arthritis: randomised, double-blind, placebo-controlled, crossover trial. Lancet 2009;373(9664):633–40.
59. McInnes I, Sieper J, Braun J, et al. Anti-interleukin 17A monoclonal antibody secukinumab reduces signs and symptoms of psoriatic arthritis in a 24-week multicenter, double-blind, randomized, placebo-controlled trial. Arthritis Rheum 2011;63(Suppl 10):779.
60. Australo-Anglo-American Spondyloarthritis Consortium, Reveille JD, Sims AM, et al. Genome-wide association study of ankylosing spondylitis identifies non-MHC susceptibility loci. Nat Genet 2010;42(2):123–7.
61. Danoy P, Pryce K, Hadler J, et al. Association of variants at 1q32 and STAT3 with ankylosing spondylitis suggests genetic overlap with Crohn's disease. PLoS Genet 2010;6(12):e1001195.
62. Karaderi T, Keidel SM, Pointon JJ, et al. Ankylosing spondylitis is associated with the anthrax toxin receptor 2 gene (ANTXR2). Ann Rheum Dis 2014;73(11):2054–8.
63. Brewerton DA, Hart FD, Nicholls A, Caffrey M, James DC, Sturrock RD. Ankylosing spondylitis and HL-A 27. Lancet 1973;1(7809):904–7.
64. Caffrey MF, James DC. Human lymphocyte antigen association with ankylosing spondylitis. Nature 1973;9(242):121.
65. Schlosstein L, Terasaki PI, Bluestone R, Pearson CM. High association of an HL-A antigen, W27, with ankylosing spondylitis. N Engl J Med 1973;288(14):704–6.
66. Hinks A, Martin P, Flynn E, et al. Subtype specific genetic associations for juvenile idiopathic arthritis: ERAP1 with the enthesitis related arthritis subtype and IL23R with juvenile psoriatic arthritis. Arthritis Res Therapy 2011;13(1):R12.
67. Tsoi LC, Spain SL, Knight J, et al. Identification of 15 new psoriasis susceptibility loci highlights the role of innate immunity. Nat Genet 2012;44(12):1341–8.
68. Franke A, McGovern DP, Barrett JC, et al. Genome-wide meta-analysis increases to 71 the number of confirmed Crohn's disease susceptibility loci. Nat Genet 2010;42(12):1118–25.
69. Kuiper JJ, Van Setten J, Ripke S, et al. A genome-wide association study identifies a functional ERAP2 haplotype associated with birdshot chorioretinopathy. Hum Molec Genet 2014;23(22):6081–7.
70. Cargill M, Schrodi SJ, Chang M, et al. A large-scale genetic association study confirms IL12B and leads to the identification of IL23R as psoriasis-risk genes. Am J Hum Genet 2007;80(2):273–90.
71. Nair RP, Ruether A, Stuart PE, et al. Polymorphisms of the IL12B and IL23R genes are associated with psoriasis. J Invest Dermatol 2008;128(7):1653–61.
72. Capon F, Di Meglio P, Szaub J, et al. Sequence variants in the genes for the interleukin-23 receptor (IL23R) and its ligand (IL12B) confer protection against psoriasis. Hum Genet 2007;122(2):201–6.
73. Liu Y, Helms C, Liao W, et al. A genome-wide association study of psoriasis and psoriatic arthritis identifies new disease loci. PLoS Genet 2008;4(3):e1000041.
74. Apel M, Uebe S, Bowes J, et al. Variants in RUNX3 contribute to susceptibility to psoriatic arthritis, exhibiting further common ground with ankylosing spondylitis. Arthritis Rheum 2013;65(5):1224–31.
75. Tsoi LC, Spain SL, Ellinghaus E, et al. Enhanced meta-analysis and replication studies identify five new psoriasis susceptibility loci. Nat Commun 2015;6:7001.
76. Bowes J, Budu-Aggrey A, Huffmeier U, et al. Dense genotyping of immune-related susceptibility loci reveals new insights into the genetics of psoriatic arthritis. Nat Commun 2015;6:6046.
77. Zhang XJ, Huang W, Yang S, et al. Psoriasis genome-wide association study identifies susceptibility variants within LCE gene cluster at 1q21. Nat Genet 2009;41(2):205–10.
78. Nair RP, Duffin KC, Helms C, et al. Genome-wide scan reveals association of psoriasis with IL-23 and NF-kappaB pathways. Nat Genet 2009;41(2):199–204.
79. Ellinghaus E, Ellinghaus D, Stuart PE, et al. Genome-wide association study identifies a psoriasis susceptibility locus at TRAF3IP2. Nat Genet 2010;42(11):991–5.
80. Sun LD, Cheng H, Wang ZX, et al. Association analyses identify six new psoriasis susceptibility loci in the Chinese population. Nat Genet 2010;42(11):1005–9.
81. Stuart PE, Nair RP, Ellinghaus E, et al. Genome-wide association analysis identifies three psoriasis susceptibility loci. Nat Genet 2010;42(11):1000–4.
82. Capon F, Bijlmakers MJ, Wolf N, et al. Identification of ZNF313/RNF114 as a novel psoriasis susceptibility gene. Hum Molec Genet 2008;17(13):1938–45.

CHAPTER 6

Immune mechanisms: HLA-B27

Robert A. Colbert and Paul Bowness

Introduction to HLA-B27

HLA-B27 is strongly associated with the development of AS. HLA-B27 is present in more than 90% of patients but less than 10% of unaffected individuals, depending on the population. However, in most circumstances HLA-B27 is probably insufficient to cause disease on its own. Indeed, more than 40 additional genes or genetic regions have now been associated with susceptibility to AS.

Currently there are two broad theories proposed to explain the role of HLA-B27 in AS pathogenesis (Fig. 6.1). The first is based on the principal immunological function of HLA-B27, which is to present peptides to cytotoxic T cells and NK cells. Like other HLA class I proteins, HLA-B27 binds short peptides within the endoplasmic reticulum (ER) and traffics to the cell surface where it displays these peptides to the immune system (Fig. 6.2). Most often the peptides are derived from self-proteins, and HLA-B27 is ignored by the immune system. However, when a cell is infected, antigenic peptides derived from the foreign organism are presented, enabling CD8+ cytotoxic T cells to recognize and kill the infected cells. It has been postulated since the early 1990s that HLA-B27 might contribute to AS by presenting peptides that become 'arthritogenic', with CD8+ T cells then triggering joint inflammation (1). A lack of evidence supporting T cell autoreactivity, together with recognition of aberrant features of HLA-B27, led to alternative proposals suggesting that this allele may stimulate the immune system in novel ways. For example, intracellular accumulation of misfolded forms of HLA-B27 (that generate ER stress) were shown to promote pro-Th17 cytokine production, and cell-surface expression of aberrant forms of the HLA-B27 heavy chain can drive proinflammatory Th17 responses through interaction with killer immunoglobulin receptors (KIR) on T and NK cells (Fig. 6.1). There is also evidence that dendritic cells expressing HLA-B27 exhibit aberrant properties that could lead to loss of immunologic tolerance, although features of HLA-B27 responsible for this phenomenon remain unclear.

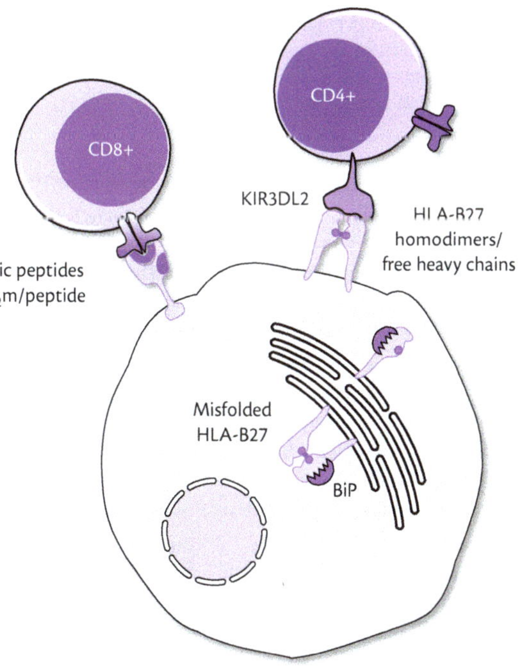

Fig. 6.1 (See colour plate section). Proposed mechanisms linking HLA-B27 to disease pathogenesis. HLA-B27 displays foreign peptides to CD8+ T cells during an infection. The T cells cross-react with self-peptides presented by HLA-B27 and thus become 'autoreactive'. Self-peptides that are specifically responsible for arthritis would be considered 'arthritogenic peptides'. HLA-B27 can form dimers on the cell surface that are capable of interacting with KIRs such as KIR3DL2, and then triggering CD4+ T cells to produce proinflammatory cytokines. HLA-B27, because of its tendency to misfold, can accumulate inside the cell where it can cause ER stress. The response to ER stress can promote proinflammatory cytokine production.

The discovery that ERAP1 influences the risk of developing AS in individuals with HLA-B27 has generated interest in the functional interaction between these gene products. ERAP1 affects the quality and quantity of peptides available for loading onto HLA class I proteins, and thus can impact upon canonical and aberrant properties of HLA-B27. The current status of research in these areas, including the interaction between HLA-B27 and ERAP1, are discussed in this chapter.

Background

AS is a common inflammatory rheumatic disease affecting up to 0.5% of the population, for which the pathogenesis is poorly understood. The association with HLA-B27 was first described in 1973 by groups in London and Los Angeles and has subsequently been confirmed in multiple studies in different countries and in different ethnic groups (2, 3). Indeed, the frequency of AS in various geographic locations around the globe correlates strongly with the prevalence of HLA-B27. Twin studies suggest that AS is largely (>90%) heritable (4), and although HLA-B27 has a dominant influence (5), approximately 95% of individuals with HLA-B27 do not develop disease, presumably because they lack sufficient additional susceptibility alleles. HLA-B27 accounts for an estimated 25% of AS heritability (6), with recently discovered genes accounting for only an additional 3% (6). Thus, while a great deal of genetic susceptibility to AS may be undefined, we focus our attention on what is known. One of the strongest genetic associations outside of the HLA region is with ERAP1 (7). This was initially reported only in HLA-B27-positive AS patients, indicating a genetic interaction

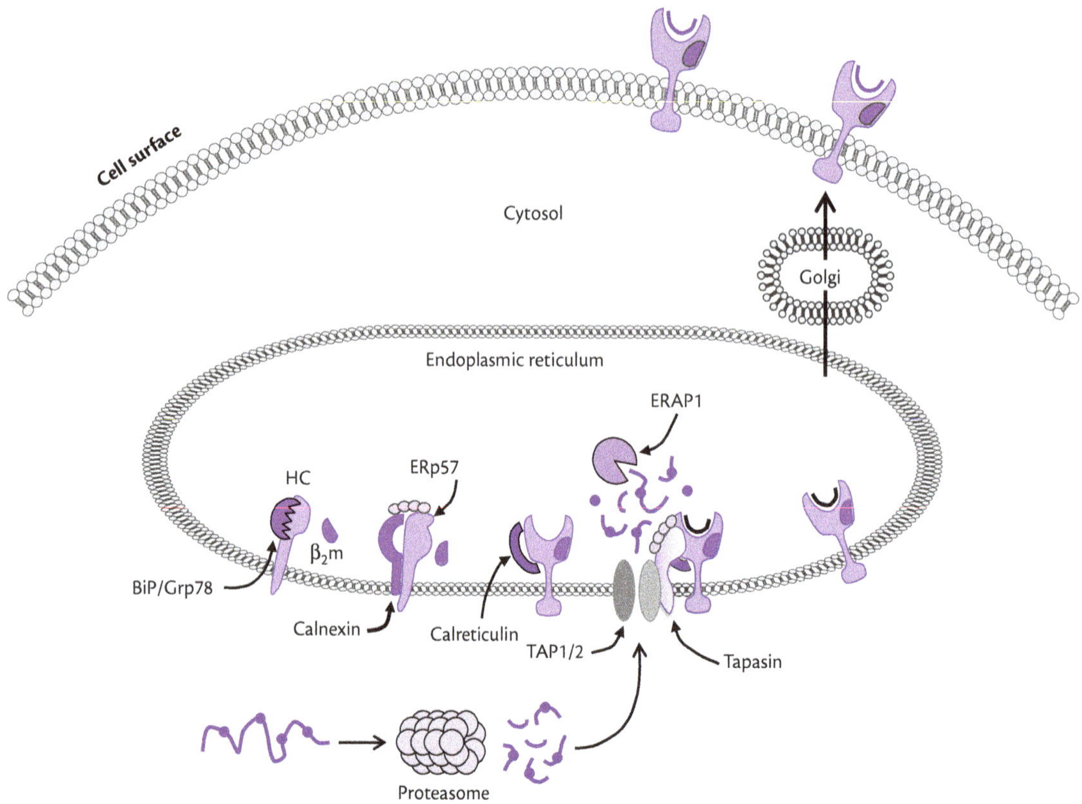

Fig. 6.2 (See colour plate section). HLA class I assembly pathway. HLA class I heavy chains are synthesized in the ER, where they interact transiently with several chaperones (binding immunoglobulin protein (BiP), calnexin, calreticulin) to facilitate folding. ERp57 is an oxidoreductase that facilitates disulphide bond formation. Folded heavy chains can bind β_2m, but remain in the ER tethered to tapasin and the peptide loading complex until optimal peptides can bind. Peptides are produced in the cytosol and transported into the ER via peptide transporters (transporter associated with antigen processing (TAP1/2), where they are further trimmed by the aminopeptidase ERAP1 (and ERAP2; not shown). Optimized HLA class I complexes are transported to the cell surface through the Golgi.

and implying that the effect of ERAP1 on disease pathogenesis was most likely mediated by its influence on ER peptide supply (8).

HLA-B27 and presentation of arthritogenic peptides

Key discoveries in the 1970s and 1980s showed that the principal natural function of MHC class I molecules including the HLA-A, B, and C proteins of humans, is to bind short peptide fragments derived largely from proteins inside cells, and to carry these to the cell surface and present them to T cells (9, 10). Indeed, the phenomenon of 'MHC restriction' describes the necessity for the T-cell receptor for antigen (or TCR) of a T lymphocyte to recognize the combination of a peptide antigen bound to a self MHC (HLA) molecule. Subsequently, the crystal structure of HLA-B27 bound to a peptide was determined by Madden et al. (11) and is shown in Fig. 6.3. The term HLA-B27 refers to the heavy chain (comprising three alpha helices) non-covalently bound to beta 2-microglobulin (β_2m) and to a small peptide. On any given cell there are many thousands of HLA-B27 molecules displaying thousands of different peptides, the majority of which are derived from self-proteins (12). Once on the cell surface, these complexes are capable of being recognized by the TCR. Classically, cytotoxic T cells recognize class I complexes including HLA-B27 in combination with the CD8 co-receptor.

HLA-B27-positive individuals have been shown to make good cytotoxic CD8+ T cell responses to a number of important human viruses, including influenza, HIV, and hepatitis C. Possession of the HLA-B27 allele may thus provide a survival advantage against serious infections (13). Indeed, there is evidence that this is the case for HIV (14, 15) and hepatitis C (16). Following the discovery of antigen presentation by MHC class I molecules, Benjamin and Parham proposed that this function, rather than postulated antibacterial cross-reactive antibodies, could lead HLA-B27 to present 'arthritogenic' peptides (1). These peptides were hypothetically derived from joint-specific proteins and would be recognized by autoreactive CD8+ T cells to cause SpA. Consistent with this notion, they demonstrated that HLA-B27 was capable of binding extracellular (in addition to intracellular-derived) peptides (1). It was also proposed that HLA-B27 itself shared short sequences with Gram-negative enteric organisms more frequently than other alleles, and that bacteria-derived peptides might fit the unique peptide binding motif required by HLA-B27. This in turn could select for robust antibacterial cross-reactive CD8+ T cell responses to initiate and promote SpA (17).

What is the evidence for and against the arthritogenic peptide hypothesis? HLA-B27 does appear to bind a unique group of peptides, characterized primarily by the presence of an arginine at position 2 (P2) from the N-terminus (12). Both pathogen-specific and autoreactive HLA-B27-restricted T cell responses have been detected in the blood of patients with SpA (18, 19).

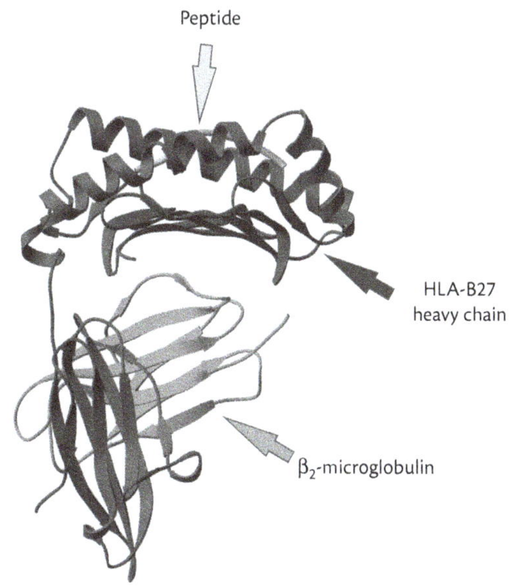

Fig. 6.3 (See colour plate section). Ribbon diagram of HLA-B27 modelled from its crystal structure. The HLA-B27 heavy chain and non-covalently attached to β_2m are arrowed. The folded heavy chain forms a peptide-binding groove, which contains a peptide, whose backbone only is shown here (arrowed). Many of the amino acids that differ between HLA-B alleles line the peptide binding groove. TCRs interact with bound peptide as regions of the HLA class I heavy chain. Only the membrane distal portion of the HLA class I molecule is shown.

HLA-B27-restricted T cell responses to *Chlamydia trachomatis* peptides have also been detected in the joints of patients with ReA using HLA-B27 peptide tetrameric complexes; however, the frequency of such responses has always been low, and presence does not imply pathogenic causality (20). If HLA-B27 were presenting specific arthritogenic peptides to pathogenic clones of CD8 T cells, one would expect to see a signature of these T cells with specific and limited or at least oligoclonal TCR. Whilst evidence of restriction of TCR repertoires exists, these have not thus far been striking (21, 22). In addition, while immunohistology of inflammatory lesions from AS patients reveals CD3+ T cell infiltrates (23, 24), CD4+ T cells often predominate rather than the CD8+ T cells that would be expected in an HLA-B27 antigen-driven process.

The strongest evidence against the arthritogenic peptide hypothesis comes from the HLA-B27 transgenic (tg) rat model of SpA. Transgenic rats overexpressing HLA-B27 and human beta 2-microglobulin (hβ_2m) develop disease resembling human SpA, with arthritis, tail and spinal involvement, gut inflammation, psoriasiform skin lesions, and epididymo-orchitis (25), while rats overexpressing HLA-B7 and hβ_2m remain healthy. Most importantly, HLA-B27 tg rats still develop disease if CD8+ T cells are ablated with either antibody treatment or by knocking out CD8 (26, 27), essentially ruling out a requirement for CD8+ T cells in rat SpA.

Recent detailed analysis of peptides from HLA-B27 subtypes that are either not associated with disease (HLA-B*27:06) or are weakly associated (B*27:09) has not revealed clear qualitative differences between disease-associated and neutral or non-associated subtypes (28). However, the lack of qualitative differences does not rule out the possibility that quantitative changes in the peptide repertoire may contribute to the risk of disease. For example, there might be an 'arthritogenic peptide repertoire' rather than a single or limited set of peptides. Notably, in addition to TCR recognition, NK cell receptors can recognize MHC class I molecules including HLA-B27, and the cognate receptor for HLA-B27 heterotrimers, KIR3DL1, is particularly sensitive to the nature of the P8 amino acid residue of peptides bound to HLA-B27 (29, 30). Thus quantitative changes in bound peptide could influence immune responses through effects on KIR signalling, although the fundamental reason that this would lead to SpA with HLA-B27 and not other KIR-interacting alleles remains unclear. Changes in the peptide repertoire might also affect both misfolding and free heavy chain or homodimer expression, as discussed in the section 'HLA-B27 misfolding and the consequences of accumulation in the endoplasmic reticulum'.

Aberrant properties of HLA-B27

In the late 1990s, the Bowness and Colbert groups independently recognized aberrant properties of HLA-B27, referred to as heavy chain 'dimerization' and 'misfolding', and proposed that they might confer non-canonical gain-of-function properties important in SpA pathogenesis (31, 32) (Fig. 6.4). Although the mechanisms by which dimerization and misfolding may contribute to disease are different, the structural features of HLA-B27 that confer these properties are similar (33, 34) and are fundamentally influenced by peptide–heavy chain interactions. More importantly, both mechanisms are linked to activation of the IL-23/IL-17 axis, which is a major pathway implicated in disease risk (35) and pathogenesis (36).

Cell-surface expression of abnormal forms of HLA-B27 and recognition by immune receptors

The observation that HLA-B27 can form β_2m-free heavy chain homodimers when expressed in cell lines (31) led to the question of whether SpA patients express such forms of HLA-B27. It is now well established that certain cell types (including monocytes) from the blood and joints of SpA patients can express increased levels of HLA class I free heavy chains (FHC) including dimers (37–39). Similarly, FHC forms of HLA-B27 are expressed by cells from HLA-B27 tg rats (40–42). These initial observations led to a search for receptors that could bind such molecules. Whilst TCRs do not (usually) bind to HLA-B27 FHC, innate immune receptors including KIR3DL2 (and the leukocyte immunoglobulin-like receptor, subfamily B, member 4 (LILRB4) as well as rodent paired immunoglobulin receptors (PIRs)) bind to HLA-B27 FHC (37) (Fig. 6.1). KIR3DL2 is expressed at higher levels compared to other KIRs on both NK cells and T cells in HLA-B27-positive SpA patients (43). Furthermore, these interactions can both promote NK and T cell survival (44) and skew T cell responses towards Th17 (Ridley et al., unpublished observations). Whilst the relative contribution of cell-surface-expressed FHC of HLA-B27 to SpA pathogenesis has not yet been established, these findings raise the possibility that SpA could in the future be treated with antibodies that target either component of the HLA-B27 FHC–KIR3DL2 interaction.

HLA-B27 misfolding and the consequences of accumulation in the endoplasmic reticulum

For MHC class I molecules to bind peptides, exit the ER, and traffic to the cell surface to be recognized by the immune system, they

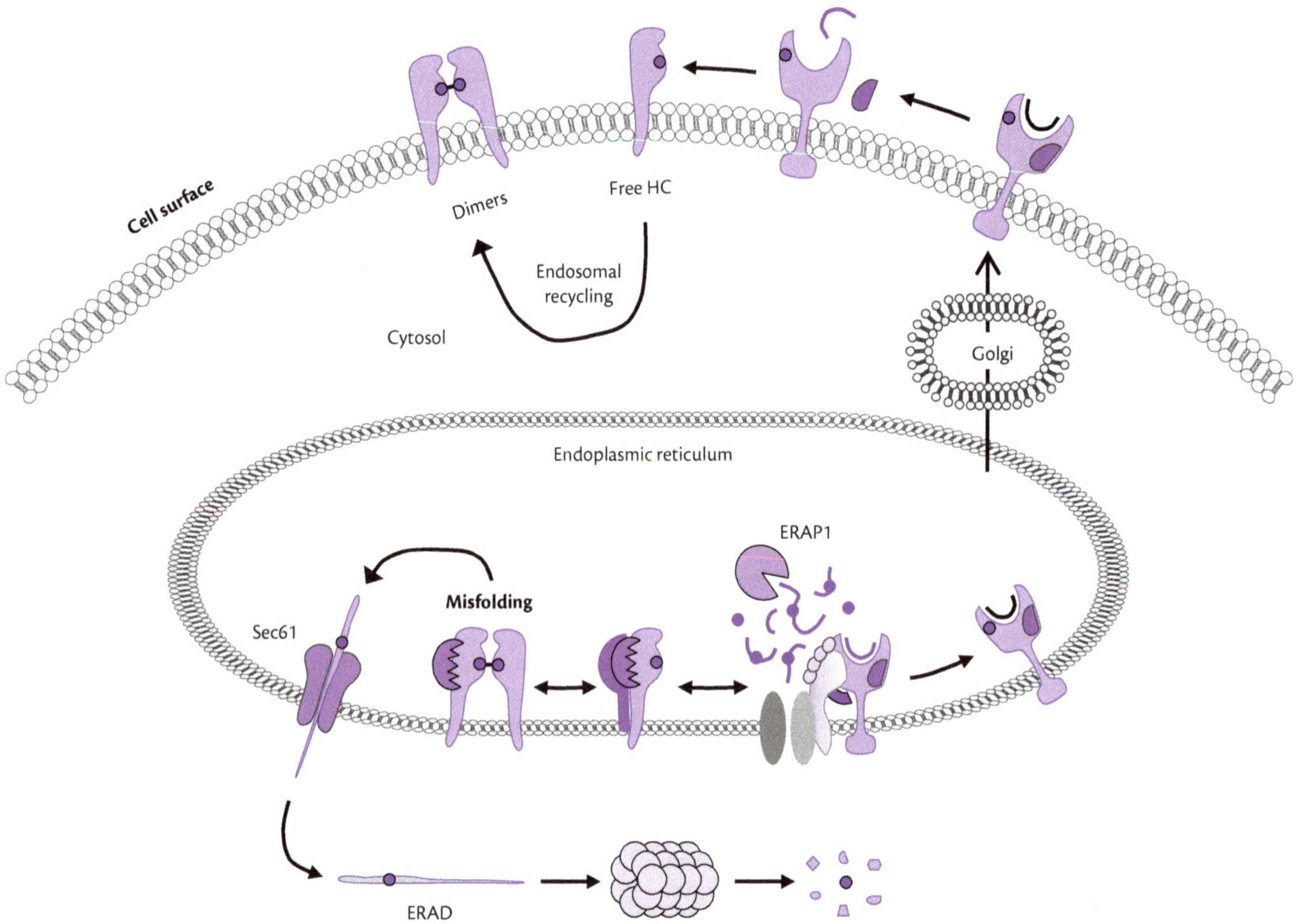

Fig. 6.4 (See colour plate section). Aberrant features of HLA-B27 cell biology. Cell surface HLA-B27 complexes can lose β_2m (and peptide) and remain as free heavy chains on the cell surface, or form disulphide-linked dimers during endosomal recycling. Newly synthesized heavy chains are slow to fold and bind β_2m in the ER, and exhibit a prolonged association with BiP. They have a tendency to dimerize due to the oxidizing environment. Accumulation of misfolded and BiP-bound heavy chains can cause ER stress.

must first fold and associate with β_2m. The HLA-B27 heavy chain exhibits a substantial delay in its progression through this pathway, which results in increased oxidation of the usually free cysteine residue at position 67 (Cys67) (32, 33). A common binding partner for the oxidized Cys67 on one heavy chain is Cys67 on another HLA-B27 heavy chain (although other binding partners have not been ruled out), resulting in the formation of disulphide-linked homodimers. Many ER chaperones assist protein folding in the ER, largely by preventing oligomerization of unfolded (or pre-folded) proteins. Like other class I molecules, the HLA-B27 heavy chain interacts with BiP, calnexin, and calreticulin, but because of its failure to fold efficiently, it can accumulate as BiP-bound complexes (40, 45). Disulphide-linked and BiP-bound heavy chains represent misfolded forms of HLA-B27 that can stress the ER if they are not eliminated, and may become terminally misfolded. Elimination of misfolded proteins usually occurs by one or both of two pathways, endoplasmic reticulum-associated degradation (ERAD) or autophagy (46). Misfolded HLA-B27 heavy chains are degraded by ERAD (32), but in certain circumstances the process may not be sufficient to prevent their accumulation. When excess misfolded HLA-B27 accumulates in the ER, such as when it is upregulated (45, 47), ER stress ensues and results in activation of a pathway known as the unfolded protein response (UPR). The UPR is often protective, enabling cells to upregulate pathways that promote the folding and secretion of ER-synthesized proteins. However, unresolved ER stress can also trigger apoptotic death of affected cells (48).

The most compelling potential link between ER stress and SpA pathogenesis is the synergistic upregulation of IL-23p19, which pairs with IL-12/23p40 to produce the active IL-23 cytokine. Synergy is seen when cells responding to ER stress are activated with Toll-like receptor (TLR) ligands (49, 50), and is attributed at least in part to the UPR target gene Ddit3 (CHOP) (51). UPR activation is robust in certain cells from transgenic rats where HLA-B27 is overexpressed, but is not seen when HLA-B7 is overexpressed in rats, consistent with the normal folding and egress from the ER observed with this allele. The level of expression and magnitude of upregulation of HLA-B27 required to activate a complete UPR has not been defined. UPR activation is not seen with baseline HLA-B27 expression or low-level upregulation either in rats or in cells from humans with SpA (45, 52–55), although cells exposed to the inflammatory milieu including IFNγ may exhibit changes (56, 57). HLA-B27 misfolding and UPR activation promotes the production of IL-1α from rat monocytes exposed to TNFα, which in turn promotes osteoclast formation (58). Interestingly, it also promotes IFNβ production (59), which has opposing effects on monocytes.

However, the dominant effect in vitro is pro-osteoclastogenic. The extent to which HLA-B27 misfolding affects other cell types that express HLA class I proteins, including mesenchymal stem cells that are precursors of bone-forming osteoblasts, remains an area of active investigation.

Definitive links between aberrant properties of HLA-B27 (FHC/homodimer expression and misfolding) and AS pathogenesis need to be better established. Both mechanisms require high expression of HLA-B27 (42, 60), suggesting that they would be most prominent during an immune response involving cytokines that upregulate HLA-B27 and the MHC class I assembly pathway. However, the level of expression required to stimulate the immune system through these mechanisms has not been established. Since MHC class I assembly pathway evolved to efficiently generate, process, and display antigenic peptides during an immune response, it is interesting that it also exacerbates expression of aberrant HLA-B27 molecules. It is also worth noting that B*27:06 and B*27:09 exhibit conformational differences from B*27:05 (the predominant disease-associated subtype) during their assembly, implicating residue 116 and possibly 114 (61). Nevertheless, a more systematic examination of FHC/homodimer expression and misfolding is needed for HLA-B*27:06 and B*27:09 in order to understand relevant differences.

ERAP1 and ankylosing spondylitis pathogenesis

While the strongest genetic association in AS is with HLA-B27, polymorphisms in ERAP1 also have significant influence on susceptibility (7). The ERAP1 association was originally reported to be restricted to HLA-B27-positive individuals (8). However, the same ERAP1 variant influences HLA-B27-negative subjects who carry HLA-B*40:01, yet no effect was seen with other HLA-B alleles that confer risk (e.g. HLA-B*47:01, B*51:01, B*40:02, and B*13:02) or protection (HLA-B*07:02 and B*57:01) (62). These studies indicate a functional interaction between ERAP1 and the HLA-B alleles B*27 and B*40:01, and raise the question of mechanism. It should also be noted that other aminopeptidases have been genetically implicated in AS but do not appear to be specifically associated with HLA-B27.

ERAP1 is localized to the ER, but can be secreted by macrophages activated by lipopolysaccharide (LPS) and IFNγ (63) or after stimulation with certain TLR agonists (64). Secreted ERAP1 can enhance macrophage phagocytic activity (63) and contribute to nitric oxide synthesis (65). The principal intracellular function of ERAP1 is to trim peptides in the ER for binding to HLA class I molecules (66–70), although it has also been implicated in cell-surface cytokine receptor shedding (71). In light of the genetic interaction between ERAP1 and HLA-B alleles in AS, it seems most likely that allelic variants influence pathogenesis either directly through alteration of the repertoire of peptides bound to HLA-B27 or indirectly by influencing the supply of peptides that are critical for the folding and stability of intracellular and/or extracellular forms of HLA-B27. Altered MHC stability and immunogenicity have been demonstrated in ERAAP (the murine equivalent of ERAP1)-deficient murine cells (70, 72), with a general reduction in MHC class I expression on the cell surface as a consequence of suboptimal peptide loading (73). The crystal structures of ERAP1 in both open and closed conformations—the latter with the protease inhibitor bestatin in the active site—have supported the concept that it acts as a 'molecular ruler' to trim N-terminal residues off peptides (74). Binding of long rather than short peptides induces a conformational change in the active site, which provides a molecular explanation for the trimming of 9–16 amino acid peptides but not shorter substrates (75). In vitro experiments show that the AS-protective single nucleotide polymorphism that substitutes arginine for lysine at position 528 (K528R) exhibits reduced trimming of long peptides, including extended peptides containing known HLA-B27 epitopes (74). This is supported by data from cell lines where expression of ERAP1 K versus R at 528 shows clear functional differences, including altered presentation of HIV-derived peptide epitopes to T cells (76, 77). However, there are multiple ERAP1 polymorphisms constituting haplotypes that encode functional allotypes (78–80). Complete ERAP1 cDNA sequencing from AS patients and healthy controls, together with functional analysis, has recently revealed the importance of assessing allotypes rather than single variants in isolation, and suggested that ERAP1 hyperfunction as well as hypofunction might be associated with AS (79).

Further evidence for critical interactions between HLA class I and ERAP1 in human disease has come with the demonstration of epistasis between ERAP1 and HLA-Cw6 in psoriasis (81), and with HLA-B*51:02 in Behçet's disease (82, 83).

ERAP1 and aberrant properties of HLA-B27

Different ERAP1 variants have been shown to alter cell-surface expression of HLA-B27 (84–86), including both increases and decreases in free heavy chains depending on the study. In one study where ERAP1 knockdown or inhibition with small molecule inhibitors reduced surface free heavy chain expression, stimulation of proinflammatory Th17 responses was also reduced (85). However, in monocytic U937 cells, ERAP1 knockdown increases expression of HLA-B27, including free heavy chains and dimers, and complexes recognized by an antibody that reacts with HLA-B27 displaying longer peptides (86). The supply of untrimmed suboptimal peptides in the ER would be expected in the absence of ERAP1, and is consistent with results from sequencing peptides eluted from HLA-B27 (76). These seemingly discrepant findings could be related to the different cell lines used, the relative expression of ERAP2 (which interacts with ERAP1) or other components of the class I assembly pathway, and/or other unrecognized variables. Clarification of these differences and how they affect disease pathogenesis will require additional patient cohorts and animal models of SpA where functional consequences of loss of ERAP1 function on HLA-B27 can be assessed. At this point it is only possible to say that ERAP1 variants most likely influence AS through peptide supply, which in turn affects the quality and/or quantity of peptides presented, heavy chain misfolding and/or trafficking in the ER, or the expression of aberrant forms of HLA-B27 on the cell surface. Further study will serve to enhance our understanding of the unusual biology of HLA-B27 in disease pathogenesis, and may help to identify novel therapeutic targets and strategies.

Other considerations for HLA-B27 and disease

The ability of HLA-B27 and hβ_2m overexpression to cause SpA-like disease in rats, together with an overwhelming amount of genetic data, provides strong evidence that it is HLA-B27 itself (and not a closely linked gene) that is pathogenic. The ability of a single risk gene associated with a complex genetic human disease to recapitulate major features of the disease in an animal model is striking and exceptional. However, rat SpA lacks ankylosis and has more prominent bowel inflammation, and thus does not phenocopy human AS, perhaps reflecting the absence of other key susceptibility alleles. Other limitations include the need to overexpress the HLA-B allele. Nevertheless, the model exhibits clear HLA class I specificity, as comparable HLA-B7 overexpression does not cause disease.

More detailed comparisons of single nucleotide polymorphisms responsible for HLA variation have recently suggested that the genetic association with HLA-B in AS may be with a particular residue (P97) or associated region of the HLA-B27 molecule (62). HLA-B27 contains an asparagine (N) at P97, while other HLA-B alleles with different P97 amino acid residues differ in AS susceptibility. For example, HLA-B7 has S at P97 (as well as 19 other amino acids that differ from HLA-B*27:05), which may be protective against AS. P97 is located in the floor of the peptide-binding groove, where it can influence peptide binding, but it also affects folding efficiency, β_2m binding, and surface expression in HLA-B27 (87) and other MHC class I molecules (88). Thus P97 is likely to influence HLA-B27 misfolding and FHC expression as well as its peptide repertoire.

In psoriasis, HLA-B27 promotes the development of arthritis (PsA), particularly the axial phenotype. Glutamic acid (Glu) at P45 and cysteine (Cys) at P67 of HLA-B, which define the classical HLA-B27 allele (B pocket), are strongly associated with arthritis (89, 90). While Glu at P45 has a dominant effect on the selection of peptides with arginine (Arg) at P2 (91), Cys at P67 probably has a minor effect. However, these residues are also critical for the aberrant properties of dimerization (31) and misfolding (32, 33), which may underlie their strong disease association.

HLA-B27 forms stable complexes with unusually long peptides (92) and has been reported to be recognized by CD4+ T cells (93), although follow-up studies of CD4+ T cell recognition have not appeared in the literature. Studies suggesting that HLA-B27 might be modified by microorganisms or have cross-reactive epitopes have not been convincingly independently replicated. More recently, it has been postulated that the microbiome might be an intermediary between HLA-B27 and disease (94). While a complete discussion of these concepts is beyond the scope of this chapter, it is of interest that HLA-B27 (as well as HLA-B7) changes the gut microbiota in transgenic rats (95), and differences in the microbiota in ileal biopsies from a small number of AS patients have recently been described (96). Changes in the microbiome might in turn promote activation of the IL-23/IL-17 axis and thus disease. However, how HLA-B27 might mediate these changes poses the same question that has plagued investigators since 1973. Clearly, further investigation is warranted.

Conclusion

HLA-B27 is an unusual HLA class I molecule, yet it dutifully and efficiently carries out its 'natural' immunological function presenting antigenic peptides to CD8+ T cells. It also has a propensity to 'misbehave', both inside cells and on the cell surface. At this point the weight of evidence suggests that these aberrant behaviours, which seem to be inextricably linked to amino acids that also influence peptide binding, are more likely than not to contribute to AS pathogenesis. However, the answer to this and other key questions requires a better understanding of differences between HLA-B27 and other alleles, and the functional consequences of the HLA-B27–ERAP1 interaction.

References

1. Benjamin RJ, Parham P. Guilt by association: HLA-B27 and ankylosing spondylitis. Immunol Today 1990;11:137–42.
2. Brewerton DA, Hart FD, Nicholls A, et al. Ankylosing spondylitis and HL-A 27. Lancet 1973;1:904–7.
3. Schlosstein L, Terasaki PI, Bluestone R, et al. High association of an HL-A antigen, W27, with ankylosing spondylitis. N Engl J Med 1973;288:704–6.
4. Brown MA, Kennedy LG, MacGregor AJ, et al. Susceptibility to ankylosing spondylitis in twins: the role of genes, HLA, and the environment. Arthritis Rheum 1997;40:1823–8.
5. Brown MA, Wordsworth BP, Reveille JD. Genetics of ankylosing spondylitis. Clin Exp Rheumatol 2002;20:S43–9.
6. Reveille JD. Genetics of spondyloarthritis—beyond the MHC. Nat Rev Rheumatol 2012;8:296–304.
7. Burton PR, Clayton DG, Cardon LR, et al. Association scan of 14,500 nonsynonymous SNPs in four diseases identifies autoimmunity variants. Nat Genet 2007;39:1329–37.
8. Evans DM, Spencer CC, Pointon JJ, et al. Interaction between ERAP1 and HLA-B27 in ankylosing spondylitis implicates peptide handling in the mechanism for HLA-B27 in disease susceptibility. Nat Genet 2011;43:761–7.
9. Zinkernagel RM & Doherty PC. Restriction of in vitro T cell-mediated cytotoxicity in lymphocytic choriomeningitis within a syngeneic or semiallogeneic system. Nature 1974;248:701–2.
10. Townsend AR, Rothbard J, Gotch FM, et al. The epitopes of influenza nucleoprotein recognized by cytotoxic T lymphocytes can be defined with short synthetic peptides. Cell 1986:44:959–68.
11. Madden DR, Gorga JC, Strominger JL, et al. The three-dimensional structure of HLA-B27 at 2.1 Å resolution suggests a general mechanism for tight peptide binding to MHC. Cell 1992;70:1035–48.
12. Jardetzky TS, Lane WS, Robinson RA, et al. Identification of self peptides bound to purified HLA-B27. Nature 1991;353:326–9.
13. Bowness P. HLA B27 in health and disease: a double-edged sword? Rheumatology (Oxford) 2002;41:857–68.
14. Goulder PJ, Phillips RE, Colbert RA, et al. Late escape from an immunodominant cytotoxic T-lymphocyte response associated with progression to AIDS. Nat Med 1997;3:212–17.
15. Goulder PJ, Brander C, Tang Y, et al. Evolution and transmission of stable CTL escape mutations in HIV infection. Nature 2001;412:334–8.
16. Neumann-Haefelin C, McKiernan S, Ward S, et al. Dominant influence of an HLA-B27 restricted CD8+ T cell response in mediating HCV clearance and evolution. Hepatology 2006;43:563–72.
17. Scofield RH, Warren WL, Koelsch G, et al. A hypothesis for the immune dysregulation in spondyloarthropathies: contributions from enteric organisms, B27 structure, peptides bound by B27 and convergent evolution. Proc Natl Acad Sci USA 1993;90:9330–4.
18. Hermann E, Yu DTY, Meyer zum Buschenfelde K-H, et al. HLA-B27-restricted CD8 T cells from synovial fluids of patients with reactive arthritis and ankylosing spondylitis. Lancet 1993;342:646–50.
19. Fiorillo MT, Maragno M, Butler R, et al. CD8+ T cell autoreactivity to an HLA-B27-restricted self-epitope correlates with ankylosing spondylitis. J Clin Invest 2000;106:47–53.
20. Appel H, Kuon W, Kuhne M, et al. Use of HLA-B27 tetramers to identify low-frequency antigen-specific T cells in *Chlamydia*-triggered reactive arthritis. Arthritis Res Ther 2004;6:R521–34.
21. Allen RL, Gillespie GM, Hall F, et al. Multiple T cell expansions are found in the blood and synovial fluid of patients with reactive arthritis. J Rheumatol 1997;24:1750–7.

22. May E, Dulphy N, Frauendorf E, et al. Conserved TCR beta chain usage in reactive arthritis; evidence for selection by a putative HLA-B27-associated autoantigen. Tissue Antigens 2002;60:299–308.
23. Braun J, Bollow M, Neure L, et al. Use of immunohistologic and in situ hybridization techniques in the examination of sacroiliac joint biopsy specimens from patients with ankylosing spondylitis. Arthritis Rheum 1995;38:499–505.
24. Braun J, Sieper J. Ankylosing spondylitis. Lancet 2007;369:1379–90.
25. Hammer RE, Maika SD, Richardson JA, et al. Spontaneous inflammatory disease in transgenic rats expressing HLA-B27 and human b_2-m: an animal model of HLA-B27-associated human disorders. Cell 1990;63:1099–112.
26. May E, Dorris ML, Satumtira N, et al. CD8ab T cells are not essential to the pathogenesis of arthritis or colitis in HLA-B27 transgenic rats. J Immunol 2003;170:1099–105.
27. Taurog JD, Dorris ML, Satumtira N., et al. Spondylarthritis in HLA-B27/human beta2-microglobulin-transgenic rats is not prevented by lack of CD8. Arthritis Rheum 2009;60:1977–84.
28. Schittenhelm RB, Sian TC, Wilmann PG, et al. Revisiting the arthritogenic peptide theory: quantitative not qualitative changes in the peptide repertoire of HLA-B27 allotypes. Arthritis Rheumatol 2015;67:702–13.
29. Peruzzi M, Wagtmann N, Long EO. A p70 killer cell inhibitory receptor specific for several HLA-B allotypes discriminates among peptides bound to HLA-B*2705. J Exp Med 1996;184:1585–90.
30. Stewart-Jones GB, di Gleria K, Kollnberger S, et al. Crystal structures and KIR3DL1 recognition of three immunodominant viral peptides complexed to HLA-B*2705. Eur J Immunol 2005;35:341–51.
31. Allen RL, O'Callaghan CA, McMichael AJ, et al. Cutting edge: HLA-B27 can form a novel beta 2-microglobulin-free heavy chain homodimer structure. J Immunol 1999;162:5045–8.
32. Mear JP, Schreiber KL, Munz C, et al. Misfolding of HLA-B27 as a result of its B pocket suggests a novel mechanism for its role in susceptibility to spondyloarthropathies. J Immunol 1999;163:6665–70.
33. Dangoria NS, DeLay ML, Kingsbury DJ, et al. HLA-B27 misfolding is associated with aberrant intermolecular disulfide bond formation (dimerization) in the endoplasmic reticulum. J Biol Chem 2002;277:23459–68.
34. Bird LA, Peh CA, Kollnberger S, et al. Lymphoblastoid cells express HLA-B27 homodimers both intracellularly and at the cell surface following endosomal recycling. Eur J Immunol 2003;33:748–59.
35. Parkes M, Cortes A, van Heel DA, et al. Genetic insights into common pathways and complex relationships among immune-mediated diseases. Nat Rev Genet 2013;14:661–73.
36. Smith JA, Colbert RA. Review: the interleukin-23/interleukin-17 axis in spondyloarthritis pathogenesis: Th17 and beyond. Arthritis Rheumatol 2014;66:231–41.
37. Kollnberger S, Bird LA, Sunm M-Y, et al. Cell surface expression and immune receptor recogntion of HLA-B27 homodimers. Arthritis Rheum 2002;46:2972–82.
38. Raine T, Brown D, Bowness P, et al. Consistent patterns of expression of HLA class I free heavy chains in healthy individuals and raised expression in spondyloarthropathy patients point to physiological and pathological roles. Rheumatology (Oxford) 2006;45:1338–44.
39. Payeli SK, Kollnberger S, Marroquin Belaunzaran O, et al. Inhibiting HLA-B27 homodimer-driven immune cell inflammation in spondylarthritis. Arthritis Rheum 2012;64:3139–49.
40. Tran TM, Satumtira N, Dorris ML, et al. HLA-B27 in transgenic rats forms disulfide-linked heavy chain oligomers and multimers that bind to the chaperone BiP. J Immunol 2004;172:5110–19.
41. Kollnberger S, Bird LA, Roddis M, et al. HLA-B27 heavy chain homodimers are expressed in HLA-B27 transgenic rodent models of spondyloarthritis and are ligands for paired Ig-like receptors. J Immunol 2004;173:1699–710.
42. McHugh K, Rysnik O, Kollnberger S, et al. Expression of aberrant HLA-B27 molecules is dependent on B27 dosage and peptide supply. Ann Rheum Dis 2014;73:763–70.
43. Chan AT, Kollnberger SD, Wedderburn LR, et al. Expansion and enhanced survival of natural killer cells expressing the killer immunoglobulin-like receptor KIR3DL2 in spondylarthritis. Arthritis Rheum 2005;52:3586–95.
44. Bowness P, Ridley A, Shaw J, et al. Th17 cells expressing KIR3DL2+ and responsive to HLA-B27 homodimers are increased in ankylosing spondylitis. J Immunol 2011;186:2672–80.
45. Turner MJ, Sowders DP, DeLay ML, et al. HLA-B27 misfolding in transgenic rats is associated with activation of the unfolded protein response. J Immunol 2005;175:2438–48.
46. Arensdorf AM, Diedrichs D, Rutkowski DT. Regulation of the transcriptome by ER stress: non-canonical mechanisms and physiological consequences. Front Genet 2013;4:256.
47. Turner MJ, Delay ML, Bai S, et al. HLA-B27 up-regulation causes accumulation of misfolded heavy chains and correlates with the magnitude of the unfolded protein response in transgenic rats: implications for the pathogenesis of spondylarthritis-like disease. Arthritis Rheum 2007;56:215–23.
48. Hetz C. The unfolded protein response: controlling cell fate decisions under ER stress and beyond. Nat Rev Mol Cell Biol 2012;13:89–102.
49. DeLay ML, Turner MJ, Klenk EI, et al. HLA-B27 misfolding and the unfolded protein response augment interleukin-23 production and are associated with Th17 activation in transgenic rats. Arthritis Rheum 2009;60:2633–43.
50. Colbert RA, DeLay ML, Klenk EI, et al. From HLA-B27 to spondyloarthritis: a journey through the ER. Immunol Rev 2010;233:181–202.
51. Goodall JC, Wu C, Zhang Y, et al. Endoplasmic reticulum stress-induced transcription factor, CHOP, is crucial for dendritic cell IL-23 expression. Proc Natl Acad Sci USA 2010;107:17698–703.
52. Smith JA, Barnes MD, Hong D, et al. Gene expression analysis of macrophages derived from ankylosing spondylitis patients reveals interferon-gamma dysregulation. Arthritis Rheum 2008;58:1640–9.
53. Zeng L, Lindstrom MJ, Smith JA. Ankylosing spondylitis macrophage production of higher levels of interleukin-23 in response to lipopolysaccharide without induction of a significant unfolded protein response. Arthritis Rheum 2011;63:3807–17.
54. Neerinckx B, Carter S, Lories RJ. No evidence for a critical role of the unfolded protein response in synovium and blood of patients with ankylosing spondylitis. Ann Rheum Dis 2014;73:629–30.
55. Kenna TJ, Lau MC, Keith P, et al. Disease-associated polymorphisms in ERAP1 do not alter endoplasmic reticulum stress in patients with ankylosing spondylitis. Genes Immun 2014;16(1):35–42.
56. Gu J, Rihl M, Marker-Hermann E, et al. Clues to the pathogenesis of spondyloarthropathy derived from synovial fluid mononuclear cell gene expression profiles. J Rheumatol 2002;29:2159–64.
57. Feng Y, Ding J, Fan CM, et al. Interferon-gamma contributes to HLA-B27-associated unfolded protein response in spondyloarthropathies. J Rheumatol 2012;39:574–82.
58. Layh-Schmitt G, Yang EY, Kwon G, et al. HLA-B27 alters the response to TNFalpha and promotes osteoclastogenesis in bone marrow monocytes from HLA-B27 transgenic rats. Arthritis Rheum 2013;65(8):2123–31.
59. Smith JA, Turner MJ, DeLay ML, et al. Endoplasmic reticulum stress and the unfolded protein response are linked to synergistic IFN-beta induction via X-box binding protein 1. Eur J Immunol 2008;38:1194–203.
60. Colbert RA, Tran TM, Layh-Schmitt G. HLA-B27 misfolding and ankylosing spondylitis. Mol Immunol 2014;57:44–51.
61. Fussell H, Nesbeth D, Lenart I, et al. Novel detection of in vivo HLA-B27 conformations correlates with ankylosing spondylitis association. Arthritis Rheum 2008;58:3419–24.
62. Cortes A, Pulit SL, Leo PJ, et al. Major histocompatibility complex associations of ankylosing spondylitis are complex and involve further epistasis with ERAP1. Nat Commun 2015;6:7146.
63. Goto Y, Ogawa K, Hattori A, et al. Secretion of endoplasmic reticulum aminopeptidase 1 is involved in the activation of macrophages

induced by lipopolysaccharide and interferon-gamma. J Biol Chem 2011;286:21906–14.
64. Goto Y, Ogawa K, Nakamura TJ, et al. TLR-mediated secretion of endoplasmic reticulum aminopeptidase 1 from macrophages. J Immunol 2014;192:4443–52.
65. Goto Y, Ogawa K, Nakamura TJ, et al. Substrate-dependent nitric oxide synthesis by secreted endoplasmic reticulum aminopeptidase 1 in macrophages. J Biochem 2015;157:439–49.
66. Serwold T, Gaw S, Shastri N. ER aminopeptidases generate a unique pool of peptides for MHC class I molecules. Nat Immunol 2001;2:644–51.
67. York IA, Chang SC, Saric T, et al. The ER aminopeptidase ERAP1 enhances or limits antigen presentation by trimming epitopes to 8-9 residues. Nat Immunol 2002;3:1177–84.
68. Saric T, Chang SC, Hattori A, et al. An IFN-gamma-induced aminopeptidase in the ER, ERAP1, trims precursors to MHC class I-presented peptides. Nat Immunol 2002;3:1169–76.
69. Hammer GE, Gonzalez F, James E, et al. In the absence of aminopeptidase ERAAP, MHC class I molecules present many unstable and highly immunogenic peptides. Nat Immunol 2007;8:101–8.
70. Hammer GE, Shastri N. Construction and destruction of MHC class I in the peptide-loading complex. Nat Immunol 2007;8:793–4.
71. Cui X, Hawari F, Alsaaty S, et al. Identification of ARTS-1 as a novel TNFR1-binding protein that promotes TNFR1 ectodomain shedding. J Clin Invest 2002;110:515–26.
72. Hammer GE, Gonzalez F, Champsaur M, et al. The aminopeptidase ERAAP shapes the peptide repertoire displayed by major histocompatibility complex class I molecules. Nat Immunol 2006;7:103–12.
73. Tran TM, Colbert RA. Endoplasmic reticulum aminopeptidase 1 and rheumatic disease: functional variation. Curr Opin Rheumatol 2015;27:357–63.
74. Kochan G, Krojer T, Harvey D, et al. Crystal structures of the endoplasmic reticulum aminopeptidase-1 (ERAP1) reveal the molecular basis for N-terminal peptide trimming. Proc Natl Acad Sci USA 2011;108:7745–50.
75. Tsujimoto M, Hattori A. The oxytocinase subfamily of M1 aminopeptidases. Biochim Biophys Acta 2005;1751:9–18.
76. Chen L, Fischer R, Peng Y, et al. Critical role of endoplasmic reticulum aminopeptidase 1 in determining the length and sequence of peptides bound and presented by HLA-B27. Arthritis Rheumatol 2014;66:284–94.
77. Sanz-Bravo A, Campos J, Mazariegos MS, et al. Dominant role of the ERAP1 polymorphism R528K in shaping the HLA-B27 peptidome through differential processing determined by multiple peptide residues. Arthritis Rheumatol 2015;67:692–701.
78. Reeves E, Edwards CJ, Elliott T, et al. Naturally occurring ERAP1 haplotypes encode functionally distinct alleles with fine substrate specificity. J Immunol 2013;191:35–43.
79. Reeves E, Colebatch-Bourn A, Elliott T, et al. Functionally distinct ERAP1 allotype combinations distinguish individuals with ankylosing spondylitis. Proc Natl Acad Sci USA 2014;111:17594–9.
80. Reeves E, Elliott T, James E, et al. ERAP1 in the pathogenesis of ankylosing spondylitis. Immunol Res 2014;60:257–69.
81. Genetic Analysis of Psoriasis Consortium, the Wellcome Trust Case Control Consortium, Strange A, et al. A genome-wide association study identifies new psoriasis susceptibility loci and an interaction between HLA-C and ERAP1. Nat Genet 2010;42:985–90.
82. Kirino Y, Bertsias G, Ishigatsubo Y, et al. Genome-wide association analysis identifies new susceptibility loci for Behçet's disease and epistasis between HLA-B*51 and ERAP1. Nat Genet 2013;45:202–7.
83. Ombrello MJ, Kastner DL, Remmers EF Endoplasmic reticulum-associated amino-peptidase 1 and rheumatic disease: genetics. Curr Opin Rheumatol 2015;27:349–56.
84. Haroon N, Tsui FW, Uchanska-Ziegler B, et al. Endoplasmic reticulum aminopeptidase 1 (ERAP1) exhibits functionally significant interaction with HLA-B27 and relates to subtype specificity in ankylosing spondylitis. Ann Rheum Dis 2012;71:589–95.
85. Chen L, Ridley A, Hammitzsch A, et al. Silencing or inhibition of endoplasmic reticulum aminopeptidase 1 (ERAP1) suppresses free heavy chain expression and Th17 responses in ankylosing spondylitis. Ann Rheum Dis 2015 June 30:pii.
86. Tran et al., manuscript submitted.
87. Blanco-Gelaz MA, Suarez-Alvarez B, Gonzalez S, et al. The amino acid at position 97 is involved in folding and surface expression of HLA-B27. Int Immunol 2006;18:211–20.
88. Smith RA, Myers NB, Robinson M, et al. Polymorphism at position 97 in MHC class I molecules affects peptide specificity, cell surface stability, and affinity for beta2-microglobulin. J Immunol 2002;169:3105–11.
89. Okada Y, Han B, Tsoi LC, et al. Fine mapping major histocompatibility complex associations in psoriasis and its clinical subtypes. Am J Hum Genet 2014;95:162–72.
90. Bowes J, Budu-Aggrey A, Huffmeier U, et al. Dense genotyping of immune-related susceptibility loci reveals new insights into the genetics of psoriatic arthritis. Nat Commun 2015;6:6046.
91. Colbert RA, Rowland-Jones SL, McMichael AJ, et al. Allele-specific B pocket transplant in class I major histocompatibility complex protein changes requirement for anchor residue at P2 of peptide. Proc Natl Acad Sci USA 1993;90:6879–83.
92. Urban RG, Chicz RM, Lane WS, et al. A subset of HLA-B27 molecules contains peptides much longer than nonamers. Proc Natl Acad Sci USA 1994;91:1534–8.
93. Boyle LH, Goodall JC, Opat SS, et al. The recognition of HLA-B27 by human CD4+ T lymphocytes. J Immunol 2001;167:2619–24.
94. Rosenbaum JT, Davey MP. Time for a gut check: evidence for the hypothesis that HLA-B27 predisposes to ankylosing spondylitis by altering the microbiome. Arthritis Rheum 2011;63:3195–8.
95. Lin P, Bach M, Asquith M, et al. HLA-B27 and human beta2-microglobulin affect the gut microbiota of transgenic rats. PLoS One 2014;9:e105684.
96. Costello ME, Ciccia F, Willner D, et al. Intestinal dysbiosis in ankylosing spondylitis. Arthritis Rheumatol 2014 Nov 21; doi 10.1002/art.38967.

CHAPTER 7

Immune mechanisms: innate immunity

Troy Noordenbos and Dominique Baeten

Introduction to innate immunity

Immune-mediated inflammatory diseases (IMIDs) can be classified in different ways based on their genetic architecture (1, 2), their organ-specific or systemic nature, the involvement of specific cytokine pathways (3), or other cellular and molecular features (Fig. 7.1). Although each of these classifications can be useful, they are also artificial and tend to oversimplify the complexity of these disorders.

A conceptually useful classification was proposed by McGonagle and McDermott (4): the authors identify two extremes with, on the one side, pure autoimmune disease caused by recognition of self-antigens by the adaptive immune system and, on the other side, autoinflammatory syndromes caused by a disproportional activation of mainly innate cytokine pathways. The extremes are represented by rare monogenic diseases. A common example for a pure autoimmune syndrome is autoimmune polyendocrine syndrome-1 (APS-1), which is caused by a loss-of-function mutation of the molecule AIRE, resulting in abnormal selection of autoreactive T and B lymphocytes. A common example of a pure autoinflammatory syndrome is TNF-receptor-associated periodic syndrome (TRAPS), caused by a mutation in TNF-receptor I.

In the continuum between these monogenic autoimmune versus autoinflammatory disorders, common polygenic IMIDs cluster roughly into two groups, based on predominant disease mechanisms. The cluster of autoimmune diseases includes rheumatic diseases such as systemic lupus erythematosus and RA. These diseases share prototypical autoimmune features such as female predominance, autoantibodies, genetic polymorphisms in B- or T-lymphocyte-related molecules (MHC class II molecules, co-stimulation, B cell receptor (BCR) and TCR, PTPN22), and clinical response to lymphocyte-targeting therapies such as blocking of T-cell co-stimulation (CTLA4-Ig) and B-cell depletion (anti-CD20). On the other side of the spectrum is a cluster of diseases that can be described as mainly autoinflammatory. Examples are gout, psoriasis, and IBD. These diseases display no female predominance, lack disease-specific autoantibodies, are genetically associated with proinflammatory cytokine pathways (TNF, IL-1, and IL-23), and respond clinically to blocking these cytokine pathways.

Over the last decade, several lines of evidence suggest that SpA belongs to the cluster of autoinflammatory diseases despite its strong genetic linkage to the MHC class I molecule HLA-B27. This association with HLA-B27, as well as more recently discovered genetic associations with genes encoding various aminopeptidases responsible for truncating peptides in preparation for MHC class I presentation, fueled the hypothesis that HLA-B27-restricted presentation of antigens (possibly autoantigens) to CD8+ cytotoxic lymphocytes is central to the pathogenesis of the disease. This hypothesis, however, has never been formally demonstrated. On the contrary, two studies showing that CD8+ cells are not required for disease development in the HLA-B27 tg rat model of SpA challenged this 'adaptive' theory (5, 6). This has initiated a large amount of research in the role of other cell types in general and in innate immune responses in particular in the pathophysiology of SpA. This chapter reviews the evidence supporting the role of innate immune alterations and autoinflammatory mechanisms in the pathogenesis of SpA. It consecutively discusses (1) the potential role of HLA-B27 in the innate immune response, (2) genetic associations with innate cytokine pathways and the role of these innate cytokine pathways in animal models of SpA, and (3) the presence and function of innate immune cells in target tissues of human SpA.

HLA-B27

Although environmental triggers might be crucial in the induction of disease, genetic risk factors are estimated to account for 80–90% of the susceptibility to AS (7). HLA-B27 confers at least 25% of this risk, indicating the central role of this molecule in the pathophysiology of SpA. Several hypotheses have been proposed to explain the association of HLA-B27 with the disease (Fig. 7.2).

Arthritogenic peptide hypothesis

HLA-B27 can, like all other MHC class I molecules, present a restricted set of peptides to cytotoxic T cells (8). The arthritogenic peptide theory proposes that HLA-B27 binds a unique peptide derived from a microorganism and elicits a cytotoxic T-cell response cross-reactive with a self-peptide in the context of HLA-B27 (9). Although HLA-B27-restricted cytotoxic T cells reactive to enteric bacteria were found in the synovial fluid of ReA patients (10, 11), the autoimmune nature of these cells has not been convincingly demonstrated. A strong argument against the arthritogenic peptide hypothesis comes from a rat model where overexpression of HLA-B27 induces spontaneous SpA-like disease (12). Genetic deletion as well as depletion of CD8+ cytotoxic T cells did not prevent or modify disease compared to wild type (5, 6). Additionally, a specific arthritogenic peptide has never been identified in human studies.

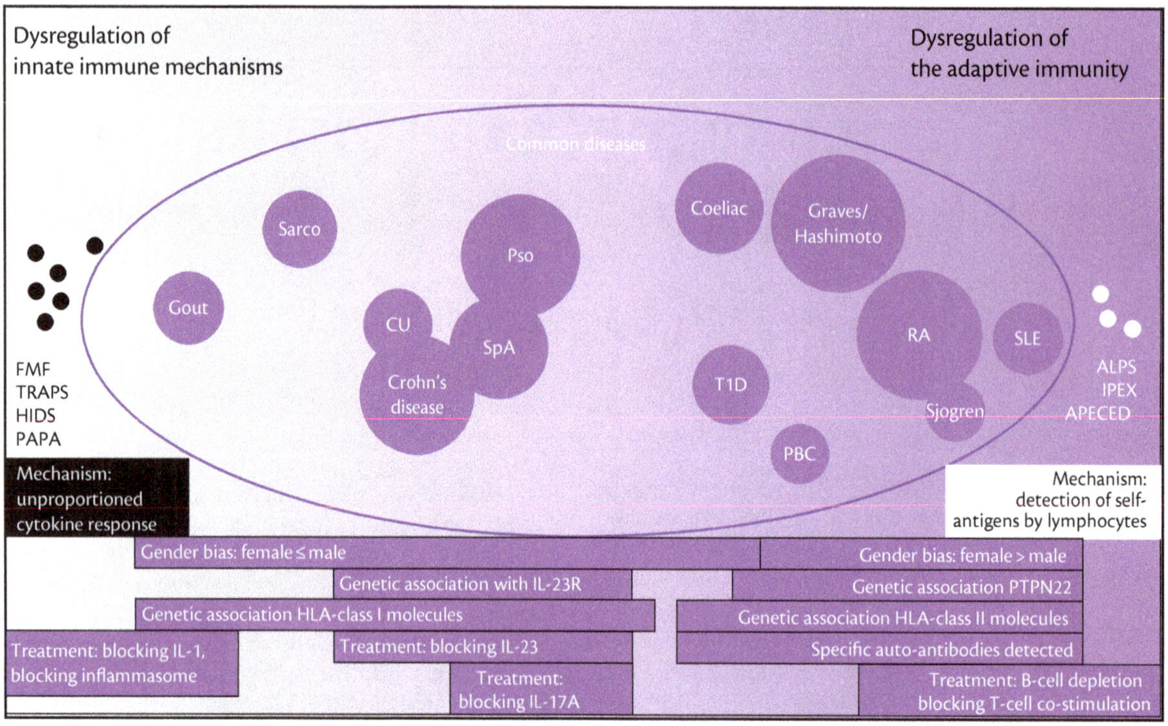

Fig. 7.1 (See colour plate section). Clustering of immune-mediated diseases based on acquired versus innate immune mechanisms. Rare monogenic diseases define the extremes of a spectrum between disease phenotypes that are caused by, on the one hand, problems in specific recognition of self-antigens by the adaptive immune system and, on the other hand, uncontrolled or inappropriate activation of innate cytokine pathways. A selection of common diseases is placed in the spectrum, based upon gender bias, genetic associations, and response to treatments. FMF, Familial Mediterranean fever; TRAPS, TNF receptor-associated periodic syndrome; HIDS, hyperimmunoglobinaemia D with periodic fever syndrome; PAPA, pyogenic arthritis pyoderma gangrenosum and severe cystic acne; ALPS, autoimmune lymphoproliferative syndrome; IPEX, immune dysregulation polyendrocrinopathy enteropathy X-linked; APECED, autoimmune polyendocrinopathy–candidiasis–ectodermal dystrophy syndrome; Sarco, sarcoidosis; CU, colitis ulcerosa; Pso, psoriasis; T1D, type I diabetes; RA, rheumatoid arthritis; PBC, primary biliary cirrhosis; SLE, systemic lupus erythematosus.

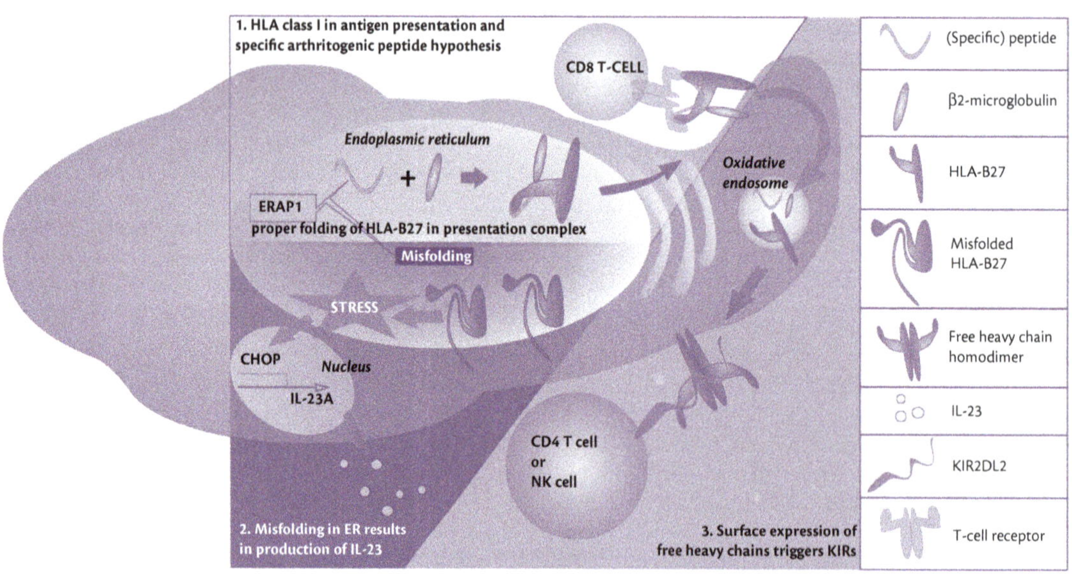

Fig. 7.2 (See colour plate section). Three theories on the contribution of HLA-B27 to SpA pathophysiology. HLA-B27 forms a heterotrimeric complex with peptide and β_2m, known as the presentation complex. The arthritogenic peptide hypothesis proposes that HLA-B27 binds a restricted peptide that is recognized by autoreactive CD8 T cells. The second theory states that misfolding of HLA-B27 occurs during formation of the presentation complex. A stress reaction is induced that is known as the unfolded protein response. This response includes upregulation of the transcription factor CHOP, which leads to expression of IL-23A. The third theory describes that the presentation complex can be internalized and that free forms of HLA-B27, including a homodimer, can be re-expressed on the cell surface. KIRs expressed on CD4+ T cells or NK cells can be triggered upon recognition of free heavy chain forms of HLA-B27. The recently discovered interaction of HLA-B27 with ERAP1, can be important for the creation of a restricted specific peptide described in the arthritogenic peptide hypothesis. Alternatively, ERAP1 is known to influence peptide availability, thus influencing the folding kinetics in the ER, which can lead to misfolding. ERAP1, Endoplasmic reticulum-associated aminopeptidase 1; CHOP, C/EBP homologous protein; IL-23, interleukin 23; KIR3DL2, killer immunoglobulin receptor 3DL2.

Recently, SNPs in the genes encoding three aminopeptidases, ERAP1, ERAP2, and aminopeptidase puromycin sensitive NPEPPS, were found to be associated with AS susceptibility (13). This finding seems to favour a role for altered antigen presentation by HLA-B27 because these molecules are important for trimming peptides for optimal loading onto MHC molecules. Alternatively, it should be considered that these molecules have a strong influence on peptide availability and thus on the kinetics of the formation of the heterotrimeric complex HLA-B27/β_2m/peptide (14–16), favouring an alternative hypothesis (see sections 'HLA-B27 misfolding and stress' and 'HLA-B27 homodimers and KIR triggering'). Interestingly, the association of ERAP1 is restricted to HLA-B27-positive AS, whereas ERAP2 is not (17). A similar interaction is seen for ERAP1 and MHC class I molecules in psoriasis (HLA-C) (18) and Behçet's disease (HLA-B*51) (19), suggesting that a similar mechanism is underlying the HLA association in the different diseases.

HLA-B27 misfolding and endoplasmatic reticulum stress

HLA-B27 has a low folding speed compared to related but not SpA-associated MHC class I molecules, which leads more frequently to misfolding (20). To avoid accumulation of misfolded proteins in the ER, continuous degradation by proteasome-dependent mechanisms takes place. When normal compensatory mechanisms cannot keep up with the load of misfolded protein, a stress response is elicited in the ER, known as the unfolded protein response. An interesting link between ER stress and SpA is that the ER-stress-induced transcription factor C/EBP homologous protein (CHOP) can directly enhance IL-23p19 expression in, for example, dendritic cells (21). As discussed in the section 'IL-23/IL-17' in detail, there is now clear pathophysiological and clinical evidence for a key role of the IL-23/IL-17 pathway in SpA.

A causative relation between HLA-B27 expression and the unfolded protein response was detected in vivo in the HLA-B27 tg rat model. In bone marrow-derived macrophages from these animals, HLA-B27 misfolding was detected (22) and this correlated with production of IL-23 (23). In SpA patients, however, the relation between HLA-B27 and the unfolded protein response is not easily detected (24–26), possibly because this process is occurring in specific cell types and in specific disease localizations. Another proposed mode of action is that HLA-B27 misfolding activates autophagy pathways (27). Interestingly, SpA is clinically and pathophysiologically related to CD, which is convincingly associated with autophagy-related genes, the strongest association of which is ATG16L1 (28). Although SNPs in ATG16L1 are not associated with AS (29), two other genes that are associated with SpA, NPEPPS and GPR37, do play a role in autophagy (13, 30). Overexpression of both molecules induces autophagy in model systems (31, 32), but the exact role of autophagy in SpA remains to be investigated in detail.

HLA-B27 homodimers and KIR triggering

Another molecular feature of HLA-B27 is that, when not properly complexed with β_2m, it can form homodimers due to its unpaired cysteine residue and this can be expressed in this conformation on the cell membrane (33, 34). Additionally, the heavy chain can be expressed on the plasma membrane as a monomer. These alternative forms of HLA-B27 heavy chains can be a ligand for innate immune receptors on myeloid cells, T cells, and NK cells. These receptors include KIR3DL1, KIR3DL2, and LILIRB2 in humans (35) and in rodent PIR (36). The interaction between KIR3DL2 and HLA-B27 has been shown to play a role in SpA as it results in direct immune activation of T cells, especially Th17 cells, and NK cells (37–39). Genetic associations with SpA were not detected for KIR3DL2, although they have been suggested for KIR3DL1 and KIR3DS1 in lower-powered studies in Asia (40). As for the unfolded protein response hypothesis, this homodimer theory proposes an antigen-independent, innate role for HLA-B27.

HLA-B27 and the microbiome

A link between GI bacteria and SpA was established several years ago. The HLA-B27-associated ReA subtype of SpA is triggered by GI infections with *Shigella*, *Salmonella*, *Yersinia*, and *Campylobacter* or urogenital infections with *Chlamydia* (41–43). Also, HLA-B27 tg rats fail to develop disease when kept in germ-free conditions (44). The underlying mechanisms are still unclear, but a direct influence of HLA-B27 on the microbiome has been recently proposed based on the concept that alterations in the microbiome can steer inflammatory diseases, possibly through promotion of Th17 responses (45, 46). In the HLA-B27 tg rat model, mono-association with *Bacteroides vulgatus*, but not with certain other strains, was sufficient to rescue the colitis phenotype in these animals. Unrestricted bacterial flora profiles were significantly different between non-tg and HLA-B27/β_2m tg rats (47). Taken together, this suggests that HLA-B27 can restrict or alter the gut microbiome.

In patients, it has been challenging to characterize the microbiome, but the first data from 16S rRNA sequencing showed dysbiosis in AS patients versus controls (48). A causative relation between altered gut microbiome and disease is still speculative and microbiota could very well be secondary to the disease process (49). Moreover, bacterial triggers in the gut could also act merely as non-specific adjuvant-like danger signals, rather than modulate the immune response in a specific way. Supporting this concept, we recently demonstrated that immunization with low amounts of TLR-ligands such as heat-killed *Mycobacterium tuberculosis* is sufficient to trigger spondylitis and arthritis, with a more than 80% incidence in HLA-B27/β_2m tg rats but not in control animals. In vitro studies using splenocytes from these rats demonstrated reactivity to innate immune stimulation by increased production of IL-1α and β (50). Independently of the exact mechanism, these data collectively indicate that bacterial stress and innate immune activation play important roles in triggering HLA-B27-associated disease.

Genetic associations with innate cytokine pathways

Genetic association with cytokines, receptors, and intracellular signalling molecules have identified IL-1, TNF, and IL-23/IL-17 as major cytokine pathways for the pathophysiology of SpA. The innate nature of these pathways is stressed by monogenic human diseases affecting these cytokine pathways in the context of a stable adaptive immune system.

IL-1

Innate triggering through pattern recognition receptors on mainly macrophages and dendritic cells stimulates the production of pro-IL-1β, which is consequently cleaved to IL-1β by the inflammasome and released to cause a proinflammatory environment. GWAS in

AS indicated an association with the *IL-1R1-IL-1R2* locus (13, 51). IL-1R1, encoding for the signalling receptor, and IL-1R2, encoding for a decoy receptor, can directly modulate the proinflammatory potential of IL-1α and IL-1β. In parallel, family-based association testing found the IL-1α locus to be associated with SpA (52). Two open-label trials blocking IL-1 signalling in SpA did not show a clinically relevant effect (53, 54), though a definite conclusion can only come from larger study populations, randomized controlled methodology, and maybe a new generation of IL-1 blockers. In mice, however, deletion of IL-1 receptor-antagonist (IL-1Ra$^{-/-}$), resulting in unopposed and thus amplified IL-1 signalling, induced erosive arthritis, aortitis, T-cell-independent psoriasis-like disease, and intervertebral disc degeneration (55–57). Interestingly, genetic deletion or neutralization of IL-17A in these mice prevented disease (58, 59) and, when crossed on an RAG2$^{-/-}$ background, these mice developed severe IL-17- mediated colitis (60). This suggests that innate induced IL-1 can fuel the IL-23/IL-17 pathway, which is discussed in the section 'IL-23/IL-17'. In a different arthritis model, the human TNF-tg mice, IL-1α and/or IL-1β mediate TNF-induced bone and cartilage destruction (61). Taken together, IL-1 is genetically linked to SpA and molecularly linked to arthritis, probably in a T-cell-independent manner.

TNF

Three genetic associations with AS were found in the TNF-pathway, TNFRSF1A (62–65), TRADD (66), and TNFSF15 (67). TNFRSF1A encodes TNFR1, an important transmembrane receptor involved in TNF signalling. TRADD is an adaptor protein that associates with the cytoplasmic domain of TNFR1, overexpression of which leads to apoptosis and activation of NFκB (68). The cytokine TNFSF15 can be induced by IL-1 and TNFα and can associate with Death receptor 3 to promote Th17-mediated disease (69, 70). Clinical inhibition of TNF is efficacious in SpA, providing the strongest evidence of the importance of the TNF pathway (71, 72).

Despite this overwhelming evidence that TNF is a central driver of the inflammatory process in SpA, it remains still largely unknown which cells produce TNF in SpA and which cells will respond to this altered TNF production. Macrophages and other myeloid cells are generally considered the major producers of TNF, but this remains to be confirmed in the context of SpA. As to the effects of TNF on other cell types, it is clear that TNF can directly and/or indirectly activate osteoclasts as TNF blockade halts joint destruction in SpA (73). However, TNF blockade fails to halt new bone formation in AS (74, 75) and the relation between TNF and osteoproliferation remains uncertain.

In this context, various animal models of TNF overexpression have provided important insights in the potential role of TNF in SpA. Mice overexpressing human TNF develop a severe systemic inflammation and destructive polyarthritis reminiscent of human RA, but do not develop SpA features (76). This destructive phenotype could be reversed by blocking DKK-1, a negative regulator of the Wnt pathway (77, 78), thereby indicating that TNF not only activates bone destruction but also impedes new bone formation through inhibitors of the Wnt pathway. The exact relevance for human SpA remains unclear, since not only TNF but also other cytokines such as IL-6 regulate DKK-1 (79). Similar to mice overexpressing human TNF, the TNFΔ ARE mice, in which murine TNF is overexpressed by modulation of mRNA stability, also demonstrate a destructive polyarthritis reminiscent of RA (80). This model, however, also develops colitis and both manifestations are dependent on TNFR1 (81). More recently, this model was also shown to develop some enthesitis and to be dependent on mechanical stress (82). Although the model fails to faithfully recapitulate key SpA features such as spondylitis and new bone formation, it does contribute to deciphering the role of TNF in the pathogenesis of SpA.

The third and most recent model consists of mice that overexpress selectively the transmembrane but not the soluble form of TNF (83). TNF is formed as a 26-kDa transmembrane molecule which is then cleaved by ADAM metallopeptidase domain 17 (ADAM17) from the membrane and released in a 17-kDa soluble form. Both soluble TNF (sTNF) and transmembrane TNF (tmTNF) can bind TNF receptors and are biologically active. Interestingly, mice overexpressing selectively tmTNF developed a completely different phenotype than the two other models: they did not show signs of systemic inflammation or destructive polyarthritis but developed spondylitis and deforming arthritis. At histology, the animals demonstrated synovitis as well as enthesitis and osteitis, which was accompanied by some bone destruction and, most interestingly, also by pronounced axial and peripheral new bone formation. Radiology confirmed progression towards total joint ankylosis. This model thus seems to phenocopy the musculoskeletal manifestations of SpA and for the first time provides a link between TNF in its transmembrane form and new bone formation. It is likely that this mechanism is also relevant for human SpA, as clearly the balance is in favour of tmTNF versus sTNF in SpA versus RA synovitis (84).

IL-23/IL-17

SNPs in IL-23R are strongly associated with AS, psoriasis, and IBD (51, 85), suggestive of a common mechanism across these diseases. In AS, the recent discovery of additional associated genes for signalling molecules directly downstream of the IL-23 receptor, TYK2, JAK2, and STAT3, provides further evidence for an involvement of the IL-23/IL-17 pathway in SpA (Fig. 7.3) (13). We previously indicated in the section 'HLA-B27' that research on the functional role of HLA-B27 has linked both HLA-B27 misfolding in the ER and HLA-B27 homodimer expression on the cell membrane to activation of the IL-23/IL-17 axis. Direct evidence for the involvement of these cytokines in the pathogenesis of SpA has now been provided by the positive results of clinical trials with targeted therapies directed towards either IL-23 or IL-17 in AS and PsA (86–90). The IL-23/IL-17 pathway has been studied in detail in animal models, where IL-23 production by myeloid cells (mainly dendritic cells) steers an IL-17 response by specialized Th17 cells. It needs to be emphasized, however, that even in animal models many different immune cells can respond to IL-23 by IL-17 production (91).

In the Introduction we discussed evidence that T cells may not be that crucial in the pathogenesis of SpA, and this raises the question of which cell types are involved in the IL-23/IL-17 axis in SpA. Il-23 consists of two subunits, p40 and p19. The p40 subunit is shared with IL-12 and p19 seems to be specific for IL-23 (92). Murine studies have revealed that deletion of either the p40 or the p19 subunit, but not the unique subunit of IL-12 (p35), protected mice from various autoimmune diseases, such as experimental autoimmune encephalomyelitis (EAE) (93, 94) and collagen-induced arthritis (CIA) (95, 96). Elegant mouse studies have identified monocytic phagocytes in the gut, such as CD11b+ dendritic cells and macrophages,

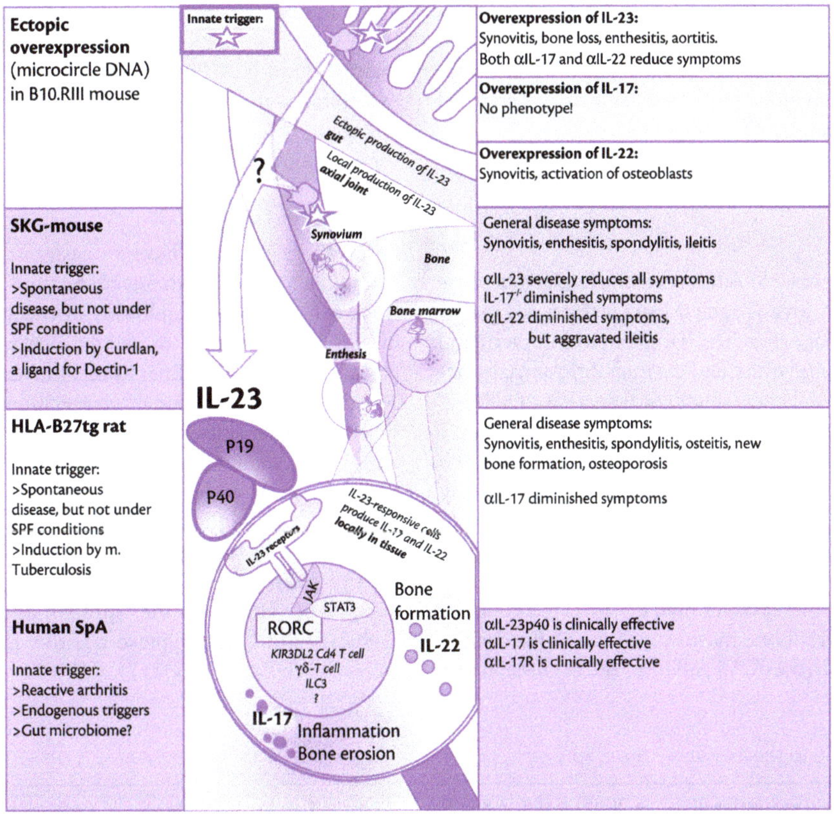

Fig. 7.3 IL-23/IL-17/IL-22 axis in experimental and human SpA. This figure summarizes the relative contribution of IL-23, IL-17, and IL-22 in various models of experimental and human SpA. The graphic models two theories on human SpA. First, IL-23 is produced ectopically, for example in the gut by monocytic phagocytes upon a bacterial trigger from the gut microbiome (concordant with the IL-23 overexpression model), or second, IL-23 is produced locally upon endogenous triggering of innate receptors and/or cellular stress (concordant with absence of systemic elevation of IL-23 in human SpA). IL-23 leads to activation of restricted responsive cells to produce locally IL-17 and/or IL-22. IL-17 can than drive inflammation and bone erosion, and IL-22 can drive bone anabolism. JAK, Janus kinase; STAT3, signal transducer and activator of transcription 3; ROR-γ, RAR-related orphan receptor gamma; ILC3, innate lymphoid cell group 3; SKG-mouse, mutation in skg-locus, fine-mapped to ZAP70; HLA-B27 tg rat, overexpression of human HLA-B27 and β_2m; αIL-23/αIL-23p40/αIL-17/αIL-17R/αIL-22, treatment with neutralizing antibodies; IL-17$^{-/-}$, animal with a deletion of the IL-17a locus.

as the natural cellular source of IL-23 during early stages of infection with *Citrobacter rodentium* (97, 98). Accordingly, it was proposed that gut-derived IL-23 may lead to increased blood levels and then act locally in target tissues on IL-23R-positive cells (99). In human SpA, however, systemic IL-23 levels are not elevated and do not correlate with disease activity (100, 101). Moreover, blood-derived macrophages and dendritic cells from SpA patients do not produce higher levels of IL-23 upon TLR stimulation than seen in healthy controls (102, 103).

Independently of the exact origin of IL-23, there is now clear experimental evidence that it plays a direct role in the pathogenesis of the disease. Systemic overexpression of IL-23 by microcircle technology induced a severe destructive polyarthritis (104) as well as enthesitis (105) in mice. In the first model, the disease appeared to be myeloid-cell dependent. In the second model, the IL-23-responsive cells appear to be entheses-resident, CD4–CD8 double-negative 'innate-like' lymphocytes. Both models thus point towards a role for innate rather than adaptive immune cells. Interestingly, the expression of the IL-23 receptor in these innate cell populations in tissues is constitutive, in contrast to the T-helper cells where the expression is restricted (106). It is hypothesized that these innate IL-23 receptor-expressing cells are important for a rapid response against various pathogens and also for gut homeostasis via the production of IL-22 (97, 98, 107).

Another animal model that has helped to better understand the role of IL-23/IL-17 in SpA is the curdlan-induced disease in SKG mice. SKG mice have a mutation in the TCR zeta chain and develop autoimmune phenomena (108). When immunized with high doses of curdlan, a TLR agonist, this mouse strain develops arthritis, enthesitis, spondylitis, and ileitis, confirming the central role of innate immune triggering which is also observed in the HLA-B27 rat model. Interestingly, preventive and therapeutic blockade of IL-23 suppressed all disease features in this model. Genetic deletion of IL-17A also had a significant, albeit limited, beneficial effect on all disease symptoms. Inhibition of another IL-23-driven cytokine, IL-22, however, only ameliorated enthesitis, had no effect on the arthritis and spondylitis, and even worsened the ileitis (109). IL-17 inhibition was also recently tested in the HLA-B27 tg rat model (110); preliminary data indicate that a preventive treatment with an IL-17A blocking antibody not only reduced clinical and histological signs of axial and peripheral inflammation but also suppressed radiographic and histological new bone formation.

Collectively, the data from genetics, experimental models, and clinical studies strongly indicate a key role for the IL-23/IL-17 pathway in SpA. In contrast to other diseases, however, it seems that the role of innate immune cells is more pronounced than that of canonical Th17 cells in this disease. This concept is further supported by analysis of human blood and tissue samples, as described in the section 'Innate immune cells in target tissue'.

Innate immune cells in target tissues

Axial tissue

Analysis of target tissue in axial SpA has been challenging, because tissue sampling is relatively invasive and is usually restricted to surgery for a clinical indication. However, tissues from intervertebral discs, SI joints, zygapophyseal joints, and the manubriosternal junction have been studied. Initial histopathological analysis of SI biopsies from patients with active disease revealed marked signals for T cells and macrophages (111, 112) and a strong signature for TNFα mRNA. In a controlled study, this T-cell infiltration was shown to be specific for AS and was present after longer disease duration in zygapophyseal joints obtained during kyphosis correction surgery (113). Later, more targeted approaches identified specific molecules in the IL-23/IL-17 axis in these tissues (Table 7.1). IL-23 could be detected in the subchondral bone marrow and in the fibrous tissue replacing the bone marrow of AS patients. The expression was found in macrophages and MPO+ cells (114). Immunostaining for IL-17A in these tissues revealed, surprisingly, that the cytokine is mainly found in MPO+ cells, CD15+ neutrophils, and to a lesser extent mast cells, as opposed to very rare in T cells. With the strong linkage to the IL-23/IL-17 axis in mind, these data from axial tissues argue for a role for innate immunity, rather than for T cells.

Peripheral tissue

Researchers generally have an easier access to tissues of peripheral joints and extra-articular structures of SpA patients and controls. Inflammatory conditions of the synovial membrane result in massive infiltration of immune cells, neovascularization, and proliferation of the intimal lining. The extent of changes related to generalized inflammation often precludes identification of disease-specific mechanisms. Using other forms of arthritis as control for SpA, like RA, gout, or osteoarthritis, effects of general inflammation can be filtered out and disease-specific cellular and molecular signatures can be identified. Surprisingly, the number of immune cells expressing cell-specific antigens like CD68 (macrophages), CD3 (T cells), and CD20 (B cells) were similar between diseases (115, 116). However, the number of CD163-expressing macrophages and C-kit/tryptase-positive mast cells was specifically increased in SpA (116, 117). CD163 is a scavenger receptor for

Table 7.1 Innate cells related to the IL-23/IL-17 axis in SpA

	Protein expression of IL-17A, IL-22, IL-23R, and ROR-γ	Contribution to pathology	Controversy
γδ-T cell (136) (FACS and ELISA)	*Peripheral blood:* Present: IL-17A, IL-23R Nr: IL-22, ROR-γ *Synovial tissue*: nr	In IL-23 minicircle overexpression in mice, enthesitis is driven by primary γδ-T cell (137)	
ILC3 (138) (FACS)	*Peripheral blood:* Present: IL-17A, IL-22, IL-23R Absent: ROR-γ *Bone marrow:* Present: IL-22, IL-23R, IL-17A Absent: IL-17A, ROR-γ *Gut:* Present: IL-17A, IL-22, IL-23R Absent: ROR-γ *Synovial tissue:* nr	Nr	The study reports on T-bet+ROR-γ-dependent production of IL-17. A cell in this state has not been observed in mice and other human studies (139)
MPO+ cell (114) (IHC)	*Synovial tissue (axial):* Present: IL-17A Nr: IL-22, IL-23R, ROR-γ	Nr	
Neutrophil 114 (IHC), (116) (IHC)	*Synovial tissue (axial and peripheral):* Present: IL-17A Nr: IL-22, IL-23R, ROR-γ	Nr	The capacity of human neutrophils to produce IL-17 is conflictingly reported (130, 131)
Mast cell (114) (IHC), (116) (IHC), (133) (Western blot, ex vivo qPCR)	*Synovial tissue (axial and peripheral):* Present: IL-17A Absent: ROR-γ Nr: IL-22, IL-23R	Mast cell blockade (nilotinib) is effective in peripheral SpA (140)	The capacity of human mast cells to produce IL-17 is conflictingly reported (132, 133). We show that human tissue mast cells can take up exogenous IL-17
Macrophage	Nr	Nr	

Nr, Not reported; ILC3, innate lymphoid cell group 3; MPO, myeloperoxidase; FACS, fluorescence activated cell sorting; ELISA, enzyme-linked immunosorbent assay; IHC, immunohistochemistry.

haemoglobin/haptoglobin complexes, binding and internalizing potentially toxic-free haem (118). CD163+ macrophages in the synovium correlated with disease activity (119) and were enriched in very early stages of disease, stressing a possible role in pathogenesis. Macrophages are very plastic and they can exert different roles, ranging from a proinflammatory phenotype (M1) to an anti-inflammatory phenotype (M2). The functional phenotype upon IL-10 polarization is considered anti-inflammatory (120). CD163+ macrophages are considered anti-inflammatory (M2), since IL-10 induces expression of CD163 in vitro (121).

This suggests that in situ CD163 macrophages induce a shift in balance towards the M2 phenotype in SpA and that these cells might be acting to counter-balance general inflammation, rather than drive inflammation. The function of this shifted balance was reflected by lower local levels of proinflammatory macrophage (M1) cytokines in the synovial fluid (122). Although clear differences in the M1–M2 balance were found between SpA and RA, conclusions should take into account that in vitro-defined classifications, like M1 and M2, do not fully apply to in situ synovial tissue macrophages (123). The exact role of these CD163+ macrophages in SpA has not been deciphered yet; moreover, the increased frequency of these cells could still be a bystander effect.

Mast cells are tissue-resident sentinel cells crucial for defence against various pathogens (124), and they are capable of modulating an immune response in the absence of pathogens (125). Due to their capacity to pre-store potent mediators, like histamine, TNF, and IL-17A, these cells have an ultra-short reaction time. Interestingly, the specific infiltration of mast cells was reproduced in a cohort of patients with short disease duration and it was not reversed by effective treatment with TNFi, suggesting that these cell types function upstream of TNF and general inflammation (116).

The IL-23/IL-17 pathway has also been analysed by immunohistochemistry in peripheral tissues. Like axial tissue, T cells expressing IL-17A were not frequently found and, as in axial tissues, both mast cells and neutrophils were identified to express IL-17A (116, 126). However, the ability of both cells types to actually produce IL-17A is debated and there are conflicting data, not only in human tissue but also in more mechanistic studies in mice. In the initial reports of the knock-in reporter mice for *IL-17a, IL-17f, IL-23R*, or *RORc*, mast cells and neutrophils were not identified among cells expressing the promotor of interest (91, 127–129). However, a recent publication detected ROR-γt and IL-17A expression in bone marrow neutrophils from reporter knock-in mice (130). Moreover, this report extended these mechanistic principles to human neutrophils isolated from peripheral blood, showing that stimulation with high levels of IL-6 in combination with IL-23 induces IL-17A production dependent on RORC. Another recent publication provides the opposite conclusion with human neutrophils isolated from peripheral blood, since investigators were not able to detect either IL-17A mRNA transcripts or IL-17A protein (131). The ability of mast cells to produce IL-17A is equally controversial. Human cord blood-derived mast cells were able to produce IL-17A in a RORC-dependent manner (132). However, our studies did not detect IL-17A mRNA transcripts in isolated mast cells from synovial tissue of SpA patients and from healthy donor tonsils. Instead, the mast cells were able to engulf exogenous IL-17A and store the cytokine for later release (133). Better understanding of the role of IL-17+ neutrophils and mast cells will be crucial for the interpretation of these data in SpA.

Potential other cell types have been identified in mouse studies and are proposed to be producers of IL-17A in human SpA, such as innate lymphoid cells and γδ-T cells. IL-17A-producing innate lymphoid cells are expanded in the gut, the blood, and the synovial fluid of SpA patients compared to healthy controls (134). Moreover, cells with the phenotypic characteristics of IL-17-producing cells were found in the synovial tissue (135). γδ-T cells are also enriched in the blood of SpA patients compared to patients with RA and healthy controls, and were shown to produce IL-17A ex vivo (136). γδ-T cells are rarely found in inflamed synovial tissue, and it is not known if they—like in the mouse—are able to drive pathology.

References

1. Parkes M, Cortes A, van Heel D, et al. Genetic insights into common pathways and complex relationships among immune-mediated diseases. Nat Rev Genet 2013;14:661–73.
2. Uddin M, Codner D, Mahmud Hasan SM, et al. Integrated genomics identifies convergence of ankylosing spondylitis with global immune mediated disease pathways. Sci Rep 2015;5:10314.
3. Schett G, Elewaut D, McInnes IB, et al. Toward a cytokine-based disease taxonomy. Nat Med 2013;19:822–4.
4. McGonagle D, McDermott MF. A proposed classification of the immunological diseases. PLoS Med 2006;3:1242–8.
5. May E, Dorris ML, Satumtira N, et al. CD8 alpha beta T cells are not essential to the pathogenesis of arthritis or colitis in HLA-B27 transgenic rats. J Immunol 2003;170:1099–105.
6. Taurog JD, Dorris ML, Satumtira N, et al. Spondylarthritis in HLA-B27/human β2-microglobulin- transgenic rats is not prevented by lack of CD8. Arthritis Rheum 2009;60:1977–84.
7. Robinson PC, Brown MA. Genetics of ankylosing spondylitis. Mol Immunol 2014;57:2–11.
8. Zinkernagel RM, Doherty PC. The discovery of MHC restriction. Immunol Today 1997;18:14–17.
9. Benjamin R, Parham P. Guilt by association: HLA-B27 and ankylosing spondylitis. Immunol Today 1990;11:137–42.
10. Hermann E, Yu DTY, Meyer zum Buschenfelde KH, et al. HLA-B27-restricted CD8 T cells derived from synovial fluids of patients with reactive arthritis and ankylosing spondylitis. Lancet 1993;342:646–50.
11. Appel H, Kuon W, Kuhne M, et al. Use of HLA B27 tetramers to identify low frequency antigen-specific T cells in *Chlamydia*-triggered reactive arthritis. Arthritis Res Ther 2004;6:R521–34.
12. Taurog JD, Maika SD, Satumtira N, et al. Inflammatory disease in HLA-B27 transgenic rats. Immunol Rev 1999;169:209–23.
13. International Genetics of Ankylosing Spondylitis C, Cortes A, Hadler J, et al. Identification of multiple risk variants for ankylosing spondylitis through high-density genotyping of immune-related loci. Nat Genet 2013;45:730–8.
14. Seregin, SS, Rastall, DPW, Evnouchidou, I, et al. Endoplasmic reticulum aminopeptidase-1 alleles associated with increased risk of ankylosing spondylitis reduce HLA-B27 mediated presentation of multiple antigens. Autoimmunity 2013; doi 10.3109/08916934.2013.819855.
15. Hammer GE, Gonzalez F, James E, et al. In the absence of aminopeptidase ERAAP, MHC class I molecules present many unstable and highly immunogenic peptides. Nat Immunol 2007;8:101–8.
16. Andrés AM, Dennis MY, Kretzschmar WW, et al. Balancing selection maintains a form of ERAP2 that undergoes nonsense-mediated decay and affects antigen presentation. PLoS Genet 2010;6:1–13.
17. Robinson PC, Costello M-E, Leo P, et al. ERAP2 is associated with ankylosing spondylitis in HLA-B27-positive and HLA-B27-negative patients. Ann Rheum Dis 2015; doi 10.1136/annrheumdis-2015-207416.
18. Strange A, Capon F, Spencer CCA, et al. A genome-wide association study identifies new psoriasis susceptibility loci and an interaction between HLA-C and ERAP1. Nat Genet 2010;42:985–90.

19. Kirino Y, Bertsias G, Ishigatsubo Y, et al. Genome-wide association analysis identifies new susceptibility loci for Behçet's disease and epistasis between HLA-B*51 and ERAP1. Nat Genet 2013;45:202–7.
20. Mear JP, Schreiber KL, Münz C, et al. Misfolding of HLA-B27 as a result of its B pocket suggests a novel mechanism for its role in susceptibility to spondyloarthropathies. J Immunol 1999;163:6665–70.
21. Goodall JC, Wu C, Zhang Y, et al. Endoplasmic reticulum stress-induced transcription factor, CHOP, is crucial for dendritic cell IL-23 expression. Proc Natl Acad Sci USA 2010;107:17698–703.
22. Turner MJ, DeLay ML, Bai S, et al. HLA-B27 up-regulation causes accumulation of misfolded heavy chains and correlates with the magnitude of the unfolded protein response in transgenic rats: implications for the pathogenesis of spondylarthritis-like disease. Arthritis Rheum 2007;56:215–23.
23. DeLay ML, Turner MJ, Klenk EI, et al. HLA-B27 misfolding and the unfolded protein response augment interleukin-23 production and are associated with Th17 activation in transgenic rats. Arthritis Rheum 2009;60:2633–43.
24. Colbert RA, Delay ML, Klenk EI, et al. From HLA-B27 to spondyloarthritis: a journey through the ER. Immunol Rev 2010;233:181–202.
25. Gu J, Rihl M, Märker-Hermann E, et al. Clues to pathogenesis of spondyloarthropathy derived from synovial fluid mononuclear cell gene expression profiles. J Rheumatol 2002;29:2159–64.
26. Dong W, Zhang Y, Yan M, et al. Upregulation of 78-kDa glucose-regulated protein in macrophages in peripheral joints of active ankylosing spondylitis. Scand J Rheumatol 37:427–34.
27. Ciccia F, Accardo-Palumbo A, Rizzo A, et al. Evidence that autophagy, but not the unfolded protein response, regulates the expression of IL-23 in the gut of patients with ankylosing spondylitis and subclinical gut inflammation. Ann Rheum Dis 2013:1–9.
28. Rioux JD, Xavier RJ, Taylor KD, et al. Genome-wide association study identifies new susceptibility loci for Crohn disease and implicates autophagy in disease pathogenesis. Nat Genet 2007;39:596–604.
29. Danoy P, Pryce K, Hadler J, et al. Association of variants at 1q32 and STAT3 with ankylosing spondylitis suggests genetic overlap with Crohn's disease. PLoS Genet 2010;6:e1001195.
30. Khor B, Gardet A, Xavier RJ. Genetics and pathogenesis of inflammatory bowel disease. Nature 2011;474:307–17.
31. Kudo LC, Parfenova L, Ren G, et al. Puromycin-sensitive aminopeptidase (PSA/NPEPPS) impedes development of neuropathology in HPSA/TAU P301L double-transgenic mice. Hum Mol Genet 2011;20:1820–33.
32. Marazziti D, Di Pietro C, Golini E, et al. Induction of macroautophagy by overexpression of the Parkinson's disease-associated GPR37 receptor. FASEB J 2009;23:1978–87.
33. Allen RL, O'Callaghan CA, McMichael AJ, et al. Cutting edge: HLA-B27 can form a novel beta 2-microglobulin-free heavy chain homodimer structure. J Immunol 1999;162:5045–8.
34. Bird LA, Peh CA, Kollnbeger S, et al. Lymphoblastoid cells express HLA-B27 homodimers both intracellularly and at the cell surface following endosomal recycling. Eur J Immunol 2003;33:748–59.
35. Kollnberger S, Bird L, Sun MY, et al. Cell-surface expression and immune receptor recognition of HLA-B27 homodimers. Arthritis Rheum 2002;46:2972–82.
36. Kollnberger S, Bird LA, Roddis M, et al. HLA-B27 heavy chain homodimers are expressed in HLA-B27 transgenic rodent models of spondyloarthritis and are ligands for paired Ig-like receptors. J Immunol 2004;173:1699–710.
37. Wong-Baeza I, Ridley A, Shaw J, et al. KIR3DL2 binds to HLA-B27 dimers and free H chains more strongly than other HLA class I and promotes the expansion of T cells in ankylosing spondylitis. J Immunol 2013;190:3216–24.
38. Chan AT, Kollnberger SD, Wedderburn LR, et al. Expansion and enhanced survival of natural killer cells expressing the killer immunoglobulin-like receptor KIR3DL2 in spondylarthritis. Arthritis Rheum 2005;52:3586–95.
39. Bowness P, Ridley A, Shaw J, et al. Th17 cells expressing KIR3DL2+ and responsive to HLA-B27 homodimers are increased in ankylosing spondylitis. J Immunol 2011;186:2672–80.
40. Harvey D, Pointon JJ, Sleator C, et al. Analysis of killer immunoglobulin-like receptor genes in ankylosing spondylitis. Ann Rheum Dis 2009;68:595–8.
41. Schwimmbeck PL, Yu DT, Oldstone MB. Autoantibodies to HLA B27 in the sera of HLA B27 patients with ankylosing spondylitis and Reiter's syndrome. Molecular mimicry with *Klebsiella pneumoniae* as potential mechanism of autoimmune disease. J Exp Med 1987;166:173–81.
42. Scofield RH, Warren WL, Koelsch G, et al. A hypothesis for the HLA-B27 immune dysregulation in spondyloarthropathy: contributions from enteric organisms, B27 structure, peptides bound by B27, and convergent evolution. Proc Natl Acad Sci USA 1993;90:9330–4.
43. van Bohemen CG, Nabbe AJ, Landheer JE, et al. HLA-B27M1M2 and high immune responsiveness to *Shigella flexneri* in post-dysenteric arthritis. Immunol Lett 1986;13:71–4.
44. Taurog JD, Richardson JA, Croft JT, et al. The germfree state prevents development of gut and joint inflammatory disease in HLA-B27 transgenic rats. J Exp Med 1994;180:2359–64.
45. Wu HJ, Ivanov II, Darce J, et al. Gut-residing segmented filamentous bacteria drive autoimmune arthritis via T helper 17 cells. Immunity 2010;32:815–27.
46. Rosenbaum JT, Davey MP. Time for a gut check: evidence for the hypothesis that HLA-B27 predisposes to ankylosing spondylitis by altering the microbiome. Arthritis Rheum 2011;63:3195–8.
47. Lin P, Bach M, Asquith M, et al. HLA-B27 and human β2-microglobulin affect the gut microbiota of transgenic rats. PLoS One 2014;9:e105684.
48. Costello M-E, Ciccia F, Willner D, et al. Intestinal dysbiosis in ankylosing spondylitis. Arthritis Rheumatol 2014 Nov 21; doi 10.1002/art.38967.
49. Rosenbaum JT, Lin P, Asquith M, et al. Does the microbiome play a causal role in spondyloarthritis? Clin Rheumatol 2014;33:763–7.
50. Van Tok M, Van Duivenvoorde L, Satumtira N, et al. FRI0164 innate immune stimulation triggers altered IL-1A/B gene expression and experimental spondyloarthritis in HLA-B27/Hu 2M transgenic rats. Ann Rheum Dis 2014;73:441.
51. Reveille JD, Sims A-M, Danoy P, et al. Genome-wide association study of ankylosing spondylitis identifies non-MHC susceptibility loci. Nat Genet 2010;42:123–7.
52. Monnet D, Kadi A, Izac B, et al. Association between the IL-1 family gene cluster and spondyloarthritis. Ann Rheum Dis 2012;71:885–90.
53. Tan AL, Marzo-Ortega H, O'Connor P, et al. Efficacy of anakinra in active ankylosing spondylitis: a clinical and magnetic resonance imaging study. Ann Rheum Dis 2004;63:1041–5.
54. Haibel H, Rudwaleit M, Listing J, et al. Open label trial of anakinra in active ankylosing spondylitis over 24 weeks. Ann Rheum Dis 2005;64:296–8.
55. Horai R, Saijo S, Tanioka H, et al. Development of chronic inflammatory arthropathy resembling rheumatoid arthritis in interleukin 1 receptor antagonist-deficient mice. J Exp Med 2000;191:313–20.
56. Matsuki T, Isoda K, Horai R, et al. Involvement of tumor necrosis factor-alpha in the development of T cell-dependent aortitis in interleukin-1 receptor antagonist-deficient mice. Circulation 2005;112:1323–31.
57. Phillips KLE, Jordan-Mahy N, Nicklin MJH, et al. Interleukin-1 receptor antagonist deficient mice provide insights into pathogenesis of human intervertebral disc degeneration. Ann Rheum Dis 2013; doi 10.1136/annrheumdis-2012-202266.
58. Koenders MI, Devesa I, Marijnissen RJ, et al. Interleukin-1 drives pathogenic Th17 cells during spontaneous arthritis in interleukin-1 receptor antagonist–deficient mice. Arthritis Rheum 2008;58:3461–70.
59. Nakae S, Saijo S, Horai R, et al. IL-17 production from activated T cells is required for the spontaneous development of destructive arthritis in mice deficient in IL-1 receptor antagonist. Proc Natl Acad Sci USA 2003;100:5986–90.
60. Akitsu A, Kakuta S, Saijo S, et al. Rag2-deficient IL-1 receptor antagonist-deficient mice are a novel colitis model in which innate

lymphoid cell-derived IL-17 is involved in the pathogenesis. Exp Anim 2014;63:235–46.
61. Zwerina J, Redlich K, Polzer K, et al. TNF-induced structural joint damage is mediated by IL-1. Proc Natl Acad Sci USA 2007;104:11742–7.
62. Corona-Sanchez EG, Muñoz-Valle JF, Gonzalez-Lopez L, et al. -383 A/C tumor necrosis factor receptor 1 polymorphism and ankylosing spondylitis in Mexicans: a preliminary study. Rheumatol Int 2012;32:2565–8.
63. Davidson SI, Liu Y, Danoy PA, et al. Association of STAT3 and TNFRSF1A with ankylosing spondylitis in Han Chinese. Ann Rheum Dis 2011;70:289–92.
64. Evans DM, Spencer CCA, Pointon JJ, et al. Interaction between ERAP1 and HLA-B27 in ankylosing spondylitis implicates peptide handling in the mechanism for HLA-B27 in disease susceptibility. Nat Genet 2011;43:761–7.
65. Karaderi T, Pointon JJ, Wordsworth TWH, et al. Evidence of genetic association between TNFRSF1A encoding the p55 tumour necrosis factor receptor, and ankylosing spondylitis in UK Caucasians. Clin Exp Rheumatol 30:110–13.
66. Pointon JJ, Harvey D, Karaderi T, et al. The chromosome 16q region associated with ankylosing spondylitis includes the candidate gene tumour necrosis factor receptor type 1-associated death domain (TRADD). Ann Rheum Dis 2010;69:1243–6.
67. Zinovieva E, Bourgain C, Kadi A, et al. Comprehensive linkage and association analyses identify haplotype, near to the TNFSF15 gene, significantly associated with spondyloarthritis. PLoS Genet 2009;5; doi 10.1371/journal.pgen.1000528.
68. Hsu H, Xiong J, Goeddel DV. The TNF receptor 1-associated protein TRADD signals cell death and NF-kappa B activation. Cell 1995;81:495–504.
69. Pappu BP, Borodovsky A, Zheng TS, et al. TL1A-DR3 interaction regulates Th17 cell function and Th17-mediated autoimmune disease. J Exp Med 2008;205:1049–62.
70. Migone TS, Zhang J, Luo X, et al. TL1A is a TNF-like ligand for DR3 and TR6/DcR3 and functions as a T cell costimulator. Immunity 2002;16:479–92.
71. Braun J, Brandt J, Listing J, et al. Treatment of active ankylosing spondylitis with infliximab: a randomised controlled multicentre trial. Lancet 2002;359:1187–93.
72. Van den Bosch F, Kruithof E, Baeten D, et al. Randomized double-blind comparison of chimeric monoclonal antibody to tumor necrosis factor α (infliximab) versus placebo in active spondylarthropathy. Arthritis Rheum 2002;46:755–65.
73. Van Der Heijde D, Kavanaugh A, Gladman DD, et al. Infliximab inhibits progression of radiographic damage in patients with active psoriatic arthritis through one year of treatment: results from the induction and maintenance psoriatic arthritis clinical trial 2. Arthritis Rheum 2007;56:2698–707.
74. van der Heijde D, Salonen D, Weissman BN, et al. Assessment of radiographic progression in the spines of patients with ankylosing spondylitis treated with adalimumab for up to 2 years. Arthritis Res Ther 2009;11:R127.
75. Heijde D van der, Landewé R, Baraliakos X, et al. Radiographic findings following two years of infliximab therapy in patients with ankylosing spondylitis. Arthritis Rheum 2008;58:3063–70.
76. Keffer J, Probert L, Cazlaris H, et al. Transgenic mice expressing human tumour necrosis factor: a predictive genetic model of arthritis. EMBO J 1991;10:4025–31.
77. Diarra D, Stolina M, Polzer K, et al. Dickkopf-1 is a master regulator of joint remodeling. Nat Med 2007;13:156–63.
78. Uderhardt S, Diarra D, Katzenbeisser J, et al. Blockade of Dickkopf (DKK)-1 induces fusion of sacroiliac joints. Ann Rheum Dis 2010;69:592–7.
79. Yeremenko N, Zwerina K, Rigter G, et al. TNF-α and IL-6 differentially regulate Dkk-1 in the inflamed arthritic joint. Arthritis Rheumatol 2015;67(8):2071–5.
80. Kontoyiannis D, Pasparakis M, Pizarro TT, et al. Impaired on/off regulation of TNF biosynthesis in mice lacking TNF AU-rich elements: implications for joint and gut-associated immunopathologies. Immunity 1999;10:387–98.
81. Kontoyiannis D, Boulougouris G, Manoloukos M, et al. Genetic dissection of the cellular pathways and signaling mechanisms in modeled tumor necrosis factor-induced Crohn's-like inflammatory bowel disease. J Exp Med 2002;196:1563–74.
82. Jacques P, Lambrecht S, Verheugen E, et al. Proof of concept: enthesitis and new bone formation in spondyloarthritis are driven by mechanical strain and stromal cells. Ann Rheum Dis 2013:1–9.
83. Alexopoulou L, Pasparakis M, Kollias G. A murine transmembrane tumor necrosis factor (TNF) transgene induces arthritis by cooperative p55/p75 TNF receptor signaling. Eur J Immunol 1997;27:2588–92.
84. van Duivenvoorde LM, Ambarus CA, Masdar H, et al. A2.15 Relative overexpression of transmembrane versus soluble TNF in human and experimental spondyloarthritis. Ann Rheum Dis 2013;72:A9–10.
85. Burton PR, Clayton DG, Cardon LR, et al. Association scan of 14,500 nonsynonymous SNPs in four diseases identifies autoimmunity variants. Nat Genet 2007;39:1329–37.
86. Mease PJ, Genovese MC, Greenwald MW, et al. Brodalumab, an anti-IL17RA monoclonal antibody, in psoriatic arthritis. N Engl J Med 2014;370:2295–306.
87. Baeten D, Baraliakos X, Braun J, et al. Anti-interleukin-17A monoclonal antibody secukinumab in treatment of ankylosing spondylitis: a randomised, double-blind, placebo-controlled trial. Lancet 2013;382:1705–13.
88. McInnes IB, Kavanaugh A, Gottlieb AB, et al. Efficacy and safety of ustekinumab in patients with active psoriatic arthritis: 1 year results of the phase 3, multicentre, double-blind, placebo-controlled PSUMMIT 1 trial. Lancet 2013;382:780–9.
89. McInnes IB, Sieper J, Braun J, et al. Efficacy and safety of secukinumab, a fully human anti-interleukin-17A monoclonal antibody, in patients with moderate-to-severe psoriatic arthritis: a 24-week, randomised, double-blind, placebo-controlled, phase II proof-of-concept trial. Ann Rheum Dis 2014;73:349–56.
90. Poddubnyy D, Hermann K-G, Callhoff J, et al. Ustekinumab for the treatment of patients with active ankylosing spondylitis: results of a 28-week, prospective, open-label, proof-of-concept study (TOPAS). Ann Rheum Dis 2014;73:817–23.
91. Awasthi A, Riol-Blanco L, Jäger A, et al. Cutting edge: IL-23 receptor gfp reporter mice reveal distinct populations of IL-17-producing cells. J Immunol 2009;182:5904–8.
92. Oppmann B, Lesley R, Blom B, et al. Novel p19 protein engages IL-12p40 to form a cytokine, IL-23, with biological activities similar as well as distinct from IL-12. Immunity 2000;13:715–25.
93. Becher B, Durell BG, Noelle RJ. Experimental autoimmune encephalitis and inflammation in the absence of interleukin-12. J Clin Invest 2002;110:493–7.
94. Cua DJ, Sherlock J, Chen Y, et al. Interleukin-23 rather than interleukin-12 is the critical cytokine for autoimmune inflammation of the brain. Nature 2003;421:744–8.
95. Murphy CA, Langrish CL, Chen Y, et al. Divergent pro- and antiinflammatory roles for IL-23 and IL-12 in joint autoimmune inflammation. J Exp Med 2003;198:1951–7.
96. Ghilardi N, Kljavin N, Chen Q, et al. Compromised humoral and delayed-type hypersensitivity responses in IL-23-deficient mice. J Immunol 2004;172:2827–33.
97. Aychek T, Mildner A, Yona S, et al. IL-23-mediated mononuclear phagocyte crosstalk protects mice from *Citrobacter rodentium*-induced colon immunopathology. Nat Commun 2015;6:6525.
98. Zheng Y, Valdez PA, Danilenko DM, et al. Interleukin-22 mediates early host defense against attaching and effacing bacterial pathogens. Nat Med 2008;14:282–9.
99. Sherlock JP, Taylor PC, Buckley CD, et al. Spondyloarthropathy: interleukin 23 and disease modification. Lancet 2015;385:2017–8.
100. Melis L, Vandooren B, Kruithof E, et al. Systemic levels of IL-23 are strongly associated with disease activity in rheumatoid arthritis but not spondyloarthritis. Ann Rheum Dis 2010;69:618–23.

101. Wendling D, Cedoz J-P, Racadot E. Serum and synovial fluid levels of p40 IL12/23 in spondyloarthropathy patients. Clin Rheumatol 2009;28:187–90.
102. Wang X, Lin Z, Wei Q, et al. Expression of IL-23 and IL-17 and effect of IL-23 on IL-17 production in ankylosing spondylitis. Rheumatol Int 2009;29:1343–7.
103. Prevosto C, Goodall JC, Gaston JSH. Cytokine secretion by pathogen recognition receptor-stimulated dendritic cells in rheumatoid arthritis and ankylosing spondylitis. J Rheumatol 2012;39:1918–28.
104. Adamopoulos IE, Tessmer M, Chao C-C, et al. IL-23 is critical for induction of arthritis, osteoclast formation, and maintenance of bone mass. J Immunol 2011;187:951–9.
105. Sherlock JP, Joyce-Shaikh B, Turner SP, et al. IL-23 induces spondyloarthropathy by acting on ROR-γt+ CD3+CD4−CD8− entheseal resident T cells. Nat Med 2012;18:1069–76.
106. Gaffen SL, Jain R, Garg AV, et al. The IL-23–IL-17 immune axis: from mechanisms to therapeutic testing. Nat Rev Immunol 2014;14:585–600.
107. Eken A, Singh AK, Treuting PM, et al. IL-23R+ innate lymphoid cells induce colitis via interleukin-22-dependent mechanism. Mucosal Immunol 2014;7:143–54.
108. Ruutu M, Thomas G, Steck R, et al. β-Glucan triggers spondylarthritis and Crohn's disease-like ileitis in SKG mice. Arthritis Rheum 2012;64:2211–22.
109. Benham H, Rehaume LM, Hasnain SZ, et al. Interleukin-23 mediates the intestinal response to microbial β-1,3-glucan and the development of spondyloarthritis pathology in SKG mice. Arthritis Rheumatol 2014;66:1755–67.
110. van Tok MN, Van Duivenvoorde LM, Krammer I, Baeten DL. OP0202 anti-IL-17A treatment blocks inflammation and new bone formation in experimental spondyloarthritis in HLA-B27 transgenic rats. Ann Rheum Dis 2015;74(2):147.3–148.
111. Braun J, Bollow M, Neure L, et al. Use of immunohistologic and in situ hybridization techniques in the examination of sacroiliac joint biopsy specimens from patients with ankylosing spondylitis. Arthritis Rheum 1995;38:499–505.
112. Bollow M, Fischer T, Reisshauer H, et al. Quantitative analyses of sacroiliac biopsies in spondyloarthropathies: T cells and macrophages predominate in early and active sacroiliitis-cellularity correlates with the degree of enhancement detected by magnetic resonance imaging. Ann Rheum Dis 2000;59:135–40.
113. Appel H, Kuhne M, Spiekermann S, et al. Immunohistologic analysis of zygapophyseal joints in patients with ankylosing spondylitis. Arthritis Rheum 2006;54:2845–51.
114. Appel H, Maier R, Wu P, et al. Analysis of IL-17(+) cells in facet joints of patients with spondyloarthritis suggests that the innate immune pathway might be of greater relevance than the Th17-mediated adaptive immune response. Arthritis Res Ther 2011;13:R95.
115. Baeten D, Kruithof E, De Rycke L, et al. Infiltration of the synovial membrane with macrophage subsets and polymorphonuclear cells reflects global disease activity in spondyloarthropathy. Arthritis Res Ther 2005;7:R359–69.
116. Noordenbos T, Yeremenko N, Gofita I, et al. Interleukin-17-positive mast cells contribute to synovial inflammation in spondylarthritis. Arthritis Rheum 2012;64:99–109.
117. Baeten D, Demetter P, Cuvelier CA, et al. Macrophages expressing the scavenger receptor CD163: a link between immune alterations of the gut and synovial inflammaton in spondyloarthropathy. J Pathol 2002;196:343–50.
118. Kristiansen M, Graversen JH, Jacobsen C, et al. Identification of the haemoglobin scavenger receptor. Nature 2001;409:198–201.
119. Baeten D, Møller HJ, Delanghe J, et al. Association of CD163+ macrophages and local production of soluble CD163 with decreased lymphocyte activation in spondylarthropathy synovitis. Arthritis Rheum 2004;50:1611–23.
120. Mosser DM, Edwards JP. Exploring the full spectrum of macrophage activation. Nat Rev Immunol 2008;8:958–69.
121. Ambarus CA, Krausz S, van Eijk M, et al. Systematic validation of specific phenotypic markers for in vitro polarized human macrophages. J Immunol Methods 2012;375:196–206.
122. Vandooren B, Noordenbos T, Ambarus C, et al. Absence of a classically activated macrophage cytokine signature in peripheral spondylarthritis, including psoriatic arthritis. Arthritis Rheum 2009;60:966–75.
123. Ambarus CA, Noordenbos T, De Hair MJ, et al. Intimal lining layer macrophages but not synovial sublining macrophages display an IL-10 polarized-like phenotype in chronic synovitis. Arthritis Res Ther 2012;14:R74.
124. Urb M, Sheppard DC. The role of mast cells in the defence against pathogens. PLoS Pathog 2012;8; doi 10.1371/journal.ppat.1002619.
125. Galli SJ, Grimbaldeston M, Tsai M. Immunomodulatory mast cells: negative, as well as positive, regulators of immunity. Nat Rev Immunol 2008;8:478–86.
126. Moran EM, Heydrich R, Ng CT, et al. IL-17A expression is localised to both mononuclear and polymorphonuclear synovial cell infiltrates. PLoS One 2011;6:e24048.
127. Eberl G, Marmon S, Sunshine M-J, et al. An essential function for the nuclear receptor RORgamma(t) in the generation of fetal lymphoid tissue inducer cells. Nat Immunol 2004;5:64–73.
128. Croxford AL, Kurschus FC, Waisman A. Cutting edge: an IL-17F-CreEYFP reporter mouse allows fate mapping of Th17 cells. J Immunol 2009;182:1237–41.
129. Price AE, Reinhardt RL, Liang H-E, et al. Marking and quantifying IL-17A-producing cells in vivo. PLoS One 2012;7:e39750.
130. Taylor PR, Roy S, Leal SM, et al. Activation of neutrophils by autocrine IL-17A-IL-17RC interactions during fungal infection is regulated by IL-6, IL-23, RORγt and dectin-2. Nat Immunol 2014;15:143–51.
131. Tamarozzi F, Wright HL, Thomas HB, et al. A lack of confirmation with alternative assays questions the validity of IL-17A expression in human neutrophils using immunohistochemistry. Immunol Lett 2014;162:194–8.
132. Hueber AJ, Asquith DL, Miller AM, et al. Mast cells express IL-17A in rheumatoid arthritis synovium. J Immunol 2010;184:3336–40.
133. Noordenbos T, Blijdorp IC, Chen S, Stap J, et al. Human mast cells, capture store and release exogenous IL-17A. J Leukoc Biol. 2016; doi 10.1189/jlb.3HI1214-542R.
134. Ciccia F, Guggino G, Rizzo A, et al. Type 3 innate lymphoid cells producing IL-17 and IL-22 are expanded in the gut, in the peripheral blood, synovial fluid and bone marrow of patients with ankylosing spondylitis. Ann Rheum Dis 2015; doi 10.1136/annrheumdis-2014-206323.
135. Al-Mossawi M, De Wit J, Kendrick B, et al. A1.1 Identification and phenotyping of innate lymphoid cells present in the diseased joints of patients with spondyloarthritis, rheumatoid arthritis and psoriatic arthritis. Ann Rheum Dis 2015;74:A1.
136. Kenna TJ, Davidson SI, Duan R, et al. Enrichment of circulating interleukin-17-secreting interleukin-23 receptor-positive γ/δ T cells in patients with active ankylosing spondylitis. Arthritis Rheum 2012;64:1420–9.
137. Sherlock JP, Joyce-Shaikh B, Turner SP, et al. IL-23 induces spondyloarthropathy by acting on ROR-γt+ CD3+CD4−CD8− entheseal resident T cells. Nat Med 2012;18:1069–76.
138. Ciccia F, Guggino G, Rizzo A, et al. Type 3 innate lymphoid cells producing IL-17 and IL-22 are expanded in the gut, in the peripheral blood, synovial fluid and bone marrow of patients with ankylosing spondylitis. Ann Rheum Dis 2015; doi 10.1136/annrheumdis-2014-206323.
139. Artis D, Spits H. The biology of innate lymphoid cells. Nature 2015; doi 10.1038/nature14189.
140. Paramarta JE, Turina MC, Noordenbos T, et al. OP0156 Targeting synovial mast cells in spondyloarthritis: a proof-of-concept study with nilotinib A tyrosine kinase inhibitor. Ann Rheum Dis 2014;73:120–1.

CHAPTER 8

Immune mechanisms: adaptive immunity

Maxime Breban and Hill Gaston

Introduction to adaptive immunity

AxSpA is currently defined by ASAS criteria which recognize radiographic and non-radiographic forms. The latter are assumed to be precursors of the former, but the proportion of nr-axSpA patients who progress to the radiographic form is not yet clearly defined. However, it seems likely that the immunopathogenesis of the two forms will be the same, with perhaps the caveat that progression might reflect a heavier 'load' of genes which increase susceptibility, or indeed other genes which do not influence susceptibility but instead affect progression itself, and the pathologic pathways that govern this. The vast majority of investigative work has been done on those with radiographic disease—that is, AS.

Adaptive immunity refers to those components of the immune system that: (1) rely on the generation and selection of a repertoire of antigen-specific receptors, and (2) have immunologic memory (i.e. respond more rapidly and more efficiently to a second encounter with an antigen). These components are classically the B and T lymphocytes. Nowadays there is some blurring of the distinction between adaptive and innate immunity, with some components of the innate system acquiring 'memory', or more accurately 'training', by accumulating epigenetic modifications (1), whilst some T-cell subsets have invariant antigen receptors and function in a similar way to effectors of the innate immune system such as natural killer (NK) cells (2). This chapter confines itself to classical B and T lymphocytes.

Insights on adaptive immunity in animal models of axial spondyloarthritis

Several models relevant to SpA, including axial pathology, have been developed in rodents since the 1990s (3). Investigations performed in those models have provided important clues for clarifying the fundamental role of adaptive immunity in this disorder.

HLA-B27 transgenic rats

Several lines of rats transgenic for HLA-B*2705 and hβ_2m genomic DNAs (B27-tg) have been produced since the early 1990s. They develop spontaneous phenotypes that recapitulate major aspects of SpA pathology, with variations dependent on the number of copies of both transgenes incorporated in the rat genome and dictating their level of expression (3). The first described phenotype combines peripheral arthritis with psoriatic skin and nail lesions, and IBD similar to UC, thus resembling more peripheral than axSpA (4). A more recently described phenotype more similar to axSpA arises in rats having integrated fewer copies of the HLA-B27 transgene. It is restricted to males and combines spondylitis with formation of syndesmophytes, sacroiliitis with osteoproliferation, peripheral erosive arthritis, and dactylitis, in the absence of extra-articular inflammation except for orchitis (5). The role of the immune system has been extensively studied, mostly in the first phenotype in which gut microbiota are required for gut and joint inflammation to happen (4, 6). One of the main conclusions was that disease expression required the presence of CD4+ T cells and that CD8+ T cells were dispensable, a finding that was rather unexpected for an MHC class I-related disorder, arguing against the classical 'arthritogenic peptide' hypothesis (7).

Indeed, CD4+ T cells with an activated phenotype tend to accumulate in lymph nodes draining inflammatory sites, such as the gut and joint (8, 9). They may be driven by gut microbiota and readily provoke disease manifestations upon transfer into B27-tg athymic nude recipients, which are otherwise protected from disease development (10, 11). The functional characterization of activated CD4+ T cells showed a predominant Th17 profile characterized by heightened production of IL-17A, IL-21, IL-22, and TNFα (9). Total production of IFNγ was not increased in CD4+ T cells, but a subset of those producing IL-17A and TNFα also produced IFNγ, corresponding to a phenotype described as polyfunctional Th1/17 that is pathogenic in inflammatory disorders and was found as enriched in SpA patients (12, 13). Such Th17 bias may also explain increased circulating IgA levels in the B27-tg rat (4, 14).

Th17 cell accumulation in the B27-tg rat can at least in part be explained by IL-23 production by myeloid cells in the gut of those animals (15). Implication of the latter cells appears consistent with the observation that SpA development could be transferred to wild-type animals by haematopoietic precursors from disease-prone B27-tg rats (16). It was intriguing to observe that antigen-presenting cells (APCs) from all disease-susceptible B27-tg lines were defective in their capacity to activate naïve T cells (17). However, the co-culture of B27-tg rat dendritic cells (DCs) with CD4+ T cells resulted in Th17 expansion bias and in reduced expression of IL-10, together with overexpression of inducible co-stimulatory molecule (ICOS) and IL-17 by regulatory T cells from B27-tg rats, providing a possible explanation for the pathogenicity of the DC (8, 9). This observation could be linked to several aberrant functions of DC from those rats, including deficiency of the CD86–CD28 co-stimulatory pathway and a decreased production of cytokines such as IFNγ, IL-10, and IL-27, known to oppose

Th17 differentiation (18, 19). Interestingly, several of those findings have also been identified in SpA patients, but the precise molecular mechanism linking HLA-B27 expression in APC to the aforementioned abnormalities remains to be clarified (15, 19, 20).

The IL-23/IL-17 axis in mouse models of axial spondyloarthritis

Transgenic expression of HLA-B27 by itself has not been conclusively shown to trigger SpA in the mouse (21). Nevertheless, several phenotypes reminiscent of SpA, including axial skeleton pathology, have been reported in other contexts.

The systemic expression of IL-23 obtained by injecting minicircle DNA and its uptake into hepatocytes of the B10.RIII mouse induces early enthesitis and entheseal new bone formation, followed by severe erosive polyarthritis (22). In this model, enthesitis affects the paws as well as the axial skeleton at the sites of attachment of the spinal ligaments to bone and the SI joint. EAMs that are characteristic of SpA (i.e. psoriasis and inflammation in the aortic root and valve) also occur. The mechanism underlying enthesitis involves a particular subset of IL-23R-positive ROR-γt+ CD3+CD4–CD8– T cells residing in the entheses and responding to IL-23 by producing IL-22 and IL-17, two cytokines that were shown to mediate entheseal inflammation and osteoproliferation.

Another SpA model was described in the SKG strain variant of the BALB/c mouse, which harbours a W163C mutation of ZAP-70, impairing T-cell receptor signaling strength and favouring T-cell-mediated autoimmunity. The SKG mouse develops polyarthritis reminiscent of RA under conventional microbial conditions, with autoantibodies, including rheumatoid factor (23). Arthritis does not occur in SKG mice raised under specific pathogen-free conditions, unless injected intraperitoneally with β-1,3-glucan (curdlan). This resulted in the induction of a thorough SpA phenotype consisting of dactylitis, Achilles tendon enthesitis, plantar fasciitis, destructive arthritis of ankles and wrists, spondylitis, sacroiliitis, and inflammation of the intervertebral discs in the tail, but without osteoproliferation. Extra-articular features comprised uveitis and late ileitis resembling CD (24). The β-1,3-glucan molecular pattern that is present in plants, fungal cell walls, and bacteria is a ligand for the dectin 1 receptor that signals through CARD9 in APC and activates the production of multiple cytokines, including IL-12 and IL-23. SKG mice do not differ from the BALB/c parental strain in their immediate response to curdlan (25).

Thus the role of adaptive immunity is presumably crucial to determine SpA pathology, as shown by the induction of arthritis, and spondylitis in immune-deficient SCID mice upon transfer of CD4+ T cells from SKG mice. A primary role of the IL-23/IL-17 axis was shown, as a consequence of microbiota-dependent induction of IL-23 in the ileum (25, 26). Hence, inhibition of IL-23 suppressed the development of peripheral arthritis and spondylitis and limited the development of ileitis, whilst osteoarticular and ileal inflammation were attenuated in IL-17A$^{-/-}$ SKG mice, as well as in germ-free animals (26). In contrast, blocking IL-22, another Th17 cytokine, only attenuated enthesitis, having no effect on arthritis or spondylitis, and resulted in aggravation of ileitis. Thus IL-22 production by local innate mononuclear cell populations in the ileum seemed to protect against inflammation in this situation. Such findings should be kept in mind when exploring inhibition of the Th17 pathway as treatment for SpA.

TNF-dependent mouse models of spondyloarthritis

Mice overexpressing TNF by deletion of the AU-rich elements in the murine TNF locus (TNF$^{\Delta ARE}$ mice) develop destructive polyarthritis, sacroiliitis, and enthesitis, without osteoproliferation, together with CD-like IBD. This model was shown to be dependent on the deregulated production of TNF by myeloid cells acting through TNF receptor type 1 on synovial and intestinal stromal cells, without the intervention of the adaptive immune system arm in the joint pathology (27, 28).

The SKG mouse was also successfully used to develop a model of *Chlamydia*-induced ReA (29). The phenotype triggered in this mouse, 5 weeks after vaginal infection with live *Chlamydia muridarum*, combined paw arthritis with spondylitis, SI, enthesitis, and psoriasiform dermatitis without intestinal inflammation. Severity of the phenotype was correlated with the degree of bacterial load. The level of specific immunoglobulin (Ig) response was unaffected, whereas decreased *Chlamydia*-specific CD4+ T-cell production of IFNγ and IL-17 was observed in the SKG mouse and thought to contribute to the systemic dissemination of *Chlamydia* via infected monocytes/macrophages. This resulted in heightened production of TNF by T cells in response to chlamydial antigen, contributing to the severity of arthritis, as shown by the effects of anti-TNF treatment (29).

Summary of insights on adaptive immunity in animal models of axial spondyloarthritis

Immunological studies performed in various animal models of SpA, whether linked to HLA-B27 or not, have shown the instrumental place of CD4+ T cells and of the Th17 pathway in driving disease appearance, presumably as a consequence of altered immune response to microbial triggers. Furthermore, TNFα and/or IL-17 appear as keynote downstream effectors of the pathogenic inflammatory response, whether dependent on the adaptive immune system or not.

Insights on adaptive immunity in human axial spondyloarthritis

B-cell immunity in axial spondyloarthritis

Autoantibodies

The designation of spondyloarthropathies as 'seronegative' correctly emphasizes the *absence* in these diseases of the kinds of autoantibodies that are a defining feature of RA and systemic lupus erythematosus (SLE). This in turn suggests that the pathogenesis of axSpA may not involve the kinds of autoantibody-mediated processes that are seen in the other conditions. Nevertheless, there have been various reports of some varieties of autoantibody in axSpA over the years. An early paper reported antibodies reactive with prostate tissue, mainly in ReA but also in AS (8/8 cases) (30). The significance of this is unknown, but genitourinary inflammation is important in one of the HLA-B27 transgenic models of SpA (see section 'HLA-B27 transgenic rats') (31).

In the 1970s, there were initial reports of autoantibodies to HLA-B27, possibly cross-reactive with *Klebsiella* (see section 'Antibodies to bacterial antigens'), but these were later refuted (32). Antibodies to heat shock proteins, again possibly cross-reactive with bacterial heat shock proteins, were reported (33). A more recent paper used protein arrays to test for antibodies to a wide variety of self-antigens (several thousand proteins) and reported that 44% of AS patients, compared to 8% of controls, had a broad autoantibody response, recognizing often more than 50 different proteins; furthermore, 60% of the antigens recognized by AS patients were not recognized by healthy controls or RA patients (34).

It is difficult to interpret these findings other than to say that they differ markedly from diseases where a relatively small number of antigens are the target of the autoimmune antibody response, for example the citrullinated proteins in RA. All healthy individuals possess autoreactive B cells at low frequency and likewise low titres of autoantibodies, so it would appear that these are boosted in a non-specific way by the chronic inflammation associated with axSpA. However, proteomic approaches also led to a recent report of autoantibodies to a single enzyme, protein phosphatase magnesium-dependent 1A (PPM1A) (35). Levels of antibodies correlated with severity of sacroiliitis; interestingly, they were also found in SpA-prone HLA-B27-tg rats. One barrier in identifying autoantibodies might be their presence as circulating immune complexes. This has been observed in the case of noggin- and sclerostin-immune complexes identified in the serum of AS patients (36).

Antibodies to bacterial antigens

Increased antibodies to *Klebsiella pneumoniae* were described by Ebringer in 1983 (37), and thanks to his tireless advocacy of the idea that there might be a causative link between this bacterium and AS/axSpA (38), further studies have been performed. The interest in antibodies was originally stimulated by reports of higher carriage of *Klebsiella* in stool of patients with active compared to inactive AS (39)—these could not be confirmed in later studies (40)—and the finding of antibodies that reacted with *Klebsiella* when rabbits were immunized with HLA-B27+ cells (41). In addition, polyclonal and some monoclonal anti-B27 antibodies were reported to react with components of *Klebsiella* (42–44). These findings led to the proposal that molecular mimicry of HLA-B27 by bacterial antigens, especially those of *Klebsiella*, was the underlying immunologic mechanism for axSpA. This was, and is, an attractive notion, but would now be seen as oversimplistic in the absence of further evidence, since molecular mimicry at both antibody and T-cell levels of recognition is exceedingly common, without necessarily breaking self-tolerance and producing inflammatory disease.

Despite the failure over many years to produce additional evidence to corroborate the idea of mimicry between HLA-B27 and *Klebsiella*, and indeed some evidence against it (45), several laboratories have independently confirmed the basic finding of increased antibodies to *Klebsiella*, especially those of the IgA class, in AS, though some have also noted elevated antibodies to other Gram-negative bacteria (46–50). The best explanation for these results would seem to lie in the significant proportion of axSpA patients who have subclinical gut inflammation (51–53). This will alter gut barrier function and allow access of organisms such as *Klebsiella* to the immune system, with the formation of antibodies, especially those of the IgA class.

Immunoregulatory role of B cells

In experimental models of arthritis it has been clearly shown that B lymphocytes can ameliorate disease. These regulatory B cells make IL-10 (53, 54). Whether such mechanisms operate in axSpA in humans is unknown; B-cell depletion is not particularly effective in the therapy of AS, but neither does it exacerbate disease (55). Combined effects of depleting both regulatory and effector B-cell subsets would complicate the analysis of the effectiveness of depletion if both were playing a role in pathogenesis. Thus assessment of any role of regulatory B cells in axSpA must await further evidence.

Summary of immunoregulatory role of B cells

The evidence for a critical role for B-cell-mediated immunity in axSpA is limited, and autoantibody formation is not a prominent feature in this disease.

T-cell immunity in axial spondyloarthritis

Studies of T-cell-mediated immunity in axSpA have mainly been carried out in peripheral blood because of the lack of access to tissue at sites of axial disease. Exceptions have included some studies on SI joint biopsies and on facet joints removed at surgery. Attention has been paid to the bone marrow subchondral infiltrates rather than synovium; these contain more CD4+ and CD8+ T cells, and to a lesser extent B cells, than control joints (56). Interestingly, the infiltrates appeared to be lost in areas where overlying cartilage was no longer present, giving rise to the hypothesis that the T-cell infiltrates might be directed against cartilage antigens (see section 'Specificity'). Immunohistochemical studies of the bone marrow infiltrates showed increased expression of IL-17+ cells compared to osteoarthritis joints, but the majority of these cells were not T cells but instead myeloperoxidase + neutrophils (57). In keeping with the role of IL-23 in driving expression of IL-17, IL-23+ cells were also more frequent in axSpA than in osteoarthritis, and more numerous than those expressing IL-12 (58).

Synovial fluid and tissue can be obtained from large joints, usually knees, of patients with axSpA, but by definition this is peripheral rather than axial disease, and synovial fluid is also more readily available from patients with psoriatic and reactive arthritis, who may or may not have axial involvement, than from those with AS. Nevertheless, studies of synovial fluid have been informative.

Properties of blood and synovial T cells in axial spondyloarthritis

Phenotype

With regard to the relative proportions of CD4+ and CD8+ T cells, there is no predominance of the CD8+ subset, despite the clear association between axSpA and the class I MHC antigen, HLA-B27. Indeed, if the B27 tg rat model of axSpA faithfully reflects human disease, there is no requirement for CD8+ cells at all (59). Nevertheless, both subsets have been investigated. Synovial fluid cells generally are of the memory phenotype (CD45R0+) and show higher levels of expression of markers of activation. This is consistent with their activation, presumably by antigen, and recruitment to the joint by the effects of integrin and chemokine receptor expression. Activation could in principle occur either outside or inside the joint—in the latter case the cells would be primed elsewhere, circulate as memory cells, and then enter the joint in response to the presence of antigen there.

In relation to cytokine expression, IFNγ+ cells are readily detected in joints and these observations were originally interpreted as implying that a Th1 polarized T-cell response was important in axSpA. However, with the discovery of the IL-17-producing T-cell subset, more recent studies have emphasized the increase in numbers of IL-17+ T cells and in IL-17 secretion in both peripheral blood and synovial fluid in axSpA (13, 60). This idea is reinforced by the associations between AS and SNPs in many genes involved in the generation and effector function of IL-17-producing cells, especially the IL-23 receptor and its downstream signals (61). Whilst most reports have described CD4+ IL-17+ cells, γδ cells making this cytokine have also been reported to be increased in axSpA (62), and it is clear that IL-17 can be made by many T-cell and non-T-cell subsets. These may include the entheseal CD3+CD4–CD8– T cell found to be responsive to IL-23 in a mouse model of axSpA (22), but a human counterpart of this cell has not yet been described.

Specificity

If T-cell-mediated immunity drives axSpA, there should be critical foreign or auto-antigens which the T cells recognize. Bacterial antigens are obvious candidates, and CD4+ and CD8+ T cells specific for the triggering infection are readily demonstrated in peripheral joints in ReA, and are also present in peripheral blood (63, 64). A specific search for *Klebsiella*-specific T cells in AS proved negative—indeed, their frequency appeared to be lower than in matched controls (65).

T cells with reactivity to undefined self-antigens are often isolated from both synovial fluid and blood when cloning procedures are undertaken (e.g. (63))—essentially such clones respond by proliferation and cytokine production to autologous antigen-presenting cells in the absence of added antigens. The significance of these cells is unknown; some may have a regulatory function, since regulatory T cells are positively selected in the thymus on the basis of their intermediate affinity for self-antigens—that is, not too high to cause death by deletion, or too low to cause death by neglect (66, 67). Whilst classical regulatory T cells are CD4+, a regulatory IL-4-producing Foxp3+ CD8+ T cell has also been described (68, 69), and higher numbers of these cells were noted in peripheral blood of AS patients than in HLA-B27– controls; HLA-B27+ controls also had higher numbers (70, 71). These cells were revealed by co-cultures of CD8+ T cells with autologous DC, whereas other forms of stimulation elicited IFNγ-producing cells. Other work suggests that the interaction between T cells and DC is defective in axSpA in both humans and the B27 tg rat (20, 72), and this may favour the generation of these cells which, whilst they had potent in vitro regulatory activity, also produced TNFα. Higher numbers of CD4+ CD25+ Foxp3+ regulatory T cells have also been reported in synovial fluid of patients with AS and other forms of SpA (73); it is known that regulatory T cells have some plasticity and may give rise to IL-17-producing cells (74).

T cells recognizing components of joints have been described in axSpA. These include HLA-B27-restricted CD8+ T cells responsive to peptides from type II and VI collagen, with synovial fluid cells responsive to the type VI peptide. However, such responses were not seen in all patients tested (4 of 7) (75), so their significance is doubtful. HLA-B27 itself has been suggested to be a target of an autoimmune response, as a source of peptides which could be mimicked by similar peptides in microorganisms. CD4+ cells that responded to 'atypical' forms of HLA-B27 have also been described (76); these forms were inhibited by the presence of high-affinity B27-binding peptides and might therefore represent free heavy chains or B27 multimers.

What role does HLA-B27 play in adaptive immunity in axial spondyloarthritis?

The most straightforward role for HLA-B27 in axSpA is its physiologic one of presenting antigenic peptides to CD8+ T cells, for example bacterial or self-antigens, as already noted. However, a second, non-classical role has emerged from reports showing, first, that HLA-B27 heavy chains have the ability to dimerize (77) and be expressed on the cell surface (78, 79), and, second, that these dimers can engage specific receptors on T cells (and also on NK cells or macrophage/monocytes) and alter their behaviour. For T cells, the high-affinity receptor for B27 multimers is KIR3DL2 (80), a member of the family of KIR which generally engage class I MHC molecules and inhibit or stimulate the activity of NK cells. For T cells, KIR3DL2 engagement by B27 homodimers and free heavy chain, but not B27/ β_2m heterodimers, results in production of IL-17 (81); thus IL-17+ cells are overrepresented amongst T cells expressing KIR3DL2, and the proportion of KIR3DL2+ cells is increased in axSpA (81).

A monoclonal antibody which appears to react with multimeric B27 stains cells from blood and joints of axSpA patients, but not controls, and reduces responses of cell lines expressing KIR3DL2 (82). The formation of the multimers seems to depend on a supply of free heavy chains, so that it is inhibited by the presence of peptides which bind strongly to B27/β_2m dimers and would therefore be expected to stabilize such complexes (83). These observations may be linked to the finding that susceptibility to axSpA is influenced by polymorphisms in the gene ERAP1 (84), which encodes an exopeptidase responsible for trimming the N-terminus of peptides which are destined to bind in the peptide groove of class I MHC molecules. Forms of ERAP1 that are inefficient at this trimming might result in an inadequate supply of tightly binding peptides, and greater availability of free B27 heavy chains to form multimers. Recent work strongly suggests that the particular 'versions'—allotypes—of ERAP1 found in axSpA have either poor or excessive trimming function (85), though earlier studies had suggested that protective forms of ERAP1 showed impaired trimming function (86).

A further unusual property of HLA-B27 is the relatively inefficient folding of the heavy chain during synthesis in the ER. This in turn can elicit the unfolded protein response, which has been shown to alter cytokine production when induced in DC (87). Importantly, the cytokine whose synthesis is favoured by the unfolded protein response is IL-23 (88, 89), and this would be predicted to increase the prevalence of IL-17-producing cells.

Implications of effective and ineffective treatments of axial spondyloarthritis

The success of blocking TNFα in the treatment of axSpA (90, 91) clearly underlines the importance of this cytokine in the disease, and the more recent evidence of efficacy in blocking IL-17 (92), and to a lesser extent IL-12/23 (93), also points to their involvement. In contrast, the conspicuous failure of antibodies neutralizing IL-6 (94), or blocking its receptor (95), seemingly excludes a major role for this cytokine—perhaps against expectations, given the role of IL-6 in the production of the Th17 subset of cells. IL-1 can also be involved in the differentiation of Th17 cells, but the reports of the use of IL-1 receptor antagonist in axSpA suggest that it is generally ineffective, except possibly in a small subgroup of patients (96, 97). The relative lack of effect of B-cell depletion has already been noted; the other major 'negative result' is the lack of efficacy of CTLA4-Ig (98). The latter might imply a lack of involvement of T-cell-mediated immunity, since CTLA4-Ig blocks the co-stimulatory signal required to activate T cells. However, it may be that once a pathogenic T-cell response has been established, it is no longer susceptible to CTLA4-Ig blockade, and the same might be true in relation to the need for IL-6/IL-1 in initial differentiation of Th17 cells, but not in their maintenance.

Summary of implications of effective and ineffective treatments of axial spondyloarthritis

Genetic evidence implicates the IL-23/IL-17 pathway in axSpA pathogenesis, and whilst this pathway is not used solely by T cells, there is evidence of Th17 cell involvement. Furthermore, several unusual properties of HLA-B27—its formation of heavy chain multimers and its inefficient folding during synthesis—favour IL-17-producing cells. There is still a dearth of information on the critical antigenic specificity of any pathogenic T cells, and whether self- or bacterial antigens are the dominant targets remains unclear.

Conclusion

Evidence from both animal and human studies strongly points to the involvement of the adaptive immune response in the pathogenesis of axSpA. Whilst the specificity of this response remains undefined—recognition of microbiota is the most likely possibility—its nature is increasingly recognized to involve the IL-23/IL-17 axis, with TNF as an important downstream inflammatory mediator. HLA-B27 has several properties that would facilitate this kind of adaptive immune response.

References

1. Saeed S, Quintin J, Kerstens HH, et al. Epigenetic programming of monocyte-to-macrophage differentiation and trained innate immunity. Science 2014;345(6204):1251086.
2. Seaman WE. Natural killer cells and natural killer T cells. Arthritis Rheum 2000;43(6):1204–17.
3. Breban M, Araujo LM, Chiocchia G. Animal models of spondyloarthritis: do they faithfully mirror human disease? Arthritis Rheum 2014;66(7):1689–92.
4. Taurog JD, Maika SD, Satumtira N, et al. Inflammatory disease in HLA-B27 transgenic rats. Immunol Rev 1999;169:209–23.
5. Tran TM, Dorris ML, Satumtira N, et al. Additional human beta(2)-microglobulin curbs HLA-B27 misfolding and promotes arthritis and spondylitis without colitis in male HLA-B27-transgenic rats. Arthritis Rheum 2006;54(4):1317–27.
6. Breban M, Hacquard-Bouder C, Falgarone G. Animal models of HLA-B27-associated diseases. Curr Mol Med 2004;4(1):31–40.
7. Benjamin R, Parham P. Guilt by association: HLA-B27 and ankylosing spondylitis. Immunol Today 1990;11:137–9.
8. Araujo LM, Fert I, Jouhault Q, et al. Increased production of interleukin-17 over interleukin-10 by treg cells implicates inducible costimulator molecule in experimental spondyloarthritis. Arthritis Rheum 2014;66(9):2412–22.
9. Glatigny S, Fert I, Blaton MA, et al. Proinflammatory Th17 cells are expanded and induced by dendritic cells in spondylarthritis-prone HLA-B27-transgenic rats. Arthritis Rheum 2012;64(1):110–20.
10. Breban M, Fernandezsueiro JL, Richardson JA, et al. T cells, but not thymic exposure to HLA-B27, are required for the inflammatory disease of HLA-B27 transgenic rats. J Immunol 1996;156:794–803.
11. Hoentjen F, Tonkonogy SL, Qian BF, Liu B, Dieleman LA, Sartor RB. CD4(+) T lymphocytes mediate colitis in HLA-B27 transgenic rats monoassociated with nonpathogenic *Bacteroides vulgatus*. Inflamm Bowel Dis 2007;13(3):317–24.
12. Duhen R, Glatigny S, Arbelaez CA, Blair TC, Oukka M, Bettelli E. Cutting edge: the pathogenicity of IFN-gamma-producing Th17 cells is independent of T-bet. J Immunol 2013;190(9):4478–82.
13. Jandus C, Bioley G, Rivals JP, Dudler J, Speiser D, Romero P. Increased numbers of circulating polyfunctional Th17 memory cells in patients with seronegative spondylarthritides. Arthritis Rheum 2008;58(8):2307–17.
14. Cao AT, Yao S, Gong B, Nurieva RI, Elson CO, Cong Y. Interleukin (IL)-21 promotes intestinal IgA response to microbiota. Mucosal Immunol 2015;8(5):1072–82.
15. Smith JA, Colbert RA. Review: the interleukin-23/interleukin-17 axis in spondyloarthritis pathogenesis: Th17 and beyond. Arthritis Rheum 2014;66(2):231–41.
16. Breban M, Hammer RE, Richardson JA, Taurog JD. Transfer of the inflammatory disease of HLA-B27 transgenic rats by bone marrow engraftment. J Exp Med 1993;178:1607–16.
17. Fert I, Glatigny S, Poulain C, et al. Correlation between dendritic cell functional defect and spondylarthritis phenotypes in HLA-B27/HUMAN beta2-microglobulin-transgenic rat lines. Arthritis Rheum 2008;58(11):3425–9.
18. Hacquard-Bouder C, Chimenti MS, Giquel B, et al. Alteration of antigen-independent immunologic synapse formation between dendritic cells from HLA-B27-transgenic rats and CD4+ T cells—selective impairment of costimulatory molecule engagement by mature HLA-B27. Arthritis Rheum 2007;56(5):1478–89.
19. Fert I, Cagnard N, Glatigny S, et al. Reverse interferon signature is characteristic of antigen-presenting cells in human and rat spondyloarthritis. Arthritis Rheum 2014;66(4):841–51.
20. Talpin A, Costantino F, Bonilla N, et al. Monocyte-derived dendritic cells from HLA-B27+ axial spondyloarthritis (SpA) patients display altered functional capacity and deregulated gene expression. Arthritis Res Ther 2014;16(4):417.
21. Kingsbury DJ, Mear JP, Witte DP, Taurog JD, Roopenian DC, Colbert RA. Development of spontaneous arthritis in beta2-microglobulin-deficient mice without expression of HLA-B27: association with deficiency of endogenous major histocompatibility complex class I expression. Arthritis Rheum 2000;43(10):2290–6.
22. Sherlock JP, Joyce-Shaikh B, Turner SP, et al. IL-23 induces spondyloarthropathy by acting on ROR-gt+ CD3+CD4–CD8– entheseal resident T cells. Nat Med 2012;18(7):1069–76.
23. Sakaguchi N, Takahashi T, Hata H, et al. Altered thymic T cell selection due to a mutation of the ZAP-70 gene causes autoimmune arthritis in mice. Nature 2003;426(6965):454–60.
24. Ruutu M, Thomas G, Steck R, et al. Beta-glucan triggers spondylarthritis and Crohn's disease-like ileitis in SKG mice. Arthritis Rheum 2012;64(7):2211–22.
25. Rehaume LM, Mondot S, Aguirre de Carcer D, et al. ZAP-70 genotype disrupts the relationship between microbiota and host, leading to spondyloarthritis and ileitis in SKG mice. Arthritis Rheum 2014;66(10):2780–92.
26. Benham H, Rehaume LM, Hasnain SZ, et al. Interleukin-23 mediates the intestinal response to microbial beta-1,3-glucan and the development of spondyloarthritis pathology in SKG mice. Arthritis Rheum 2014;66(7):1755–67.
27. Armaka M, Apostolaki M, Jacques P, Kontoyiannis DL, Elewaut D, Kollias G. Mesenchymal cell targeting by TNF as a common pathogenic principle in chronic inflammatory joint and intestinal diseases. J Exp Med 2008;205(2):331–7.
28. Jacques P, Lambrecht S, Verheugen E, et al. Proof of concept: enthesitis and new bone formation in spondyloarthritis are driven by mechanical strain and stromal cells. Ann Rheum Dis 2014;73(2):437–45.
29. Baillet AC, Rehaume L, Benham H, et al. High *Chlamydia* burden promotes TNF-dependent reactive arthritis in SKG mice. Arthritis Rheum 2015;67(6):1535–47.
30. Grimble A. Auto-immunity in Reiter's syndrome. Br J Vener Dis 1963;39:246–7.

31. Taurog JD, Rival C, van Duivenvoorde LM, et al. Autoimmune epididymoorchitis is essential to the pathogenesis of male-specific spondylarthritis in HLA-B27-transgenic rats. Arthritis Rheum 2012;64(8):2518–28.
32. de Vries DD, Dekker-Saeys AJ, Gyodi E, Bohm U, Ivanyi P. Absence of autoantibodies to peptides shared by HLA-B27.5 and *Klebsiella pneumoniae* nitrogenase in serum samples from HLA-B27 positive patients with ankylosing spondylitis and Reiter's syndrome. Ann Rheum Dis 1992;51(6):783–9.
33. Lakomek H, Plomann M, Specker C, Schwochau M. Ankylosing spondylitis: an autoimmune disease? Ann Rheum Dis 1991;50(11):776–81.
34. Wright C, Sibani S, Trudgian D, et al. Detection of multiple autoantibodies in patients with ankylosing spondylitis using nucleic acid programmable protein arrays. Mol Cell Proteomics 2012;11(2):M9 00384.
35. Kim YG, Sohn DH, Zhao X, et al. Role of protein phosphatase magnesium-dependent 1A and anti-protein phosphatase magnesium-dependent 1A autoantibodies in ankylosing spondylitis. Arthritis Rheum 2014;66(10):2793–803.
36. Tsui FW, Tsui HW, Las Heras F, Pritzker KP, Inman RD. Serum levels of noggin- and sclerostin-immune complexes are elevated in ankylosing spondylitis. Ann Rheum Dis 2014;73(10):1873–9.
37. Ebringer A, Cox N, Abuljadayel I, et al. *Klebsiella* antibodies in ankylosing spondylitis and *Proteus* antibodies in rheumatoid arthritis. Br J Rheumatol 1988;27(Suppl 2):72–85.
38. Ebringer A. Ankylosing spondylitis is caused by *Klebsiella*. Evidence from immunogenetic, microbiologic, and serologic studies. Rheum Dis Clin N Am 1992;18(1):105–21.
39. Ebringer R, Cooke D, Cawdell DR, Cowling P, Ebringer A. Ankylosing spondylitis: *Klebsiella* and HL-A B27. Rheumatol Rehabil 1977;16(3):190–6.
40. Eastmond CJ, Willshaw HE, Burgess SE, Shinebaum R, Cooke EM, Wright V. Frequency of faecal *Klebsiella aerogenes* in patients with ankylosing spondylitis and controls with respect to individual features of the disease. Ann Rheum Dis 1980;39(2):118–23.
41. Welsh J, Avakian H, Cowling P, et al. Ankylosing spondylitis, HLA-B27 and *Klebsiella*. I. Cross-reactivity studies with rabbit antisera. Br J Exp Pathol 1980;61(1):85–91.
42. Avakian H, Welsh J, Ebringer A, Entwistle CC. Ankylosing spondylitis, HLA-B27 and *Klebsiella*. II. Cross-reactivity studies with human tissue typing sera. Br J Exp Pathol 1980;61(1):92–6.
43. van Bohemen CG, Grumet FC, Zanen HC. Identification of HLA-B27M1 and -M2 cross-reactive antigens in *Klebsiella, Shigella* and *Yersinia*. Immunology 1984;52(4):607–10.
44. Ellis SA, Taylor C, McMichael A. Recognition of HLA-B27 and related antigen by a monoclonal antibody. Hum Immunol 1982;5(1):49–59.
45. DeVries D, Dekker SA, Gyodi E, Bohm U, Ivanyi P. Absence of autoantibodies to peptides shared by HLA B27.5 and *Klebsiella pneumoniae* nitrogenase in serum samples from HLA B27 positive patients with ankylosing spondylitis and Reiter's syndrome. Ann Rheum Dis 1992;51(6):783–9.
46. Maki-Ikola O, Lehtinen K, Granfors K. Similarly increased serum IgA1 and IgA2 subclass antibody levels against *Klebsiella pneumoniae* bacteria in ankylosing spondylitis patients with/without extra-articular features. Br J Rheumatol 1996;35:125–8.
47. Makiikola O, Nissila M, Lehtinen K, Leirisalorepo M, Granfors K. IgA1 and IgA2 subclass antibodies against *Klebsiella pneumoniae* in the sera of patients with peripheral and axial types of ankylosing spondylitis. Ann Rheum Dis 1995;54(8):631–5.
48. Blankenberg-Sprenkels SH, Fielder M, Feltkamp TE, Tiwana H, Wilson C, Ebringer A. Antibodies to *Klebsiella pneumoniae* in Dutch patients with ankylosing spondylitis and acute anterior uveitis and to *Proteus mirabilis* in rheumatoid arthritis. J Rheumatol 1998;25(4):743–7.
49. Ahmadi K, Wilson C, Tiwana H, Binder A, Ebringer A. Antibodies to *Klebsiella pneumoniae* lipopolysaccharide in patients with ankylosing spondylitis. Br J Rheumatol 1998;37(12):1330–3.
50. Nissila M, Lahesmaa R, Leirisalo-Repo M, Lehtinen K, Toivanen P, Granfors K. Antibodies to *Klebsiella pneumoniae, Escherichia coli,* and *Proteus mirabilis* in ankylosing spondylitis: effect of sulfasalazine treatment. J Rheumatol 1994;21(11):2082–7.
51. Mielants H, Veys EM, De Vos M, et al. The evolution of spondyloarthropathies in relation to gut histology. I. Clinical aspects. J Rheumatol 1995;22(12):2266–72.
52. Mielants H, Veys EM, Goemaere S, Cuvelier C, Devos M. A prospective study of patients with spondyloarthropathy with special reference to HLA-B27 and to gut histology. J Rheumatol 1993;20(8):1353–8.
53. Mauri C, Gray D, Mushtaq N, Londei M. Prevention of arthritis by interleukin 10-producing B cells. J Exp Med 2003;197(4):489–501.
54. Carter NA, Vasconcellos R, Rosser EC, et al. Mice lacking endogenous IL-10-producing regulatory B cells develop exacerbated disease and present with an increased frequency of Th1/Th17 but a decrease in regulatory T cells. J Immunol 2011;186(10):5569–79.
55. Song IH, Heldmann F, Rudwaleit M, et al. Different response to rituximab in tumor necrosis factor blocker-naive patients with active ankylosing spondylitis and in patients in whom tumor necrosis factor blockers have failed: a twenty-four-week clinical trial. Arthritis Rheum 2010;62(5):1290–7.
56. Appel H, Kuhne M, Spiekermann S, et al. Immunohistologic analysis of zygapophyseal joints in patients with ankylosing spondylitis. Arthritis Rheum 2006;54(9):2845–51.
57. Appel H, Maier R, Wu P, et al. Analysis of IL-17(+) cells in facet joints of patients with spondyloarthritis suggests that the innate immune pathway might be of greater relevance than the Th17-mediated adaptive immune response. Arthritis Res Ther 2011;13(3):R95.
58. Appel H, Maier R, Bleil J, et al. In situ analysis of interleukin-23- and interleukin-12-positive cells in the spine of patients with ankylosing spondylitis. Arthritis Rheum 2013;65(6):1522–9.
59. May E, Dorris ML, Satumtira N, et al. CD8 alpha beta T cells are not essential to the pathogenesis of arthritis or colitis in HLA-B27 transgenic rats. J Immunol 2003;170(2):1099–105.
60. Shen H, Goodall JC, Gaston JS. Frequency and phenotype of T helper 17 cells in peripheral blood and synovial fluid of patients with reactive arthritis. J Rheumatol 2010;37(10):2096–9.
61. Thomas GP, Brown MA. Genetics and genomics of ankylosing spondylitis. Immunol Rev 2010;233(1):162–80.
62. Kenna TJ, Davidson SI, Duan R, et al. Enrichment of circulating interleukin-17-secreting interleukin-23 receptor-positive gamma/delta T cells in patients with active ankylosing spondylitis. Arthritis Rheum 2012;64(5):1420–9.
63. Hermann E, Yu DTY, Meyer zum Buschenfelde KH, Fleischer B. HLA-B27-restricted CD8 T-cells derived from synovial fluids of patients with reactive arthritis and ankylosing spondylitis. Lancet 1993;342:646–50.
64. Viner N, Bailey L, Life P, Bacon P, Gaston J. Isolation of *Yersinia* specific T cell clones from the synovial membrane and synovial fluid of a patient with reactive arthritis. Arthritis Rheum 1991;34(9):1151–7.
65. Hermann E, Sucke B, Droste U, Meyer zum Buschenfelde KHM. *Klebsiella pneumoniae*-reactive T cells in blood and synovial fluid of patients with ankylosing spondylitis: comparison with HLA-B27+ healthy control subjects in a limiting dilution study and determination of the specificity of synovial fluid T cell clones. Arthritis Rheum 1995;38(9):1277–82.
66. Sakaguchi S. Regulatory T cells: key controllers of immunologic self-tolerance. Cell 2000;101(5):455–8.
67. Jordan M, Boesteanu A, Reed A, et al. Thymic selection of CD4+CD25+ regulatory T cells induced by an agonist self-peptide. Nat Immunol 2001;2:301–6.
68. Jarvis LB, Matyszak MK, Duggleby RC, Goodall JC, Hall FC, Gaston JS. Autoreactive human peripheral blood CD8+ T cells with a regulatory phenotype and function. Eur J Immunol 2005;35(10):2896–908.
69. Jarvis LB, Goodall JC, Gaston JS. Human leukocyte antigen class I-restricted immunosuppression by human CD8+ regulatory T cells requires CTLA-4-mediated interaction with dendritic cells. Hum Immunol 2008;69(11):687–95.
70. Baek HJ, Zhang L, Jarvis LB, Gaston JS. Increased IL-4+ CD8+ T cells in peripheral blood and autoreactive CD8+ T cell lines of

patients with inflammatory arthritis. Rheumatology (Oxford) 2008;47(6):795–803.

71. Zhang L, Jarvis LB, Baek HJ, Gaston JS. Regulatory IL4+CD8+ T cells in patients with ankylosing spondylitis and healthy controls. Ann Rheum Dis 2009;68(8):1345–51.
72. Stagg AJ, Breban M, Hammer RE, Knight SC, Taurog JD. Defective dendritic cell (DC) function in a HLA-B27 transgenic rat model of spondyloarthropathy (SpA). Adv Exp Med Biol 1995;378:557–9.
73. Appel H, Wu P, Scheer R, et al. Synovial and peripheral blood CD4+FoxP3+ T cells in spondyloarthritis. J Rheumatol 2011;38(11):2445–51.
74. Komatsu N, Mariotti-Ferrandiz ME, Wang Y, Malissen B, Waldmann H, Hori S. Heterogeneity of natural Foxp3+ T cells: a committed regulatory T-cell lineage and an uncommitted minor population retaining plasticity. Proc Natl Acad Sci USA 2009;106(6):1903–8.
75. Atagunduz P, Appel H, Kuon W, et al. HLA-B27-restricted CD8+ T cell response to cartilage-derived self peptides in ankylosing spondylitis. Arthritis Rheum 2005;52(3):892–901.
76. Boyle LH, Goodall JC, Opat SS, Gaston JSH. The recognition of HLA-B27 by human CD4(+) T lymphocytes. J Immunol 2001;167(5):2619–24.
77. Allen RL, O'Callaghan CA, McMichael AJ, Bowness P. Cutting edge: HLA-B27 can form a novel beta(2)- microglobulin-free heavy chain homodimer structure. J Immunol 1999;162(9):5045–8.
78. Kollnberger S, Bird L, Sun MY, et al. Cell-surface expression and immune receptor recognition of HLA-B27 homodimers. Arthritis Rheum 2002;46(11):2972–82.
79. Bird LA, Peh CA, Kolinberger S, Elliott T, McMichael AJ, Bowness P. Lymphoblastoid cells express HLA-B27 homodimers both intracellularly and at the cell surface following endosomal recycling. Eur J Immunol 2003;33(3):748–59.
80. Wong-Baeza I, Ridley A, Shaw J, et al. KIR3DL2 binds to HLA-B27 dimers and free H chains more strongly than other HLA class I and promotes the expansion of T cells in ankylosing spondylitis. J Immunol 2013;190(7):3216–24.
81. Bowness P, Ridley A, Shaw J, et al. Th17 cells expressing KIR3DL2+ and responsive to HLA-B27 homodimers are increased in ankylosing spondylitis. J Immunol 2011;186(4):2672–80.
82. Payeli SK, Kollnberger S, Marroquin Belaunzaran O, et al. Inhibiting HLA-B27 homodimer-driven immune cell inflammation in spondylarthritis. Arthritis Rheum 2012;64(10):3139–49.
83. McHugh K, Rysnik O, Kollnberger S, et al. Expression of aberrant HLA-B27 molecules is dependent on B27 dosage and peptide supply. Ann Rheum Dis 2014;73(4):763–70.
84. International Genetics of Ankylosing Spondylitis Consortium, Cortes A, Hadler J, et al. Identification of multiple risk variants for ankylosing spondylitis through high-density genotyping of immune-related loci. Nat Genet 2013;45(7):730–8.
85. Reeves E, Colebatch-Bourn A, Elliott T, Edwards CJ, James E. Functionally distinct ERAP1 allotype combinations distinguish individuals with ankylosing spondylitis. Proc Natl Acad Sci USA 2014;111(49):17594–9.
86. Chen L, Fischer R, Peng Y, et al. Critical role of endoplasmic reticulum aminopeptidase 1 in determining the length and sequence of peptides bound and presented by HLA-B27. Arthritis Rheum. 2014;66(2):284–94.
87. Colbert RA. The immunobiology of HLA-B27: variations on a theme. Curr Mol Med 2004;4(1):21–30.
88. DeLay ML, Turner MJ, Klenk EI, Smith JA, Sowders DP, Colbert RA. HLA-B27 misfolding and the unfolded protein response augment interleukin-23 production and are associated with Th17 activation in transgenic rats. Arthritis Rheum 2009;60(9):2633–43.
89. Goodall JC, Wu C, Zhang Y, et al. Endoplasmic reticulum stress-induced transcription factor, CHOP, is crucial for dendritic cell IL-23 expression. Proc Natl Acad Sci USA 2010;107:17698–703.
90. Braun J, Brandt J, Listing J, et al. Treatment of active ankylosing spondylitis with infliximab: a randomised controlled multicentre trial. Lancet 2002;359(9313):1187–93.
91. Brandt J, Haibel H, Cornely D, et al. Successful treatment of active ankylosing spondylitis with the anti-tumor necrosis factor alpha monoclonal antibody infliximab. Arthritis Rheum 2000;43(6):1346–52.
92. Baeten D, Baraliakos X, Braun J, et al. Anti-interleukin-17A monoclonal antibody secukinumab in treatment of ankylosing spondylitis: a randomised, double-blind, placebo-controlled trial. Lancet 382(9906):1705–13.
93. Poddubnyy D, Hermann KG, Callhoff J, Listing J, Sieper J. Ustekinumab for the treatment of patients with active ankylosing spondylitis: results of a 28-week, prospective, open-label, proof-of-concept study (TOPAS). Ann Rheum Dis 2014;73(5):817–23.
94. Sieper J, Braun J, Kay J, et al. Sarilumab for the treatment of ankylosing spondylitis: results of a phase II, randomised, double-blind, placebo-controlled study (ALIGN). Ann Rheum Dis 2014;74(6):1051–7.
95. Sieper J, Porter-Brown B, Thompson L, Harari O, Dougados M. Assessment of short-term symptomatic efficacy of tocilizumab in ankylosing spondylitis: results of randomised, placebo-controlled trials. Ann Rheum Dis 2014;73(1):95–100.
96. Bennett AN, Tan AL, Coates LC, Emery P, Marzo-Ortega H, McGonagle D. Sustained response to anakinra in ankylosing spondylitis. Rheumatology (Oxford) 2008;47(2):223–4.
97. Haibel H, Rudwaleit M, Listing J, Sieper J. Open label trial of anakinra in active ankylosing spondylitis over 24 weeks. Ann Rheum Dis 2005;64(2):296–8.
98. Song IH, Heldmann F, Rudwaleit M, et al. Treatment of active ankylosing spondylitis with abatacept: an open-label, 24-week pilot study. Ann Rheum Dis 2011;70(6):1108–10.

CHAPTER 9

Infection and spondyloarthritis

Marjatta Leirisalo-Repo and John D. Carter

Introduction to infection and spondyloarthritis

SpA is the designation encompassing a group of inflammatory diseases with several features in common. The patients have mono- or oligoarthritis with or without inflammatory back symptoms. Distinctive extra-articular inflammatory symptoms also characterize the diseases. The diagnostic subgroups in the SpA family include ReA, AS, arthritis associated with IBD, PsA, and some forms of juvenile-onset arthritis. These diseases share a strong association with a genetic marker, HLA-B27, absence of rheumatoid factor, tendency to family aggregation, and frequently occurring EAMs.

This chapter discusses the role of infections, either as triggering of the disease, most evident in the case of ReA, or as possibly contributing factors in the development of chronic forms of SpA and AS.

Reactive arthritis

It has been recognized for many years that venereal infections can trigger a systemic inflammatory arthritis in certain individuals. Because the clinical features of post-enteric ReA and post-venereal ReA are congruent and they cannot be differentiated on clinical features alone, the literature often lumps these together, despite the fact that they have different aetiologic triggers. Indeed, the nomenclature for both is the same—that is, ReA. Although ReA is the preferred term, the literature includes a variety of names to describe this same condition. Perhaps most notable is Reiter syndrome. This eponym was first coined in 1942 when two Harvard researchers, Bauer and Engelmann, noted that Hans Reiter described a classic case of ReA in 1916 (1). Reiter described a German soldier who developed the clinical triad of arthritis, non-gonococcal urethritis, and conjunctivitis after an episode of bloody diarrhoea (2).

Although Reiter is often given credit for describing the first case of ReA, there are several examples of researchers describing ReA many years before Reiter. Reiter's case was a rather clear case of post-enteric ReA. In 1507, Pierre van Forest documented a case of 'secondary arthritis and urethritis' (3). However, patients with post-enteric ReA can sometimes develop urethritis, as documented in Reiter's case, so the aetiologic trigger in Forest's case cannot be accurately determined. In 1818, Sir Benjamin Brodie described the clinical symptoms of ReA most eloquently in his book (4). There he described five patients with a 'train of symptoms' consisting of urethritis, arthritis, and conjunctivitis. However, the potential link to infectious triggers was largely unexplored. The most definitive descriptions of *Chlamydia*-induced ReA (CiReA) date to the 1800s. In 1806, Yvan described a French captain who developed 'ophthalmia' and inflammatory arthritis primarily of the lower extremities 15 days after a venereal infection (5). Eighteen years later, in 1824, Cooper also proposed the concept of the relationship between venereal infection and arthritis, particularly of the lower extremities (6). While both sound typical of CiReA, Yvan and Cooper each surmised that the trigger was *Neisseria gonorrhoea*.

ReA is a classic example of interaction between an environmental factor (infection) and arthritis. The triggering infection is usually in the GI or urogenital tract. The term reactive arthritis was first used by Ahvonen, Sievers, and Aho (7). They described ReA as arthritis that develops soon after or during infection elsewhere in the body, but in which the microorganism cannot be recovered from the joint. The description was used in association with enteric infection caused by *Yersinia enterocolitica* (7), but other Gram-negative microbes causing enteric infections and associated with ReA include *Yersinia pseudotuberculosis* (8, 9), different serovars of *Salmonella enterica* (10, 11), *Campylobacter jejuni* (12,13) and *Campylobacter lari* (14), *Shigella flexneri* (15,16), *Shigella sonnei* (17), and *Shigella dysenteriae* (18), and *Clostridium difficile* (19), and the urogenital pathogen *Chlamydia trachomatis* (20). In about 60% of ReA patients, evidence of previous infection can be detected either by serology or by cultures from urogenital or stool samples (21). In other cases, the role of infection is less distinct and the aetiology can remain undetected. In such cases, the diagnosis is based on clinical features supported by a history of preceding infection.

Reactive arthritis associated with enteric infections

About 1–5% of patients with Gram-negative microbes causing enteric infections are at risk for musculoskeletal symptoms. The total incidence has been estimated to be 10–30 per 100 000 (22, 23–25), with an annual incidence of ReA of 1.3 per 100 000 in *Shigella* (15), 1.8 per 100 000 in *Salmonella* (11), and 4.3 per 100 000 in *Campylobacter* (12) infections.

There is usually a span of 1–4 weeks from the start of infection to the onset of musculoskeletal symptoms. The triggering infection can also be asymptomatic (26, 27). The patients are usually young adults, with a mean age of about 30–40 years; in children the disease is uncommon (28–30). Male and female patients have similar risk for the development of ReA induced by GI infection.

Clinical features of reactive arthritis

The clinical features of post-enteric ReA and CiReA are generally congruent. Typical features of ReA are asymmetric oligoarthritis, often affecting the joints of the lower extremities. In addition to arthritis, patients can have other features common to SpA, such as enthesitis, dactylitis, tendonitis, inflammatory low back pain, arthritis of sternoclavicular joints, skin and nail lesions mimicking psoriasis, and conjunctivitis or AAU.

In terms of the inflammatory joint symptoms of ReA, it is primarily felt to be a peripheral arthritis (18). The most common joints involved tend to be the large joints of the lower extremity. About 50% of patients have arthritis also in their upper limbs. A mild polyarticular form of arthritis in small joints can also occur. The axial system can definitely be involved; indeed, axial involvement might be underrecognized. One of the earliest efforts to analyse a large number of patients with ReA demonstrated that 49% of patients with ReA have back pain as part of their initial presenting symptoms (31). As a comparison from the same study, 28% of patients with PsA had this same complaint. Similarly, 14% of patients with ReA presented with sacroiliitis compared to 7% with PsA in this same analysis. Another study demonstrated that 32% of patients with ReA had axial and upper limb involvement by whole-body scintigraphy; 68% had lower limb involvement (32).

Enthesitis is a term used to describe inflammation at tendon, ligament, and joint capsule insertions. The presence of enthesitis in patients with all types of SpA correlates with axial and peripheral joint involvement (33). Patients can also have dactylitis. Data suggest that enthesitis is more common and dactylitis is less common in ReA compared to PsA (34, 35). It has been suggested that enthesitis is more common than synovitis in ReA (36). Enthesitis and bursitis can occur either in association with arthritis or as the only reactive complication. Other EAMs of SpA include eye symptoms, usually conjunctivitis, less frequently AAU, various skin symptoms, including pustular eruption, erythema nodosum, and keratodermia blenorrhagica, a pustular skin lesion usually observed in the soles of the feet. Circinate balanitis is most frequently associated with *Chlamydia* arthritis but can also occur in ReA with other aetiologies. Erythema nodosum is usually associated with *Yersinia* infection, especially in HLA-B27-negative female patients. In prolonged or chronic cases, onycholysis of the nails resembling those seen in psoriasis can occur.

In a Finnish study, the average duration of ReA was 3–5 months, and about 15% of patients developed chronic sequelae or proceeded into chronic SpA (26). At the 4th International workshop on ReA in 1999, it was suggested that if the symptoms persist longer than 6 months, then the disease should be considered chronic (37). A prolonged (>1-year) extension of the acute arthritis has been described in about 4% of *Yersinia* arthritis, in 19% of *Salmonella* arthritis, in 19% of *Shigella* arthritis, and in 17% of *Chlamydia* arthritis patients (21, 26, 38, 39). In some studies, chronicity has been reported in the vast majority of patients with post-dysentery ReA (40).

An association between ReA and antigen HLA-B27 is well known. In hospital-based series, about 60–80% of the patients carry HLA-B27. Its presence is associated with a more severe arthritis and occurrence of EAMs, and it predicts a prolonged disease. In studies of defined outbreaks and in epidemiological surveys at population level, the picture is different. The disease is usually mild, oligo- or polyarticular, and there is only a slight or no increased frequency of HLA-B27 (41).

Pathophysiology of reactive arthritis

The classical bacteria capable of triggering ReA are Gram-negative obligate and facultative intracellular aerobic bacteria with a lipopolysaccharide-containing outer membrane. They are invasive and cause primary infection of GI mucosa (enteric pathogens) and urogenital mucosa (*C. trachomatis*). The invasiveness of the bacteria is probably affected by genetic factors (HLA-B27), but there is abundant evidence in favour of the hypothesis of an impaired elimination of the microbes in the infected host. In patients with ReA, bacterial antigens seem to disseminate in the body, and *Chlamydia, Yersinia, Salmonella*, and *Shigella* antigens and *Chlamydia* and *Yersinia* DNA (42) and RNA (43) have been detected in synovial fluid and synovial tissue (44–47). As for enterobacteria, however, whether the joint is infected directly is still under debate (48). The pathophysiology of synovial-based *Chlamydiae* is discussed further in the section '*Chlamydia*-induced reactive arthritis'.

An imbalance in the production of proinflammatory cytokines by peripheral blood mononuclear cells during acute arthritis (low TNF production) has been observed (49, 50). Interestingly, IL10. G12 microsatellite polymorphism is associated with reduced risk for the development of ReA, while IL10.G8 polymorphism is a marker of chronicity (51).

According to a hypothesis proposed by Gaston and Lillicrap (52), after invasion via the mucosal route, the microbes persist either in the epithelium or within associated lymphoid tissues, liver, and spleen. The viable organisms or bacterial antigens are disseminated to the joint, causing a local inflammatory response there. A CD4+ T-cell response to the invading microorganism may drive the arthritic process, supported probably also by CD8+ T-cell response. A deviating/poor Th2 cytokine response may favour the persistence of the microbes/microbial antigens and contribute to the poor elimination of the antigens in the host.

While HLA-B27 is not required for the development of ReA, its presence is contributory to the chronicity of the disease. A favourite hypothesis is a cross-reaction between microbial structures and HLA-B27, or that HLA-B27 itself might be a target of the immune response. In general, molecular mimicry as a pathogenic mechanism has been difficult to prove. Nevertheless, the persistence of microbial structures in the host could be explained by an impaired elimination of the microbes by deficient cytokine reaction or defective/aberrant function of HLA-B27 (53). This might also explain the more chronic course of ReA in HLA-B27-positive patients.

Chlamydia-induced reactive arthritis

CiReA represents the classic interplay of host and environment in much the same way as the post-enteric variety. There are, however, some unique features in CiReA, which are addressed here.

In the 1960s and 1970s, it started to become apparent that *C. trachomatis* was indeed an aetiologic trigger of ReA. However, the stealthy role that this bacterium potentially plays in CiReA disease persistence or propagation remains unresolved. ReA in general, and CiReA specifically, was termed a 'sterile arthritis' in the 1970s and 1980s because traditional culture techniques failed to demonstrate live chlamydial organisms in the synovial fluid (20, 54). However, electron microscope (EM) studies performed during that same time period did show what appeared to be intact *Chlamydiae* along with elementary bodies and/or reticulate bodies from synovial samples of patients with a prior infection of that same organism (55, 56). Research in the 1990s began to show that *Chlamydiae* can enter a 'persistent state' in vivo in chronic CiReA; these same organisms can be induced to 'persistence' in in vitro model systems as well (57–60). Recently, the term itself—that is, 'persistence'—has been called into question, as it relates to Chlamydiae, specifically (61). An improved and universal definition of the downregulated, yet viable state of *Chlamydiae* in vivo and its role in disease sequelae is needed.

Clinical features of CiReA

Because the literature often lumps post-venereal ReA and post-enteric ReA as one, it is difficult to determine if the clinical features vary to some degree. Compared with post-enteric ReA, CiReA is more frequently diagnosed in male patients. The incubation time from the infection to the onset of joint symptoms might be longer than in post-enteric ReA. Approximately 5% of patients who experience an acute *C. trachomatis* infection will develop CiReA within about 1–6 weeks of their initial infection (34). It was initially felt that the classic triad of symptoms was arthritis, urethritis, and conjunctivitis, as described by Reiter. However, it is now known that the majority of patients do not present with the classic triad (34). It is important to note that, as in the case of post-enteric ReA, the majority of cases of CiReA spontaneously remit, but the exact percentage has been debated. The disease course of chronic CiReA tends to wax and wane.

Data suggest that patients with chronic CiReA might be more likely to have axial involvement. A study in 2005 assessed the lumbosacral radiographic findings of 95 patients with chronic ReA, demonstrating that 23% of these patients had grade 2–4 sacroiliitis and 14% had syndesmophytes (62). Interestingly, sacroiliitis and syndesmophyte formation were both significantly more common in post-venereal ReA compared to the post-dysentery variant. In a different study involving CiReA patients with an average disease duration of more than 10 years, it was demonstrated that 76% of these patients had axial arthritis and 90% had evidence of at least grade 2 unilateral sacroiliitis (63). The association of the HLA-B27 antigen with ReA, and CiReA specifically, is well established. It has been suggested that HLA-B27 should be considered a risk factor for both chronic disease and axial involvement, rather than a susceptibility factor for CiReA (64).

Enthesitis and dactylitis seem to be more prevalent in CiReA compared with post-enteric ReA. Active enthesitis has been documented in between 50% and 60% of patients with chronic CiReA, specifically (63, 65). Taken together, these data also might suggest that axial involvement is more common in CiReA and ReA in general compared to PsA.

Because CiReA is a type of SpA, it shares the majority of the EAMs with the entire group. One feature that is somewhat specific for ReA and that differentiates it from other types of SpA is conjunctivitis. In a Russian cohort of over 250 patients with ReA, 51% suffered from conjunctivitis (66). Uveitis is another common EAM of ReA, more so than other types of peripheral SpA, such as PsA. In this same Russian cohort, uveitis was more common in patients with chronic ReA (66). Urethritis or cervicitis occurs rather frequently in CiReA, but these same symptoms are rarely seen in the post-enteric variety (26). However, the absence of these symptoms does not rule out ReA; data suggest that asymptomatic initial chlamydial infections are capable of triggering ReA (63, 65). It should also be noted that ReA is associated with specific cutaneous findings—that is, keratoderma blennorrhagicum and circinate balanitis. These can occur also in enteric-triggered ReA, but are more frequently associated with CiReA. Although many consider these to be unique features of ReA that occur in a minority of these patients, these cutaneous lesions cannot be differentiated from pustular psoriasis (37).

Pathophysiology of CiReA

Chlamydia trachomatis is known to be the aetiologic agent for a number of important human diseases. In the setting of CiReA, the infecting *Chlamydiae* are clearly responsible for disease genesis, but some have argued that the initial elicitation of disease by *Chlamydiae* during primary infection might simply be a preliminary for the establishment of a longer term habitation of the host. In CiReA, these infecting *Chlamydiae* undergo transcriptional transformation. When this transformation occurs is not completely understood, but it likely takes place before dissemination. They travel from the initial site of infection via peripheral blood monocytes and then establish residence in the synovial tissue and possibly other organ systems. Others argue that these synovial-based *Chlamydia* simply represent colonization after having triggered an autoinflammatory response.

Although debate continues regarding the true significance of synovial-based *Chlamydiae* in terms of CiReA propagation, much is known about persistent *Chlamydiae*. Chlamydial persistence is well documented by PCR and real-time (RT)-PCR analyses of synovial samples from patients with CiReA (58, 65). The pattern of gene expression is attenuated and significantly different from that seen during normal active infection (67). The evidence of increased IL-10- and TGF-β-secreting cells in the synovial membrane of patients with CiReA compared with RA can also be interpreted as indirect evidence in favour of ineffective elimination of the microbes in the joint thus permitting the prolongation of arthritis (68).

PCR and RT-PCR data demonstrating *Chlamydiae* in the synovial tissue are not unique to patients with CiReA. Reports have described similar findings in a small percentage of patients with osteoarthritis and even normal controls (69–71). These data have called into question the pathologic importance of synovial-based *Chlamydiae* in patients with CiReA. However, the prevalence of *Chlamydiae* in the synovial tissue of patients with other conditions is significantly less compared to synovial tissue of patients with CiReA (65, 66). Surprising recent data have demonstrated that persistent *Chlamydiae* detected in the synovial tissue of patients with CiReA uniquely belong to the ocular, not genital, serovars (72). This perplexing observation might explain two puzzling features of ReA. First, ocular serovars are rarely included as part of the inoculum in genital infections (1–5% of the time); this might explain the attack rate. Second, patients with CiReA often develop ocular symptoms.

Whether these viable synovial-based *Chlamydiae* in the setting of CiReA are the true stimulus of the inflammatory arthritis or have simply triggered a host response remains to be defined; however, the concept of CiReA as a 'sterile arthritis' needs to be revised. Details regarding which genes among the more than 200 in the *C. trachomatis* genome also might contribute to elicitation of the inflammatory response remain to be determined. Chronic synovial pathogenesis and its consequent inflammation must result from a complex process of host–pathogen interaction.

Treatment of reactive arthritis

NSAIDs, corticosteroids, DMARDs, and antibiotics have been assessed as potential therapeutic options for patients with ReA. However, the majority of the therapeutic clinical trials make little effort to separate CiReA from the post-enteric variant. Given the probable differences in the pathophysiology between the two, as outlined in this chapter, this could be a fatal flaw. NSAIDs and corticosteroids are only used for symptomatic relief and there are published studies on their use. The vast majority of treatment data with ReA pertain to the use of antibiotics. These clinical trials have produced apparent conflicting results.

Our understanding the role the causative organisms play in the synovial-based pathophysiology has taught us that in the case of persistent synovial-based *Chlamydiae*, specifically, these organisms exist in a viable, albeit aberrant, state. This important apparent difference in the pathophysiology of post-chlamydial versus post-enteric ReA suggests that these two clinically indistinct entities might need to be considered different in terms of therapeutic approach. The first prospective trial assessing antibiotics as a therapeutic option was performed in 1991 (73). In this trial, patients with both post-chlamydial and post-enteric acute ReA were treated with either lymecycline or placebo in a double-blind fashion for 3 months. Interestingly, lymecycline significantly decreased the duration of illness in those subjects with post-chlamydial ReA, but not those with the post-enteric variety. Critics cited the potential anti-inflammatory effect of lymecycline as the possible explanation of efficacy (74); however, if true, both groups should have fared equally well.

In 2006, Putschky et al. (75) compared in a double-blind controlled study the effect of doxycycline 100 mg bid for 10 days versus 4 months in ReA patients with post-chlamydial ReA. There, the prolonged treatment for 4 months was not superior to short-term treatment. Subsequent studies with various antibiotics suggested no therapeutic benefit, but little effort was made to separate CiReA patients, and all of these trials assessed antibiotic monotherapy (76–79). Furthermore, a double-blind, randomized, placebo-controlled study of 3-month treatment with a combination of ofloxacin and roxithromycin had no advantage over placebo in patients with early active ReA followed up to 6 months (80). Most (84%) of the patients had post-enteric ReA. So the effect of this treatment on CiReA could not be evaluated. A more recent study suggested that a prolonged course of combination antibiotics which included rifampin + doxycycline or rifampin + azithromycin for 6 months in patients with chronic CiReA can not only ameliorate the symptoms but also clear the synovial-based chlamydial infection (81). If the inflammatory process in patients with CiReA can be terminated with combination antibiotics, it could be argued that CiReA meets a reasonable definition of septic arthritis rather than ReA.

The only traditional DMARD that has been assessed as a potential treatment for ReA is SSZ. In a European 6-month, randomized, placebo-controlled double-blind study of patients with SpA treated with SSZ (3 g daily) included also 81 patients with chronic ReA (82). In the whole group of SpA patients, there was a statistically significant difference in favour of SSZ for the patients' overall assessment. The most distinct effect was observed in PsA. ReA patients had considerable treatment response, both in the SSZ and placebo arms, without statistically significant differences between the treatment arms. Another prospective, placebo-controlled trial assessing SSZ at a dose of 2 g/day was assessed in 134 subjects with chronic ReA in a Department of Veterans Affairs Cooperative Study (83). The projected sample size of 240 subjects was not achieved. Using the last observation carried forward technique, the response rates were 62.3% in the SSZ group and 47.7% in the placebo group ($p = 0.089$). A longitudinal analysis did reveal improvement in the subjects taking SSZ compared to placebo ($p = 0.02$). SSZ was analysed in a third double-blind, placebo-controlled study of 6 months' duration (84). In this trial, SSZ was tested in 79 subjects at a dose of 2–3 g per day. An important difference with this trial compared to the previously mentioned SSZ trials was that the study subjects in this trial had acute ReA with mean disease duration of 4.7 months in the SSZ group and 3.9 months in the placebo group. Intention-to-treat analysis revealed no significant difference between the two groups.

There are no randomized trials in ReA to accurately assess the efficacy of TNFi therapy. Several case reports and a small open-label study suggest clinical benefit with these drugs in the treatment of ReA. The limited clinical data we have regarding the TNFi in ReA suggest possible therapeutic benefit (87, 88) without evident reactivation of the inciting infection.

The treatment of chronic CiReA can be challenging. Clinical trial data suggest limited benefit with SSZ and there are no data to show whether the treatment effect might differ in CiReA versus post-enteric ReA. The data with TNFi are very limited, but suggest benefit; however, there is no reason to expect eradication of the root cause in CiReA with this treatment approach. Combination antibiotics which include rifampin, an antibiotic that has effect on *Chlamydia*, might treat the symptoms and the root cause. Interesting data from a CiReA-induced animal model mirror these findings in that TNFi can treat the symptoms and combination antibiotics can prevent the disease (89).

Axial spondyloarthritis

Chronic reactive arthritis or spondyloarthritis?

During acute ReA, inflammatory low back pain is common and a minority of the patients present with radiological sacroiliitis during the first known attack of arthritis (26, 27). During the ensuing years after acute ReA, mild joint pain or enthesopathy is common in patients with previous ReA. Also, one-third of the patients have occasional attacks of low back pain (26, 90, 91). In patients with previous post-enteric ReA, signs and symptoms of chronic SpA occur in 14% (92). The long-term outcome of acute ReA during the following 10–20 years is dependent on the triggering infection and on the follow-time: chronic arthritis is observed in 2–18% (38, 39), sacroiliitis in 14–49% (26, 38, 39), and AS in 12–26% (39, 40). Patients with HLA-B27 have a worse prognosis (26). It is still uncertain to what extent ReA contributes to the development of sacroiliitis or AS, or whether SI changes would have developed in a subject with the appropriate genetic background even in the absence of intervening ReA.

As reviewed in the section 'Pathophysiology of reactive arthritis', bacteria seem to persist for prolonged periods and trigger immune response in patients with acute ReA. The crucial question is whether the assumed autoimmune disease runs an independent course after the initial bacterial trigger, or whether a chronic interaction of the immune system with persisting bacteria is necessary to result in a chronic immune response against self-antigens. For a prolonged/chronic course of ReA and the development of SpA, the interaction between microbial antigens and HLA-B27 seems to be important. The arthritogenic peptide hypothesis is one of the most favoured to explain the association, and HLA-B27-restricted peptides from *Chlamydia* and *Yersinia* have been identified; the peptides are stimulatory for CD8+ T cells derived from patients with ReA. In addition to aberration in the T-cell immune response, defective innate immunity has been suggested to be playing a role in the first-line defence and clearing of the infection (93).

Role of infection in the development of chronic spondyloarthritis

Factors determining the progression of acute ReA to chronic SpA are incompletely known, but persistent or recurrent urogenital infection or chronic inflammatory focus in the gut could be candidates. *Yersinia* structures have been shown to persist in submucosa of the gut (94), and in lymph nodes of patients with prolonged or chronic *Yersinia* arthritis (95, 96). *Chlamydia trachomatis* persists for prolonged period in the infected host. There is evidence for the presence of whole *Chlamydiae* in the synovial fluid and/or tissue in patients with seronegative arthritis with persisting synovitis for months or even for years (97–99).

In concert with the infection, the presence of HLA-B27 is also an important factor in the progression of the disease to chronic SpA or AS.

Gut and microbes in the pathogenesis of spondyloarthritis

IBD and Gram-negative microbial infections in the gut are well known to be associated with SpA and ReA. It is also now recognized that about half of the SpA patients show microscopic gut inflammation. If chronic, they associate with an increased risk for the progression of SpA to AS, as reviewed by De Wilde et al. (100). Interestingly, recent studies have shown that SpA patients have gut inflammation already early in the SpA, and the lesions correlate with disease activity and degree of SI joint inflammation, as shown by MRI (100). AS patients have increased gut permeability, and this has been proposed as a mechanism for dissemination of microbial antigens to the host. Interestingly, in Mexican patients with juvenile-onset SpA (JoSpA), a very severe form of arthritis, the presence of microbial DNA of *Salmonella, Shigella, Campylobacter*, and *Mycobacterium tuberculosis* has been detected (101). For the rest of the patients with SpA, there is also some evidence for the contribution of milieu factors in the pathogenesis/symptoms of the patients. HLA-B27 is probably the link between increased permeability and enhanced inflammatory response. This is evidenced by the HLA-B27 tg rats, which develop gut and joint inflammation. However, if the animals are housed in germ-free conditions, they do not develop such features (100). In addition to HLA-B27, animal models have shown the importance of the IL-23/IL-17 pathway in the development of chronic inflammatory conditions mimicking SpA and IBD. An increased load of Gram-negative pathogens probably also contributes to the peripheral and axial arthritis in patients with IBD.

A newer concept suggests that the microbiome, or microbiota, can potentially be aetiologic for several different types of inflammatory arthritis, including SpA (102–104). The human microbiome is the population of more than 100 trillion microorganisms that live in the gut, mouth, skin, and elsewhere in our bodies. The microbiome can lead to dysbiosis, which, in turn, may set the stage for a range of human diseases. Interestingly, the gut microbiome seen in patients with PsA is similar to that of patients with IBD (104).

Patients with active SpA and AS are often treated with TNFi. An increased risk for infections is a common feature of these drugs when used to treat patients with rheumatic conditions. The limited data to date about the flare of the background infections in SpA in this context are reassuring. In an uncontrolled study, infection rate was 3.93 per 100 patient years. Out of the patients who developed infections, nine (4%) presented with a relapse and 21 (9.3%) with a single infection episode (105). Compared with SpA patients treated conventionally, the use of TNFi therapy was not associated with higher rates of infections (106). Furthermore, when comparing the biological register data of patients with RA and SpA, no significant increase was observed in SpA patients in the incidence of severe infections (107).

Ankylosing spondylitis

The debate regarding the potential role that bacteria play in the aetiology and pathophysiology of SpA has been, perhaps, the most contested with AS.

The best evidence in favour is in the case of ReA and the long-term outcome of such patients. As discussed in the section 'Clinical features of reactive arthritis', after preceding bacterial infections of the gut with enterobacteriae or the urogenital tract with *C. trachomatis*, ReA occurs in 1–5% of these patients, 30–70% of these patients being positive for HLA-B27. About 20–40% of these patients develop, if they are positive for HLA-B27, the full clinical picture of AS, which can develop 10–20 years after the initial infection (108).

In less than 10% of AS patients is a preceding infection or IBD evident, but infections with ReA-associated bacteria and gut lesions in patients with IBD are often subclinical (109). The question whether asymptomatic or uncomplicated infection would lead to the development of AS has not been rigorously answered yet. There are some reports that would speak in favour of the hypothesis. Interestingly, 2 out of 94 patients with acute uncomplicated gut infection with *Yersinia enterocolitica* outbreak when examined 13 years later had AS, both HLA-B27 positive (110). Also, patients with pelvic inflammatory disease due to *C. trachomatis* can develop sacroiliitis. HLA-B27-positive patients have higher frequency of symptomatic sacroiliitis (111). Also, a higher frequency of positive *Chlamydia* antibodies has been reported in patients with AS of long duration (33%) compared with patients with RA (8%) or controls (18%) (112). In the AS patients, the presence of *Chlamydia* antibodies was associated with a history of acute anterior uveitis, whereas active *Chlamydia* infection was as common in AS patients as in matched controls (113). From these results it can be interpreted that an infection might be able to trigger the pathogenic mechanisms, which later manifest themselves as 'primary AS'. Thus, at least in some of the AS patients, a bacterial trigger plays a role in the pathogenesis of the disease.

In established AS or chronic SpA, a flare of the disease is not usually suspected to be related to an infection. However, interestingly, Martínez et al. (114) described the relationship between the disease activity and a history of recent infection, especially enteric infection in SpA patients. Furthermore, Lange et al. (115) reported *Chlamydia*-induced urethral syndrome in 15 out of 32 female AS patients; the infected patients had higher incidence of enthesopathy, involvement of the spine, and higher ESR and CRP levels compared with the rest of the patients. A recent case report describes the development of acute arthritis and severe bilateral anterior uveitis in an AS patient 6 weeks after infection with urethral *C. trachomatis*. The AS had been well controlled with ETN and MTX for 3 years (116).

It has been suggested that *Klebsiella pneumoniae* (Kp) is responsible for disease initiation in AS (117). Early reports suggesting that Kp is aetiologic for AS demonstrated increase prevalence of Kp in the stool microflora of patients with this condition; this same study suggested a correlation with Kp and AS disease activity (117). Proponents continue to cite several reasons for this association, including molecular mimicry between *Klebsiella* and the HLA-B27 antigen and increased antibodies to *Klebsiella* in AS patients (118). Other studies indicate that CD4+ and CD8+ T cells are stimulated by *Klebsiella* HSP60 in the majority of patients with AS, whereas this response was absent in normal controls (119). HLA-B27+ and HLA-B27− AS patients both recognize the same epitope of Kp; however, there is a different quantitative response (120). Conversely, early data questioned the relationship between *Klebsiella* and AS (121), and more recent data suggest no differences in cellular or humoral immune responses with respect to *Klebsiella* in patients with AS, unaffected family members, or normal controls (122).

The arthritogenic peptide theory has been proposed as a key pathogenic mechanism in AS. The presentation of pathogenic antigens, either self-antigens or peptides derived from intracellular pathogens, bound to HLA-B27, activates cytotoxic lymphocytes, which cross-react on molecularly similar self-peptides. This hypothesis was also recently approached by analysing more than 7500 self-peptides presented by eight different HLA-B27 allotypes. The study did not confirm but did not completely exclude the theory. It revealed considerable overlap between all alleles independent of disease association. Allelic polymorphisms resulting in changes in the amino acid composition of the antigen-binding cleft manifested largely as quantitative changes in the peptide cargo of these molecules (123).

More recently, another stool microflora, specifically *Bacteroides*, has been implicated as a possible aetiologic agent for AS (124). A significantly higher prevalence of sulphate-reducing bacteria was demonstrated in 15 AS patients compared to 15 controls. In addition, there was indication of a possible loss of immunological tolerance to *Bacteroides*. This same group performed follow-up studies suggesting that reduced IL-10 production in response to stimulation with autologous *Bacteroides* allows inflammation to develop and persist in AS patients (125).

The possibility remains that *Bacteroides*, or *Klebsiella*, or other enteric organisms could play a role in shaping the gut microbiome. A recent study investigated whether the AS gut carries a distinct microbial signature (126). Microbial profiles from terminal ileal biopsies from subjects with recent-onset, TNFi-naïve AS and healthy controls were generated using culture-independent 16S rRNA gene sequencing and analysis techniques. The terminal ileal microbial communities of patients with AS differed significantly from healthy controls. Recent animal data have also demonstrated that HLA-B27 is associated with altered caecal microbiota (127). Perhaps the definitive missing link lies in the newly discovered genetic contributions of AS and how these genes might interact with HLA-B27 in the presence of certain stool microflora.

Conclusion

In conclusion, infections do play an important role in SpA, as triggers of ReA, and can contribute to the development of chronic musculoskeletal diseases. The eradication of the triggering microbe has been very challenging from the point of cure of the arthritis. The recent advances in use of combination antibiotic therapies to eradicate *Chlamydia* and the recognition of the role of the gut microbiome in the immunopathogenesis of SpA open up new opportunities for the future.

References

1. Bauer W, Engelmann EP. Syndrome of unknown aetiology characterized by urethritis, conjunctivitis, and arthritis (so-called Reiter's Disease). Trans Assoc Am Physics 1942;57:307–8.
2. Reiter H. Uber eine bisher unerkannate Spirochateninfektion (Spirochetosis arthritica). Dtsch Med Wochenschr 1916;42:1535–6.
3. Sharp JT. Reiter's syndrome. In: Hollander JH, McCarthy DJ (eds) Arthritis and Allied Conditions, 8th edn. Philadelphia, Lea and Febiger, 1979, pp. 1223–9.
4. Brodie BC. Pathological and Surgical Observations on Diseases of the Joints. London, Longman, 1818, p.54.
5. Yvan AU. Observation sur une metastase de gonorrhee. Ann Soc Med Prat Montpellier 1806:119–25.
6. Cooper A. On gonorrhoeal rheumatism. On gonorrhoeal ophthalmia. Lancet 1824;2:273–4.
7. Ahvonen P, Sievers K, Aho K. Arthritis associated with *Yersinia enterocolitica* infection. Acta Rheum Scand 1969;15:232–53.
8. Tertti R, Granfors K, Lehtonen O-P, et al. An outbreak of *Yersinia pseudotuberculosis* infection. J Infect Dis 1984;149:245–50.
9. Hannu T, Mattila L, Nuorti JP, et al. Reactive arthritis after an outbreak of *Yersinia pseudotuberculosis* serotype O:3 infection. Ann Rheum Dis 2003;62:866–9.
10. Mäki-Ikola O, Granfors K. *Salmonella*-triggered reactive arthritis. Scand J Rheumatol 1992;21:265–70.
11. Tuompo R, Hannu T, Mattila L, Siitonen A, Leirisalo-Repo M. Reactive arthritis following *Salmonella* infection: a population-based study. 2013. Scand J Rheumatol 2013;42:196–202.
12. Hannu T, Mattila L, Rautelin H, et al. *Campylobacter*-triggered reactive arthritis: a population-based study. Rheumatology 2002;41:312–18.
13. Peterson MC. Clinical aspects of *Campylobacter jejuni* infections in adults. West J Med 1994;161:148–52.
14. Goudswaard J, Sabbe L, te Winkel W. Reactive arthritis as a complication of *Campylobacter lari* enteritis (letter). J Infection 1995;31:171–6.
15. Hannu T, Mattila L, Siitonen A, Leirisalo-Repo M. Reactive arthritis attributable to *Shigella* infection: a clinical and epidemiological nationwide study. Ann Rheum Dis 2005;64:594–8.
16. Paronen I. Reiter's disease. A study of 344 cases observed in Finland. Acta Med Scand 1948;131(Suppl 212):1–113.
17. Lauhio A, Lähdevirta J, Janes R, Kontiainen S, Repo H. Reactive arthritis associated with *Shigella sonnei* infection. Arthritis Rheum 1988;31:1190–3.
18. Mazumder RN, Salam MA, Ali MA, Bhattacharya MK. Reactive arthritis associated with *Shigella dysenteriae* type I infection. J Diarrhoel Dis Res 1997;15:21–4.
19. Putterman C, Rubinow A. Reactive arthritis associated with *Clostridium difficile* pseudomembranous colitis. Semin Arthritis Rheum 1993;22:420–6.
20. Keat A, Thomas B, Dixey J, Osborn M, Sonnex C, Taylor-Robinson D. *Chlamydia trachomatis* and reactive arthritis: the missing link. Lancet 1987; :72–4.
21. Keat A. Reiter's syndrome and reactive arthritis in perspective. N Engl J Med 1983;309:1606–15.
22. Savolainen E, Kaipiainen-Seppanen O, Kroger L, Luosujarvi R. Total incidence and distribution of inflammatory joint diseases in a defined population: results from the Kuopio 2000 arthritis survey. J Rheumatol 2003;30:2460–8.
23. Isomaki H, Raunio J, von Essen R, Hameenkorpi R. Incidence of inflammatory rheumatic diseases in Finland. Scand J Rheumatol 1978;7:188–92.
24. Kvien TK, Glennas A, Melby K, et al. Reactive arthritis: incidence, triggering agents and clinical presentation. J Rheumatol 1994;21:115–22.
25. Soderlin MK, Borjesson O, Kautiainen H, Skogh T, Leirisalo-Repo M. Annual incidence of inflammatory joint diseases in a population based study in southern Sweden. Ann Rheum Dis 2002;61:911–15.

26. Leirisalo M, Skylv G, Kousa M, et al. Followup study on patients with Reiter's disease and reactive arthritis, with special reference to HLA-B27. Arthritis Rheum 1982;25:249–59.
27. Hannu TJ, Leirisalo-Repo M. Clinical picture of reactive *Salmonella* arthritis. J Rheumatol 1988;15:1668–71.
28. Mattila L, Leirisalo-Repo M, Koskimies S, Granfors K, Siitonen A. Reactive arthritis following an outbreak of *Salmonella* infection in Finland. Br J Rheumatol 1994;33:1136–41.
29. Mattila L, Leirisalo-Repo M, Pelkonen P, Koskimies S, Granfors K, Siitonen A. Reactive arthritis following an outbreak of *Salmonella bovismorbificans* infection. J Infect 1998;36:289–95.
30. Rudwaleit M, Richter S, Braun J, Sieper J. Low incidence of reactive arthritis in children following a *Salmonella* outbreak. Ann Rheum Dis 2001;60:1055–7.
31. Willkens RF, Arnett FC, Bitter T, et al. Reiter's syndrome: evaluation of proposed criteria. Ann Rheum Dis 1979;38(Suppl 1):8–11.
32. Kim SH, Chung SK, Bahk YW, Park YH, Lee SY, Sohn HS. Whole-body and pinhole bone scintigraphic manifestations of Reiter's syndrome: distribution patterns and early and characteristic signs. Eur J Nucl Med 1999;26:163–70.
33. Carneiro S, Bortoluzzo A, Gonçalves C, et al. Effect of enthesitis on 1505 Brazilian patients with spondyloarthritis. J Rheumatol 2013;40:1719–25.
34. Carter JD, Hudson AP. Reactive arthritis: clinical aspects and medical management. Rheum Dis Clin North Am 2009;35:21–44.
35. Pavlica L, Mitrović D, Mladenović V, Popović M, Krstić S, Anđelković Z. Reiter's syndrome—analysis of 187 patients. Vojnosanit Pregl 1997;54:437–46.
36. Townes JM, Deodhar AA, Laine ES, et al. Reactive arthritis following culture-confirmed infections with bacterial enteric pathogens in Minnesota and Oregon: a population-based study. Ann Rheum Dis 2008;67:1689–96.
37. Braun J, Kingsley G, van der Heijde D, Sieper J. On the difficulties of establishing a consensus on the definition of and diagnostic investigations for reactive arthritis. Results and discussion of a questionnaire prepared for the 4th International Workshop on Reactive Arthritis, Berlin, 3–6 July 1999. J Rheumatol 2000;27:2185–92.
38. Leirisalo-Repo M, Suoranta H. Ten year follow-up study of patients with *Yersinia* arthritis. Arthritis Rheum 1988;31:533–7.
39. Leirisalo-Repo M, Helenius P, Hannu T, et al. Long-term prognosis of reactive *Salmonella* arthritis. Ann Rheum Dis 1997;56:516–20.
40. Sairanen E, Paronen I, Mahonen H. Reiter's syndrome: a follow-up study. Acta Med Scand 1969;185:57–63.
41. Leirisalo-Repo M, Hannu T, Mattila L. Microbial factors in spondyloarthropathies: insights from population studies. Curr Opin Rheumatol 2003;15:408–12.
42. Wilkinson NZ, Kingsley GH, Jones HW, Sieper J, Braun J, Ward ME. The detection of DNA from a range of bacterial species in the joints of patients with a variety of arthritides using a nested, broad-range polymerase chain reaction. Rheumatology (Oxford) 1999;38:260–6.
43. Cox CJ, Kempsell KE, Gaston JS. Investigation of infectious agents associated with arthritis by reverse transcription PCR of bacterial rRNA. Arthritis Res Ther 2003;5:R1–8.
44. Granfors K, Jalkanen S, von Essen R, et al. *Yersinia* antigens in synovial-fluid cells from patients with reactive arthritis. N Engl J Med 1989;320:216–21.
45. Granfors K, Jalkanen S, Lindberg AA, et al. *Salmonella* lipopolysaccharide in synovial cells from patients with reactive arthritis. Lancet 1990;335:685–8.
46. Keat AC, Thomas BJ, Taylor-Robinson D, Pegrum GD, Maini RN, Scott JT. Evidence of *Chlamydia trachomatis* infection in sexually acquired reactive arthritis. Ann Rheum Dis 1980;39:431–7.
47. Granfors K, Jalkanen S, Toivanen P, Koski J, Lindberg AA. Bacterial lipopolysaccharide in synovial fluid cells in *Shigella* triggered reactive arthritis. J Rheumatol 1992;19:500.
48. Rihl M, Klos A, Köhler L, Kuipers JG. Infection and musculoskeletal conditions. Reactive arthritis. Best Pract Res Clin Rheumatol 2006;20:1119–37.
49. Braun J, Yin Z, Spiller I, et al. Low secretion of tumor necrosis factor alpha, but no other Th1 or Th2 cytokines, by peripheral blood mononuclear cells correlates with chronicity in reactive arthritis. Arthritis Rheum 1999;42:2039–44.
50. Butrimiene I, Jarmalaite S, Ranceva J, Venalis A, Jasiuleviciute L, Zvirbliene A. Different cytokine profiles in patients with chronic and acute reactive arthritis. Rheumatology (Oxford) 2004;43:1300–4.
51. Kaluza W, Leirisalo-Repo M, Marker-Hermann E, et al. IL10.G microsatellites mark promoter haplotypes associated with protection against the development of reactive arthritis in Finnish patients. Arthritis Rheum 2001;44:1209–14.
52. Gaston HJS, Lillicrap MS. Arthritis associated with enteric infection. Best Pract Res Clin Rheumatol 2003;17:219–39.
53. McMichael A, Bowness P. HLA-B27: natural function and pathogenic role in spondyloarthritis. Arthritis Res 2002;4(Suppl 3):S153–8.
54. Gordon FB, Quan AL, Steinman TI, Philips RN. Chlamydial isolates from Reiter's syndrome. Br J Vener Dis 1973;49:376–8.
55. Norton WL, Lewis D, Ziff M. Light and electron microscopic observation on the synovitis of Reiter's disease. Arthritis Rheum 1966;9:747–57.
56. Ishikawa H, Ohno O, Yamasaki K, Ikuta S, Hirohata K. Arthritis presumably caused by *Chlamydia* in Reiter's syndrome. Case report with electron microscopic studies. J Bone Joint Surg 1986;68:777–9.
57. Köhler L, Nettelnbreker E, Hudson AP, et al. Ultrastructural and molecular analysis of the persistence of *Chlamydia trachomatis* (serovar K) in human monocytes. Microb Pathogen 1997;22:133–42.
58. Gerard HC, Branigan PJ, Schumacher HR Jr, Hudson AP. Synovial *Chlamydia trachomatis* in patients with reactive arthritis/Reiter's syndrome are viable but show aberrant gene expression. J Rheumatol 1998;25:734–42.
59. Beatty WL, Morrison RP, Byrne GI. Persistent *Chlamydiae*: from cell culture to a paradigm for chlamydial pathogenesis. Microbiol Rev 1994;58:686–99.
60. Moulder JW. Interaction of *Chlamydiae* and host cells in vitro. Microbiol Rev 1991;55:143–90.
61. Bavoil PM. What's in a word: the use, misuse, and abuse of the word 'persistence' in *Chlamydia* biology. Front Cell Infect Microbiol 2014;4:27.
62. Mannoja A, Pekkola J, Hämäläinen M, Leirisalo-Repo M, Laasonen L, Kivisaari L. Lumbosacral radiographic signs in patients with previous enteroarthritis or uroarthritis. Ann Rheum Dis 2005; 64:936–9.
63. Carter JD, Espinoza LR, Inman RD, et al. Combination antibiotics as a treatment for chronic *Chlamydia*-induced reactive arthritis: a double-blind, placebo-controlled, prospective study. Arthritis Rheum 2010;62:1298–307.
64. Zeidler H, Kuipers J, Köhler L. *Chlamydia*-induced arthritis. Curr Opin Rheumatol 2004;16:380–92.
65. Carter JD, Gérard HC, Espinoza LR, et al. *Chlamydiae* as etiologic agents in chronic undifferentiated spondylarthritis. Arthritis Rheum 2009;60:1311–16.
66. Kovalev IuN, Il'in II. Ophthalmological aspects of Reiter's disease. Vestn Oftalmol 1990;106:65–9.
67. Gerard HC, Whittum-Hudson JA, Schumacher HR, Hudson AP. Differential expression of three *Chlamydia trachomatis* hsp60-encoding genes in active vs. persistent infections. Microb Pathog 2004;36:35–9.
68. Appel H, Neure L, Kuhne M, Braun J, Rudwaleit M, Sieper J. An elevated level of IL-10- and TGF beta-secreting T cells, B cells and macrophages in the synovial membrane of patients with reactive arthritis compared to rheumatoid arthritis. Clin Rheumatol 2004;23:435–40.
69. Wilkinson NZ, Kingsley GH, Jones HW, et al. The detection of DNA from a range of bacterial species in the joints of patients with a variety of arthritidies using a nested, broad-range polymerase chain reaction. Rheumatology 1999;38:260–6.
70. Schumacher HR, Arayssi T, Crane M, et al. *Chlamydia trachomatis* nucleic acids can be found in synovium of some asymptomatic volunteers. Arthritis Rheum 1999;42:1281–4.

71. Olmez N, Wang GF, Li Y, Zhang H, Schumacher HR. Chlamydial nucleic acids in synovium in osteoarthritis: what are the implications? J Rheumatol 2001;28:1874–80.
72. Gerard HC, Stanich JA, Whittum-Hudson JA, Schumacher HR, Carter JD, Hudson AP. Patients with *Chlamydia*-associated arthritis have ocular (trachoma), not genital, serovars of *C. trachomatis* in synovial tissue. Microb Pathog 2010;48:62–8.
73. Lauhio A, Leirisalo-Repo M, Lahdevirta J, Saikku P, Repo H. Double-blind, placebo-controlled study of three-month treatment with lymecycline in reactive arthritis, with special reference to *Chlamydia* arthritis. Arthritis Rheum 1991;34:6–14.
74. Sadowski T, Steinmeyer J. Minocycline inhibits the production of inducible nitric oxide synthase in articular chondrocytes. J Rheumatol 2001;28:336–40.
75. Putschky N, Pott HG, Kuipers JG, Zeidler H, Hammer M, Wollenhaupt J. Comparing 10-day and 4-month doxycycline courses for treatment of *Chlamydia* trachomatis-reactive arthritis: a prospective, double-blind trial. Ann Rheum Dis 65:1521–4.
76. Kvien TK, Gaston JS, Bardin T, et al. Three-month treatment of reactive arthritis with azithromycin: a EULAR double-blind, placebo-controlled study. Ann Rheum Dis 2004;63:1113–19.
77. Smieja M, MacPherson DW, Kean W, et al. Randomised, blinded, placebo controlled trial of doxycycline for chronic seronegative arthritis. Ann Rheum Dis 2001;60:1088–94.
78. Wakefield D, McCluskey P, Verma M, Aziz K, Gatus B, Carr G. Ciprofloxacin treatment does not influence course or relapse rate of reactive arthritis and anterior uveitis. Arthritis Rheum 1999;42:1894–7.
79. Yli-Kerttula T, Luukkainen R, Yli-Kerttula U, et al. Effect of a three month course of ciprofloxacin on the outcome of reactive arthritis. Ann Rheum Dis 2000;59:565–70.
80. Kuuliala A, Paimela L, Peltomaa R, et al. Double-blind, placebo-controlled study of three-month treatment with the combination of ofloxacin and roxithromycin in recent-onset reactive arthritis. Rheumatol Int 2013;33:2723–9.
81. Carter JD, Espinoza LR, Inman RD, et al. Combination antibiotics as a treatment for chronic *Chlamydia*-induced reactive arthritis: a double-blind, placebo-controlled, prospective trial. Arthritis Rheum 2010;62:1298–307.
82. Dougados M, van der Linden S, Leirisalo-Repo M, et al. Sulfasalazine in the treatment of spondylarthropathy: a randomized, multi-center, double-blind, placebo-controlled study. Arthritis Rheum 1995;38:618–27.
83. Clegg DO, Reda DJ, Weisman MH, et al. Comparison of sulfasalazine and placebo in the treatment of reactive arthritis (Reiter's syndrome). A Department of Veterans Affairs Cooperative Study. Arthritis Rheum 1996;39:2021–7.
84. Egsmose C, Hansen TM, Andersen LS, et al. Limited effect of sulfasalazine treatment in reactive arthritis. A randomized double blind placebo controlled trial. Ann Rheum Dis 1997;56:32–6.
85. Flagg SD, Meador R, Hsia E, Kitumnuaypong T, Schumacher HR Jr. Decreased pain and synovial inflammation after etanercept therapy in patients with reactive and undifferentiated arthritis: an open-label trial. Arthritis Rheum 2005;53:613–17.
86. Oili KS, Niinisalo H, Korpilahde T, Virolainen J. Treatment of reactive arthritis with infliximab. Scand J Rheumatol 2003;32:122–4.
87. Schrafranski MD. Infliximab for reactive arthritis secondary to *Chlamydia trachomatis* infection. Rheumatol Int 2010;30:679–80.
88. Meyer A, Chatelus E, Wendling D, et al. Safety and efficacy of anti-tumor necrosis factor α therapy in ten patients with recent-onset refractory reactive arthritis. Arthritis Rheum 2011;63:1274–80.
89. Baillet AC, Rehaume L, Benham H, et al. High *Chlamydia* burden promotes TNF-dependent reactive arthritis in SKG mice. Arthritis Rheum 2015;67:1535–47.
90. Fox R, Calin A, Gerber RC, Gibson D. The chronicity of symptoms and disability in Reiter's syndrome. An analysis of 131 consecutive patients. Ann Intern Med 1979;91:190–3.
91. Good AE. Reiter's syndrome: long-term follow-up in relation to development of ankylosing spondylitis. Ann Rheum Dis 1979;38(Suppl 1): 39–45.
92. Kruger K, Schattenkirchner M. [Reactive arthritis—clinical aspects and course.] Wien Klin Wochenschr 1983;95:884–9.
93. Zhang X, Glogauer M, Zhu F, Kim TH, Chiu B, Inman RD. Innate immunity and arthritis: neutrophil Rac and toll-like receptor 4 expression define outcomes in infection-triggered arthritis. Arthritis Rheum 2005;52:1297–304.
94. Hoogkamp-Korstanje JA. Antibiotics in *Yersinia enterocolitica* infections. J Antimicrob Chemother 1987;20:123–31.
95. Hoogkamp-Korstanje JA, de Koning J, Heesemann J. Persistence of *Yersinia enterocolitica* in man. Infection 1988;16:81–5.
96. Hoogkamp-Korstanje JA, de Koning J, Heesemann J, Festen JJ, Houtman PM, van Oyen PL. Influence of antibiotics on IgA and IgG response and persistence of *Yersinia enterocolitica* in patients with *Yersinia*-associated spondylarthropathy. Infection 1992;20:53–7.
97. Bas S, Griffais R, Kvien TK, Glennas A, Melby K, Vischer TL. Amplification of plasmid and chromosome *Chlamydia* DNA in synovial fluid of patients with reactive arthritis and undifferentiated seronegative oligoarthropathies. Arthritis Rheum 1995;38:1005–13.
98. Sieper J, Braun J, Brandt J, et al. Pathogenetic role of *Chlamydia, Yersinia* and *Borrelia* in undifferentiated oligoarthritis. J Rheumatol 1992;19:1236–42.
99. Gerard HC, Branigan PJ, Schumacher HR Jr, Hudson AP. Synovial *Chlamydia trachomatis* in patients with reactive arthritis/Reiter's syndrome are viable but show aberrant gene expression. J Rheumatol 1998;25:734–42.
100. De Wilde K, Debusschere K, Beeckman S, Jacques P, Elewaut D. Integrating the pathogenesis of spondyloarthritis: gut and joint united? Curr Opin Rheumatol 2015;27:189–96.
101. Pacheco-Tena C, Alvarado DLB, Lopez-Vidal Y, et al. Bacterial DNA in synovial fluid cells of patients with juvenile onset spondyloarthropathies. Rheumatology (Oxford) 2001;40:920–7.
102. Scher JU, Abramson SB. The microbiome and rheumatoid arthritis. Nat Rev Rheumatol 2011;7:569–78.
103. McLean MH, Dieguez D Jr, Miller LM, Young HA. Does the microbiota play a role in the pathogenesis of autoimmune diseases? Gut 2015;64:332–41.
104. Scher JU, Ubeda C, Artacho A, et al. Decreased bacterial diversity characterizes the altered gut microbiota in patients with psoriatic arthritis, resembling dysbiosis in inflammatory bowel disease. Arthritis Rheum 2015;67:128–39.
105. Modesti V, Ramonda R, Ortolan A, et al. Infection relapse in spondyloarthritis treated with biological drugs: a single-centre study. Scand J Rheumatol 2012; 41:490–1.
106. Wallis D, Thavaneswaran A, Haroon N, Ayearst R, Inman RD. Tumour necrosis factor inhibitor therapy and infection risk in axial spondyloarthritis: results from a longitudinal observational cohort. Rheumatology (Oxford) 2015;54:152–6.
107. Sampaio-Barros PD, van der Horst-Bruinsma IE. Adverse effects of TNF inhibitors in SpA: are they different from RA? Best Pract Res Clin Rheumatol 2014;28:747–63.
108. Leirisalo-Repo M. Prognosis, course of disease, and treatment of the spondyloarthropathies. Rheum Dis Clin North Am 1998;24:737–51, viii.
109. Sieper J, Braun J. Pathogenesis of spondylarthropathies. Persistent bacterial antigen, autoimmunity, or both? Arthritis Rheum 1995;38:1547–54.
110. Lindholm H, Visakorpi R. Late complications after a *Yersinia enterocolitica* epidemic: a follow up study. Ann Rheum Dis 1991;50:694–6.
111. Szanto E, Hagenfeldt K. Sacro-iliitis in women—a sequela to acute salpingitis. A follow-up study. Scand J Rheumatol 1983;12:89–92.
112. Lehtinen K. 76 patients with ankylosing spondylitis seen after 30 years of disease. Scand J Rheumatol 1983;12:5–11.
113. van der Paardt M, van Denderen JC, van den Brule AJ, et al. Prevalence of *Chlamydia trachomatis* in urine of male patients

with ankylosing spondylitis is not increased. Ann Rheum Dis 2000;59:300–2.

114. Martinez A, Pacheco-Tena C, Vazquez-Mellado J, Burgos-Vargas R. Relationship between disease activity and infection in patients with spondyloarthropathies. Ann Rheum Dis 2004;63:1338–40.

115. Lange U, Berliner M, Ludwig M, et al. Ankylosing spondylitis and infections of the female urogenital tract. Rheumatol Int 1998;17:181–4.

116. Kim GT. Acute exacerbation of ankylosing spondylitis after chlamydial infection in a patient well-controlled with etanercept. Int J Rheum Dis 2012;15:e113.

117. Ebringer R, Cooke D, Cawdell DR, Cowling P, Ebringer A. Ankylosing spondylitis: *Klebsiella* and HL-A B27. Rheumatol Rehabil 1977;16:190–6.

118. Rashid T, Ebringer A. Ankylosing spondylitis is linked to *Klebsiella*—the evidence. Clin Rheumatol 2007;26:858–64.

119. Zambrano-Zaragoza F, García-Latorre E, Domínguez-López ML, Cancino-Díaz ME, Burgos-Vargas R, Jiménez-Zamudio L. CD4 and CD8 T cell response to the rHSP60 from *Klebsiella pneumoniae* in peripheral blood mononuclear cells from patients with ankylosing spondylitis. Rev Invest Clin 2005;57:555–62.

120. Cancino-Díaz M, Ayala-Narváez H, Burgos-Vargas R, et al. Recognition of B cells epitopes of the *Klebsiella pneumoniae* GroEL-like protein by HLA-B27 positive subjects. Microb Pathog 2000;28:211–20.

121. Kinsella TD, Fritzler MJ, Lewkonia RM. Normal anti-*Klebsiella* lymphocytotoxicity in ankylosing spondylitis. Arthritis Rheum 1986;29:358–62.

122. Stone MA, Payne U, Schentag C, Rahman P, Pacheco-Tena C, Inman RD. Comparative immune responses to candidate arthritogenic bacteria do not confirm a dominant role for *Klebsiella* pneumonia in the pathogenesis of familial ankylosing spondylitis. Rheumatology (Oxford) 2004;43:148–55.

123. Schittenhelm RB, Sian TC, Wilmann PG, Dudek NL, Purcell AW. Revisiting the arthritogenic peptide theory: quantitative not qualitative changes in the peptide repertoire of HLA-B27 allotypes. Arthritis Rheum 2015; 67:702–13.

124. Stebbings S, Munro K, Simon MA, et al. Comparison of the faecal microflora of patients with ankylosing spondylitis and controls using molecular methods of analysis. Rheumatology (Oxford) 2002;41:1395–401.

125. Stebbings SM, Taylor C, Tannock GW, Baird MA, Highton J. The immune response to autologous bacteroides in ankylosing spondylitis is characterized by reduced interleukin 10 production. J Rheumatol 2009;36:797–800.

126. Costello ME, Ciccia F, Willner D, et al. Intestinal dysbiosis in ankylosing spondylitis. Arthritis Rheum 2014 Nov 21;doi 10.1002/art.38967.

127. Lin P, Bach M, Asquith M, et al. HLA-B27 and human β2-microglobulin affect the gut microbiota of transgenic rats. PLoS One 2014;9(8):e105684.

CHAPTER 10

Pathology: bone

Rik J. Lories and Georg Schett

Introduction to bone pathology

The cumbersome clinical presentation witnessed in some patients with long-standing axSpA represents a fearful prospect for patients in whom the diagnosis has recently been established. Progressive disease is characterized by spinal stiffness and loss of mobility leading to reduced flexion, extension, rotation, and side-ward bending. Imaging of the skeleton reveals extensive osteoproliferation in the spine, leading to the formation of syndesmophytes, with a steady evolution towards bridging of the vertebrae and ankylosis of the SI joints. In some patients, additional deformities occur, such as the deformity of vertebral bodies due to osteoporotic fractures. Bone apposition, apparent in radiographic examination of the spine may not be the sole contributor to loss of function in axSpA patients, with persisting inflammation and associated muscle stiffness also playing a role, but it does represent a daunting challenge for patients and physicians. Osteoproliferation may represent the most striking feature of skeletal damage in axSpA, but loss of bone and inflammation-associated osteoporosis should not be underestimated. From the scientific perspective, the simultaneous occurrence of bone growth in the cortical bone and bone loss in the trabecular bone represent an enormous scientific challenge to understand the cellular and molecular events underlying these phenomena, in particular as opposing processes appear to take place in adjacent anatomical structures.

The introduction of novel treatments for axSpA more than a decade ago that have unprecedented effects on inflammation gradually shifted the attention of the research community towards these specific structural disease manifestations of axSpA and their clinical consequences. This chapter introduces the key concepts of bone biology that appear to be of specific relevance for the different structural bone changes in axSpA, summarizing current knowledge about the pathophysiologic concepts and how these changes contribute to the burden of disease. Emerging insights into the molecular mechanisms of both bone loss and osteoproliferation are discussed, in an effort to translate experimental data into a clinically relevant context, as are current concepts and hypotheses dealing with the complex relationship between inflammation and structural damage, in particular osteoproliferation leading to axial ankylosis. Current treatment strategies are revisited concerning their effects on structural disease progression in axSpA. Finally, the authors use this information to develop a patient-centred perspective of disease modification in axSpA that goes beyond the assessment of progressive osteoproliferation and ankylosis.

Bone biology and its importance for axial spondyloarthritis

Bone formation and bone turnover are very interesting biological processes that are tightly regulated under developmental and homeostatic conditions. Rheumatic diseases have shown to profoundly impact local and systemic bone turnover, highlighting the disease-relevant interactions between bone biology and the rheumatology field (1). In particular, better appreciation of the close interactions between bone and the immune system, commonly termed osteoimmunology, helps to understand the mechanisms of structural bone changes in axSpA. Hence it is essential to revisit the fundamental concepts of bone biology in this chapter to better describe the mechanisms of structural bone changes in patients with axSpA (Fig. 10.1).

Effectively, osteoproliferation can be understood as a consequence of loss of local bone homeostasis and an effort to repair damage. Therefore this process should be clearly distinguished from skeletal modelling and remodelling, two key aspects of physiological bone biology. Bone modelling is a developmental process that determines the shape and structure of the skeleton. Basic principles, key cells, and molecular signalling pathways of bone modelling are well conserved during evolution, allowing the use of rodent models to understand human skeletal development. Modelling of bone is a well-orchestrated and tightly regulated process in which progenitor cell populations differentiate through indirect endochondral bone formation or direct bone formation. The former process typically lays out a temporary cartilage template that is subsequently replaced by bone, whereas the latter is characterized by direct differentiation of progenitor cells into bone cells. Endochondral bone formation is particularly important for limb development and is at least partially recapitulated during fracture healing. Direct bone formation is critical for the cranial bones and for the formation of the cortical parts of the long bones. During endochondral bone formation, different cell populations can be identified: proliferating chondrocytes, pre- and hypertrophic chondrocytes, and finally osteoblasts. In direct bone formation the progenitors directly differentiate into osteoblasts. In contrast to bone modelling, remodelling of bone refers to the critical continuous renewal of the skeletal tissue by a unique population of bone-resorbing cells (osteoclasts, derived from the monocytic lineage) and bone-forming osteoblasts (of mesenchymal origin). Fully differentiated osteoblasts are entrapped in their self-produced matrix and become mechanosensing osteocytes that have an important function in directing the bone remodelling process.

In contrast to these physiological processes, osteoproliferation in axSpA is a disease-associated and therefore pathological bone remodelling process. It can easily be distinguished from physiological bone remodelling, as it does not respect the existing or original anatomic boundaries. This is also in sharp contrast with new bone formation seen during fracture healing, a repair process that restores the original shape of the bone, albeit by going through the callus-building proliferative phase, in which the fracture is initially

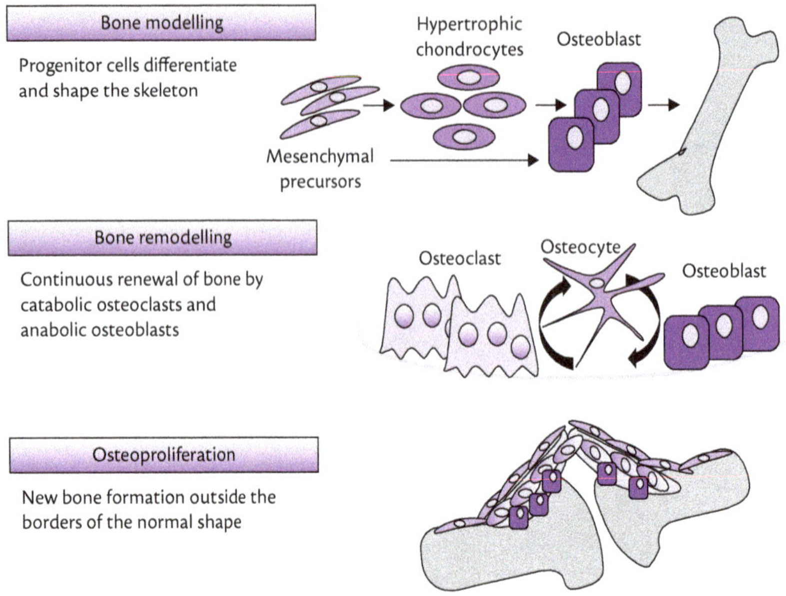

Fig. 10.1 (See colour plate section). Concepts of bone formation. Bone modelling is a developmental process that determines the shape and structure of the skeleton. In this well-orchestrated process, progenitors differentiate by endochondral or direct bone formation. Bone remodelling refers to the continuous renewal of the skeleton by bone-resorbing osteoclasts (multinucleated cells) and bone-forming osteoblasts. The osteocytes are mechanosensitive cells and orchestrate the bone remodelling cycle. Bone modelling in SpA is a disease-associated process, in which new bone formation occurs outside the original borders of the skeleton.

Reprinted from Rheum Dis Clin North Am, 38, 3, Lories, R, Schett G. Pathophysiology of new bone formation and ankylosis in spondyloarthritis, 555–67. Copyright (2012) with permission from Elsevier.

bridged outside of the defined anatomic boundaries. Taking this perspective into account, it is possible to define the structural bone changes in axSpA as two different processes: on the one hand, new bone formation leading to ankylosis is orchestrated by proliferation, differentiation, maturation, and most likely also migration of mesenchymal cells. The term 'osteoproliferation' has been introduced in this regard, although semantically it may not exactly reflect the complex cellular and molecular processes involved. Osteoproliferation leading to ankylosis occurs in connection with the existing bone but clearly extends beyond the original physiological border, often following the adjacent ligamental structures. On the other hand, patients with axSpA paradoxically develop osteoporosis in the vertebral bodies due to excess of osteoclast activity in the trabecular bone of the vertebral bodies (Fig. 10.2). It is clear that such different types of bone changes in cortical and trabecular bone support the concept that pathological bone remodelling in axSpA is fundamentally different from physiological bone turnover.

Clinical burden of osteoproliferation in axial spondyloarthritis

If structural damage becomes a prominent feature in patients with axSpA, it clearly resembles a major contributor to the burden of disease. A fully ankylosed spine, classically referred to as bamboo spine, severely limits mobility of the spine in all axes and strongly increases the risk of spinal fracture, with severe neurological consequences, including paralysis and paraplegia even after minor trauma. Similarly, vertebral insufficiency fractures are a common cause of severe pain. The importance of structural damage

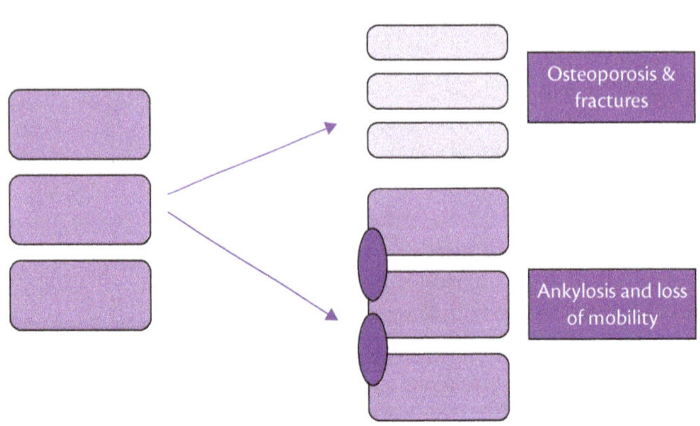

Fig. 10.2 The bone paradox in axSpA. Inflammation of the spine is associated with both trabecular bone loss, leading to osteoporosis and fractures, and cortical new bone formation, leading to ankylosis. Each rectangle represents a vertebral body and the intensity of the purple colour correlates with the grade of bone density.

as a critical determinant of morbidity has been well documented. Whereas in early disease stages, patient burden is largely dependent on the degree of inflammation, this situation changes rapidly over time, with structural damage appearing to be a major precipitating factor. In addition, however, relatively limited structural damage may have more serious consequences than one anticipates. In humans, the mobility of the SI joint is limited and therefore consequences of SI joint ankylosis are often small. Nevertheless, loss of mobility in these joints connecting the spine and the limbs can profoundly affect the biomechanics of the entire spine, resulting in increased back pain. Despite the fact that this type of back pain will likely be more mechanical than inflammatory in its character, it is a major diagnostic and therapeutic challenge in patients with axSpA.

Concepts of osteoproliferation in axial spondyloarthritis

A major limitation to the study of bone pathology in patients with axSpA is the difficulty of collecting relevant patient tissues. Spine and SI biopsies are invasive procedures that are extremely rarely performed. Post-surgery specimens may have become damaged during surgical procedures, whereas autopsy materials usually are only representative of end-stage disease. From a translational perspective these issues are difficult to overcome, and much of the human data that have been collected results from a limited number of autopsy studies performed decades ago (2, 3). Nevertheless, in the last decade it has been possible to collect more of these precious samples after spine surgery, which has helped to shed better light on the process of pathological bone remodelling in patients with axSpA (4, 5). Current concepts suggest that both endochondral bone formation with the cartilage template as well as direct bone formation contribute to osteoproliferation and spinal ankylosis. As compared to developmental, homeostatic remodelling and fracture healing, bone remodelling in axSpA appears less well orchestrated and controlled. In addition to morphological features resembling endochondral and direct bone formation, cartilage metaplasia has been described in certain lesions, which is defined by the presence of cartilage cells within a calcified extracellular matrix.

It seems conceivable that osteoproliferation in axSpA depends on the presence of progenitor cell populations in the joint or bone environment that can commit towards either chondro- or osteogenic differentiation, depending on specific local growth factor gradients. Effectively, progenitor cell populations have been described in different tissues, including the bone marrow, synovium, and periosteum. The potential role of other cells types such as pericytes and of transdifferentiation processes such as endothelial–mesenchymal transition remain to be defined. Moreover, the type of bone formation as well as the cell populations that are primarily involved may also be dependent on the specific site of new bone formation. For instance, a detailed study of the ankylosed zygoapophysygeal joints in axSpA has suggested that cells originating from the underlying bone marrow lesions play critical roles in pathological bone remodelling (4).

Mechanisms of osteoproliferation in axial spondyloarthritis

As mentioned in the section 'Concepts of osteoproliferation in axial spondyloarthritis', direct access to the tissues involved in axSpA is difficult. The limited amount of histology data available from such patients suggest that both endochondral and membranous bone formation contribute to ankylosis (4–8). Although formal proof is lacking, it appears likely that skeletal progenitor populations commit towards differentiation into either chondrocytes or osteoblasts in axSpA. Indeed, the multilineage potential of cell types, such as synovial, periosteal, and bone marrow cells, has been demonstrated (9–11). Nevertheless, other cells involved in bone formation may be circulating fibrocytes (12) or vessel-associated pericytes (13), as well as local endothelial–mesenchymal transition (14). At the molecular level, osteoproliferation in axSpA appears to be directed by bone morphogenetic proteins (BMPs), Wnt proteins, hedgehog proteins, and fibroblast growth factors (FGFs) and their respective cascades. BMPs, Wnts, and hedgehogs have been studied in animal models and to some extent also in axSpA patient samples, as discussed below.

BMPs were originally identified as protein factors isolated from a decalcified bone matrix that can ectopically induce a full cascade of endochondral bone formation, when injected intramuscularly or subcutaneously in vivo (15). Moreover, this type of potent growth factor was subsequently demonstrated to play an important role not only in skeletal development but also in body patterning and in the development of other organ systems. Increasing evidence suggests that BMPs have homeostatic or regulatory roles in different organ systems, including the skeleton (bone and cartilage), the kidney, and the endocrine system postnatally. Interestingly, the orthopaedic community has adopted BMPs as treatment for non-union fractures and to obtain spinal ankylosis in patients with intervertebral disk degeneration (16). BMPs are part of a large family of ligands related to transforming growth factor beta. The different ligands and promiscuous receptor associations lead to the activation of distinct signalling cascades, thereby allowing distinct BMPs to have wide-ranging effects on specific cell types. Regulatory mechanisms include the expression of endogenous extracellular and intracellular antagonists and the complex interactions of coactivator and corepressors at the level of transcription. Such interactions are essential for the fine-tuning of this signalling system. In skeletal development, BMPs play an essential role in the early phases of chondrogenesis by stimulating chondrogenic differentiation, including the late hypertrophic stages of chondrogenesis (15). Different BMPs have also direct positive effects on osteoblast differentiation.

The role of the BMP pathway in osteoproliferation was studied in animal models of SpA (17, 18). The spontaneous arthritis model in aging male DBA/1 mice is characterized by a short phase of acute inflammation, followed by extensive bone remodelling originating from the entheses, potentially leading to joint ankylosis (18). Microscopic assessment of the model shows ectopic endochondral bone formation, with consecutive phases of chondrocyte proliferation, condensation, differentiation, hypertrophy, and ultimately replacement of the cartilage template by bone. Different BMPs are expressed in this mouse model and activation of intracellular BMP signalling molecules is found in the early phases of the disease (17). When overexpressing noggin, an endogenous BMP antagonist that interferes with ligand-receptor binding, osteoproliferation and ankylosis could be inhibited in both preventive and therapeutic settings (17) (Fig. 10.3).

Wnt proteins were originally identified in cancer biology and fruit fly development and have been associated with a diversity of

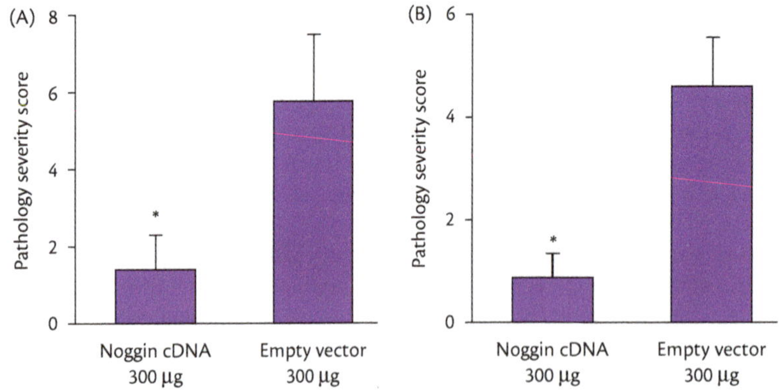

Fig. 10.3 Noggin gene transfer ameliorated the pathological cascade in ankylosing enthesitis in mice. Noggin or empty vector control gene transfer was performed either as a preventive strategy (A) or as a therapeutic strategy immediately after the first symptoms appeared (B). Noggin gene transfer significantly reduced pathological disease severity in treated animals compared with empty vector-treated controls. *Mann-Whitney U test, $p < 0.05$. Data are shown as mean ± SEM of the cumulative score of all interphalangeal and metacarpophalangeal joints from the hind feet; each group consisted of eight mice, except the noggin cDNA-treated group in B ($n = 6$).
Lories RJ, Derese I and Luyten FP. Modulation of bone morphogenetic protein signaling inhibits the onset and progression of ankylosing enthesitis. J Clin Invest 2005;115:1571–9.

effects, ranging from early developmental processes to postnatal tissue homeostasis and disease (19, 20). The Wnt family mediates its effects by using complex ligand–receptor interactions, as well as activation of different intracellular signalling cascades. Canonical Wnt signalling primarily involves β-catenin translocation to the nucleus. In skeletal development and biology, Wnts stimulate bone formation and their expression appears regulated by the mechanosensing osteocytes. Wnts stimulate new bone formation by direct effects on osteoblasts. Moreover, Wnt proteins tightly regulate articular cartilage homeostasis, and shifts in the balance between Wnt ligands and endogenous antagonists appear important in osteoarthritis (20).

The link between Wnt signalling and ankylosis in SpA came from observations in the human TNF tg mouse model of arthritis (21, 22) (Fig. 10.4). In this model, induction of Wnt signalling by neutralization of the Wnt antagonist dickkopf-1 (DKK1), previously linked to systemic bone loss, resulted in osteoproliferation and and ankylosis in peripheral and axial joints. This local phenomenon was accompanied by a systemic gain of bone mass, indicating that enhancing Wnt signalling in this model affects bone remodelling in addition to bone modelling. DKK1 is a factor induced by proinflammatory cytokines such as TNF (21).

Hedgehog proteins also importantly contribute to skeletal development and are key mediators of an essential feedback loop that controls bone growth (23). This feedback loop is established with parathyroid hormone-related protein (PTHrP). Indian hedgehog (IHH) defines the rate of chondrocyte proliferation and hypertrophy. IHH binds to the Smoothened and Patched receptor complex and leads to an activation of the GLI transcription factors. GLI1 and GLI2 are considered transcriptional activators, while GLI3 acts as a transcriptional repressor. A small compound that inhibits hedgehog signalling by directly interfering with Smoothened limits osteoproliferation in a model of inflammatory arthritis (24). Of particular interest, this effect appeared specific for pathological osteoproliferation, while no inhibitory effects were noted on physiological bone remodelling. While BMPs and Wnts have multiple effects in different organ systems postnatally and blockade of these pathways may thus be associated with toxicity, hedgehog signalling appears to be more restricted to developing bone and may thus have less general toxicity issues in inhibiting osteoproliferation.

Recently the presence of antibodies against BMP antagonist noggin and Wnt antagonist sclerostin was reported in axSpA (25). Although this intriguing observation requires confirmation in additional cohorts, it may explain some of the specific features of the disease. The presence of these antibodies could be due to the release of these factors from the extracellular matrix secondary to tissue damage. When exposed to the immune cells, neoepitopes may be present, eventually due to binding to extracellular matrix fragments and the development of secondary immune responses.

Clinical concepts of osteoproliferation

Triggered by data from animal models and by cohort studies that failed to show a structural effect of TNFi over a 2-year period (26–29), the relationship between inflammation and ankylosis has been debated. The cohort data following the initial clinical trials do not completely exclude an effect of anti-inflammatory therapies on osteoproliferation, although, if present, it may be very mild. More data from early axSpA are awaited, which may shed more light on the kinetics of the interaction of inflammation and osteoproliferation in axSpA. Better diagnosis, classification, and prognostic insights into patients without existing radiographic damage—the so-called nr-axSpA—will likely contribute to further develop and refine concepts of the natural disease course in axSpA.

The negative data on the effect of TNFα inhibitors on osteoproliferation in SpA contrast with the accumulating evidence that treatment with NSAIDs may slow down this process (30–32). First demonstrated in a landmark study with specific cyclooxygenase 2 inhibitor celecoxib (30), newer data demonstrate that this important feature is most likely a general effect of NSAIDs, provided that they are used continuously or in sufficiently high doses (31, 32).

Different views on the relationship between inflammation and new bone formation in axSpA have been developed (33). A direct link between inflammation and new bone formation has been questioned (34). MRI studies have rather suggested that active inflammatory lesions later evolve into 'remodelling' lesions characterized by mesenchymal tissue responses. These lesions have

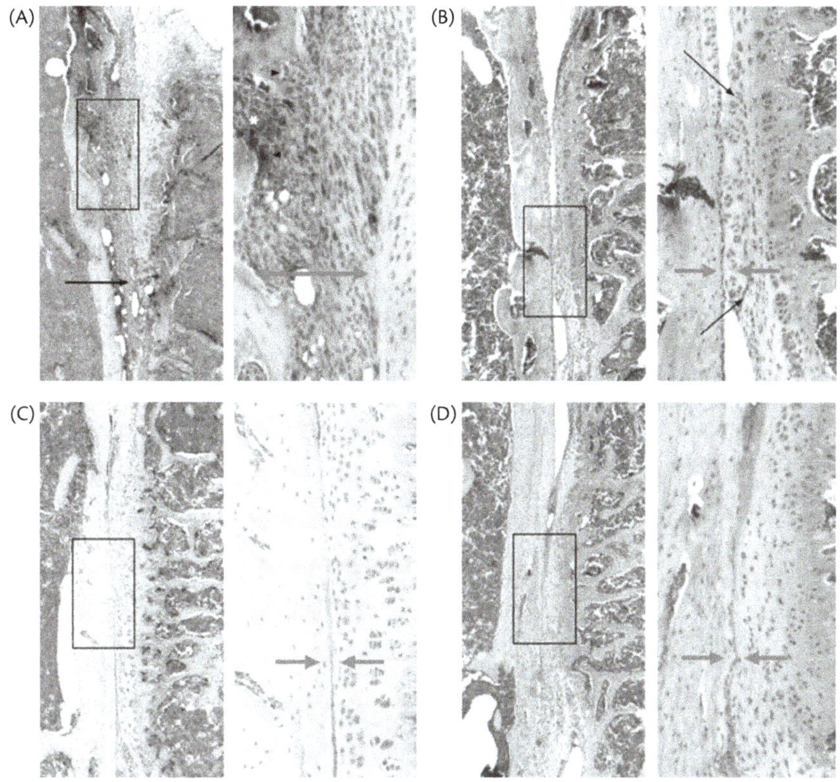

Fig. 10.4 (See colour plate section) Blockade of Dickkopf (DKK)-1 leads to ankylosis of SI joints. Microphotographs of tartrate-resistant acid phosphatase (TRAP)-stained sections counterstained with haematoxylin of SI joints of TNF tg mice. Framed inserts within left pictures show regions depicted in close-up pictures on the right. (A) Vehicle-treated TNF tg mouse with marked synovial inflammation in the SI joint (arrow) and multiple osteoclasts (arrowheads) and bone erosion (star). (B–D) Various degrees of bony proliferations and joint ankylosis after treatment with anti-DKK antibody: (B) localized chondro-osteophyte leading to narrowing of the joint gap (arrows); (C) bone and hypertrophic cartilage filling the entire joint gap; (D) bony ankylosis. Original magnification 5× (left), 20× (right). Purple dots represent osteoclasts and orange arrows mark the joint gap.

been identified as the preferred sites for new bone formation (35). Some authors have suggested that active inflammation, including cytokines such as TNFα, may temporarily act as a brake of bone formation by inducing molecules such as DKK1 that inhibit bone formation (36, 37). Upon resolution of inflammation and the decline of cytokine levels, new bone formation may then become apparent. This view has a dual impact on the clinical concepts of disease treatment: first, it suggests that the use of TNFα inhibitors, despite being highly effective to control inflammation, may result in accelerated bone formation. Although increased bone formation has not been seen in any of the cohort studies on TNFα inhibitors until now, such effect may be masked by the anti-inflammatory effects of TNFi, which suppress the development of the primary inflammatory lesions. Second, this concept suggests that an early and likely sustained intervention will have an impact on radiographic progression by preventing the development of such primary lesions.

An alternative view puts forward that inflammation and new bone formation are linked, but largely uncoupled, processes in terms of molecular pathways driving the effects (38, 39). Accordingly, inflammation and new bone formation should be considered as complementary targets for the treatment of the disease. This concept is supported by the observation that TNFα inhibitors do not affect radiographic progression in either a positive or a negative way, and by MRI data demonstrating that the majority of syndesmophytes appear at sites in which no preceding inflammation had been documented. This hypothesis suggests that biomechanical factors, such as entheseal strain and microdamage, or infections may trigger both inflammation and bone modelling at entheseal sites, and that both processes together may determine the phenotype of axSpA (40–42). It appears that IL-23 plays a critical role in triggering inflammation and bone formation at mechano-sensitive sites of the body, such as the entheses (41, 42). In this context, it is noteworthy that patients with high tissue turnover as measured by tissue turnover biomarkers show more structural damage (43). This concept suggests that the rate and extent of new bone formation depends on the degree of damage and that new bone formation represents a sort of stabilizing effort. This view appears to reconcile the existing differences in the concepts and also explains the pattern of osteoproliferation starting in the SI joints and the lower spine. In this perspective, early intervention, even before active signs of damage can be recognized, will likely result in long-term structural benefits.

Biomarkers for osteoproliferation

In axSpA there is still a relatively large gap between animal model data and clinical practice, in particular with regards to the prediction of structural damage and the identification of patients that are at high risk for osteoproliferation. Two different and contrasting features are found in the skeleton of patients with axSpA (44).

Inflammation is associated with trabecular bone loss and osteoporosis, while at the same time, and in close proximity, new bone formation and even ankylosis occurs. Therefore any assessment of specific bone markers should be considered in this complex setting, not only in cross-sectional analyses but also when the effect of a therapeutic intervention is evaluated in a longitudinal setting. This challenge affects not only the classical markers of bone and cartilage turnover, such as collagen breakdown and synthesis products, but also new markers associated with the pathways highlighted that have recently been studied or proposed.

Some examples highlight this complexity. Data obtained before the introduction of TNFα inhibitors indicated that patients with axSpA show increased bone and cartilage degradation (urinary pyridinium crosslinks) with normal ranges of bone formation markers (alkaline phosphatase and osteocalcin) (45). Other work showed increased cartilage turnover that was correlated with higher CRP levels, and which could either indicate increased turnover of articular cartilage and intervertebral disks or reflect the ongoing process of endochondral bone formation (46). Similar views can be derived from the analysis of type II collagen telopeptide, a marker of cartilage degradation (47). Treatment with TNFα inhibitors increased bone formation markers, reflected by higher levels of bone-specific alkaline phosphatase, and decreased bone resorption, reflected by lower type I collagen telopeptide levels (48). Tissue turnover reflected by matrix metalloproteinase 3 (MMP3) levels was earlier identified as a biomarker for radiographic progression in AS (43).

Different groups have tried to translate the animal model data into human biomarkers development. With regards to Wnt signalling, the initial study on DKK1 in mice included an analysis of DKK1 levels in SpA patients, controls, and RA patients (21). Based on a functional assay (binding to the LRP6 Wnt receptor), levels of DKK1 were consistently lower in axSpA patients. Interestingly, within the German Spondyloarthritis Inception Cohort (GESPIC), those patients with low levels of DKK1 showed increased radiographic progression compared to those with higher levels (49). These data were also based on the functional assay. Surprisingly, a classical sandwich enzyme-linked immunosorbent assay (ELISA) using two anti-Dkk1 antibodies demonstrated that patients with axSpA had significantly increased levels of Dkk1 (50). Levels further increased upon treatment with TNFα inhibitors, but Dkk1 itself was dysfunctional in a cell-based assay, explaining the discrepancy between both types of ELISA used (50). Low levels of sclerostin, an osteocyte-specific Wnt antagonist, were also strongly associated with radiographic progression in axSpA patients (Fig. 10.5) and correlated well with functional Dkk1 levels (51).

Consistent data on BMPs as markers of radiographic progression are relatively rare and have not provided clear insights until now. Patients with radiographic signs of ankylosis have higher serum levels of different BMPs compared to axSpA patients without signs of new bone formation and healthy controls (52). However, other studies have not reproduced these results (53, 54). The latter phenomenon highlights one of the particular challenges in the field of biomarkers, in particular with regards to progression of ankylosis in axSpA patients.

Clinical burden of osteoporosis in axial spondyloarthritis

At first sight, bone loss seems a paradoxical event in a disease like axSpA, which is characterized by excessive local bone formation (44).

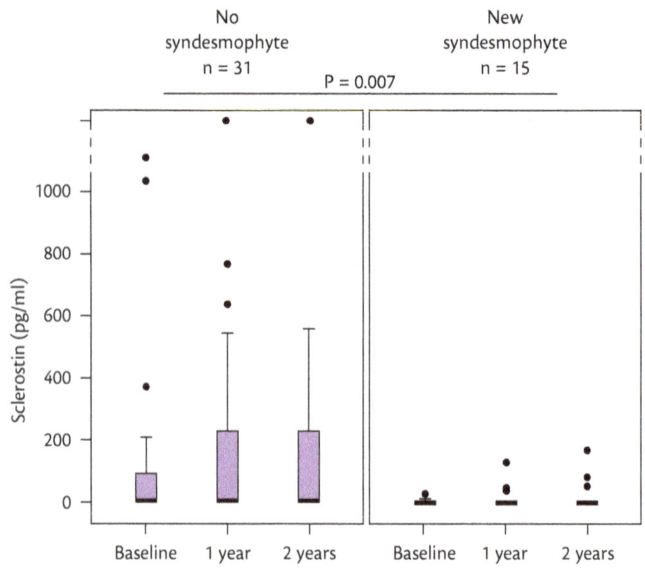

Fig. 10.5 Relationship between low serum levels of sclerostin and new bone formation in patients with AS. Serum levels of sclerostin over time were significantly higher in patients with no syndesmophyte growth than in patients with new syndesmophyte growth. Values are the mean and SEM.
Appel H, Ruiz-Heiland G, Listing J et al., Altered skeletal expression of sclerostin and its link to radiographic progression in ankylosing spondylitis, 2009, Wiley.

Nevertheless, bone loss is a consistent feature of inflammation and inflammatory disease. Diseases like RA and PsA, SLE, and IBD are associated with secondary osteoporosis, and axSpA is no different. Osteoporosis of the spine is often recognized as an early disease event (55–57). However, there are large discrepancies in the reported incidence, varying between 18.7% and 62% (58). Some of these differences between cohorts can be explained by the intrinsic difficulties that are encountered when measuring bone mineral density (BMD) in axSpA patients. The accuracy of BMD measurements in the presence of syndesmophytes and hyperossification is limited. Consequently, measurements at alternative sites, such as the femoral neck, are required in order to assess BMD in patients with advanced axSpA. Assessment of BMD at the femoral neck is considered to be more reliable in axSpA and also correlates well with vertebral fracture risk and the degree of inflammation (59). To date, the majority of studies report decreased BMD at the femoral neck in both early and late axSpA, with bone loss even more prevalent in patients developing syndesmophytes, suggesting that both bone loss and new bone formation could be considered markers of more severe disease (59).

Mechanisms of osteoporosis in axial spondyloarthritis

The specific aetiology of trabecular bone loss and consequent osteoporosis in axSpA is complex and involves several factors. One early hypothesis suggested that immobility associated with pain, stiffness, and eventual ankylosis is the likely cause of increased bone turnover and bone loss. The concept was built around the theory that the extraspinal bone in advanced disease dispersed gravitational, motional, and compressive stresses in the vertebral trabeculae, resulting in decreased trabecular density. However, as trabecular bone loss and even osteoporosis is also present in patients with early disease long before new bone formation has changed the biomechanics of the spine, it is likely that systemic inflammatory factors relevantly contribute to bone loss. Nevertheless, the loss of mobility seen in patients with axSpA is not exclusively due to the structural damage itself, but also related to inflammation, and therefore inflammation and immobility may go hand-in-hand in precipitating trabecular bone loss in axSpA. Importantly, fracture risk is increased in patients with axSpA (60, 61).

Several studies have shown significant correlations between markers of bone turnover, proinflammatory cytokines, and acute phase reactants in axSpA (45, 47, 62), suggesting a direct link between inflammation and bone loss. These findings support the view that systemic inflammatory mediators play a role in modulating bone loss in axSpA. More specifically, TNFα, IL-1, and IL-6 levels have been shown to correlate with several bone turnover markers (pyridinoline (PYD), deoxypyridinoline (DPYD), osteocalcin) as well as standard measures of inflammation (ESR, CRP) in other rheumatic diseases.

IL-17 is another important cytokine that is relevantly expressed in axSpA patients and could therefore be implicated in the development of the disease-associated osteoporosis. IL-17 stimulates TNFα production and can mediate osteoclast activation via shifting receptor activator of nuclear factor κB ligand (RANKL)/osteoprotegerin (OPG) balance towards RANKL. As OPG functions as a soluble receptor for RANKL, serving to neutralize RANKL and osteoclast formation, it is not surprising that low serum levels of OPG have been associated with osteopaenia in AS (63). Nonetheless, consistent associations with disease progression have yet to be demonstrated. Several other factors can influence the development of osteoporosis in axSpA (64). Such factors likely include sex hormones as, for instance, positive correlations between BMD and levels of sex hormones have been reported. Although remaining to be confirmed, genetic variations in the vitamin D gene, associated with BMD differences, appear to be related to both bone metabolism and inflammation in patients with axSpA (65). Furthermore, vitamin D levels and calcium metabolism may be affected in axSpA patients due to the presence of subclinical IBD.

Treatment of osteoporosis in axial spondyloarthritis

Currently, there is no general consensus for treating osteoporosis in axSpA patients. The goals of treatment need to be more clearly defined, as the consequences of bone loss and the associated risk for fracture are far less understood and predictable than in women with postmenopausal osteoporosis. Taking the link between inflammation and bone loss into account, it is easy to anticipate that inhibition of inflammation, and in particular the inhibition of TNF, can be considered as the most effective approach for reducing the impact of inflammation on trabecular bone loss in patients with axSpA. Although there is evidence that TNFα inhibitors influence trabecular bone loss in axSpA (66), very few studies have directly investigated the effect of anti-TNF on bone, thus providing only circumstantial evidence for a specific disease-defined therapeutic approach to inhibit trabecular bone loss in axSpA. Bisphosphonates are widely used to treat osteoporosis in the general population and may also be suitable to improve bone quality in axSpA. However, there are still limited data regarding the specific use of bisphosphonates in axSpA. Considering the deleterious link between inflammation and bone loss, it appears important to define the burden of inflammation in patients with axSpA early in the disease course, in order to maintain or even increase BMD by timely and effective anti-inflammatory therapy and to prevent advanced stages of trabecular bone loss, as well as spinal immobility due to syndesmophyte formation.

Conclusion

Our understanding of osteoproliferation in axSpA is still limited. Concepts from developmental biology have found their way towards understanding disease and its pathological mechanisms. In addition, novel insights into some of the molecular pathways have been gained that trigger new bone formation in axSpA. However, most of these insights need further work and confirmation in human disease and additional molecular specification in terms of the ligands, receptors, and pathways involved. The opposing views on the relationship between inflammation and new bone formation are likely to become merged into a common concept as further data accumulate. It appears likely that early intervention can result in a better outcome, but the costs and toxicity may warrant such approach only for patients that are at risk for severe disability. However, current markers and predictors, including genetics, are not yet ready for use in clinical practice and require large population confirmation and validation.

Developing specific therapies against osteoproliferation and ankylosis remains a challenge with regards to effectiveness, but also toxicity and long-term side-effects, taking into account the pleiotropic effects of signalling cascades such as BMPs and Wnts. In this context, the importance of the effect of NSAIDs on osteoproliferation should not be underestimated. The eventual continued use of these drugs in patients with good disease control but a high risk for structural damage is a matter of debate. Exciting new data such as the discovery of growth factor pathway stimulating antibodies and increasing attention towards the impact of biomechanical forces are likely to further boost the field. Finally, the concept of disease modification that is commonly used in RA, and that is specifically determined by radiographic scores, may not be ideal for use in axSpA. The impact of TNFα inhibitors on signs and symptoms of disease but also on short- and long-term functionality is of such magnitude that it should be considered as prognosis and therefore disease modifying, even in the absence of classical radiographic structural effects.

References

1. Schett G, Saag KG, Bijlsma JW. From bone biology to clinical outcome: state of the art and future perspectives. Ann Rheum Dis 2010;69:1415–19.
2. Cruickshank B. Histopathology of diarthrodial joints in ankylosing spondylitis. Ann Rheum Dis 1951;10:393–404.
3. Bollow M, Fischer T, Reisshauer H, et al. Quantitative analyses of sacroiliac biopsies in spondyloarthropathies: T cells and macrophages predominate in early and active sacroiliitis—cellularity correlates with the degree of enhancement detected by magnetic resonance imaging. Ann Rheum Dis 2000;59:135–40.
4. Appel H, Kuhne M, Spiekermann S, et al. Immunohistologic analysis of zygapophyseal joints in patients with ankylosing spondylitis. Arthritis Rheum 2006;54:2845–51.

5. Appel H, Loddenkemper C, Grozdanovic Z, et al. Correlation of histopathological findings and magnetic resonance imaging in the spine of patients with ankylosing spondylitis. Arthritis Res Ther 2006;8:R143.
6. Appel H, Maier R, Loddenkemper C, et al. Immunohistochemical analysis of osteoblasts in zygapophyseal joints of patients with ankylosing spondylitis reveal repair mechanisms similar to osteoarthritis. J Rheumatol 2010;37:823–8.
7. Francois RJ, Gardner DL, Degrave EJ, et al. Histopathologic evidence that sacroiliitis in ankylosing spondylitis is not merely enthesitis. Arthritis Rheum 2000;43:2011–24.
8. Francois RJ. Some pathological features of ankylosing spondylitis as revealed by microradiography and tetracycline labelling. Clin Rheumatol 1982;1:23–9.
9. De Bari C, Dell'Accio F, Tylzanowski P, et al. Multipotent mesenchymal stem cells from adult human synovial membrane. Arthritis Rheum 2001;44(8):1928–42.
10. De Bari C, Dell'Accio F, Luyten FP. Human periosteum-derived cells maintain phenotypic stability and chondrogenic potential throughout expansion regardless of donor age. Arthritis Rheum 2001;44:85–95.
11. Jones EA, English A, Henshaw K, et al. Enumeration and phenotypic characterization of synovial fluid multipotential mesenchymal progenitor cells in inflammatory and degenerative arthritis. Arthritis Rheum 2004;50:817–27.
12. Lories RJ, Luyten FP. Activated fibrocytes: circulating cells that populate the arthritic synovium? Rheumatology (Oxford) 2010;49:617–18.
13. Kurth TB, Dell'accio F, Crouch V, et al. Functional mesenchymal stem cell niches in adult mouse knee joint synovium in vivo. Arthritis Rheum 2011;63:1289–300.
14. Medici D, Shore EM, Lounev VY, et al. Conversion of vascular endothelial cells into multipotent stem-like cells. Nat Med 2010;16:1400–6.
15. Hogan BL. Bone morphogenetic proteins: multifunctional regulators of vertebrate development. Genes Dev 1996;10:1580–94.
16. Axelrad TW, Einhorn TA. Bone morphogenetic proteins in orthopaedic surgery. Cytokine Growth Factor Rev 2009;20:481–8.
17. Lories RJ, Derese I, Luyten FP. Modulation of bone morphogenetic protein signaling inhibits the onset and progression of ankylosing enthesitis. J Clin Invest 2005;115:1571–9.
18. Lories RJ, Matthys P, de Vlam K, et al. Ankylosing enthesitis, dactylitis, and onychoperiostitis in male dba/1 mice: a model of psoriatic arthritis. Ann Rheum Dis 2004;63:595–8.
19. Clevers H, Nusse R. Wnt/beta-catenin signaling and disease. Cell 2012;149:1192–205.
20. Luyten FP, Tylzanowski P, Lories RJ. Wnt signaling and osteoarthritis. Bone 2009;44:522–7.
21. Diarra D, Stolina M, Polzer K, et al. Dickkopf-1 is a master regulator of joint remodeling. Nat Med. 2007;13:156–63.
22. Uderhardt S, Diarra D, Katzenbeisser J, et al. Blockade of Dickkopf (DKK)-1 induces fusion of sacroiliac joints. Ann Rheum Dis 2010;69:592–7.
23. Hui CC, Angers S. Gli proteins in development and disease. Annu Rev Cell Dev Biol 2011;27:513–37.
24. Ruiz-Heiland G, Horn A, Zerr P, et al. Blockade of the hedgehog pathway inhibits osteophyte formation in arthritis. Ann Rheum Dis 2012;71:400–7.
25. Tsui FW, Tsui HW, Las Heras F, Pritzker KP, Inman RD. Serum levels of novel noggin and sclerostin-immune complexes are elevated in ankylosing spondylitis. Ann Rheum Dis 2014;73:1873–9.
26. van der Heijde D, Salonen D, Weissman BN, et al. Assessment of radiographic progression in the spines of patients with ankylosing spondylitis treated with adalimumab for up to 2 years. Arthritis Res Ther 2009;11:R127.
27. van der Heijde D, Landewe R, Baraliakos X, et al. Radiographic findings following two years of infliximab therapy in patients with ankylosing spondylitis. Arthritis Rheum 2008;58:3063–70.
28. van der Heijde D, Landewe R, Einstein S, et al. Radiographic progression of ankylosing spondylitis after up to two years of treatment with etanercept. Arthritis Rheum 2008;58:1324–31.
29. Schett G, Landewe R, van der Heijde D. TNF blockers and structural remodeling in ankylosing spondylitis: what is reality and what is fiction? Ann Rheum Dis 2007;66:709–11.
30. Wanders A, Heijde D, Landewe R, et al. Nonsteroidal antiinflammatory drugs reduce radiographic progression in patients with ankylosing spondylitis: a randomized clinical trial. Arthritis Rheum 2005;52:1756–65.
31. Kroon F, Landewe R, Dougados M, et al. Continuous NSAID use reverts the effects of inflammation on radiographic progression in patients with ankylosing spondylitis. Ann Rheum Dis 2012; doi 10.1136/annrheumdis-2012-201370.
32. Poddubnyy D, Rudwaleit M, Haibel H, et al. Effect of non-steroidal anti-inflammatory drugs on radiographic spinal progression in patients with axial spondyloarthritis: Results from the german spondyloarthritis inception cohort. Ann Rheum Dis 2012;71(10):1616–22.
33. Maksymowych WP, Elewaut D, Schett G. Motion for debate: the development of ankylosis in ankylosing spondylitis is largely dependent on inflammation. Arthritis Rheum 2012;64(6):1713–19.
34. Van der Heijde D, Machado P, Braun J, et al. MRI inflammation at the vertebral unit only marginally predicts new syndesmophyte formation: a multilevel analysis in patients with ankylosing spondylitis. Ann Rheum Dis 2012;71:369–73.
35. Chiowchanwisawakit P, Lambert RG, Conner-Spady B, Maksymowych WP. Focal fat lesions at vertebral corners on magnetic resonance imaging predict the development of new syndesmophytes in ankylosing spondylitis. Arthritis Rheum 2011;63:2215–25.
36. Maksymowych WP. Disease modification in ankylosing spondylitis. Nat Rev Rheumatol 2010;6:75–81.
37. Maksymowych WP, Morency N, Conner-Spady B, et al. Suppression of inflammation and effects on new bone formation in ankylosing spondylitis: evidence for a window of opportunity in disease modification. Ann Rheum Dis 2013;72(1):23–8.
38. Lories RJ, Derese I, De Bari C, Luyten FP. Evidence for uncoupling of inflammation and joint remodeling in a mouse model of spondylarthritis. Arthritis Rheum 2007;56:489–97.
39. Lories RJ, de Vlam K, Luyten FP. Are current available therapies disease-modifying in spondyloarthritis? Best Pract Res Clin Rheumatol 2010;24(5):625–35.
40. Benjamin M, McGonagle D. The enthesis organ concept and its relevance to the spondyloarthropathies. Adv Exp Med Biol 2009;649:57–70.
41. Sherlock JP, Joyce-Shaikh B, Turner SP, et al. Il-23 induces spondyloarthropathy by acting on ROR-γt(+) CD3(+)CD4(−)CD8(−) entheseal resident T cells. Nat Med 2012;18:1069–76.
42. Lories RJ, McInnes IB. Primed for inflammation: enthesis-resident T cells. Nat Med 2012;18:1018–19.
43. Maksymowych WP, Landewe R, Conner-Spady B, et al. Serum matrix metalloproteinase 3 is an independent predictor of structural damage progression in patients with ankylosing spondylitis. Arthritis Rheum 2007;56:1846–53.
44. Carter S, Lories RJ. Osteoporosis: a paradox in ankylosing spondylitis. Curr Osteoporos Rep 2011;9:112–15.
45. Marhoffer W, Stracke H, Masoud I, et al. Evidence of impaired cartilage/bone turnover in patients with active ankylosing spondylitis. Ann Rheum Dis 1995;54:556–9.
46. Kim TH, Stone M, Payne U, et al. Cartilage biomarkers in ankylosing spondylitis: relationship to clinical variables and treatment response. Arthritis Rheum 2005;52:885–91.
47. Vosse D, Landewe R, Garnero P, et al. Association of markers of bone- and cartilage-degradation with radiological changes at baseline and after 2 years follow-up in patients with ankylosing spondylitis. Rheumatology (Oxford) 2008;47:1219–22.
48. Appel H, Janssen L, Listing J, et al. Serum levels of biomarkers of bone and cartilage destruction and new bone formation in different cohorts of patients with axial spondyloarthritis with and without tumor necrosis factor-alpha blocker treatment. Arthritis Res Ther 2008;10:R125.

49. Heiland GR, Appel H, Poddubnyy D, et al. High level of functional dickkopf-1 predicts protection from syndesmophyte formation in patients with ankylosing spondylitis. Ann Rheum Dis 2012;71:572–4.
50. Daoussis D, Liossis SN, Solomou EE, et al. Evidence that dkk-1 is dysfunctional in ankylosing spondylitis. Arthritis Rheum 2010;62:150–8.
51. Appel H, Ruiz-Heiland G, Listing J, et al. Altered skeletal expression of sclerostin and its link to radiographic progression in ankylosing spondylitis. Arthritis Rheum 2009;60:3257–62.
52. Chen HA, Chen CH, Lin YJ, et al. Association of bone morphogenetic proteins with spinal fusion in ankylosing spondylitis. J Rheumatol 2010;37:2126–32.
53. Park MC, Park YB, Lee SK. Relationship of bone morphogenetic proteins to disease activity and radiographic damage in patients with ankylosing spondylitis. Scand J Rheumatol 2008;37:200–4.
54. Wendling D, Cedoz JP, Racadot E, et al. Serum IL-17, BMP-7, and bone turnover markers in patients with ankylosing spondylitis. Joint Bone Spine 2007;74:304–5.
55. Will R, Bhalla A, Palmer R, Ring F, Calin A. Osteoporosis in early ankylosing spondylitis; a primary pathological event? Lancet 1989;23:1483–5.
56. van der Weijden MA, Claushuis TA, Nazari T, Lems WF, Dijkmans BA, van der Horst-Bruinsma IE. High prevalence of low bone mineral density in patients within 10 years of onset of ankylosing spondylitis: a systematic review. Clin Rheumatol 2012;31:1529–35.
57. Briot K, Durnez A, Paternotte S, Miceli-Richard C, Dougados M, Roux C. Bone oedema on MRI is highly associated with low bone mineral density in patients with early inflammatory back pain: results from the DESIR cohort. Ann Rheum Dis 2013;72:1914–19.
58. Geusens P, Vosse D, van der Linden S. Osteoporosis and vertebral fractures in ankylosing spondylitis. Curr Opin Rheumatol 2007;19:335–9.
59. Klingberg E, Geijer M, Göthlin J, et al. Vertebral fractures in ankylosing spondylitis are associated with lower bone mineral density in both central and peripheral skeleton. J Rheumatol 2012;39:1987–95.
60. Toussirot E, Ricard-Blum S, Dumoulin G, Cedoz JP, Wendling D. Relationship between urinary pyridinium cross-links, disease activity and disease subsets of ankylosing spondylitis. Rheumatology (Oxford) 1999;38:21–7.
61. Ralston SH, Urquhart GD, Brzeski M, Sturrock RD. Prevalence of vertebral compression fractures due to osteoporosis in ankylosing spondylitis. BMJ 1990;300:563–5.
62. Spencer D, Park W, Dick H, et al. Radiologic manifestations in 200 patients with ankylosing spondylitis; correlations with clinical features and HLA-B27. J Rheumatol 1979;6:305.
63. Franck H, Meurer T, Hofbauer LC. Evaluation of bone mineral density, hormones, biochemical markers of bone metabolism, and osteoprotegerin serum levels in patients with ankylosing spondylitis. J Rheumatol 2004;31:2236–41.
64. Wendling D. Bone loss in ankylosing spondylitis: can we put the puzzle together? J Rheumatol 2005;32:1184–5.
65. Obermayer-Pietsch BM, Lange U, Tauber G, et al. Vitamin D receptor initiation codon polymorphism, bone density and inflammatory activity of patients with ankylosing spondylitis. Osteoporos Int 2003;14:995–1000.
66. Visvanathan S1, van der Heijde D, Deodhar A, et al. Effects of infliximab on markers of inflammation and bone turnover and associations with bone mineral density in patients with ankylosing spondylitis. Ann Rheum Dis 2009;68:175–82.
67. Lories, R, Schett G. Pathophysiology of new bone formation and ankylosis in spondyloarthritis. Rheum Dis Clin North Am 2012; 38(3):555–67.

CHAPTER 11

Clinical features

Muhammad Asim Khan

Introduction to clinical features

The leading chronic progressive inflammatory rheumatic disease involving the SI joints and the spinal column is traditionally known as ankylosing spondylitis (AS) (1–4). It is a prototype of related forms of arthritis grouped under the term spondyloarthritis or spondyloarthropathy (SpA) (4–9). This clinical entity is strongly associated with HLA-B27, a normal gene that is also present in a small percentage of the general population (1, 10, 11). The term SpA traditionally includes, in addition to AS, PsA, enteropathic arthritis (associated with CD and UC), ReA, and undifferentiated SpA (uSpA) (5, 7, 8, 9). This chapter deals with the clinical features of axSpA, a relatively recently proposed clinical entity that encompasses patients with AS (12).

AxSpA is not an uncommon rheumatic disease (13); this subject is reviewed in detail in Chapter 2. Most of the existing knowledge about the clinical picture of axSpA comes from long-standing experience with patients who suffer from AS. There is a predilection for the inflammation to affect sites where the tendons and ligaments attach to the bones (entheses), especially in the SI joints and the spinal column (14–17). The enthesitis can result in gradual and progressive spinal ankylosis, with resultant physical deformity in patients with severe forms of AS, as shown in Fig. 11.1.

Axial spondyloarthritis versus ankylosing spondylitis

Patients with SpA are now subgrouped into those with predominantly axial disease (axSpA) and those with predominantly peripheral disease, according to the ASAS classification criteria (Fig. 11.2) (12, 18). Patients with axSpA are further subdivided into those with radiographic evidence of sacroiliitis ('r-axSpA') and those with 'spondylitis disease without radiographic evidence of sacroiliitis' (19), which is currently more often termed 'nr-axSpA' (1, 2, 13) (Figs 11.2 and 11.3). These classification criteria were developed to facilitate earlier detection of the disease in patients with chronic back pain that began before age 45, and since they were developed for in a 'specialized' clinical setting, they may not be useful for large epidemiologic studies, one of the intended purpose of any classification criteria (20). Moreover, it has not yet been firmly established that nr-axSpA and AS represent one single entity (21–24). An unknown, but probably not an insignificant proportion of patients with nr-axSpA may never develop structural damage in the SI joints, just as not every patient with sacroiliitis progresses to spinal ankylosis (Fig. 11.3). A prospective long-term follow-up of large cohorts may help in clarifying whether nr-axSpA is simply an early stage in the spectrum of SpA, evolving into AS over time, or if there is an inherent difference between them (24).

The term AS is more restrictive, as it requires X-ray evidence of sacroiliitis, which may take years to develop. Incidentally, strictly speaking, AS is not identical with the new term r-axSpA because—while the radiographic criteria are the same—the two terms differ in the additional clinical or laboratory criteria that have to be fulfilled; for example, the latter term (i.e., r-axSpA) does not require the patient's chronic back pain to have inflammatory features (25). Requirement for X-ray evidence of sacroiliitis is one of the reasons that the diagnosis is often delayed by 3–11 years (or even longer) from the onset of symptoms, and this delay in diagnosis also

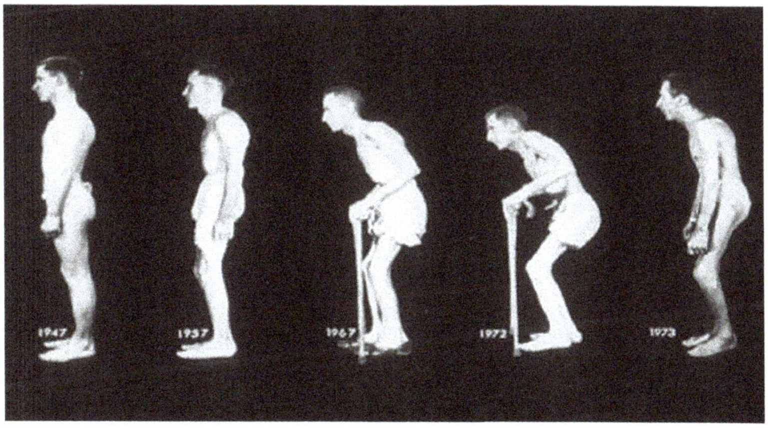

Fig. 11.1 Progressive deformity due to AS in a patient whose illness began in 1946 when he was 21 years old. In 1972 total hip replacements were performed and he regained 3 inches in height. Interestingly, this patient developed psoriasis and then psoriatic dactylitis and nail changes 26 years after the onset of his AS. He died in September 1973 from cervical cord compression resulting from upward subluxation of the axis.

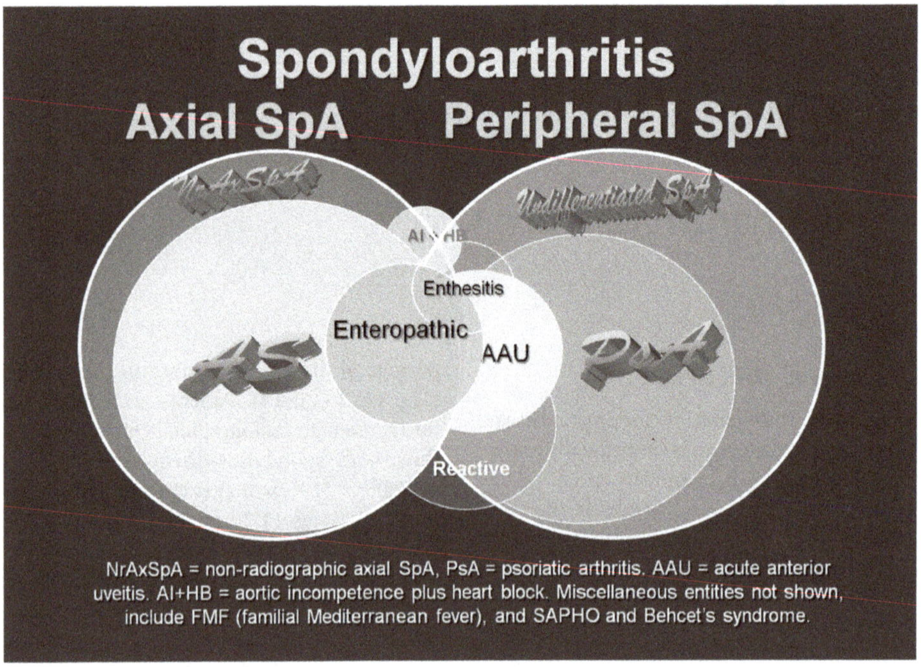

Fig. 11.2 Venn diagram showing clinical overlap of various types of SpA, but they can be broadly divided into predominantly axial and predominantly peripheral forms. The two main types of axSpA are AS and nr-axSpA. Other miscellaneous forms include SpA associated with hidradenitis suppurativa, acne conglobata and dissecting cellulitis of the scalp.
Ozgocmen S, Khan MA. Current concept of spondyloarthritis: Special emphasis on early referral and diagnosis. Curr Rheumatol Rep. 2012, Oct;14(5):409–14. Erratum: 2012 Dec;14(6):624.

depends on the type of the patient's presenting symptoms and the clinical training of the physician seeing the patient (26–31). During this period, many patients may undergo unnecessary or even invasive investigations and receive inappropriate treatment. Detection of SI joint involvement (sacroiliitis) on musculoskeletal imaging (X-ray or MRI) in the presence of typical clinical manifestations is virtually diagnostic. The average delay in the diagnosis is relatively longer in women than in men, in children and adolescents than in older patients, and in HLA-B27-negative patients (27, 32). The longer the diagnosis is delayed, the worse the functional outcome, especially with juvenile-onset AS (32).

Classic AS with radiographic changes of sacroiliitis has been considered to be more common in males than females, but this gender gap has markedly decreased with better recognition of this condition in females, and currently the male:female ratio is considered to be closer to 2:1(1). There has been in the past a greater degree of underdiagnosis and delayed recognition of AS among women because the disease was wrongly considered to be much

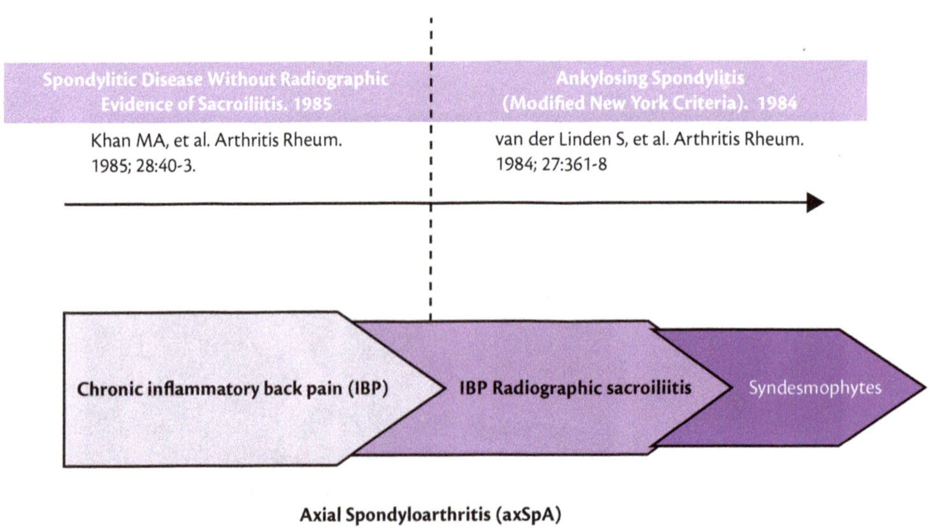

Fig. 11.3 The wide spectrum of predominantly axSpA shows that not everyone suffering from nr-axSpA or 'spondylitic disease without radiographic evidence of sacroiliitis' progresses to ankylosing spondylitis.
Rudwaleit M, Khan MA, Sieper J. Arthritis Rheum 2005;52:1000–8, with permission from John Wiley & Sons.

more common in men. For example, only 10% of the patients diagnosed around 1960 in Germany were females, but this percentage has increased in the subsequent decades to reach 46% among those diagnosed since 1990 (27). With the introduction of the Amor and the ESSG classification criteria, and more recently the ASAS classification criteria for axSpA, and the use of MRI for detecting spinal inflammation early, the demographics of this clinical entity has shifted remarkably (2, 32). The disease seems to progress to radiographic sacroiliitis relatively more slowly in women than in men, and that may be one of the reasons why women are relatively overrepresented compared to men among patients with 'spondylitis disease without radiographic evidence of sacroiliitis' (19), now called nr-axSpA (33).

Musculoskeletal manifestations

Symptoms resulting from inflammation of the sacroiliac joints and the spine

The disease symptoms usually start during the late teens or early twenties. Data from developed countries indicate that the average age of onset is around 24 years and approximately 15% have disease onset in childhood (before age 16), but this percentage may be as high as 40% in some developing countries (34). The average age at onset does not differ significantly among males and females, but is significantly younger in HLA-B27-positive patients versus those who lack this gene (27, 35, 36). The disease starts insidiously, and the presenting clinical manifestations during the early stage of the disease can often be non-specific and wide ranging. Thus a variety of healthcare professionals (such as primary care physicians, physiatrists, orthopaedists, chiropractors, podiatrists, dermatologists ophthalmologists, and gastroenterologists, as well as other medical and surgical specialists) first see such patients, and the diagnosis is often missed or markedly delayed.

Pain resulting from inflammation of the SI joints is usually the earliest symptom. The pain is of insidious onset, and is usually dull in character, difficult to localize, felt initially deep pain in the sacroiliac joints or gluteal/intrapelvic area. It can sometimes be intermittent and also affect one side and later alternate from side to side before it becomes bilateral chronic pain (2, 4, 5). The inflammatory process gradually progresses to involve the lumbar spine, causing chronic low back pain and stiffness that worsens late at night and early morning or after prolonged inactivity, but is alleviated to a variable extent with physical activity or exercise, hot showers, or use of NSAIDs (2, 4, 5). The pain is not alleviated with rest, unlike the mechanical low back pain. A teenager or a young adult presenting with chronic back pain and stiffness is a very typical clinical presentation, but since back pain in general is very prevalent in the population, axSpA is not the most common cause of back pain.

The features suggesting the inflammatory nature of the patient's back pain, as proposed by Calin et al. (37), include insidious onset before the age of 45 years, with a duration of at least 3 months, worsening with inactivity, improving with physical exercise, and being associated with spinal morning stiffness. Most recently, it has been defined by having at least four of the following five characteristics: 1: insidious onset, 2: onset before age 40 years, 3: pain at night (with improvement upon getting up), 4: improvement with exercise, and 5: no improvement with rest. According to the best trade-off, if at least four of these five parameters are fulfilled, this definition has 80% sensitivity and 72% specificity (33, 38). It is rare for the disease to begin after the age of 45, but there is a small percentage of patients with well-documented late-onset AS (39, 40). Some may have had minimal symptoms progression (41) or had been pain-free for long periods of time (42), and some may finally present with back pain due to osteoporosis-related microfractures rather than due to inflammation.

IBP and stiffness is a very important presenting clinical symptom suggesting axSpA. However, it is not specific for AS/axSpA because approximately 80% of SpA patients versus about 20% of control groups (such as patients with mechanical back pain) also report the same symptoms. Occasionally, back pain may be absent or too mild to impel the patient to seek medical care. Some patients may complain only of back stiffness, fleeting muscle aches, or musculotendinous tender spots. These symptoms may become worse on exposure to cold or dampness, and some of these patients may be misdiagnosed with fibromyalgia (4). Sometimes pain and stiffness in the mid-thoracic or the cervical region or anterior chest wall pain and tenderness may be the initial symptom, rather than the more typical low backache. This may be a more common presentation in women. Moreover, women tend to have a milder disease course or atypical presentation and therefore may not be as easily diagnosed as men. However, this delay in diagnosis of AS in women, as in men, is decreasing as a result of greater awareness of this disease by many healthcare providers (43). Radiographic evidence of sacroiliitis and spinal ankylosis may progress more slowly in women than in men, but functional outcome, as analysed by studying activities of daily living, is similar. However, when it comes to pain and the need for drug therapy, female patients tend to be worse off, possibly because of slower (or a relatively incomplete) progression of spinal fusion and resultant decrease in inflammatory pain, or the problem of any concomitant fibromyalgia-like symptoms.

Tenderness and stiffness of the paraspinal muscles often accompany the inflammation of the axial skeleton. With disease progression, there is a gradual loss of spinal mobility, along with flattening of the lumbar spine, wasting of gluteal muscles. Later there is exaggerated thoracic spinal kyphosis and progressive spinal fusion that follows the inflammatory process involving the discovertebral junctions and the facet joints, as well as the costovertebral, and the costotransverse joints, and the paravertebral ligamentous attachments. Measures of spinal mobility, such as modified Schober's test and lateral spinal flexion, are important in the assessment of AS, but are often late findings. Involvement of the costovertebral and costotransverse joints leads to a gradual decrease in chest expansion, with resultant greater diaphragmatic breathing. Inability to fully expand the chest on inspiration may sometimes be the presenting complaint to the physician, or the patient may complain about chest pain and exertional dyspnoea. The chest expansion is normally at least 5 cm in healthy young individuals at the level of the xiphisternum, below the breasts. In patients with severe disease there is gradual limitation of neck mobility due to progressive syndesmophyte formation and fusion of facet joints, with forward stooping of the neck. Spontaneous atlantoaxial subluxation and vertical subluxation of axis can rarely occur (44, 45).

Involvement of the hip and the shoulder joints

The hip and shoulder joints, the so-called girdle joints, are affected in at least one-third of AS patients over the course of their disease. Hip joint involvement is usually bilateral and insidious (gradual) in onset; the pain is usually felt in the groin, although some patients feel it in the knee or the front of the thigh on the same side. Sometimes the first symptoms may result from involvement of the hip and shoulders joints. Hip joint involvement has been correlated with early age at onset of AS and is an indicator for a bad prognosis (4, 32). There is a gradual destruction and thinning of the joint cartilage and it is accompanied by gradual limitation of joint motion. However, some degree of contracture of the hip joints is not uncommon at later stages of the disease even without hip joint involvement, giving rise to a characteristic rigid gait, with the patient keeping the knees bent a little in an attempt to maintain an erect posture (4). There is usually some atrophy and weakness of thigh and buttock muscles due to their lack of use in patients with advanced disease. Involvement of the hip joints in a patient with a rigid spine, including the neck, is potentially more crippling and can lead to greater disability, but total hip joint replacement can minimize those limitations. Shoulder joint involvement is generally mild, with some limitation of full range of motion.

Peripheral joint involvement

Involvement of the peripheral joints other than the hips and shoulders in 'primary' AS (without associated psoriasis or IBD) is uncommon, and may affect knees more so than other joints. It is rarely persistent or destructive and tends to resolve without any residual joint deformity. However, more prominent and/or widespread peripheral joint involvement, tendinitis, bursitis, tenosynovitis, and dactylitis are more often observed in patients with concomitant IBD and psoriasis, and this is discussed in Chapters 17 and 18, respectively. Inflammation can also affect structures adjacent to the joints, such as tendons and bursae, resulting in tendonitis and bursitis. Inflammation of the temporomandibular joint is uncommon; it causes pain, tenderness, or some limitation in fully opening the mouth, but rarely can result in more severe limitation.

Enthesitis

The entheses, the site of bony insertion of ligaments and tendons, are among the major affected sites in AS, especially those in the axial skeleton, including the pelvis and girdle joints (hip and shoulders) (46–48). These aspects are discussed in detail in Chapter 10. Enthesitis can result in tenderness over vertebral spinal processes, iliac crest, anterior chest wall, calcaneus (plantar fasciitis and/or Achilles tendinitis), ischial tuberosities, greater trochanters, and sometimes patella and tibial tubercles. Pain and tenderness of the anterior chest wall due to enthesitis at costosternal junctions and inflammation of the manubriosternal junction, and sternoclavicular and costoclavicular joints can occur early in the disease course. Some of these patients present with chest pain that is usually accentuated on coughing or sneezing and at times may even mimic symptoms of atypical angina or pericarditis (4). Many patients give a history of having complained of chest pain to a physician before AS was diagnosed. Some patients can present with pain at the insertions of the plantar fascia and Achilles tendon into the calcaneum, or patellar tendon insertion into the tibial tubercle. Enthesitis most frequently occurs at sites that are subject to greater physical stress (46). It may be detected radiographically, but not in early stages, while ultrasonography and MRI, on the other hand, can detect early inflammatory changes even before they appear on conventional radiographs (46).

Osteoporosis, spinal ankylosis, and risk of fracture

Patients with AS are more likely to develop osteoporosis, which can contribute to progressive spinal kyphosis (49, 50). There is paradoxical occurrence of osteoproliferation and osteoporosis, and this is discussed in detail in Chapter 10. Spinal osteoporosis is caused in part by the ankylosis and lack of mobility, but it can also occur relatively early in the disease, possibly due to high disease activity with increased level of proinflammatory cytokines and an alteration in vitamin D metabolism, causing increased bone resorption (51, 52). Patients with a rigid osteoporotic spine are prone to spinal fracture with relatively minor physical trauma, which may not even be recalled by some patients (4, 7). Therefore spinal fracture needs to be ruled out in any patient with advanced AS who has new onset of neck or back pain, even in the absence of a history of trauma. Transverse displaced fractures of the neck are associated with significant morbidity and mortality and can result in quadriplegia. Patients with AS have a five-fold higher risk of clinical spine fracture and a 35% increased risk of non-vertebral fracture (50).

Extra-articular manifestations

AxSpA/AS is associated with many extra-articular manifestations (EAMs) (Fig. 11.4) (53–72). The most common such manifestation is the occurrence of one or more episodes of acute anterior uveitis in 25–40% of patients with AS during the course of the disease, and sometimes this can be the presenting manifestation that triggers a further rheumatological diagnostic evaluation (53). Occurrence of uveitis is significantly less common among patients lacking HLA-B27 (35, 53). Uveitis is covered in detail in Chapter 16. SpA also shows association with CD and UC (54) (see Chapter 17) and psoriasis (see Chapter 18).

Mild constitutional symptoms, such as anorexia, malaise, weight loss, and low-grade fever, may occur in some patients in the early stages of the disease; these are more common among patients with juvenile-onset AS, especially in developing countries. In many patients, daytime fatigue and getting tired easily, as well as sleep disturbance are major complaints. Many patients complain of lack of adequate uninterrupted sleep because of back pain and stiffness that is worse at night.

Increased cardiovascular morbidity and mortality have been observed in AS because of accelerated atherosclerosis (62, 63). Increased incidence of diastolic left ventricular dysfunction has been known for a long time and it probably serves as a precursor to chronic heart failure and may cause morbidity and mortality (64–67). Some of the relatively uncommon extraskeletal features include aortic insufficiency and cardiac conduction disturbances or heart block (68, 70).

Inflammation at the aortic root (aortitis) can lead to fibrosis that is often haemodynamically insignificant, and some patients might develop aortic incompetence due to a dilated aortic ring and changes in the aortic valve (70). Extension of the inflammation and fibrosis to the atrioventricular conduction system can cause a variable degree of heart block.

Pulmonary, renal, and neurological comorbidities in AS patients have recently been reviewed (69). Limitation of chest expansion can impair pulmonary function, but lung involvement in the form of a slowly progressive bilateral apical pulmonary fibrobullous disease or cavitations (with rare fungal infection) is a rare and late manifestation of AS in 1–2% of patients. However, the use of newer

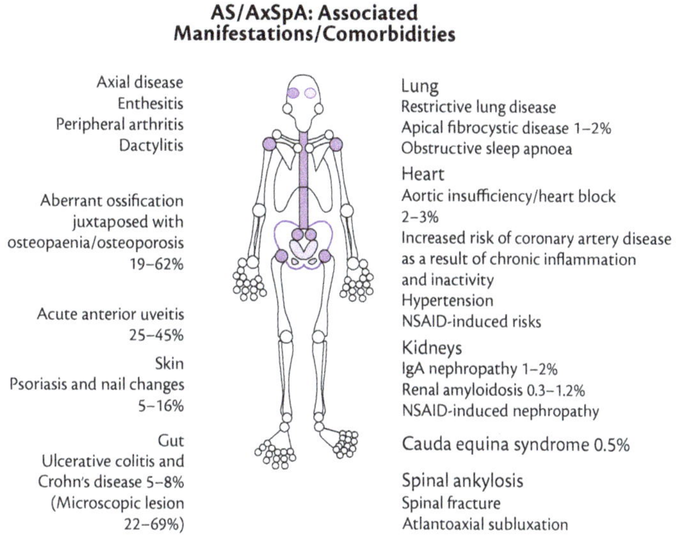

Fig. 11.4 Articular and extra-articular features and comorbidities of AS/AxSpA.

imaging modalities, such as high-resolution computed tomography (HRCT), suggest a higher incidence of interstitial lung disease than previously thought (71). In addition to ventilatory restriction from reduced chest wall movement, there is increased occurrence of obstructive sleep apnoea in patients with advanced disease with ankylosed forward-stooping cervical spine (69). Renal amyloidosis, IgA nephropathy and nephrolithiasis are uncommon occurrences, and NSAID-related nephropathy can also occur (13, 72).

Patients with AS are also subject to neurologic manifestations that are often related to spinal fracture dislocation. The fracture usually occurs in the cervical spine (81%), and neurologic deficits are often subtle on initial presentation, resulting being missed because of a low index of suspicion and poor visualization of lower cervical fractures on conventional radiographs (73). Extension of the ankylosed kyphotic cervical spine during conventional immobilization or for radiologic procedures can result in or worsen neurologic deficits and make stable fracture unstable (73–75). Aseptic spondylodiscitis can occur, mostly in the mid-thoracic spine, and is more commonly seen in patients with advanced disease. It is usually asymptomatic, and can occur with minimal or no history of physical trauma (76, 77).

Cauda equina syndrome, characterized by dull pain in the lower back and upper buttock region, analgesia in the buttocks, genitalia, or thighs (saddle area), and a disturbance of bowel and bladder function, is a rare and late complication of AS. It probably results from chronic adhesive arachnoiditis, which results from fibrous entrapment and scarring of the sacral and lower lumbar nerve roots (78, 79). Spontaneous atlantoaxial subluxation as well as upward subluxation of axis has also been reported in patients with AS (44, 45, 80). There are several case reports of co-occurrence of AS and demyelination, possibly multiple sclerosis, but a true link remains to be established (81, 82).

Physical findings

A careful and thorough physical examination should be conducted in order to look for signs that support the diagnosis and/or determine the severity of the disease. This includes looking for tenderness over the SI joints or eliciting SI joint pain by manoeuvres to stress the joints. These include hip flexion, FABERE (flexion, abduction, external rotation, and extension) Patrick's tests, Gaenslen' smanoeuvres, lateral pelvic compression, and anteroposterior (AP) pelvic compression tests (Box 11.1). They have been illustrated elsewhere (83, 84). Clinical indicators of enthesitis include tenderness over the SI joints, spinal processes, heels, iliac crest, anterior chest wall, and other bony prominences. Anterior chest wall tenderness can be localized over costochondral areas, manubriosternal junction, or sternoclavicular joints. Pain and stiffness in the cervical spine generally tend to develop after some years but occasionally occur in the early stages of the disease, and some patients may have recurrent severe episodes of stiff neck (torticollis).

Measures of spinal mobility (such as modified Schober's test and lateral spinal flexion) may be better clinical indicators of AS than limitation of chest expansion. Tools to assess and monitor SpA have recently been reviewed in detail (85). There is gradual flattening of the anterior chest wall, shoulders become 'stooped', the abdomen becomes protuberant, and breathing becomes increasingly diaphragmatic (Fig. 11.1). Occiput-to-wall or tragus-to-wall distances measure forward stooping deformity of the cervical spine (86). Involvement of the cervical spine can gradually result in progressive limitation of the ability to turn or fully extend or laterally bend the neck. The rate and pattern of spinal ankylosis development varies among patients. The typical spinal limitation of mobility and physical deformities usually evolve after at least 10 years. However, the disease may occasionally remain limited to SI joints, and spinal ankylosis may not occur at all in some patients with very mild disease (87). Syndesmophyte formation with resultant spinal ankylosis may progress more slowly in women than in men, but functional outcome, as analysed by studying activities of daily living, is similar. Mild to moderate limitation of chest expansion can be an early physical finding in some patients with AS, whereas severe limitation is typically a late physical finding. However, it has limited sensitivity for the diagnosis.

Importance of early diagnosis

Early diagnosis and management are crucial in SpA (88). The disease symptoms start insidiously, and symptoms can often be mild

Box 11.1 SI joint stress manoeuvres

Patrick's test or FABERE

- The patient lies supine on the examining table, one hip is flexed, abducted, externally rotated, then extended, to form a figure-4 with the ankle on the contralateral knee.
  - This manoeuvre stresses the ipsilateral SI joint.
  - If this manoeuvre causes posterior hip pain, mostly overlying the SI joint area, sacroiliitis should be suspected.

  The test is repeated on the contralateral side.

Gaenslen's test

- The patient lies supine on the examination table, with the side to be tested projecting over the side of the table.
  - The patient draws his or her knees to the chest.
  - The physician stabilizes the patient, while the lower extremity of the side being tested is left to drop off the table to fully extending the hip joint.
  - If this manoeuvre causes pain in the SI joint area, sacroiliitis should be suspected.

  The test can then be repeated on the contralateral side.

Lateral pelvic compression test

- The patient lies on his or her side on a firm examining table.
  - The physician applies pressure on the iliac crest to compress the pelvis down toward the table top.
  - Pain elicited in the SI joint area on either or both sides may be indicative of sacroiliitis.

AP pelvic compression test

- The patient lies supine on a firm examining table.
  - The physician applies pressure on the anterior superior iliac spine bilaterally to compress the pelvis.
  - Pain elicited in the SI joint area on either or both sides may be indicative of sacroiliitis.

Box 11.2 Clinical parameters ('red flags'), laboratory tests, and imaging that suggest presence of axSpA

IBD (CD and UC)
Good symptomatic response to NSAIDs
Acute anterior uveitis
Family history of SpA
Psoriasis
Dactylitis
Enthesitis (heels)
Peripheral arthritis (often asymmetric and in lower extremities)
Elevated CRP
Presence of HLA-B27
Imaging

and less specific during the early stage of the disease. Physical signs on clinical examination may sometimes be minimal in the early stages of the disease. Therefore clinical assessment of a patient with suspected axSpA should include a detailed clinical history, including a family history (and inquiry about smoking), assessment of the patient's spinal and hip and shoulder mobility, chest expansion, examination for peripheral arthritis, and a search for signs of enthesitis. Important physical findings due to enthesitis, which are present in many patients but are often overlooked, include tenderness over SI joints, vertebral spinal processes, the iliac crests, anterior chest wall, calcaneus (plantar fasciitis and/or Achilles tendinitis), ischial tuberosities, greater trochanters, and sometimes patella and tibial tubercles. Box 11.2 lists the clinical parameters or 'red flags' that help clinicians to recognize such patients at an earlier stage (29).

A teenager or a young adult presenting with chronic back pain is a very typical presentation, but back pain is very prevalent in the general population, and AS or other related SpA are not the most common cause of back pain. Moreover, in many patients with AS, it may take years from the onset of IBP to the development of radiographic sacroiliitis, despite the presence of inflammation as detected by MRI and the presence of some of the other clinical manifestations (42). Availability of MRI has confirmed that active inflammation of the SI joints and/or the spine is present long before the appearance of unequivocal sacroiliitis on plain radiography (89).

As the need for an early diagnosis becomes more and more important, as a result of the availability of more effective therapies which may even be more effective if given early, new strategies are being developed that will assist primary care physicians in screening for these patients, so that they can be referred to a rheumatologist when the disease is in its early stages (90–92). Proposals for improving the referral of patients with a possible diagnosis of axSpA include clinical parameters, imaging parameters, and HLA-B27 test (90–92).

Effect on lifespan

There is, in general, a gradual progression of the disease over the years, leading to worsening physical function. However, some patients have slow disease progression and can be minimally symptomatic, or almost pain-free for long periods of time (41, 42). The disease burden is discussed in detail in Chapters 25 and 26. Previous reports had reported increased mortality in AS, possibly resulting from cardiovascular disease (CVD), pulmonary diseases, smoking, spinal fractures due to physical trauma, alcohol-related injury, GI bleeding, and miscellaneous conditions (such as associated diseases, radiation treatment, and amyloidosis) (93–95). More recent studies have confirmed previous reports of increased mortality in AS (96–98). The most recent study, comprising patients from Sweden, Norway, and Denmark, also confirms increased mortality in AS (99), showing increased mortality for both men (age-adjusted hazard ratio (HR) = 1.53, 95% CI 1.36–1.72) and women (age-adjusted HR = 1.83, 95% CI 1.50–2.22). Within the AS cohort, statistically significant predictors for death were a lower level of education, general comorbidities (diabetes, infections, cardiovascular, pulmonary, and malignant diseases) and previous hip replacement surgery. An earlier smaller study from Norway (96) reported that parameters associated with reduced survival include the duration and intensity of inflammation, and the factors independently associated with reduced survival were diagnostic delay (OR 1.05), increasing levels of CRP (OR 2.68), work disability (OR 3.65), and not using any NSAIDs (OR 4.35). Thus there is a need for early disease detection and anti-inflammatory treatment, as well management and prevention of comorbidities (100).

References

1. Braun J, Sieper J. Ankylosing spondylitis. Lancet 2007;369(9570):1379–90.
2. van Tubergen A. The changing clinical picture and epidemiology of spondyloarthritis. Nat Rev Rheumatol 2015;11(2):110–18.
3. Khan MA. Ankylosing Spondylitis. PCI (Professional Communications, Inc.) 2016 (in press).
4. Khan MA. Clinical features of ankylosing spondylitis. In: Hochberg MC, Silman AJ, Smolen JS, Weinblatt ME, Weisman MH (eds) Rheumatology, 3rd edn. London, Mosby, 2003, pp. 1161–81.
5. Khan MA. Update on spondyloarthropathies. Ann Intern Med 2002;136(12):896–907.
6. Dougados M, Baeten D. Spondyloarthritis. Lancet 2011 18;377(9783):2127–37.
7. Khan MA. Spondyloarthropathies. In: Hunder GG (ed) Atlas of Rheumatology. Philadelphia, Current Medicine, 2002, pp. 141–67.
8. Khan MA, van der Linden SM. A wider spectrum of spondyloarthropathies. Semin Arthritis Rheum 1990;20(2):107–13.
9. Zeidler H, Mau W, Khan MA. Undifferentiated spondyloarthropathies. Rheum Dis Clin North Am 1992;18:187–202.
10. Brewerton DA. Discovery: HLA and disease. Curr Opin Rheumatol 2003;15(4):369–73.
11. Khan, MA. HLA and spondyloarthropathies. In: Mehra NK (ed) The HLA Complex in Biology and Medicine. A Resource Book. New Delhi, Jaypee Brothers Medical Publishers, 2010, pp. 259–75.
12. Rudwaleit M, Khan MA, Sieper J. The challenge of diagnosis and classification in early ankylosing spondylitis: do we need new criteria? Arthritis Rheum 2005;52:1000–8.
13. Akkoc N, Khan MA. Epidemiology of ankylosing spondylitis and related spondyloarthropathies. In: Weisman MH, Reveille JD, van der Heijde D (eds) Ankylosing Spondylitis and the Spondyloarthropathies: A Companion to Rheumatology. London, Mosby, 2006, pp. 117–31.
14. McGonagle D, Khan MA, Marzo-Ortega H, O'Connor P, Gibbon W, Emery P. Enthesitis in ankylosing spondylitis and related spondyloarthropathies. Curr Opin Rheumatol 1999;11:244–50.
15. François RJ, Braun J, Khan MA. Entheses and enthesitis: a histopathological review and relevance to spondyloarthropathies. Curr Opin Rheumatol 2001;13:255–64.
16. Jacques P, Lambrecht S, Verheugen E, et al. Proof of concept: entheses and new bone formation in spondyloarthritis are driven by mechanical strain and stromal cells. Ann Rheum Dis 2014;73(2)437–45.
17. Ronneberger M, Schett G. Pathophysiology of spondyloarthritis. Curr Rheumatol Rep 2011;13(5)416–20.
18. Sieper J, Rudwaleit M, Khan MA, Braun J. Concepts and epidemiology of spondyloarthritis. Best Pract Res Clin Rheumatol 2006;20:401–17.
19. Khan MA, van der Linden SM, Kushner I, Valkenburg HA, Cats A. Spondylitic disease without radiological evidence of sacroiliitis in relatives of HLA B27 positive patients. Arthritis Rheum 1985;28:40–3.
20. Stolwijk C, Boonen A, van Tubergen A, Reveille JD. Epidemiology of spondyloarthritis. Rheum Dis Clin North Am 2012;38(3):441–76.
21. Robinson PC, Wordsworth BP, Reveille JD, Brown MA. Axial spondyloarthritis: a new disease entity, not necessarily early ankylosing spondylitis. Ann Rheum Dis 2012;72(2):162–4.
22. Akkoc N, Khan, MA. Looking into the new ASAS classification criteria for axial spondyloarthritis through the other side of the glass. Curr Rheumatol Rep 2015;17(6):515.
23. van der Linden S, Akkoc N, Brown MA, Robinson PC, Khan MA. The ASAS criteria for axial spondyloarthritis: strengths, weaknesses and proposals for a way forward. Curr Rheumatol Rep 2015;17(9):535.
24. Malaviya AN, Kalyani A, Rawat R, Gogia SB. Comparison of patients with ankylosing spondylitis (AS) and non-radiographic axial SpA (nr-axSpA) from a single rheumatology clinic in New Delhi. Int J Rheum Dis 2015;18(7):736–41.
25. Akkoc N, Khan MA. Radiographic axial spondyloarthritis versus ankylosing spondylitis. Clin Exp Rheumatol 2016 March–April;34(1 Suppl 95):7. (Epub 2015 Aug 27)
26. Seo MR, Baek HL, Yoon HH, et al. Delayed diagnosis is linked to worse outcomes and unfavourable treatment responses in patients with axial spondyloarthritis. Clin Rheumatol 2015;34(8):1397–405.
27. Feldtkeller E, Khan MA, van der Linden S, van der Heijde D, Braun J. Age at disease onset and diagnosis delay in HLA-B27 negative vs. positive patients with ankylosing spondylitis. Rheumatol Int 2003; 23:61–6.
28. Khan MA. Thoughts concerning the early diagnosis of ankylosing spondylitis and related diseases. Clin Exp Rheumatol 2002;20(Suppl 28):S6–10.
29. Rudwaleit M, van der Heijde D, Khan MA, Braun J, Sieper J. How to diagnose axial spondyloarthritis early. Ann Rheum Dis 2004;63:535–43.
30. Song IH, Sieper J, Rudwaleit M. Diagnosing early ankylosing spondylitis. Curr Rheumatol Rep 2007;9(5):367–74.
31. Martindale J, Goodacre L. The journey to diagnosis in AS/axial SpA: the impact of delay. Musculoskeletal Care 2014;12(4):221–31.
32. Stone M, Warren RW, Bruckel J, Cooper D, Cortinovis D, Inman RD. Juvenile-onset ankylosing spondylitis is associated with worse functional outcomes than adult-onset ankylosing spondylitis. Arthritis Rheum 2005;53(3):445–51.
33. Rudwaleit M, Haibel H, Baraliakos X, et al. The early disease stage in axial spondylarthritis: results from the German Spondyloarthritis Inception Cohort. Arthritis Rheum 2009;60(3):717–27.
34. Malaviya AN, Sawhney S, Mehra NK, Kanga U. Seronegative arthritis in South Asia: an up-to-date review. Curr Rheumatol Rep 2014;16(4):413.
35. Khan MA, Kushner I, Braun WE. Comparison of clinical features of HLA B27 positive and negative patients with ankylosing spondylitis. Arthritis Rheum 1977;20:909–12.
36. Reynolds TL, Khan MA, van der Linden S, Cleveland RP. Differences in HLA B27 positive and negative patients with ankylosing spondylitis: study of clinical disease activity and levels of serum IgA, C reactive protein, and haptoglobin. Ann Rheum Dis 1991;50:154–7.
37. Calin A, Porta J, Fries JF, Schurman DJ. Clinical history as a screening test for ankylosing spondylitis. JAMA 1977;237:2613–14.
38. Sieper J, van der Heijde D, Landewé R, et al. New criteria for inflammatory back pain in patients with chronic back pain: a real patient exercise by experts from the Assessment of SpondyloArthritis international Society (ASAS). Ann Rheum Dis 2009;68(6):784–8.
39. Toussirot E. Late-onset ankylosing spondylitis and spondylarthritis: an update on clinical manifestations, differential diagnosis and pharmacological therapies. Drugs Aging 2010;27(7):523–31.
40. Olivieri I, D'Angelo S, Padula A, Leccese P, Palazzi C. Spondyloarthritis with onset after age 45. Curr Rheumatol Rep 2013;15:374.
41. Carette S, Graham D, Little H, Rubenstein J, Rosen P. The natural disease course of ankylosing spondylitis. Arthritis Rheum 1983;26(2):186–90.
42. Mau W, Zeidler H, Mau R, et al. Clinical features and prognosis of patients with possible ankylosing spondylitis. Results of a 10-year followup. J Rheumatol 1988;15(7):1109–14.
43. Salvadorini G, Bandinelli F, Delle Sedie A, et al. Ankylosing spondylitis: how diagnostic and therapeutic delay have changed over the last six decades. Clin Exp Rheumatol 2012;30:561–5.
44. Shim SC, Yoo DH, Lee JK, et al. Multiple cerebellar infarction due to vertebral artery obstruction and bulbar symptoms associated with vertical subluxation and atlanto-occipital subluxation in ankylosing spondylitis. J Rheumatol 1998;25(12):2464–8.
45. Thompson GH, Khan MA, Bilenker RM. Spontaneous atlantoaxial subluxation as a presenting manifestation of juvenile ankylosing spondylitis. Spine 1982;7:78–9.
46. Francois RJ, Braun J, Khan MA. Entheses and enthesitis: a histopathologic review and relevance to spondyloarthritides. Curr Opin Rheumatol 2001;13:255–64.
47. McGonagle D, Khan MA, Marzo-Ortega H, O'Connor P, Gibbon W, Emery P. Enthesitis in ankylosing spondylitis and related spondyloarthropathies. Curr Opin Rheumatol 1999;11:244–50.

48. Gladman DD, Inman RD, Cook RR, et al. International Spondyloarthritis Inter-observer Reliability Exercise—the INSPIRE Study: II. Assessment of peripheral joints, enthesitis and dactylitis. J Rheumatol 2007; 34(8):1740–5.
49. Prieto-Alhambra D, Munoz-Ortego J, De Vries F, et al. Ankylosing spondylitis confers substantially increased risk of clinical spine fracture: a nationwide case-control study. Osteoporosis Int 2015;26(1):85–91.
50. Magrey M, Khan MA. Osteoporosis in ankylosing spondylitis. Curr Rheumatol Rep 2010;12:332–6.
51. Magrey MN, Lewis S, Khan MA. Utility of DXA scanning and risk factors for osteoporosis in ankylosing spondylitis—A prospective study. Semin Arthritis Rheum 2016 (in press).
52. Gratacós J, Collado A, Pons F, et al. Significant loss of bone mass in patients with early, active ankylosing spondylitis: a followup study. Arthritis Rheum 1999;42(11):2319–24.
53. Khan MA, Haroon M, Rosenbaum JT. Acute anterior uveitis and spondyloarthritis: more than meets the eye. Curr Rheum Rep 2015:17(9):59.
54. Jacques P, Elewaut D. Spondyloarthritis: gut inflammation in SpA: flagellin joins the dance? Nat Rev Rheumatol 2014;10(1):5–6.
55. Rodrigues CE, Vieira WP, Bortoluzzo AB, et al. Low prevalence of renal, cardiac, pulmonary, and neurological extra-articular clinical manifestations in spondyloarthritis: analysis of the Brazilian Registry of Spondyloarthritis. Rev Bras Rheumatol 2012;52(3):375–83.
56. Solak O, Fidan F, Dündar U, et al. The prevalence of obstructive sleep apnea syndrome in ankylosing spondylitis patients. Rheumatology (Oxford) 2009;48(4):433–5.
57. El Maghraoui A. Extra-articular manifestations of ankylosing spondylitis: prevalence, characteristics and therapeutic implications. Eur J Intern Med 2011;22(6):554–60.
58. Jacquet A, Francois H, Frangie C, et al. IgA nephropathy associated with ankylosing spondylitis is not controlled by infliximab therapy. Nephrol Dial Transplant 2009;24(11):3540–2.
59. Jakobsen AK, Jacobsson LT, Patschan O, Askling J, Kristensen LE. Is nephrolithiasis an unrecognized extra-articular manifestation in ankylosing spondylitis? A prospective population-based Swedish national cohort study with matched general population comparator subjects. PLoS One 2014;9(11):e113602.
60. Mercieca C, van der Horst-Bruinsma IE, Borg AA. Pulmonary, renal and neurological comorbidities in patients with ankylosing spondylitis; implications for clinical practice. Curr Rheumatol Rep 2014;16(8):434.
61. Lautermann D, Braun J. Ankylosing spondylitis—cardiac manifestations. Clin Exp Rheum 2002;6(Suppl 28):S11–15.
62. Lin CW, Huang YP, Chiu YH, et al. Increased risk of ischemic stroke in young patients with ankylosing spondylitis: a population-based longitudinal follow-up study. PLoS One 2014;9(4):e94027.
63. Gupta N, Saigal R, Goyal L, et al. Carotid intima media thickness as a marker of atherosclerosis in ankylosing spondylitis. Int J Rheumatol 2014;2014:839135.
64. Khan MA, Sun JP, Bahler RC. Echocardiographic evidence of altered cardiac diastolic function in ankylosing spondylitis. Lancet 1987; i:1501.
65. Rowe IF, Gibson DG, Keat AC, Brewerton DA. Echocardiographic diastolic abnormalities of the left ventricle in inflammatory joint disease. Ann Rheum Dis 1991;50(4):227–30.
66. Sun JP, Khan MA, Farhat AZ, Bahler RC. Alterations in cardiac diastolic function in patients with ankylosing spondylitis. Int J Cardiol 1992;37:65–72.
67. Heslinga SC, Van Dongen CJ, Konings TC, et al. Diastolic left ventricular dysfunction in ankylosing spondylitis—a systematic review and meta-analysis. Semin Arthritis Rheum 2014;44(1):14–19.
68. Forsblad-d'Elia H, Wallberg H, Klingberg E, Carlsten H, Bergfeldt L. Cardiac conduction system abnormalities in ankylosing spondylitis: a cross-sectional study. BMC Musculoskelet Disord 2013;14:237.
69. Merciaca C, van der Horst-Bruinsma IE, Borg AA. Cardiovascular and cerebrovascular diseases in ankylosing spondylitis; current insights. Curr Rheumatol Rep 2012;14(85):415–21.
70. Klingberg E, Sveälv BG, Täng MS, et al. Aortic regurgitation is common in ankylosing spondylitis: time for routine echocardiography evaluation? Am J Med 2015;128(11):1244–50.
71. Turetschek K, Ebner W, Fleischmann D, et al. Early pulmonary involvement in ankylosing spondylitis: assessment with thin-section CT. Clin Radiol 2000;55(8):632–6.
72. Donmez S, Pamuk ON, Pamuk GE, Aydogdu E, Inman R. Secondary amyloidosis in ankylosing spondylitis. Rheumatol Int 2013;33(7):1725–9.
73. Thumbikat P, Hariharan RP, Ravichandran G, McClelland MR, Mathew KM. Spinal cord injury in patients with ankylosing spondylitis: a 10-year review. Spine 2007;32(26):2989–95.
74. Westerveld LA, VerlaanJJ, Oner FC. Spinal fractures in patients with ankylosing spinal disorders: a systematic review of the literature on treatment, neurological status and complications. Eur Spine J 2009;18(2):145–56.
75. Alaranta H, Luoto S, Konttinen YT. Traumatic spinal cord injury as a complication to ankylosing spondylitis. An extended report. Clin Exp Rheumatol 2002;20(1):66–8.
76. Langlois S, Cedoz JP, Lohse A, Toussirot E, Wendling D. Aseptic discitis in patients with ankylosing spondylitis: a retrospective study of 14 cases. Joint Bone Spine 2005;72(3):248–53.
77. Little H, Urowitz MB, Smythe HA, Rosen PS. Asymptomatic spondylodiscitis. An unusual feature of ankylosing spondylitis. Arthritis Rheum 1974;17(4):487–93.
78. Bilgen IG, Yunten N, Ustun EE, Oksel F, Gumusdis G. Adhesive arachnoiditis causing cauda equina syndrome in ankylosing spondylitis: CT and MRI demonstration of dural calcification and a dorsal dural diverticulum. Neuroradiology 1999;41(7):508–11.
79. Ginsburg WW, Cohen MD, Miller GM, Bartleson JD. Posterior vertebral body erosion by arachnoid diverticula in cauda equina syndrome: an unusual manifestation of ankylosing spondylitis. J Rheumatol 1997;24(7):1417–20.
80. Little H, Swinson DR, Cruickshank B. Upward subluxation of the axis in ankylosing spondylitis. A clinical pathologic report. Am J Med 1976;60(2):279–85.
81. Khan MA, Kushner I. Ankylosing spondylitis and multiple sclerosis: a possible association. Arthritis Rheum 1979;22:784–6.
82. Whitman GJ, Khan MA. Unusual occurrence of ankylosing spondylitis and multiple sclerosis in a black patient. Cleve Clin J Med 1989;56:819–22.
83. Khan MA. Ankylosing Spondylitis: The Facts. Oxford, Oxford University Press, 2002, pp.1–193.
84. Elyan M, Khan MA. Diagnosing ankylosing spondylitis. J Rheumatol 2006;78:12–23.
85. Landewé R, van Tubergen A. Clinical tools to assess and monitor spondyloarthritis. Curr Rheumatol Rep 2015;17(7):47.
86. Heuft-Dorenbosch L, Vosse D, Landewé R, et al. Measurement of spinal mobility in ankylosing spondylitis: comparison of occiput-to-wall and tragus-to-wall distance. J Rheumatol 2004;31(9):1779–84.
87. Brophy S, Mackay K, Al-Saidi A, Taylor G, Calin A. The natural history of ankylosing spondylitis as defined by radiological progression. J Rheumatol 2002;29(6):1236–43.
88. Wendling D, Claudepierre P, Prati C. Early diagnosis and management are crucial in axial SpA. Joint Bone Spine 2013;80(6):582–5.
89. Oostveen J, Prevo R, den Boer J, van de Laar M. Early detection of sacroiliitis on magnetic resonance imaging and subsequent development of sacroiliitis on plain radiography. A prospective, longitudinal study. J Rheumatol 1999;26(9):1953–8.
90. Braun J, Baraliakos X, Reqel A, Klitz U. Assessment of spinal pain. Best Pract Res Clin Rheumatol 2014;28(6):875–87.
91. Rudwaleit M, Sieper J. Early diagnosis of spondyloarthritis with special attention to the axial forms. Z Rheumatol 2005;64(8):524–30.
92. van Hoeven L, Luime J, Han H, Vergouwe Y, Weel A. Identifying axial spondyloarthritis in Dutch primary care patients, ages 20–45 years, with chronic low back pain. Arthritis Care Res (Hoboken) 2014;66(3):446–53.

93. Khan MA, Khan MK, Kushner I. Survival among patients with ankylosing spondylitis: a life-table analysis. J Rheumatol 1981;8(1):86–90.
94. Myllykangas-Luosujarvi R, Aho K, Lehtinen K, et al. Increased incidence of alcohol-related deaths from accidents and violence in subjects with ankylosing spondylitis. Br J Rheumatol 1998;37(6):688–90.
95. Lehtinen K. Mortality and causes of death in 398 patients admitted to hospital with ankylosing spondylitis. Ann Rheum Dis 1993;52(3):174–6.
96. Bakland G, Gran JT, Nossent JC. Increased mortality in ankylosing spondylitis is related to disease activity. Ann Rheum Dis 2011;70(11):1921–5.
97. Haroon NN, Paterson JM, Li P, Inman RD, Haroon N. Patients with ankylosing spondylitis have increased cardiovascular and cerebrovascular mortality: A population-based study. Ann Intern Med 2015;163(6):409–16.
98. Walsh JA, Zhou X, Clegg DO, Teng C, Cannon GW, Sauer B. Mortality in American Veterans with the HLA-B27 gene. J Rheumatol 2015;42(4):638–44.
99. Exarchou S, Lie E, Lindström U, et al. Mortality in ankylosing spondylitis: results from a nationwide population-based study. Ann Rheum Dis 2015;Sep 2. pii: annrheumdis-2015-207688. doi: 10.1136/annrheumdis-2015-207688. (Epub ahead of print.)
100. Ward MM, Deodhar A, Aki EA, et al. American College of Rheumatology/Spondylitis Association of America/Spondyloarthritis Research and Treatment Network 2015 Recommendations for the treatment of ankylosing spondylitis and nonradiographic axial spondyloarthritis. Arthritis Rheumatol 2016;68(2):282–98.

CHAPTER 12

Clinical outcomes

Astrid van Tubergen and Robert Landewé

Introduction to clinical outcomes

It is often difficult to define what the 'outcome' of a disease means. While the term 'outcome parameter' is frequently used in the context of clinical trials (and is synonymous to 'endpoint'), in order to describe a situation that should either be achieved (e.g. low disease activity) or be prevented (e.g. mortality), outcome has a slightly different connotation in chronic conditions such as rheumatic diseases. In rheumatology we usually talk about (long-term) outcome as the situation that will be reached after, for example, 20–30 years of disease, under the assumption that a patient is not actively treated for that disease—that is, the natural course of the disease. Therefore examples of broadly accepted long-term outcomes of a disease such as RA include 'premature death', 'joint destruction', 'job loss', and 'disability'. With subtle modifications, these long-term outcomes also pertain to other rheumatic diseases such as axSpA.

It is impossible nowadays to reliably measure and predict the long-term consequences of inflammatory diseases for the simple reason that we are rather successful in treating patients with these conditions. We start treatment early, apply tailor treatment strategies based on prognostication algorithms, and monitor patients carefully during the treatment. Considering the group of patients with inflammatory diseases, these treatment techniques have proven efficacy with regard to positively influencing long-term outcome.

Unfortunately, groups of patients (e.g. in RCTs) are not the same as individual patients (e.g. in clinical practice): the fact that a particular drug works well in terms of relieving symptoms in the actively treated arm of an RCT with axSpA patients may indicate a higher likelihood of a positive response in an individual patient with axSpA, but does not provide certainty! This is a principle that is often ignored in clinical medicine. The only way to find out if a patient will respond to a particular treatment (sequence) is to follow that patient over time. Subsequently, treatment can be adjusted if the clinical situation requires such a change. Therefore it is pivotal to somehow describe the patient's clinical situation, preferably in an unbiased manner, which means that such a description 'makes sense' and is unequivocal in its content. Measurement instruments are essential to achieve these goals, and we have a multitude of measurement instruments available to measure different aspects of the same disease. We tend to talk about 'outcome measures' when we describe these instruments that are used to follow patients over time, either in RCTs, observational studies, or clinical practice. It is important to realize that such 'real-time outcome measures' do not truly measure the long-term outcome of the disease itself, but that we justify their application by the fact that they are associated to some extent with the long-term consequences of the disease: these 'outcome measures' should have predictive validity.

The underlying principle of 'real-time measurement' in rheumatology is that assessing these 'outcome measures' provides us with a picture of long-term outcome without the need to measure that outcome itself. Consequently, the assumption is that if we base our therapeutic actions on the results of that intermediate outcome measure, we may influence that long-term outcome in a positive manner.

Note that it may have immediate as well as delayed value to influence a 'real-time outcome' by treatment: treating a patient with active axSpA with an effective drug may reduce signs and symptoms of inflammation (i.e. immediate success; improved status) *and*, for example, reduce the likelihood of syndesmophyte formation (or bamboo spine) over time (i.e. delayed success; improved prognosis).

While the simplest means of measurement is a judgmental statement in the patient's record, such as 'the patient is doing better', modern medicine requires a more transparent, objective, and reliable description of the patient's actual status, and many instruments have been developed over time to measure several aspects (domains) of the disease. Rheumatology as a medical discipline has truly been 'running ahead of the troops' with regard to the development of (principles of) measurement(s). Expert organizations such as OMERACT and the disease-specific ASAS have boosted the development of validated instruments to better measure diseases such as axSpA.

OMERACT has spelled out the requirements for appropriate measurement instruments in their OMERACT filter (1): instruments should be 'truthful', 'reliable', and 'feasible'. 'Truthful' refers to measuring what they intend to measure; 'reliable' implies that instruments can properly discriminate between several stages of the disease, but also between different treatments (or placebo) in an RCT; 'feasible' refers to 'ease of use' and applicability.

Instruments propagated by OMERACT are instruments that have successfully passed that filter: they have been properly validated for their specific purpose, and are thought to have predictive validity. Note that this purpose may be application in clinical trials or in observational research, but also, for example, monitoring in clinical practice, and that several settings may require different instruments. OMERACT has been instrumental in the development of so-called core sets of outcome measures for several settings and ASAS has been responsible for the development of such core-sets for research and clinical practice in the field of axSpA (2, 3).

This chapter gives an overview of the most important outcomes in axSpA and the most commonly used instruments to measure these, as recommended in the core set by ASAS. It also addresses some additional measures, which are frequently used but not (yet) included in the core set, and describes several sets of response criteria applied in axSpA research. Furthermore, we provide some guidance in which setting (research versus practice) and with which frequency these measures can be used.

ASAS/OMERACT core set of outcome measures

In 1999, ASAS, under the auspice of OMERACT, defined a core set of variables to be measured in patients with AS, by applying the OMERACT filter for use in clinical trials and daily practice (2–4). The ASAS/OMERACT core set of outcome measures defines the minimum of information that should be collected for three different settings (Fig. 12.1).

The inner circle of the ASAS/OMERACT core set describes the domains that should be assessed in patients receiving 'symptom-modifying antirheumatic drugs' (SMARDs) and/or physical therapy. An example of a SMARD in axSpA is treatment with NSAIDs. The core set of clinical record keeping includes the same domains as the previous core set and additionally the domains 'peripheral joints and entheses' and 'acute phase reactants'. The core set of 'disease-controlling antirheumatic treatment' (DC-ART) includes the same domains as the previous core set and additionally the domain 'spine radiograph'. An example of a DC-ART in axSpA is treatment with TNFα inhibitors.

For each domain included in the core set, specific instruments are selected (Table 12.1). Depending on the research question or clinical presentation of a patient, additional instruments, for example on comorbidity or work participation, may also be relevant to apply. Most instruments have been developed in patients with AS, but they can also be applied in patients with nr-axSpA (5). More information can also be found on the website of the ASAS (http://www.ASAS-group.org).

Table 12.1 ASAS/OMERACT core domains

Domain	Instrument
Function	BASFI
Pain	NRS/VAS (last week/spine/at night due to axSpA) *and* NRS/VAS (last week/spine due to axSpA)
Spinal mobility	Chest expansion *and* modified Schober *and* occiput to wall distance *and* cervical rotation *and* lateral spine flexion or BASMI
Patient global	NRS/VAS (global disease activity last week)
Peripheral joints and entheses	Number of swollen joints (44-joint count) Validated enthesitis scores, such as MASES, San Francisco, and Berlin
X-ray spine	Lateral lumbar spine and lateral cervical spine
Stiffness	NRS/VAS (duration of morning stiffness/spine/last week)
Acute phase reactants	CRP or ESR
Fatigue	Fatigue question from BASDAI

AxSpA, Axial spondyloarthritis; BASDAI, Bath Ankylosing Spondylitis Disease Activity Index; BASFI, Bath Ankylosing Spondylitis Functional Index; BASMI, Bath Ankylosing Spondylitis Metrology Index; CRP, C-reactive protein; ESR, erythrocyte sedimentation rate; MASES, Maastricht Ankylosing Spondylitis Enthesitis Score; NRS, numerical rating scale; VAS, visual analogue scale.

Source: Reprinted with permission from the Journal of Rheumatology, Van der Heijde et al., J Rheumatol 1999; 26(4).

Physical function

Physical function refers to the degree of functional limitation. In early axSpA, physical function is primarily affected by the activity of the disease, whereas in later disease, structural damage of the spine may play a larger role (6). However, it may be difficult to differentiate between these two in an individual patient.

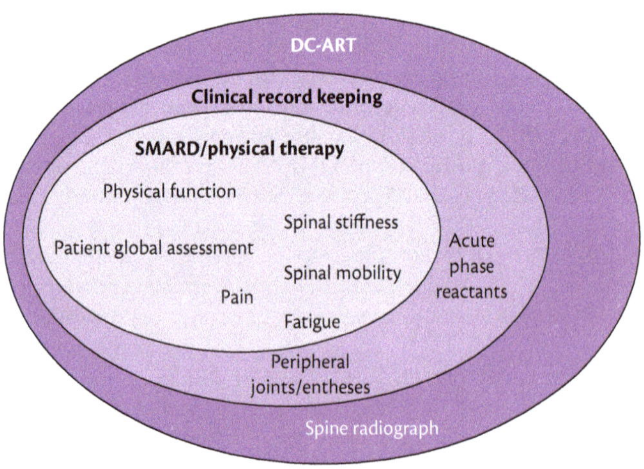

Fig. 12.1 ASAS/OMERACT core domains for AS. DC-ART, Disease-controlling antirheumatic treatment; SMARD, symptom-modifying antirheumatic drugs. Reprinted with permission from the Journal of Rheumatology, Van der Heijde et al., J Rheumatol 1999; 26(4).

Physical function tests are used in both research and practice. For daily practice, it is recommended to measure physical function at least once per year in every patient. In the ASAS/OMERACT core set, the BASFI is recommended for measuring function (7). The BASFI consists of ten questions: eight refer to the functional anatomy of the patients, and two assess the patient's ability to cope with everyday life. All questions are answered, preferably, on an 11-point numerical rating scale (NRS) or, alternatively, on a 10-cm visual analogue scale (VAS), with two anchors 'easy' and 'impossible' at either side. The mean of the ten questions defines the final score, ranging from 0 (best) to 10 (worst). Up to three missing items are allowed in the BASFI, which can be imputed by the average of the remaining items (8).

Disease activity

Disease activity in patients with axSpA can be measured in several ways. Single-item questions on, for example, pain, stiffness, and global well-being can give an impression of these single parameters. It is, however, recommended to measure disease activity with an instrument addressing all the important aspects that represent the activity of a disease. Two instruments are available: the BASDAI (9) and Ankylosing Spondylitis Disease Activity Score (ASDAS) (10). The BASDAI is fully patient reported, whereas the ASDAS also includes an objective measure of inflammation. For this reason, and also because the ASDAS showed better test characteristics over the BASDAI, the ASDAS is preferred for use in both clinical practice and trials. In case acute phase reactants have not been assessed, the BASDAI can be used. It is recommended to assess disease activity at least twice per year, and more frequently in the case of active disease.

Spinal stiffness

Spinal stiffness is assessed by the question: 'How long does your morning stiffness last from the time you wake up?' The answer is recorded, preferably, on an NRS or, alternatively, on a 10-cm VAS with three anchors: '0 hours', '1 hour', and '2 or more hours'. Score ranges from 0 (none) to 10 (severe).

Pain

Pain is assessed by two questions: (1) 'How much pain of your spine due to axSpA do you have?' and (2) 'How much pain of your spine due to axSpA do you have at night?' The answer is recorded, preferably, on an NRS or, alternatively, on a 10-cm VAS with two anchors, 'no pain' and 'most severe pain', at either side. Score ranges from 0 (no pain) to 10 (most severe pain).

Patient global assessment

Patient global assessment is assessed by the question: 'How active was your axSpA last week?' The answer is recorded, preferably, on an NRS or, alternatively, on a 10-cm VAS with two anchors, 'not active' and 'very active', at either side. Score ranges from 0 (not active) to 10 (very active).

Physician global assessment

Physician global assessment reflects the physician's perspective of global disease activity and can be assessed by the question: 'How active do you consider the patient's axSpA last week?' The answer is recorded, preferably, on an NRS or, alternatively, on a 10-cm VAS with two anchors, 'not active' and 'very active', at either side. Score ranges from 0 (not active) to 10 (very active).

Bath Ankylosing Spondylitis Disease Activity Index

The BASDAI consists of six questions on fatigue, spinal pain, pain and/or swelling of the peripheral joints, localized tenderness, intensity of morning stiffness, and duration of morning stiffness (9). Each question is scored, preferably, on an NRS or, alternatively, on a 10-cm VAS with two anchors, 'none' and 'very severe', on either side for the first five questions, and three anchors, '0 hours', '1 hour', and '2 or more hours', for the duration of morning stiffness. The mean of the items on morning stiffness counts as one variable. The mean of the five items defines the final score. The score ranges from 0 (no disease activity) to 10 (very active disease). A cut-off of 4 is frequently used to define active disease, but this cut-off level does not have a firm justification. One missing questions is allowed in the BASDAI, which can be imputed by the average of the remaining items (8).

Ankylosing Spondylitis Disease Activity Score

The ASDAS is a score that combines patient reported outcomes on back pain, peripheral pain/swelling, and duration of morning stiffness (derived from the BASDAI), as well as patient global assessment, together with either the erythrocyte sedimentation rate (ASDAS-ESR) or C-reactive protein (ASDAS-CRP) as an objective measure of inflammation (10). The total score can be calculated with the following formulae:

$$\text{ASDAS-CRP: } 0.121 \times \text{total back pain} + 0.110 \times \text{patient global} + 0.073 \times \text{peripheral pain/swelling} + 0.058 \times \text{duration of morning stiffness} + 0.579 \times \text{Ln}(\text{CRP} + 1).$$

$$\text{ASDAS-ESR: } 0.113 \times \text{patient global} + 0.293 \times \sqrt{\text{ESR}} + 0.086 \times \text{peripheral pain/swelling} + 0.069 \times \text{duration of morning stiffness} + 0.079 \times \text{total back pain}.$$

The ASAS prefers the use of the ASDAS-CRP over the ASDAS-ESR, both in clinical practice and in clinical trials. An ASDAS value below 1.3 is considered low disease activity, between 1.3 and 2.1 as moderate disease activity, between 2.1 and 3.5 as high disease activity, and above 3.5 as very high disease activity, with no maximum (Fig. 12.2) (11).

Fatigue

A substantial number of patients with axSpA suffer from fatigue. Fatigue may be related to the activity of the disease (pain and stiffness), functional ability, global well-being, and metal health status (12). In order to get an impression about the level of fatigue in a patient, it is often sufficient to ask the question 'How would you describe the overall level of fatigue/tiredness you have experienced?', which corresponds to the first question from the BASDAI. The answer is recorded, preferably, on an NRS or, alternatively, on a 10-cm VAS with two anchors, 'none' and 'very severe', at either side. The score ranges from 0 (none) to 10 (very severe).

Quality of life

Health-related quality of life (HRQoL) and disability, a concept that includes social functioning and adaptation, are not disease specific. However, QoL can be measured by both generic- and disease-specific instruments. Generic instruments are useful for comparison across different interventions and different diseases. Examples of generic instruments applied to patients with axSpA are the 36-item Short-Form Health Survey (SF-36) (13) and the EuroQol Five Dimensions questionnaire (EQ-5D) (14). A potential disadvantage of a generic instrument is that not all questions may apply to the patient category under investigation, whilst other relevant questions may be lacking. A disease-specific instrument specifically developed for axSpA is the ASQoL (15). QoL in axSpA may

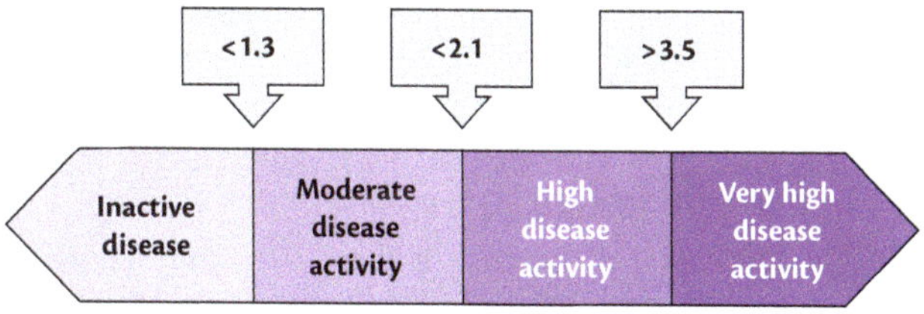

Fig. 12.2 (See colour plate section). ASDAS cut-offs for status scores.
Reproduced from Ann Rheum Dis, Machado P, Landewe R, Lie E, Kvien TK, Braun J, Baker D, et al. 70, 47–53, 2011 with permission from BMJ Publishing Group Ltd.

be affected by several factors, such as disease activity and physical function, but also by fatigue and ability to cope with the disease. Outcome measures on QoL are used in both research and practice. For clinical practice, it is often sufficient to asses QoL only once per year.

36-item Short-Form Health Survey

The SF-36 consists of 36 Likert-formatted questions covering eight domains: vitality, physical functioning, bodily pain, general health perceptions, physical role functioning, emotional role functioning, social role functioning, and mental health (13). A summarized Physical Component Score (PCS) and Mental Component Score (MCS) can be calculated, each with a scoring range of 0 (worse) to 100 (best).

EuroQol Five Dimensions questionnaire

The EQ-5D measures QoL in five dimensions: mobility, self-care, daily activities, pain/discomfort, and anxiety/depression (14). Each domain is scored based on the perceived level of problems by the patient, ranging from 'no problems' to 'extreme problems'. The levels for each dimension are combined into one health state. The score ranges from 0 (worse) to 100 (best).

Ankylosing Spondylitis Quality of Life Questionnaire

The Ankylosing Spondylitis Quality of Life Questionnaire (ASQoL) consists of 18 questions, which can be answered with yes (score 1) or no (score 0) (15). The total score is calculated by summing the scores for each question, and ranges from 0 (best) to 18 (worst).

ASAS Health Index

The main complaints indicated by patients with axSpA are pain, stiffness, fatigue, and limitation in activities and social participation (16–18). For the assessment of patients with axSpA, many instruments have been developed that focus predominantly on specific aspects of health and measure specific concepts, such as physical function. However, the overall picture of impairments, limitations, and restrictions in activities and social participation of patients with axSpA is not adequately assessed by these axSpA-specific questionnaires (19). The ASAS has developed an instrument, the ASAS Health Index (ASAS HI) (20), which assesses health as operationalized by the International Classification of Functioning, Disability, and Health (ICF) core set for AS (21). The whole range of functioning and disability of patients with axSpA is captured, and the ASAS HI also includes items that were proposed by patients, which were not captured by other published indices on function and disability. The ASAS HI contains 17 dichotomous items addressing categories of pain, emotional functions, sleep, sexual functions, mobility, self-care, community life, and employment. The score ranges from 0 to 17. The real-life performance of the ASAS HI is currently tested in clinical trials and clinical practice.

Spinal mobility

Spinal mobility may be affected in many patients with axSpA. Different instruments are available to assess spinal mobility, of which some are recommended by the ASAS and some are included in the BASMI (Table 12.2). The BASMI is a composite index of five measures of spinal mobility. Age-specific reference intervals and percentiles for 11 spinal mobility measures have been established (22) and are also available through the ASAS website (http://www.asas-group.org). The reference intervals may guide clinicians in the assessment of individual patients. Population-based reference values from the US for a selection of spinal mobility measures have also been published (23). Spinal mobility measures are used in both research and practice. In daily practice, it is recommended to assess spinal mobility once per year.

Table 12.2 Spinal mobility measures

Spinal mobility measure	Recommended by ASAS	Included in BASMI
Chest expansion	X	
Modified Schober	X	X
Occiput-to-wall distance	X	
Tragus-to-wall distance		X
Cervical rotation	X	X
Lateral spinal flexion	X*	X
Intermalleolar distance		X
Internal hip rotation‡		

*As an alternative for lateral spinal flexion, BASMI can be used.

‡Internal hip rotation is included neither in the ASAS recommendation nor in the BASMI.

Chest expansion

To measure chest expansion, the patient is asked to rest his or her hands on or behind the head. The difference between maximal inspiration and expiration is measured at the fourth intercostal level anteriorly in centimetres to the nearest 0.1 cm. Chest expansion is measured twice, and the better of two tries is recorded.

Modified Schober

The modified Schober is measured with the patient standing erect. An imaginary line, connecting both posterior superior iliac spines, is marked. A second mark is placed 10 cm above the first mark. The patient is asked to bend forward maximally, and the distance between the two marks is measured. The increase in centimetres to the nearest 0.1 cm is recorded. The modified Schober is measured twice, and the better of two tries is recorded.

Occiput-to-wall distance and tragus-to-wall distance

For measuring the occiput-to-wall distance (OWD) and tragus-to-wall distance (TWD), the patient stands with the heels and back resting against the wall, with the hips and knees as straight as possible. The chin should be held at the usual carrying level. The patient is asked to make maximal effort to touch the head against the wall. For the OWD the distance between the occiput and wall is measured in centimetres to the nearest 0.1 cm. The OWD is measured twice, and the better of two tries is recorded. For the TWD, the distance between the tragus and wall is measured twice in centimetres to the nearest 0.1 cm on the left side, and the better of two tries is recorded. The same procedure is followed for the right side. The final TWD is calculated by averaging the best value for the left and the right side.

The OWD and TWD were found to be equally reliable in assessing thoracic spine extension (24). A limitation of the TWD is that it can vary with the size of the head. However, the TWD is less influenced by inclination of the cervical spine. Although the TWD is in general easier to perform, the OWD is recommended by the ASAS, because a value of 0 in the OWD measurement easily distinguishes patients with normal thoracic spine extension from kyphosed patients (24).

Cervical rotation

Cervical rotation is measured with the patient sitting straight on a chair and the chin at the normal carrying level. The assessor places a goniometer at the top of the head in line with the nose. The patient is asked to rotate the neck maximally to the left, and the assessor follows with the goniometer. The angle between the first sagittal plane and the new plane after rotation is measured in degrees. The better of two tries is recorded. The same procedure is followed for the right side. The final score for cervical rotation is calculated by averaging the best values for the left and the right side and is recorded in degrees.

Lateral spinal flexion

The lateral spinal flexion is measured with the patient standing with the heels and back resting against the wall, without flexion in the knees and without bending forward. A first mark is placed on the right thigh, at the level of the patient's middle fingertip. The patient is then asked to bend sideward to the right as far as possible without bending the knees or lifting the heels, and a second mark is placed again at the level of the patient's middle fingertip. The distance between the two marks is measured in centimetres to the nearest 0.1 cm. The better of two tries is recorded. The same procedure is followed for the left side. The score for lateral spinal flexion is calculated by averaging the best values for the left and the right side.

Hip function

The intermalleolar distance (IMD) is preferably measured with the patient lying supine with the legs separated as far as possible, the knees straight, and the toes pointing upwards. The distance between the medial malleoli is measured in centimetres. Alternatively, the IMD is measured with the patient standing erect and the legs separated as far as possible. The better of two tries is recorded.

Because measuring the IMD is frequently found uncomfortable for patients, an alternative measurement for hip function has been proposed, the internal rotation of the hip (IHR), which is part of the Edmonton Ankylosing Spondylitis Metrology Index (EDASMI) (25). For measuring the IHR, the subject is seated on an examining table with the knees and hips flexed at 90 degrees and the knees together clasping a piece of card paper. The subject is asked to move the ankles apart as far as possible without releasing the card paper from between the knees. The distance between the medial malleoli is recorded in centimetres.

The IMD and IHR are only weakly correlated, indicating that they measure different aspects of hip mobility (26). Therefore the IHR cannot be used as a substitute for the IMD to quantify hip function in patients with axSpA.

BASMI

The BASMI combines five measures of spinal mobility (Table 12.2). Three scoring methods for the BASMI are available: BASMI-2, BASMI-10, and BASMI-linear. In the original BASMI, called BASMI-2, all continuous measurements were converted into a three-point scale (0 to 2) using a conversion table (27). The final BASMI-2 score is calculated by summing the individual converted scores, and ranges from 0 to 10. Because much information is lost when converting a continuous scale into a nominal scale with only three categories, a different conversion table with 11 categories was proposed, called the BASMI-10 (28). The final BASMI-10 score is calculated by the mean of all five converted scores.

Disadvantages of converting continuous measurements into nominal scales are that small changes in the assessments can as well be suppressed as lead to large jumps in the resulting BASMI. However, even small changes may be of importance in, for instance, clinical trials. For this reason, the BASMI-linear was proposed, in which the continuous scores are converted into a linear scale using five equations (29). The BASMI-linear score is calculated by the mean of the five linear scores and ranges from 0 to 10. The BASMI-linear has shown to be more sensitive to change in clinical trials compared with the BASMI-2 and BASMI-10 (30). ASAS recommends using either the BASMI-10 or the BASMI-linear. Importantly, scores from the BASMI-10 and BASMI-linear are not interchangeable with the BASMI-2.

Peripheral joints

Approximately one-third of the patients with axSpA suffer from peripheral joint involvement. In clinical practice, the joints are usually examined on indication at each visit. In research, the joints can be systematically assessed by the 44-joint count. The joints are assessed for the presence of swelling and tenderness. Included joints are: humeroscapular joints, acromioclavicular joints, sternoclavicular joints, elbows, wrists, metacarpophalangeal joints, proximal interphalangeal joints, knees, ankles, and metatarsophalangeal joints. There is no grading and the total score varies from 0 to 44.

Entheses

Entheses are sites where the ligaments, tendons, and joint capsules attach to the bone. Enthesitis—inflammation at these sites—is frequently seen in patients with axSpA. Enthesitis is often difficult to assess clinically and does not always correspond with findings by ultrasound (31). Several instruments are available for measuring enthesitis in axSpA. The use of such indices is not recommended in daily clinical practice by the ASAS, because they may be time consuming or may not encompass all entheseal sites. For practice, it is recommended to ask at each visit for entheseal complaints, and to examine these entheses on indication.

The Mander Enthesitis Index (MEI) is the first instrument developed for measuring enthesitis (32). The MEI measures the patient's response to pain following local pressure to 66 entheseal sites, and is scored 0 (no pain), 1 (mild tenderness), 2 (moderate tenderness), or 3 (tenderness severe enough to elicit a wince or withdrawal). Because the MEI is time consuming and therefore not useful in practice, alternative indices have been proposed which examine importantly fewer entheseal sites (Table 12.3). These include the San Francisco Enthesitis Index (SFI) (33), the Berlin Enthesitis Index (BEI) (34), and the Maastricht Ankylosing Spondylitis Enthesitis Score (MASES) (35). These instruments were found to reliably measure enthesitis in axSpA (36) and are included in the ASAS/OMERACT core set for DC-ARTs. The SFI examines 17 sites, with a

Table 12.3 Entheses included in each enthesitis index

Anatomical region	MEI (range 0–90)	SFI (range 0–51)	BEI (range 0–12)	MASES (range 0–13)	SPARCC (range –16)	LEI (range 0–6)
Front side						
Manubriosternal joint (bilateral)	X					
All costochondral joints (bilateral)	X					
1st costochondral joints (bilateral)				X		
7th costochondral joints (bilateral)				X		
Symphysis pubis		X				
Iliac crest (bilateral)	X		X	X		
Anterior superior iliac spine (bilateral)	X	X		X		
Greater trochanter femur (bilateral)	X	X	X		X	
Greater tuberosity of the humerus bilateral	X				X	
Pelvic abductor origin bilateral		X				
Medial condyle of the femur (bilateral)	X		X			X
Lateral condyle of the femur (bilateral)	X		X			
Lateral epicondyle of the humerus (bilateral)	X				X	X
Medial epicondyle of the humerus (bilateral)	X				X	
Quadriceps insertion on patella (bilateral)					X	
Patellar ligament insertion inferior pole of patella or tibial tubercle (bilateral)					X	
Back side						
Nuchal crest (bilateral)	X					
All cervical spinous processes	X					
Spinous process C1/C2		X				
Spinous process C7/T1		X				
All thoracic spinous processes	X					
Spinous process T12/L1		X				
All lumbar spinous processes	X					
5th lumbar spinous process		X		X		
Ischial tuberosity (bilateral)	X	X				
Posterior superior iliac spine (bilateral)	X			X		
Achilles tendon insertion calcaneus (bilateral)	X	X	X	X	X	X
Plantar fascia insertion calcaneus (bilateral)	X	X	X		X	

SFI, San Francisco Enthesitis Index; BEI, Berlin Enthesitis Index; MASES, Maastricht Ankylosing Spondylitis Enthesitis Score; SPARCC, Spondyloarthritis Research Consortium of Canada Enthesitis Index; LEI, Leeds Enthesitis Index.

scoring identical to the MEI. The final score ranges from 0 to 51 (37). The BEI examines 12 sites (34). The sites are scored as 0 (absent) or 1 (present), without grading; the score ranges from 0 to 12. The MASES examines 13 sites, also with a binary scoring system, and ranges from 0 to 13 (35). Alternative indices have been developed, although not (yet) included in the ASAS/OMERACT core set: the Spondyloarthritis Research Consortium of Canada (SPARCC) Enthesitis Index (16 sites) (38) and the Leeds Enthesitis Index (LEI) (six sites) (39). Both indices are scored dichotomously for the presence (score 1) or absence (score 0) of tenderness. Scores range from 0 to 16 for the SPARCC Enthesitis Index and from 0 to 6 for the LEI.

Acute phase reactants

ESR and CRP are the sole laboratory parameters included in the core set of clinical record keeping. Acute phase reactants are elevated in less than 50% of patients with active disease; therefore normal values do not rule out inflammation. In concomitant peripheral involvement and bowel disease, the acute phase reactants are more likely to be elevated (40). Elevated ESR and CRP are predictors of a favourable response to treatment (41).

For clinical practice, it is recommended to test CRP and/or ESR at least once a year, preferably together with other outcome measures of disease activity, such as the BASDAI or ASDAS.

Radiographic assessment of the spine

Radiographic damage of the spine is frequently seen in patients with axSpA. Different scoring methods are available for assessing this. The most frequently used, and recommended by the ASAS, is the modified Stoke Ankylosing Spondylitis Spinal Score (mSASSS) (42). In the mSASSS, the anterior parts of the cervical and lumbar spine at a lateral view are scored for the presence of squaring and/or erosion and/or sclerosis (1 point), non-bridging syndesmophytes (2 points), and/or bridging syndesmophytes (3 points). The total score ranges from 0 to 72.

An alternative scoring method, the Radiographic Ankylosing Spondylitis Spinal Score (RASSS), has been proposed (43). The RASSS includes, besides the cervical and lumbar spine, the lower thoracic vertebrae, under the assumption that most progression occurs here. However, in a study comparing the two scoring methods, the RASSS did not perform better and, therefore, does not justify the additional scoring efforts (44).

Because radiographic progression in axSpA occurs slowly, the ASAS recommends not to order new spinal radiographs within a 2-year period, unless other features are present, for example acute spinal pain, which may be suggestive for an (osteoporotic) fracture (45). The ASAS does not recommend the use of the mSASSS in daily practice.

Comorbidities

In axSpA, besides EAMs, comorbidities may occur. EAMs are co-existing conditions that are clearly part of the concept of SpA, for example acute anterior uveitis, IBD, and psoriasis. Comorbidities are co-existing diseases that occur in patients with axSpA but are not part of the concept of SpA, for example CVD and diabetes mellitus. The presence of a comorbidity may have consequences for the treatment, prognosis, and outcome of the disease. Therefore, when studying health outcomes, it is recommended to take comorbidities and/or EAMs into account. In daily practice, the presence of a comorbidity or EAM adds complexity to patient care, and treatment decisions may be affected by this.

Information on the presence of comorbidities can be collected either by recording individual diseases (e.g. breast cancer, kidney failure) or by summarizing this into a comorbidity index. The use of a comorbidity index has the advantage that co-existing diseases and their impact are expressed in a single score, allowing comparison across patients and diseases. Different instruments are available to measure comorbidity, depending on the outcome of interest, and can be record-based or self-reported.

Elixhauser et al. comorbidity measure

The Elixhauser et al. comorbidity measure uses administrative data to identify 30 comorbidities that have a major impact on short-term outcome in hospitalized patients (46). The score ranges from 0 to 30.

Charlson comorbidity index

The Charlson comorbidity index is a record-based comorbidity index (47). It is developed to predict mortality in hospitalized patients. The index consists of 19 conditions with specific weighting for each condition, based on the mortality risk. The score ranges from 0 to 33.

Self-administered comorbidity questionnaire

The self-administered comorbidity questionnaire is a generic, self-report questionnaire with 13 common medical conditions and an option to list three other, non-specified medical problems (48). It was developed to adjust for the impact of comorbidity on functional status. The patient is asked to indicate for each condition whether this is present (yes/no), is currently treated (yes/no), and imposes functional limitations (yes/no). Every 'yes' is given 1 point, with a maximum score of 45.

Rheumatic Diseases Comorbidity Index

The Rheumatic Diseases Comorbidity Index (RDCI) is a self-report comorbidity index (49). It was developed for outpatients with four rheumatic diseases (RA, osteoarthritis, SLE, and fibromyalgia) in order to predict several outcomes, including functional status and health resource utilization (50). The RDCI includes 11 weighted conditions. The score ranges from 0 to 9.

Work

Work is an important outcome in axSpA from both the perspective of the patient and society. The ability to work is in many patients affected by their condition, and costs associated with work disability and sick leave constitute the largest part of the cost-of-illness (51).

Different levels of impact of disease on work can be distinguished. 'Presenteeism' refers to the restrictions that patients can face when they attend work despite being ill. 'Absenteeism' is defined as not being at work due to either sick leave (when still having an employment contract) or work disability (when a patient has lost his or her employment contract).

Many patient-reported instruments are available to assess absenteeism and/or presenteeism, of which most focus on the measurement of presenteeism (52). Two constructs can be distinguished, one addressing the '*ability*', reflecting patient experience, and the other addressing the '*productivity*' perspective, reflecting possible economic consequences when the loss of productivity of the sick employee is not compensated by him-/herself or colleagues in usual work hours.

For assessment of presenteeism, the Work Limitations Questionnaire (WLQ-25) and the Workplace Activity Limitations Scale (WALS) can be used. These multidimensional instruments address different types of limitations. Also the presenteeism items (asking about productivity) from the Rheumatoid Arthritis Specific Work Productivity Survey (WPS-RA) and the Work Productivity and Activity Impairment (WPAI) can be used (52). The WPS-RA and WPAI have the advantage that they also address absenteeism. Furthermore, the WPS-RA also assesses restrictions in other social roles.

The use of outcome instruments on work is restricted to research; ASAS does not recommend their use in daily practice.

Response and remission criteria

Several criteria have been developed for the evaluation of an individual's response to treatment. The ASAS, BASDAI, and ASDAS improvement criteria can be used for defining improvement and treatment response in both clinical practice and research.

ASAS 20 improvement criteria

The ASAS 20 improvement criteria include four domains: patient global, pain, function (assessed by the BASFI), and inflammation (mean of the BASDAI questions 5 and 6) (53). In order to meet an ASAS 20 response, three of the four domains should improve by at least 20% and a minimum of one unit on a scale from 0 to 10. In the remaining domain, there should be no worsening of more than 20% and a minimum of 1 unit, on a 0 to 10 scale.

ASAS 40 improvement criteria

The ASAS 40 improvement criteria include the same domains as the ASAS 20 improvement criteria (54). In order to meet an ASAS 40 response, three of the four domains should improve by at least 40% and a minimum of two units on a scale from 0 to 10. In the remaining domain there should be no worsening of more than 20% and a minimum of 1 unit, on a 0 to 10 scale.

ASAS 5/6 improvement criteria

The ASAS 5/6 improvement criteria include six domains: patient global, pain, function (assessed by the BASFI), inflammation (mean of the BASDAI questions 5 and 6), CRP, and spinal mobility (assessed by the lateral spinal flexion) (54). In order to meet an ASAS 5/6 improvement, there should be an improvement of at least 20% in at least five of these six domains.

ASAS partial remission

ASAS has defined a state of partial remission, which reflects very low disease activity (53). In order to fulfill an ASAS partial remission state, a value of 2 (on a 0 to 10 scale) or less should be present in each of the following domains: patient global, pain, function (BASFI), and inflammation (mean of the BASDAI questions 5 and 6).

BASDAI 50 response

The BASDAS 50 response is defined as an improvement of at least 50% in the BASDAI-score or an absolute change of 2 units (on a 0 to 10 scale) after 3 months of treatment with TNFα inhibitors, together with an expert opinion compatible with improvement (55).

ASDAS improvement criteria

An improvement of $\geq$1.1 in the ASDAS score, for example after initiation of treatment, is considered a clinically important improvement, and a change score of $\geq$2.0 as a major improvement (11).

ASDAS inactive disease

ASAS has defined cut-offs for disease activity states, using the ASDAS score (11). A value below 1.3 is considered inactive disease (Fig. 12.2).

Conclusion

Whilst pathophysiological research, or research aiming at better treatments, is usually mentioned as 'scientific research', the research underlying the assessment of outcome in chronic inflammatory diseases such as axSpA is often somewhat neglected and pejoratively laid aside as representing only 'low hanging fruit'. That is inaccurate. We dare to defend the thesis that the development of proper outcome assessment has contributed as much to the improved treatment of chronic inflammatory diseases such as RA and axSpA as the improved treatments themselves have. What is often overlooked in disease such as axSpA is that outcome is multifaceted, wealthy if you like, and cannot be described by a sole and parsimonious set of measures. Whoever wants to understand axSpA in all its facets needs to be informed about the heterogeneity of its manifestations. Many have understood this heterogeneity of outcomes in the past, which has resulted in more than 100 different instruments measuring all thinkable aspects of the disease. Organizations such as OMERACT and ASAS have brought the badly needed parsimony in this pleiotropic mine-field by defining core sets and domains and selecting only the best instruments for measuring outcome. These core sets have facilitated the clinical trials with biologicals and their regulatory approval, so that patients suffering from axSpA can now be successfully treated by their rheumatologist.

Increasingly, the core sets of outcome will fulfil a slightly different role in the practice of rheumatology. Where possible, they will be used to monitor patients with axSpA being treated with often effective but always costly treatments: outcome measures will be applied in clinical practice to justify to society, payers, and/or government the deployment of expensive treatments.

It is obvious that the application of an outcome instrument in the context of a clinical trial, where its results are expressed as group means, differs from its application in individual patients, where subtle changes occurring in individual patients are cautiously interpreted.

In this chapter we have described all relevant aspects of outcome assessment in both contexts: the clinical trial as well as the clinical practice. Often, preferred outcome instruments are similar; sometimes distinctions should be made. However, the reader of this chapter can be certain that the most up-to-date status of outcome assessment in axSpA is presented here.

References

1. Boers M, Brooks P, Strand CV, Tugwell P. The OMERACT filter for outcome measures in rheumatology. J Rheumatol 1998;25(2):198–9.
2. van der Heijde D, Calin A, Dougados M, Khan MA, van der Linden S, Bellamy N. Selection of instruments in the core set for DC-ART, SMARD, physical therapy, and clinical record keeping in ankylosing spondylitis. Progress report of the ASAS Working Group. Assessments in ankylosing spondylitis. J Rheumatol 1999;26(4):951–4.
3. van der Heijde D, van der Linden S, Bellamy N, Calin A, Dougados M, Khan MA. Which domains should be included in a core set for endpoints in ankylosing spondylitis? Introduction to the ankylosing spondylitis module of OMERACT IV. J Rheumatol 1999;26(4):945–7.
4. van der Heijde D, van der Linden S, Dougados M, Bellamy N, Russell AS, Edmonds J. Ankylosing spondylitis: plenary discussion and results of voting on selection of domains and some specific instruments. J Rheumatol 1999;26(4):1003–5.
5. van Tubergen A, Black PM, Coteur G. Are patient-reported outcome instruments for ankylosing spondylitis fit for purpose for the axial

spondyloarthritis patient? A qualitative and psychometric analysis. Rheumatology 2015;54(10):1842–51.
6. Landewe R, Dougados M, Mielants H, van der Tempel H, van der Heijde D. Physical function in ankylosing spondylitis is independently determined by both disease activity and radiographic damage of the spine. Ann Rheum Dis 2009;68(6):863–7.
7. Calin A, Garrett S, Whitelock H, et al. A new approach to defining functional ability in ankylosing spondylitis: the development of the Bath Ankylosing Spondylitis Functional Index. J Rheumatol 1994;21(12):2281–5.
8. Ramiro S, van Tubergen A, van der Heijde D, van den Bosch F, Dougados M, Landewe R. How to deal with missing items in BASDAI and BASFI. Rheumatology 2014;53(2):374–6.
9. Garrett S, Jenkinson T, Kennedy LG, Whitelock H, Gaisford P, Calin A. A new approach to defining disease status in ankylosing spondylitis: the Bath Ankylosing Spondylitis Disease Activity Index. J Rheumatol 1994;21(12):2286–91.
10. van der Heijde D, Lie E, Kvien TK, et al. ASDAS, a highly discriminatory ASAS-endorsed disease activity score in patients with ankylosing spondylitis. Ann Rheum Dis 2009;68(12):1811–18.
11. Machado P, Landewe R, Lie E, et al. Ankylosing Spondylitis Disease Activity Score (ASDAS): defining cut-off values for disease activity states and improvement scores. Ann Rheum Dis 2011;70(1):47–53.
12. van Tubergen A, Coenen J, Landewe R, et al. Assessment of fatigue in patients with ankylosing spondylitis: a psychometric analysis. Arthritis Rheum 2002;47(1):8–16.
13. Ware JE Jr, Sherbourne CD. The MOS 36-item short-form health survey (SF-36). I. Conceptual framework and item selection. Med Care 1992;30(6):473–83.
14. EuroQol Group. EuroQol—a new facility for the measurement of health-related quality of life. Health Policy 1990;16(3):199–208.
15. Doward LC, Spoorenberg A, Cook SA, et al. Development of the ASQoL: a quality of life instrument specific to ankylosing spondylitis. Ann Rheum Dis 2003;62(1):20–6.
16. Machado P, Landewe R, Braun J, et al. A stratified model for health outcomes in ankylosing spondylitis. Ann Rheum Dis 2011;70(10):1758–64.
17. van Echteld I, Cieza A, Boonen A, et al. Identification of the most common problems by patients with ankylosing spondylitis using the international classification of functioning, disability and health. J Rheumatol 2006;33(12):2475–83.
18. Ward MM. Health-related quality of life in ankylosing spondylitis: a survey of 175 patients. Arthritis Care Res 1999;12(4):247–55.
19. Sigl T, Cieza A, van der Heijde D, Stucki G. ICF based comparison of disease specific instruments measuring physical functional ability in ankylosing spondylitis. Ann Rheum Dis 2005;64(11):1576–81.
20. Kiltz U, van der Heijde D, Boonen A, et al. Development of a health index in patients with ankylosing spondylitis (ASAS HI): final result of a global initiative based on the ICF guided by ASAS. Ann Rheum Dis 2015;74(5):830–5.
21. Cieza A, Hilfiker R, Boonen A, van der Heijde D, Braun J, Stucki G. Towards an ICF-based clinical measure of functioning in people with ankylosing spondylitis: a methodological exploration. Disab Rehab 2009;31(7):528–37.
22. Ramiro S, van Tubergen A, Stolwijk C, van der Heijde D, Royston P, Landewe R. Reference intervals of spinal mobility measures in normal individuals: the mobility study. Ann Rheum Dis 2015;74(6):1218–24.
23. Assassi S, Weisman MH, Lee M, et al. New population-based reference values for spinal mobility measures based on the 2009–2010 National Health and Nutrition Examination Survey. Arthritis Rheum 2014;66(9):2628–37.
24. Heuft-Dorenbosch L, Vosse D, Landewe R, et al. Measurement of spinal mobility in ankylosing spondylitis: comparison of occiput-to-wall and tragus-to-wall distance. J Rheumatol 2004;31(9):1779–84.
25. Maksymowych WP, Mallon C, Richardson R, et al. Development and validation of the Edmonton Ankylosing Spondylitis Metrology Index. Arthritis Rheum 2006;55(4):575–82.
26. Stolwijk C, Ramiro S, Vosse D, Landewe R, van der Heijde D, van Tubergen A. Comparison of tests for lumbar flexion and hip function in patients with and without axial spondyloarthritis. Arthritis Care Res 2015;67(4):538–45.
27. Jenkinson TR, Mallorie PA, Whitelock HC, Kennedy LG, Garrett SL, Calin A. Defining spinal mobility in ankylosing spondylitis (AS). The Bath AS Metrology Index. J Rheumatol 1994;21(9):1694–8.
28. Jones SD, Porter J, Garrett SL, Kennedy LG, Whitelock H, Calin A. A new scoring system for the Bath Ankylosing Spondylitis Metrology Index (BASMI). J Rheumatol 1995;22(8):1609.
29. van der Heijde D, Landewe R, Feldtkeller E. Proposal of a linear definition of the Bath Ankylosing Spondylitis Metrology Index (BASMI) and comparison with the 2-step and 10-step definitions. Ann Rheum Dis 2008;67(4):489–93.
30. van der Heijde D, Deodhar A, Inman RD, Braun J, Hsu B, Mack M. Comparison of three methods for calculating the Bath Ankylosing Spondylitis Metrology Index in a randomized placebo-controlled study. Arthritis Care Res 2012;64(12):1919–22.
31. Balint PV, Kane D, Wilson H, McInnes IB, Sturrock RD. Ultrasonography of entheseal insertions in the lower limb in spondyloarthropathy. Ann Rheum Dis 2002;61(10):905–10.
32. Mander M, Simpson JM, McLellan A, Walker D, Goodacre JA, Dick WC. Studies with an enthesis index as a method of clinical assessment in ankylosing spondylitis. Ann Rheum Dis 1987;46(3):197–202.
33. Clegg DO, Reda DJ, Weisman MH, et al. Comparison of sulfasalazine and placebo in the treatment of ankylosing spondylitis. A Department of Veterans Affairs Cooperative Study. Arthritis Rheum 1996;39(12):2004–12.
34. Braun J, Brandt J, Listing J, et al. Treatment of active ankylosing spondylitis with infliximab: a randomised controlled multicentre trial. Lancet 2002;359(9313):1187–93.
35. Heuft-Dorenbosch L, Spoorenberg A, van Tubergen A, et al. Assessment of enthesitis in ankylosing spondylitis. Ann Rheum Dis 2003;62(2):127–32.
36. Gladman DD, Inman RD, Cook RJ, et al. International spondyloarthritis interobserver reliability exercise—the INSPIRE study: II. Assessment of peripheral joints, enthesitis, and dactylitis. J Rheumatol 2007;34(8):1740–5.
37. Gorman JD, Sack KE, Davis JC Jr. Treatment of ankylosing spondylitis by inhibition of tumor necrosis factor alpha. New Engl J Med 2002;346(18):1349–56.
38. Maksymowych WP, Mallon C, Morrow S, et al. Development and validation of the Spondyloarthritis Research Consortium of Canada (SPARCC) Enthesitis Index. Ann Rheum Dis 2009;68(6):948–53.
39. Healy PJ, Helliwell PS. Measuring clinical enthesitis in psoriatic arthritis: assessment of existing measures and development of an instrument specific to psoriatic arthritis. Arthritis Rheum 2008;59(5):686–91.
40. Spoorenberg A, van der Heijde D, de Klerk E, et al. Relative value of erythrocyte sedimentation rate and C-reactive protein in assessment of disease activity in ankylosing spondylitis. J Rheumatol 1999;26(4):980–4.
41. Arends S, van der Veer E, Kallenberg CG, Brouwer E, Spoorenberg A. Baseline predictors of response to TNF-alpha blocking therapy in ankylosing spondylitis. Curr Opin Rheumatol 2012;24(3):290–8.
42. Creemers MC, Franssen MJ, van't Hof MA, Gribnau FW, van de Putte LB, van Riel PL. Assessment of outcome in ankylosing spondylitis: an extended radiographic scoring system. Ann Rheum Dis 2005;64(1):127–9.
43. Baraliakos X, Listing J, Rudwaleit M, Sieper J, Braun J. Development of a radiographic scoring tool for ankylosing spondylitis only based on bone formation: addition of the thoracic spine improves sensitivity to change. Arthritis Rheum 2009;61(6):764–71.
44. Ramiro S, van Tubergen A, Stolwijk C, et al. Scoring radiographic progression in ankylosing spondylitis: should we use the modified Stoke Ankylosing Spondylitis Spine Score (mSASSS) or the Radiographic

Ankylosing Spondylitis Spinal Score (RASSS)? Arthritis Res Ther 2013;15(1):R14.
45. Braun J, van den Berg R, Baraliakos X, et al. 2010 update of the ASAS/EULAR recommendations for the management of ankylosing spondylitis. Ann Rheum Dis 2011;70(6):896–904.
46. Elixhauser A, Steiner C, Harris DR, Coffey RM. Comorbidity measures for use with administrative data. Med Care 1998;36(1):8–27.
47. Charlson ME, Pompei P, Ales KL, MacKenzie CR. A new method of classifying prognostic comorbidity in longitudinal studies: development and validation. J Chronic Dis 1987;40(5):373–83.
48. Sangha O, Stucki G, Liang MH, Fossel AH, Katz JN. The Self-Administered Comorbidity Questionnaire: a new method to assess comorbidity for clinical and health services research. Arthritis Rheum 2003;49(2):156–63.
49. Michaud K, Wolfe F. Comorbidities in rheumatoid arthritis. Best Practice Res Clin Rheumatol 2007;21(5):885–906.
50. Wolfe F, Michaud K, Li T, Katz RS. Chronic conditions and health problems in rheumatic diseases: comparisons with rheumatoid arthritis, noninflammatory rheumatic disorders, systemic lupus erythematosus, and fibromyalgia. J Rheumatol 2010;37(2):305–15.
51. Franke LC, Ament AJ, van de Laar MA, Boonen A, Severens JL. Cost-of-illness of rheumatoid arthritis and ankylosing spondylitis. Clin Exp Rheum 2009;27(4 Suppl 55):S118–23.
52. Escorpizo R, Bombardier C, Boonen A, et al. Worker productivity outcome measures in arthritis. J Rheumatol 2007;34(6):1372–80.
53. Anderson JJ, Baron G, van der Heijde D, Felson DT, Dougados M. Ankylosing spondylitis assessment group preliminary definition of short-term improvement in ankylosing spondylitis. Arthritis Rheum 2001;44(8):1876–86.
54. Brandt J, Listing J, Sieper J, Rudwaleit M, van der Heijde D, Braun J. Development and preselection of criteria for short term improvement after anti-TNF alpha treatment in ankylosing spondylitis. Ann Rheum Dis 2004;63(11):1438–44.
55. Braun J, Davis J, Dougados M, et al. First update of the international ASAS consensus statement for the use of anti-TNF agents in patients with ankylosing spondylitis. Ann Rheum Dis 2006;65(3):316–20.

CHAPTER 13

Imaging: sacroiliac joints

Walter P. Maksymowych and Robert G.W. Lambert

Introduction to sacroiliac joints

SpA comprises a group of inflammatory disorders that primarily affect the SI joints and structures of the spine and are associated with the HLA-B27 gene. Recent advances in imaging of the SI joints have been driven by recognition that more information is required to evaluate active inflammation within soft tissues and bone, and not merely the structural damage that is a consequence of inflammation, in order to recognize and manage early disease, to assist the basic scientist in the examination of immunopathological events in early disease, and to develop internationally validated outcome assessment tools to assist the clinical researcher in the evaluation of therapeutic interventions and prognostic indicators. Four principal methods are currently used to evaluate the SI joints of patients with SpA: plain radiography, CT, scintigraphy, and MRI. There has also been limited evaluation using sonography. This chapter examines the advantages and limitations of each imaging modality for its ability to influence diagnostic and therapeutic decisions for the practicing clinician and the potential of each method as an outcome assessment tool for the basic and clinical researcher.

Plain radiography

Early features of spondyloarthritis in sacroiliac joints

Plain radiography of the SI joints is still the cornerstone of diagnosis, evaluation, and classification of SpA, but its inability to visualize soft tissue abnormalities within bone marrow means that it can only depict the consequences of inflammation and the enhanced turnover of joint tissue. In the context of the SI joints, radiographic abnormalities are therefore limited to cancellous and/or cortical bone and include focal or diffuse changes of osteoporosis, sclerosis or erosion, and changes related to the diameter of the space between the bones (joint space) or ankylosis. The earliest abnormality indicative of inflammation in the SI joints is visible as a loss of distinctness of the subchondral bone of the lower one-third of the iliac bone, leading to the classic depiction of the serrated postage stamp (Fig. 13.1). This probably reflects early inflammation in the subchondral bone marrow of the cartilaginous portion of the joint. Limited histopathological evaluation of SI joints in early disease has shown that a prominent feature is subchondral inflammation eroding through the overlying cartilage (1). This is followed by more obvious erosion and apparent widening of the radiographic joint space as the inflammation becomes more extensive, and erosion may affect both articular surfaces. Progressive sclerosis and joint space ankylosis represent late features of disease.

Diagnostic evaluation using radiography

A major challenge to early diagnosis using radiography is the complex anatomy of the joint. The cartilaginous portion, which is the region primarily affected in early disease, is convex antero-inferiorly in the anterior one-third of the joint. In addition, the joint cavity is curved and obliquely orientated, with the posterior aspect located medially and the anterior part located laterally. This creates

(A)

(B)

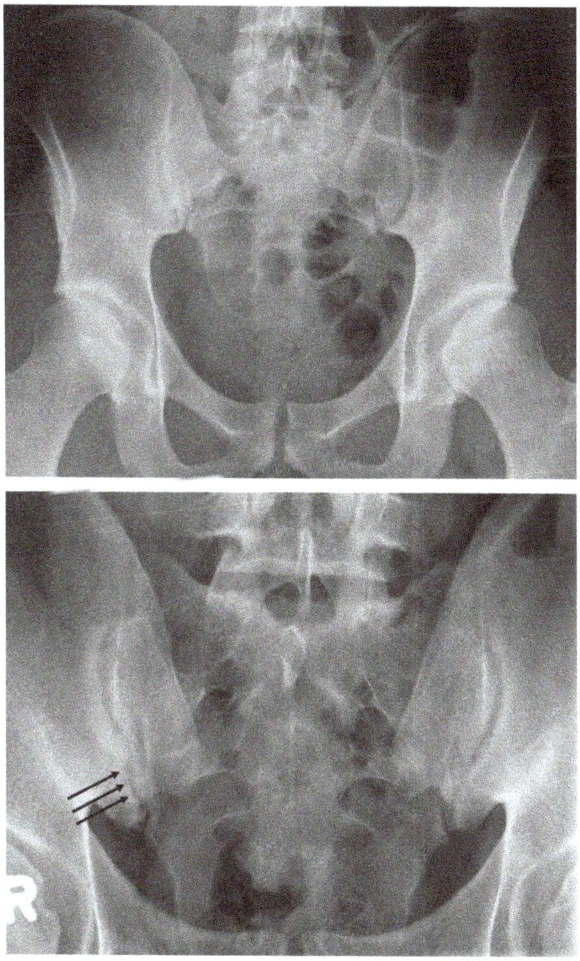

Fig. 13.1 AP radiograph of the pelvis (A) and dedicated view of the SI joints (Ferguson view (B)) in a young man with nr-SpA. The inferior half of the right SI joint is less well defined than normal. Small erosions (arrows) are better seen on the Ferguson view and mild subchondral sclerosis is present (right SI joint: grade 2; left SI joint: grade 1). No erosion is visible on the left side. Erosions are harder to see on the AP radiograph (right SI joint: grade 1; left SI joint: grade 0), and in other cases may be completely obscured by overlying gas and stool in the colon.

(A) (B) (C)

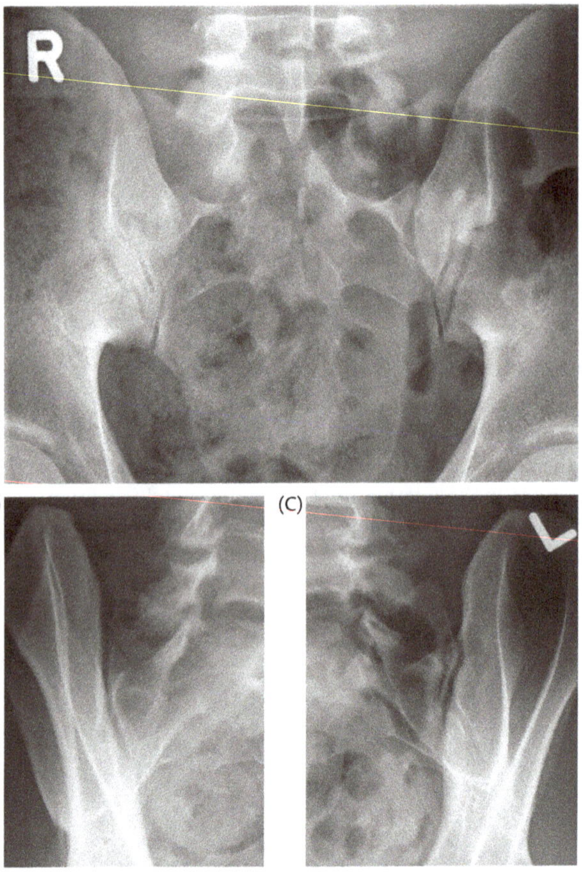

Fig. 13.2 Dedicated radiographs of SI joints in a normal subject. These may include an AP view with 25–30 degrees cranial angulation (Ferguson view (A)) and/or oblique views with 25–30 degrees of patient rotation (B, C). The tilted orientation of the SI joint and its complex undulating contour may make it difficult to interpret SI joint radiographs, and the standard pelvic view may be supplemented by a dedicated view of the SI joints. However, there is little evidence that the oblique projections provide significant additional information and these views tend to obscure the lower one-third of the SI joints, which is the critical area for evaluation of early disease. Because of the significant additional radiation exposure, it is recommended that oblique views should not be performed.

difficulty in the interpretation of early subchondral changes using the conventional AP view. Overlying bowel gas further confounds detection of abnormalities. Erosion may therefore be quite severe in the SI joints before being reliably detected, because either it is not in profile or it is obscured by other structures. Radiographic sacroiliitis is not reliably detected in early SpA, even amongst experienced readers (2). This has led to the use of various radiographic methodologies in clinical practice to optimize assessment of the SI joints (Fig. 13.2).

Oblique views of individual SI joints are aimed at superimposing the anterior and posterior joint margins and are taken at 25–30 degrees of patient rotation. In the Ferguson view, the patient is in the same position as for the AP pelvis, but the tube is angled 30–35 degrees cranial and is centred to the mid-portion of the pelvis. With this projection, the symphysis pubis overlaps the sacrum below the SI joints without obscuring it and this has been proposed as an approach that more directly visualizes the joint. The postero-anterior (PA) view of the pelvis is sometimes used in preference to the AP view in order to take advantage of radiographic beam divergence, producing an image more closely parallel to the surface of the SI joints in the PA projection.

Data comparing the diagnostic accuracy of these methodologies are limited. One report described the assessment of 43 consecutive patients referred with clinical suspicion of IBP (3). Each patient had four views of the SI joints taken and CT was conducted on 35 unselected patients as the gold standard evaluation. Individual views had comparable diagnostic accuracy, and obtaining additional views when findings were equivocal on a single view enhanced diagnostic accuracy in only 10–15%. Additional data confirm these observations (4). Consequently, there is little evidence to support the use of specific SI joints views over the conventional AP pelvis, and there is minimal additional diagnostic utility to the use of specific SI joints views where the AP of the pelvis is equivocal for sacroiliitis, which come at the expense of additional radiation exposure. In the setting of early SpA where a radiograph is reported as equivocal for SpA, MRI of the pelvis is a more useful option than additional radiography (vide infra).

Several prospective studies have assessed development of radiographic sacroiliitis in patients presenting with clinical features of SpA but without radiographic sacroiliitis (5–9). These have shown that only 10–15% develop radiographic sacroiliitis after 2 years, about 40% after 5 years, and about 60% after 10 years. These studies highlight the important limitations in the diagnostic sensitivity of radiography in patients who are symptomatic even in the presence of objective features of inflammation in the SI joints. In addition, it does not appear worthwhile to repeat radiographic examination where earlier examinations were conducted within the previous 5 years, and especially if there is access to MRI.

Classification of spondyloarthritis using radiography

The mNY classification criteria represent a major advance in the field for defining this disease and rely substantially on the finding of radiographic sacroiliitis (10). Radiographic changes are graded according to the degree of severity of abnormalities in the SI joints. At least bilateral grade 2, defined by small localized areas with erosion or sclerosis without alteration in joint width, or unilateral grade 3, defined by one or more of erosions, sclerosis, widening, narrowing, or partial ankylosis, must be present for classification of disease as being AS.

Radiography of the sacroiliac joint in juvenile spondyloarthritis

Onset of SpA before age 16 is termed juvenile spondyloarthritis (JoSpA) and up to 20% of cases of SpA may have a juvenile onset. SI joint radiography in children is usually performed with a single AP projection collimated to the SI joints to minimize radiation exposure. Interpretation of findings may be challenging because of the immature skeleton. In the child, the bone surface is normally irregular and the radiographic joint space appears much wider because the cartilage is comprised of both the articular surface and the centres of growth for the ilium and sacral ala. Erosion and sclerosis are the more common findings and are seen with similar frequency (about 70% of subjects), but erosion is more specific and more reliably detected (11). SI joint space narrowing also has high specificity for JoSpA but does not occur often, and SI joint ankylosis is quite rare in the juvenile population. A negative result does not rule out disease, as half of all JoSpA patients never develop sacroiliitis at any stage.

Differential diagnosis of radiographic sacroiliitis

Many conditions can affect the SI joints but not many of them start in the SI joints. Degenerative changes may be seen in 23.8% of primary care patients, with back pain and osteophytes the most common observation (12). These are seen twice as often in women and are more often bilateral. Degenerative changes in the SI joints become increasingly frequent over the age of 50, and, on CT scanning, joint space narrowing and intra-articular gas are often seen, but these features are much harder to identify on radiographs. Subchondral cyst formation may occur, but the contour of the subchondral bone remains smooth and well defined, and erosion is rarely seen in SI joint osteoarthritis.

The single most important differential diagnosis to exclude is a septic arthritis. The radiographic findings are unilateral, with erosion of subchondral bone and joint space widening most often seen. The majority of cases are subacute or chronic, and so reactive sclerosis is also frequently seen but it is seldom pronounced. Osteitis condensans ilii (OCI) is a condition in which the iliac side of the SI joints becomes densely sclerotic. It occurs more often in past-partum female patients. On radiography, the subchondral sclerosis is usually the only observation, occurring in a characteristic triangular distribution, being narrowest at the top and widest at the bottom of the SI joint. Erosion or alteration of joint space width is rarely seen and the radiographic findings may completely resolve over time. Other arthropathies and systemic disorders can affect the SI joints; however, they do not start in the SI joints and the clinical context will usually direct radiographic interpretation.

Computed tomography

As for radiography, observations with CT are mainly restricted to abnormalities of cancellous or cortical bone. For the SI joints, however, CT is easier to interpret without overlapping structures and erosion is detectable at an earlier stage (Fig. 13.3). CT has been reported to show greater sensitivity and specificity in the diagnosis of sacroiliitis than radiography, although studies included small numbers of patients. The SI joints were examined by radiography and CT over a 2-year period in a retrospective study of 910 patients with back pain (13). Agreement between these methods was only fair, but 41% of radiographic reports provided a false answer. Moreover, definitive diagnosis of sacroiliitis was reported over twice as frequently with CT (25%) as with plain radiography (11%). In a French cohort of 489 patients with suspected SpA, definite sacroiliitis was ascertained on radiographs in six patients (3.5%) and on CT scans in 32 patients (18.5%) (14). Studies comparing radiography, CT, and MRI in the same populations found that MRI was more sensitive for detecting sacroiliitis than the other two methods (15, 16). The primary limitation of pelvic CT is higher radiation dose, although this may be less using a protocol of discontiguous slices or specific low-dose techniques. The use of CT in routine practice appears to be limited to the diagnostic evaluation of IBP where plain radiography shows normal SI joints and access to MRI is limited.

Isotopic imaging

Scintigraphy relies upon abnormal uptake of radiotracer in areas of increased bone turnover. This test is often positive earlier than X-ray in patients with sacroiliitis, but the complex shape of the joint makes interpretation of planar images difficult. Inflammatory lesions in bone marrow are not directly visualized and the scintigraphic activity reflects the impact of inflammation on bone turnover. Erosion, cartilage lesions, and reparative lesions such as fat metaplasia or ankylosis are not detected. Quantitative scanning of the SI joints has been evaluated as a diagnostic tool, although cut-offs that reliably distinguish patients from controls have proved difficult to establish. Sensitivity has ranged from 29% to 40%, while specificity was usually less than 80%. One prospective study compared quantitative radionuclide scanning with MRI of the SI joints in patients with IBP but normal plain radiographs (17). Of 21 patients, 20 had MRI evidence of SI inflammation, whereas only

(A)

(B)

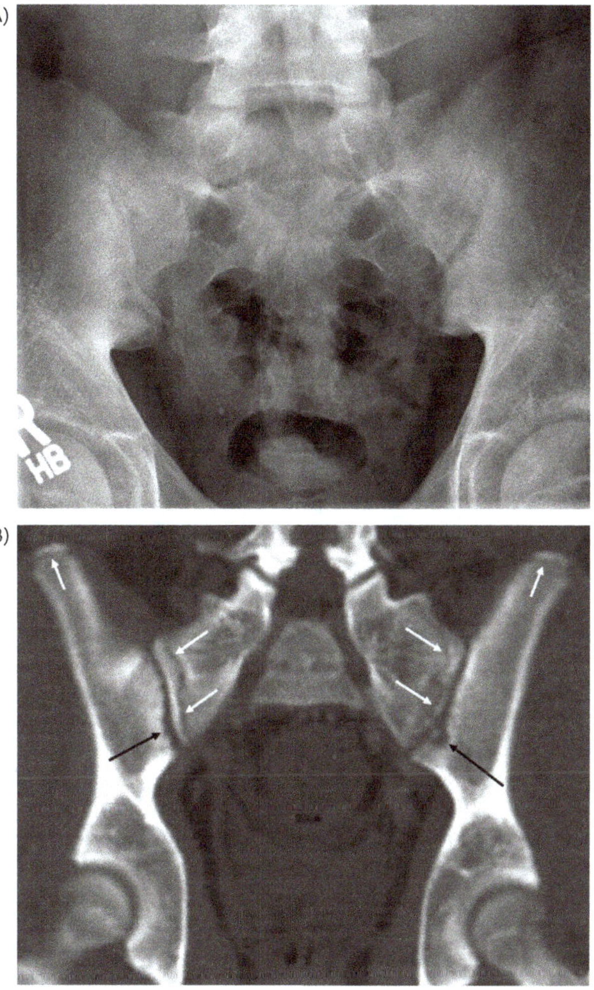

Fig. 13.3 Ferguson view of the SI joints (A) and coronal CT scan (B) in a 15 year old with JoSpA. Normal borders of the SI joint are less well seen in younger children because the apparent joint space seems wider on account of the large depth of cartilage, especially on the sacral side, which includes both articular cartilage and physeal cartilage of the growing bone. Typical radiographic features of SpA are seen in this case with subchondral sclerosis and poor definition of the margins of the SI joints (right SI joints: grade 3; left SI joints: grade 2). Focal erosion of subchondral bone is visible in the radiograph but is hard to see clearly and appears worse on the right. CT scan confirms erosion of subchondral bone (black arrows) with broad shallow erosion on the right, but in fact erosion is deeper on the left side. CT also clearly shows multiple physeal centres of bone growth, as represented by linear areas of radiolucent cartilage paralleling the sacral articular surface and iliac crests (white arrows).

ten had radionuclide scan evidence of sacroiliitis. A recent systematic review concluded that isotopic imaging of the SI joints had low diagnostic utility for evaluation of IBP (18). Consequently, this technique is increasingly used for diagnostic evaluation of SpA only in centres that lack access to MRI.

Ultrasound

The dorsal joint capsule and the dorsal enthesis can be detected using ultrasound (US) and have been assessed in several studies to detect sacroiliitis or to guide injections into the SI joint. Preliminary studies have also used colour and pulsed Doppler US to detect arterial vascularity within and around SI joints and paraspinal areas in patients with AS. Arterial vascularity as measured by the resistive index was significantly greater in patients with clinically defined active inflammation and decreased in response to anti-TNF therapy (19). A subsequent study compared microbubble contrast-enhanced colour Doppler US with MRI of the SI joints in 103 patients with IBP, 75% of whom had SpA, and showed that contrast-enhanced colour Doppler US showed a sensitivity of 94% and specificity of 86% (20). However, results in patients with inactive AS were similar to controls, indicating that this approach is likely to be of limited diagnostic value, though it may be useful as an objective parameter of disease activity. In addition, contrast enhancement is limited in duration due to collapse of microbubbles. A second-generation contrast enhancement technique has been evaluated using grey-scale US (contrast-enhanced ultrasound, CEUS) in which the microbubbles are more stable, allowing more prolonged US scanning and maximization of contrast and spatial resolution. A cross-sectional comparison of 42 patients with SpA and 21 controls showed that CEUS detected enhancement in all clinically active SI joints, while inactive joints were correctly classified (21). The reliability of the technique and its comparative performance with other imaging modalities requires further study in unselected cohorts of patients with undiagnosed back pain.

Magnetic resonance imaging

A major advance in the field has been the development of MRI for SpA because of its ability to permit earlier diagnosis, which until now has relied primarily on radiography. It is superior to radiography and CT through its ability to visualize soft tissue inflammation and inflammatory lesions within bone in three dimensions. It therefore provides objective features of active inflammation, which may not be readily assessed by clinical or laboratory evaluation, particularly if disease is confined to the axial joints. Quantitative assessment by MRI of SI joint inflammation and structural changes has now become possible and has been shown to facilitate evaluation of new therapeutics in clinical trials. Despite this, many clinicians and radiologists still remain unfamiliar with the spectrum of acute and chronic MRI features in SpA and appropriate indications for the use of MRI in diagnostic evaluation.

Technical considerations

T1W images readily detect the signal from fat, which appears bright, whilst fluid appears grey and bone appears dark. T2W MRI sequences detect the signal from water, as may be observed in cysts, inflammatory infiltrates, and highly vascularized tissues such as tumours. With these sequences, fluid is very bright, whilst fat is less bright, and bone is black. Fat-suppressed sequences, such as STIR, are particularly useful in SpA where inflammatory lesions are characteristically present in subchondral bone and adjacent to entheses. With this technique, the signal from bone marrow fat is suppressed so that the marrow appears dark whilst fluid remains bright, allowing visualization of oedema, cysts, tumours, and inflammatory infiltration.

An alternative approach to the detection of inflammation is with contrast enhancement after intravenous administration of gadolinium (Gd). For this, a T1 sequence with fat suppression is used. Gd accumulates at sites of increased vascularity and capillary permeability, where it alters the magnetic properties of surrounding soft tissues. This process can be followed over time, where both the rate and degree of Gd enhancement provide quantitative information on the severity of inflammation. This is termed dynamic MRI. Gd-enhanced MRI therefore offers the possibility of quantifying inflammation in terms of the intensity (peak), the maximal rate (slope), and the time to peak enhancement.

Normal appearance of the sacroiliac joint

Imaging of the SI joints has to address the fact that the region of interest in the SI joint, the cartilaginous portion, is convex shaped, with the apex facing antero-inferiorly. Consequently, consecutive images are obtained in the semicoronal orientation along the long axis of the sacral bone, which allows visualization of this portion of the joint (Fig. 13.4). Axial sections may allow superior evaluation of ligamentous structures in the posterosuperior portion of the joint and are orientated perpendicular to semicoronal sections (Fig. 13.4). On a T1W spin echo (SE) sequence, bone marrow fat in the iliac and sacral bones appears bright, whilst subchondral bone lining the joint cavity is dark (Fig. 13.5). When evaluating the joint from anterior to posterior slices, there is a transitional slice defined as the first slice in the cartilaginous portion that has a visible portion of the ligamentous joint, which appears bright because of the presence of fat surrounding the ligaments (Fig. 13.5). Further posteriorly, in the ligamentous compartment there is both bright signal, indicating fat, and dark signal, indicating ligaments between iliac and sacral bones.

On T2W fat-suppressed images of the normal SI joint the bone marrow is dark, and bright signal is detected from presacral veins on anterior coronal slices through the joint (Fig. 13.5). Further posteriorly, bright signal can be seen in the spinal canal, reflecting cerebrospinal fluid. An initial study for diagnostic evaluation should consist of a semicoronal T1SE and either a STIR or fat-saturated T2W (T2FS) sequence, since they provide complementary information, and one sequence in the semiaxial plane, most often STIR or T2FS. Questionable abnormalities can be further analysed using fat-saturated Gd-enhanced imaging.

Early MRI features of spondyloarthritis in sacroiliac joints

Several inflammatory lesions have been described on T2W and/or contrast-enhanced MRI in patients with early sacroiliitis, namely capsulitis, synovitis, and subchondral bone marrow inflammation (22, 23) (Fig. 13.6). Subchondral BME was noted in the first detailed description of the MR appearances of sacroiliitis in a study of 27 consecutive patients with symptoms suggestive of sacroiliitis and 11 healthy controls (24). To enhance the sensitivity of MRI in the detection of early sacroiliitis, subsequent studies used dynamic MR imaging with Gd enhancement (25). Examination of patients clinically characterized as having inflammatory low back pain but

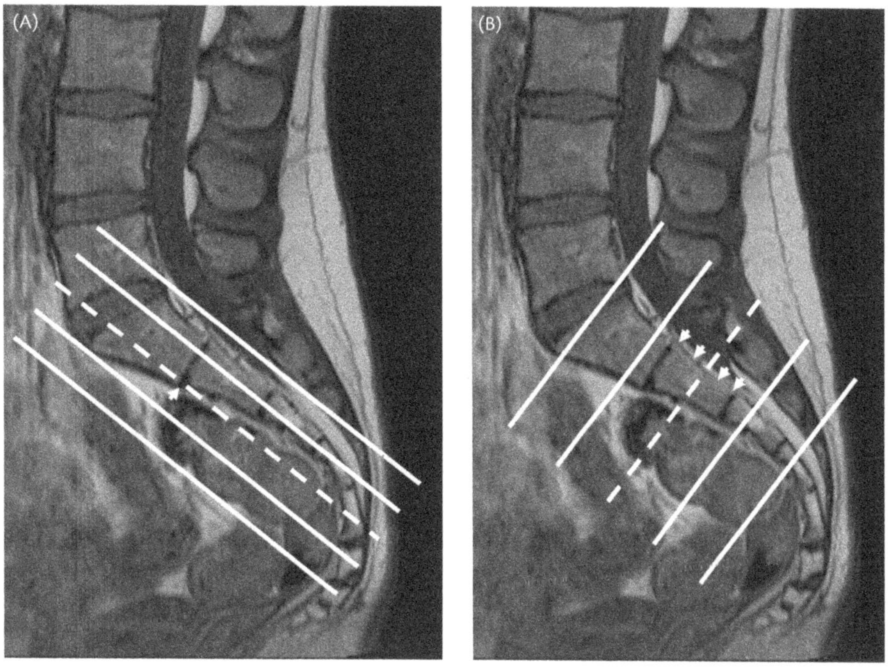

Fig. 13.4 Sagittal T1W MR images of the lumbosacral spine for planning of SI joint sequences. SI joints are best visualized on semicoronal and semiaxial sequences orientated parallel and perpendicular to the long axis of the second sacral vertebra. The semicoronal sequence should be planned (A) so that the centre (dashed line) of a stack of 12–15 images 4 mm thick (or 15–19 images 3 mm thick) is positioned at the anterior border of the sclerotic line, representing the junction of the 1st and 2nd sacral segments (arrowhead). Orientation of the semicoronal sequence is parallel to the dorsal cortex of the S2 vertebra. The semiaxial sequence should be planned (B) so that the centre (dashed line) of a stack of 15–19 images 4 mm thick (or 19–23 images 3 mm thick) is positioned at the centre of the S2 vertebra. Orientation of the semiaxial sequence is perpendicular to the dorsal cortex of the S2 vertebra (arrowheads). The semicoronal sequence must include one or two slices anterior to the SI joint and all of the cartilage compartment. The semiaxial sequence must include all of the first three sacral vertebrae.

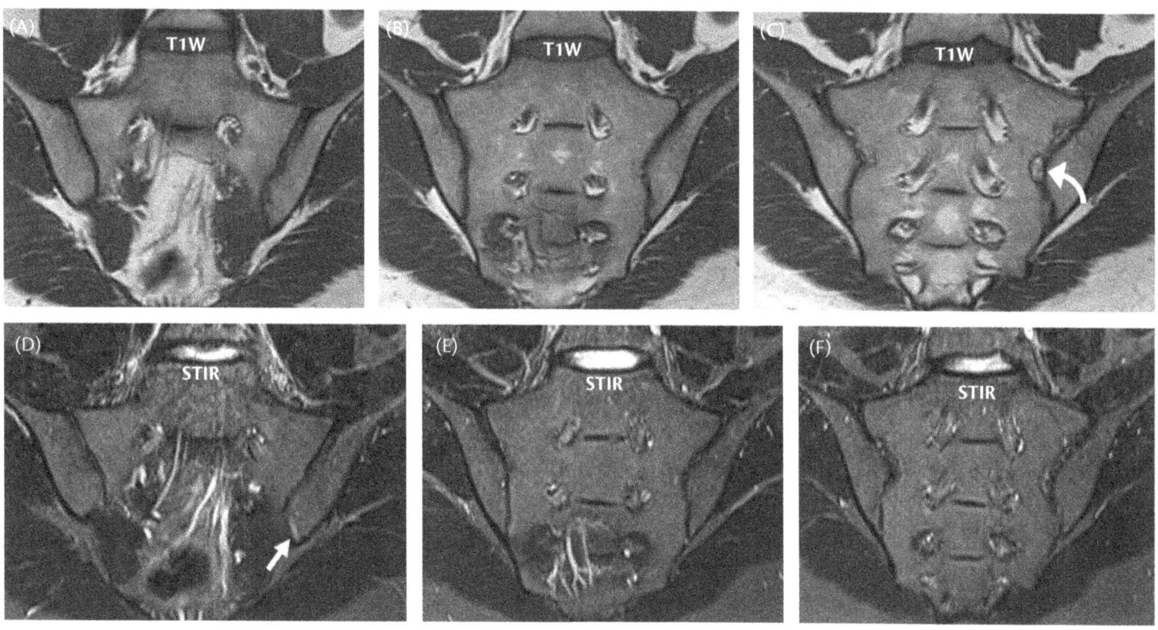

Fig. 13.5 MRI of SI joints in a healthy young subject. Semicoronal images are orientated to the long axis of the sacrum and T1W spin echo images (A–C) and STIR images (D, E) are most often acquired. On T1, fat is very bright and bone marrow is brighter than muscle because of the higher fat content in bone marrow. On STIR, fat signal is suppressed, bone marrow appears darker, and fluid signal is very bright. The SI joints extend further anteriorly than sacral vertebral bodies, so anterior parts of the cartilage compartment are visualized on anterior slices (A, D), along with presacral soft tissues. On a centre slice (B, E), the entire length of the cartilage compartment is well seen. Posterior to this, a transitional slice represents the start of the ligamentous compartment (C, F). The transitional slice is best identified on T1 (C) when fat is seen in the centre of the joint (curved arrow) representing fat surrounding SI ligaments. Note that on any water-sensitive sequence, small blood vessels are frequently observed adjacent to the perimeter of the joint or even within bone at these locations. Although usually easily recognized (arrow in D), this may mimic small foci of BME.

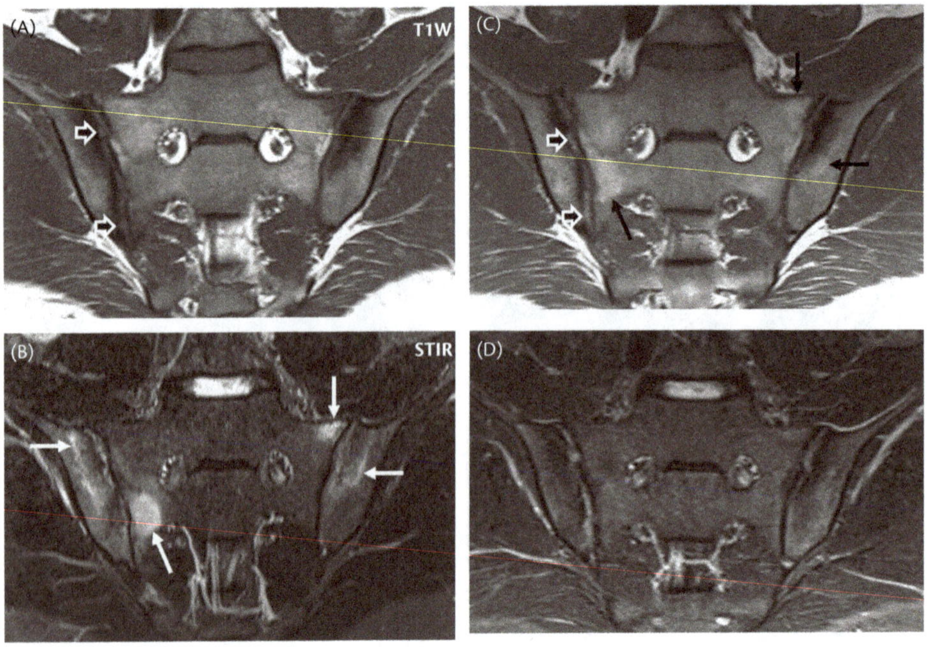

Fig. 13.6 MRI SI joints with coronal T1W and STIR images, at two time points, before and after biologic therapy, in a young man with axSpA. On the first STIR image (B), typical foci of BME are present (white arrows) and are more prominent in the sacrum where disease is at an earlier stage. On T1 (A), small erosions (arrows) are seen in the right ilium, with bilateral iliac sclerosis also clearly visible. Note that in the ilium, BME is seen around the perimeter of the sclerosis. After treatment, most of the BME has resolved (D). On T1 (C), bone marrow that was previously oedematous is now increased in signal, with fat metaplasia replacing BME (long arrows). At the site of the erosion in the right ilium, erosion is less apparent and increased signal is also seen in that location (short arrows). Although it is not known exactly what tissue this represents, the phenomenon of articular erosion being replaced by tissue that is bright on T1 is termed 'backfill'.

normal radiographs revealed enhancement of the joint capsule, synovium, and subchondral bone marrow in a significant proportion of patients, especially in the posterocaudal portion of the synovial part of the joint where the capsule attaches to bone. Subsequent studies using fat suppression techniques and higher magnetic field strength that led to improvements in resolution of images have consistently noted subchondral BME as an important component of the early pathology of sacroiliitis.

Validation of early MRI abnormalities in the SI joints according to clinical and pathological features of SpA has been limited. One group quantified Gd enhancement in the SI joints by measuring maximal enhancement compared to baseline values, and showed that a grading scheme for severity of inflammation correlated with disease activity, as determined by clinical parameters (26). Direct CT-guided biopsy of the SI joints has also demonstrated significant correlations between the degree of Gd enhancement on MRI of the SI joints and the histopathological grade of inflammation (27).

MRI features in established spondyloarthritis of sacroiliac joints

As the BME lesion evolves, there is erosion of the subchondral bony plate. Erosions do not develop marginally, as typically seen in peripheral arthritis, but adjacent to the joint space and are visible as loss of subarticular bone with decreased fat signal on T1W images, reflecting loss of marrow matrix adjacent to eroded bone (Fig. 13.7). Erosion may evolve from a circumscribed breach of the cortical bone and loss of adjacent bone marrow matrix signal to confluence of multiple erosions, resulting in extended erosion along the entire

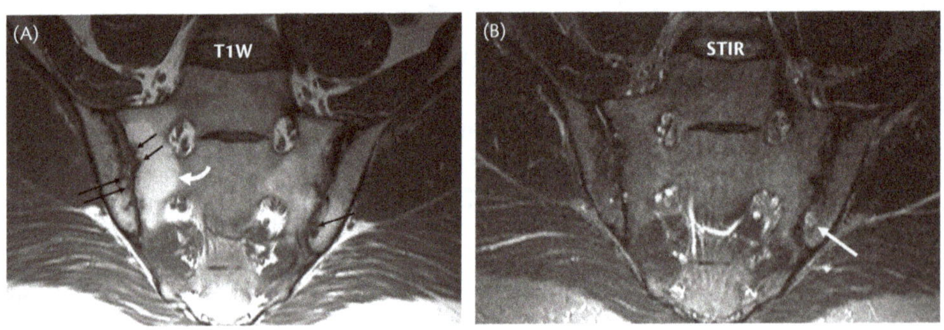

Fig. 13.7 MRI SI joints—coronal T1W and STIR—in a patient with axSpA with advanced structural damage. Multiple small foci of erosion (black arrows) are clearly seen in the subchondral bone in both joints, more apparent on the right side. Focal defects are associated with loss of normal outline of bone cortex of the articular surface and loss of normal bone marrow signal within the erosion. A large area of fat metaplasia (curved arrow) in the right sacrum is consistent with post-inflammatory change extending to the articular surface and a sharp medial border. Most of the erosions are inactive, with only a small focus of BME in the left lower ilium (white arrow).

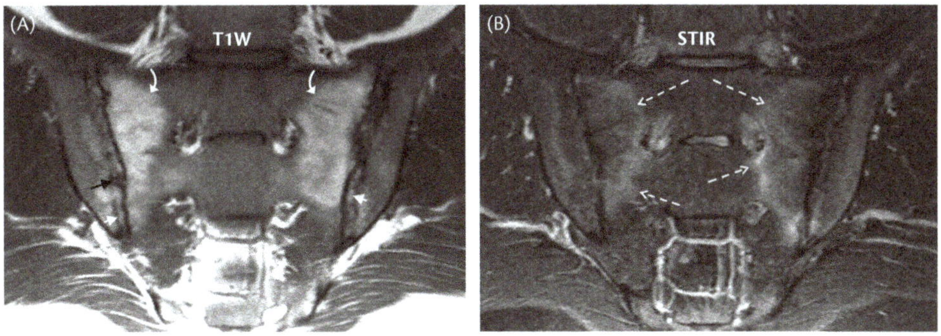

Fig. 13.8 MRI SI joints—coronal T1W and STIR. Established inflammatory sacroiliitis in a patient with axSpA. Evidence of healing of extensive SI erosion is present on MRI scan with backfill (white arrowheads) seen in the subarticular bone of the ilium in both SI joints. This is represented by bright signal on a T1W sequence, consistent with fatty tissue that is seen in the location of previous erosion. A dark line beneath the backfill represents sclerosis at the deep margin of the original erosion. This image also shows a small persistent defect due to erosion (black arrow) in the right ilium and bilateral post-inflammatory fat metaplasia of sacral bone marrow (curved white arrows). On STIR, some residual BME (dashed white arrows) is still visible at the perimeter of the fat metaplasia and in the lowest part of the left SI joint.

vertical height of the iliac cortical bone, leading to the appearance of pseudo-widening of the joint space. The STIR/T2FS sequence shows increased signal at the site of erosion when inflammation is still active. When inflammation resolves, new tissue with high signal intensity appears on the T1W sequence both in the erosion cavity and in the adjacent subchondral bone marrow (Fig. 13.7). This reflects accumulation of fatty acids and has therefore been termed fat metaplasia. Prospective assessment of MRI scans has confirmed this sequence of events (28). The histopathological counterpart to this reparative lesion is unknown. When this reparative tissue is observed in the excavated area caused by erosion it has been termed backfill (Fig. 13.8) (29). A multivariate analysis of 147 patients followed over 2 years has shown that reduction in erosions and increase in fat metaplasia on MRI are each independently associated with the development of new ankylosis (28). Fat metaplasia therefore appears to be an inherent characteristic of the tissue response following resolution of inflammation in the axial skeleton in SpA, and supports the hypothesis that resolution of erosion progresses to a stage of ankylosis through this key intermediary tissue.

Additional structural changes include the development of bone sclerosis, characterized by low signal intensity on both T1W and T2W sequences, and ankylosis, which is evident as bone marrow signal on T1W sequences extending between the sacral and iliac bone marrow, with full-thickness loss of the dark appearance of the iliac and sacral cortical bone (Fig. 13.9).

Diagnostic evaluation using MRI

Subchondral BME can be observed on STIR/T2FS MRI sequences within a few weeks of presentation of IBP (30) and can be reliably detected. An online training module for assessment of BME in the SI joints has been developed (available at http://www.carearthritis.com/MRI_scoring_modules.php). There has been relatively limited study of the sensitivity and specificity of MRI abnormalities of the SI joints in patients with early SpA, especially unselected patients presenting with chronic back pain that may resemble SpA clinically. This has been problematic because the gold standard for diagnosis requires plain radiographic features of sacroiliitis, which means that such evaluations must be prospective to allow time for radiographic abnormalities to appear. One group that used Gd contrast-enhanced MRI demonstrated sensitivity of 83% and specificity of 93% for clinically defined IBP (31). A second study evaluated fat-suppressed MRI in a cohort of 68 patients with IBP of less than 2 years' duration, of whom 57 and 14 fulfilled ESSG and mNY criteria, respectively (32). Inflammation in the SI joints could be detected in only about one-third of the patients, but it was sufficient to look for subchondral BME alone as a sign of inflammation, since only one patient had inflammation that was restricted to joint capsule and ligaments. It is important to point out that symptoms of IBP are common in patients with mechanical causes of back pain, so that selection of patients for MRI studies based largely on clinical criteria will inevitably result in varying estimates for sensitivity and specificity.

There has been limited diagnostic evaluation of MRI sequences used in routine clinical practice where the study cohort included age- and sex-matched scans from healthy controls and back conditions resembling SpA. Five readers assessed scans from 187 subjects less than 45 years of age in one study (33). Cases included 75 patients with AS and symptom duration less than 10 years, 27 patients with IBP of symptom duration 29 months but without radiographic sacroiliitis, 26 patients with non-specific back pain, and 59 healthy

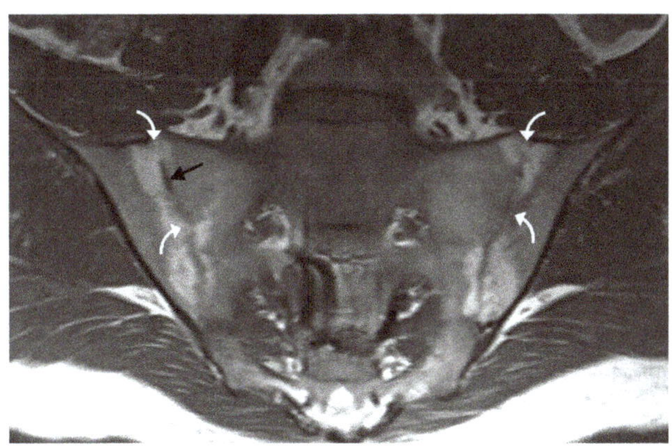

Fig. 13.9 MRI SI joints—coronal T1. Extensive ankylosis of the SI joint is common in end-stage inflammatory sacroiliitis. On T1W sequences, this is seen as obliteration of the dark lines that represent the subchondral cortices and cartilage of 'joint space'. Bright lipid signal from fatty bone marrow is seen crossing between bones (curved white arrows). Signal intensity may be equal to normal marrow or may be even brighter due to post-inflammatory fat metaplasia. A faint remnant of the joint may be visible, but the dark lines are lost except where erosion was incomplete, and small remnants of joint (black arrow) may be seen surrounded by ankylosis.

controls. Diagnostic utility was high for all five readers, both for patients with AS (sensitivity 0.90, specificity 0.97, positive likelihood ratio (LR) 44.6) and for patients with non-radiographic IBP (sensitivity 0.51, specificity 0.97, positive LR 26.0).

A second study assessed MRI scans from two independent inception cohorts of consecutive patients aged ≤ 50 years with back pain (34). One cohort of 69 cases comprised patients with back pain and symptom duration of 1.3 years referred by primary care physicians for further evaluation of clinically suspected SpA. The second cohort of 88 cases comprised patients who presented with acute anterior uveitis and were referred for assessment of SpA if they indicated past or present back pain for at least 3 months. Mean duration of back pain symptoms was 10 years. The study cohort included 20 age- and sex-matched healthy controls. Sensitivity and specificity of MRI for nr-SpA, defined according to rheumatologist expert opinion, compared to non-specific back pain was 74%/44% and 95%/83%, respectively, for the first and second cohorts, respectively. Analysis of concordant MRI data from an inception cohort of 40 patients with high clinical suspicion of SpA and IBP of 24 weeks' duration, nine patients with mechanical back pain, and nine healthy controls showed that sensitivity was 66% and specificity was 94% for the clinical diagnosis of SpA (LR+ 11.8, LR– 0.4) (35). A study of patients suspected of having SpA but without radiographic sacroiliitis that combined MRI and histopathological assessment of SI joints after needle biopsy showed that specificity of MRI for sacroiliitis was 100% while sensitivity was only 38%, using inflammation in immunohistology as the gold standard (36). This was a 10-year follow-up study and since this report there have been substantial refinements in MRI scanning technology.

Lengthy follow-up is required for predictive validation of abnormalities observed on MRI according to radiographic sacroiliitis. Longitudinal studies with plain radiographic endpoints are limited in both numbers of patients studied and duration of follow-up. One study evaluated 17 patients with IBP of 3–14 months' duration but normal pelvic X-ray who were followed for 1½–2½ years (8). Virtually all patients had abnormalities on baseline MRI that persisted on follow-up MRI 2–30 months later and 11 developed plain radiographic features of sacroiliitis. In a study of 29 patients with nr-radiographic SpA followed for 7.7 years, baseline MRI had 100% sensitivity for subsequent radiographic sacroiliitis, although specificity was only 56% (35). Severity of MRI inflammation in subchondral bone has been identified as a prognostic factor for radiographic sacroiliitis (9, 36).

An expert taskforce of EULAR concluded, on the basis of 13 studies that evaluated the diagnostic utility of MRI, that assessment of the SI joints should be conducted if the diagnosis of axSpA cannot be established based on clinical features and conventional radiography, and axSpA is still suspected (37). MRI of the SI joints is most useful diagnostically in those patients with a clinical suspicion of IBP who are HLA-B27-positive, have a normal or equivocal radiograph of the SI joints, and have an insufficient symptomatic response to NSAIDs and are considered candidates for more intensive therapy.

Classification of spondyloarthritis using MRI

The enhanced sensitivity of MRI over radiography for detection of early SpA together with the unreliability of radiographic assessment of the SI joints were amongst the key factors that provided impetus to the development of the new ASAS classification criteria for SpA. The inclusion of MRI necessitated the further step of defining what constituted a positive MRI for the purposes of classification. The first proposal has been generated by a consensus exercise conducted by rheumatologist and radiologist experts in the field. This definition is based primarily on the imaging features of active sacroiliitis on MRI, and although several different inflammatory lesions of the SI joints can be detected on MRI, the clear presence of BME/osteitis in subchondral bone on a fat-suppressed sequence is considered to be the defining observation (38). This definition by ASAS includes a quantitative component, which specifies that the definition is met when there are at least two lesions on a single semicoronal slice or when a single lesion is present on two consecutive slices. However, subsequent controlled studies revealed the prevalence of BME in the SI joints of up to 30% of mechanical back pain patients and healthy controls, causing doubt as to whether MRI detection of SI joints BME is a specific enough criterion to enable discrimination between SpA patients and patients with other causes of back pain (33, 34, 39). (For the use of MRI in a diagnostic approach in axSpA patients see Chapter 3.) The BME lesions in patients with non-specific back pain and healthy controls tend to be small, evident on only one or two slices, and have only mildly increased signal intensity compared to background signal on STIR/T2FS MRI sequences. The presence of subchondral BME on at least three semicoronal slices substantially increases specificity for SpA (34). False positive signal on fat-suppressed MRI may also be observed in the sacrum on the most anterior slice that includes the joint or in the postero-inferior iliac bone due to partial volume averaging with blood vessels located in close proximity to the joint at these locations (Fig. 13.5).

Structural lesions on T1W MRI, especially erosions, may contribute to the decision by the observer that inflammatory lesions are genuinely due to SpA (34). Erosions can be reliably detected and have been detected in about 60% of patients with nr-SpA compared to just 8% of patients with non-specific causes of back pain or healthy controls (29). The combined presence of erosion and BME enhanced specificity for classification of SpA in one controlled study (34) and training of readers to reliably detect structural lesions enhanced the diagnostic utility of MRI (40).

Fat metaplasia in the SI joints has also been evaluated for classification and diagnostic utility. It has been long recognized that fat infiltration may be observed in healthy individuals distributed in a heterogeneous manner in the central sacrum. Post-inflammatory fat metaplasia is typically evident adjacent to subchondral bone, has a distinct border from adjacent marrow matrix, displays a homogeneous increase in T1W signal, and is often associated with other MRI features of SpA, such as erosions, sclerosis, and BME (Figs 13.6–13.8). SI joint fat metaplasia per se is not of clinical utility in recognition of nr-axSpA, however, because of its strong association with concomitant BME or erosion. Appropriate evaluation of an MRI scan of the SI joints for both diagnosis and classification of axSpA should always include simultaneous assessment of T1W and fat-suppressed sequences, since each sequence provides complementary information.

Contrast-enhanced MRI of the sacroiliac joint

The potential use of Gd-enhanced sequences to improve detection of active MRI lesions in the SI joints has often been advocated and it has been considered superior to fat-suppressed MRI for detection of synovitis and resultant fluid in the joint cavity (2). This method may cause discomfort to patients because it requires the patient to lie still for up to 1 hour during the course of MRI examination. It requires intravenous administration of contrast and is costly. A Danish study revealed that active bone marrow abnormalities of the SI joints in 40 SpA patients with 3–14 years of symptom duration were detected equally well by use of STIR and by use of Gd-enhanced fat-suppressed T1 sequences (41). This conclusion was confirmed in a cohort of 127 early-SpA patients with symptom duration of less than 2 years (42). Synovitis, capsulitis, and enthesitis visualized by use of Gd administration were observed only in the presence of BME detected by use of STIR alone (Fig. 13.10). Consequently, it is highly questionable whether this technique is necessary for routine diagnostic evaluation.

MRI of the sacroiliac joint in juvenile spondyloarthritis.

The principles of MRI evaluation of the SI joints in children are much the same as in adults. However, MRI of the immature skeleton does confer some additional challenges, and a T1W sequence with fat suppression (T1FS) following intravenous contrast enhancement with Gd (T1FS + Gd) is often used (Fig. 13.10). Enthesopathy and hip disease are more frequent in JoSpA than adults, and the routine SI joint MRI protocol may be adjusted with expansion of the field of view and/or the number of slices in one of the acquisition planes so as to include the hips and entheses.

The normal axial skeleton in children has a higher proportion of erythropoietic bone marrow than in adults, resulting in several effects. With less fat content, bone marrow appears darker on T1W images, and on STIR or T2FS, the erythropoietic component may be slightly brighter than in adults, making BME harder to detect. This is compounded by the appearance of a 'subchondral flare' of brighter signal on STIR or T2FS in the subchondral bone due to the normal accentuation of vascularity at sites of bone growth. For this reason, T1FS + Gd may be preferred for detection of SI joint inflammation, although it comes at the price of additional cost, time, and the need for injection, and the additional diagnostic utility of T1FS + Gd in addition to standard sequences has been repeatedly questioned. A recent study of 51 patients showed that fluid-sensitive sequences had identical sensitivity to T1FS + Gd and were only marginally less specific (43). Since fatty replacement of normal marrow is not a feature of the juvenile axial skeleton, post-inflammatory fat metaplasia in subchondral bone has much higher specificity (specificity 0.91) than in adults (11). Erosion is often seen (sensitivity 0.58) and is quite specific (specificity 0.91), but may be harder to observe in some cases as the normal bone–cartilage interface is very irregular in younger children. Alterations of joint space width are hardest of all to observe consistently in children because the bone lacks a smooth surface and the 'joint space' includes the cartilage of the growth centre and the joint. Subchondral sclerosis is one of the most frequent findings on MRI in JoSpA, but the density of the normal subchondral bone is variable so the diagnostic utility of this observation is not as good. Evidence of capsulitis/synovitis is well demonstrated on T1FS + Gd and is seen quite often with this sequence. Other findings typical of JoSpA may also be observed in the pelvis, such as enthesopathy at ligamentous and tendinous insertions, and hip joint inflammation.

Differential diagnosis of spondyloarthritis lesions on MRI of the sacroiliac joint

The most common abnormality to affect the SI joint is degenerative change. Osteoarthritis of the SI joints becomes increasingly frequent with age and it is very common over age 45. However, even under age 45, minor changes due to osteoarthritis are still common, more so in women. The typical findings are seen somewhere at or near the perimeter of the joint. The typical MRI features are small foci of sclerosis and/or BME without erosion and seldom with significant fat metaplasia. Joint space narrowing and osteophytosis are associated but are harder to discern on MRI. In some cases, osteoarthritis is hard to distinguish from osteitis condensans ilii (OCI), and both of these conditions may cause broad areas of diffuse or dense sclerosis in subchondral bone, predominantly on the iliac side (Fig. 13.11). Mild BME may be seen, usually as a thin rim of BME surrounding the sclerotic bone. With specific sequences, cartilage thinning may be seen, and a thin well-defined bright line throughout the joint space on STIR/T2FS typically represents joint fluid in a degenerate joint. Other signs of inflammation in capsule or soft tissues are usually not associated with degenerative change.

The most crucial differential diagnosis of a unilateral sacroiliitis is septic arthritis. The acute septic joint reveals much more widespread inflammation on MRI which does not respect anatomical boundaries and is seen extending far from the joint in bone marrow and soft tissues with periostitis, capsulitis, joint effusion, and abscess formation. In subacute cases, the inflammatory signs are still prominent, but destruction of joint surface and subchondral bone may be

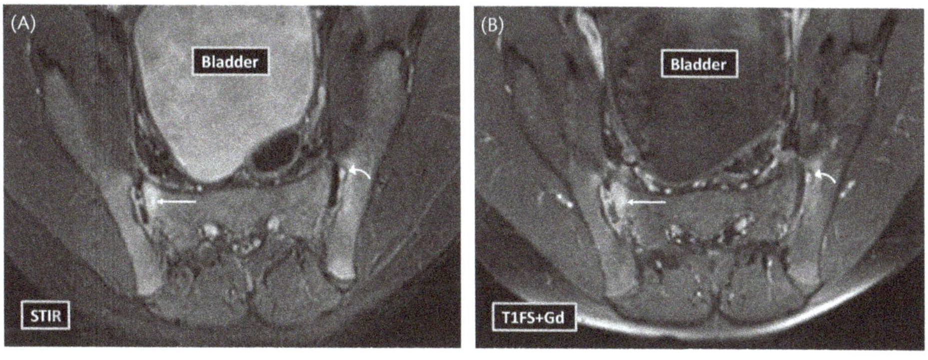

Fig. 13.10 MRI in a young adolescent—axial images of SI joints with STIR and T1W fat saturation following contrast enhancement with intravenous Gd (T1FS + Gd) sequences. Bilateral sacroiliitis is seen equally well with both sequences. BME/osteitis is most prominent in the right sacral ala (straight arrow) and focal bone erosion is best seen in the left ilium (curved arrow). These and other images in the series showed capsulitis/synovitis to varying degrees.

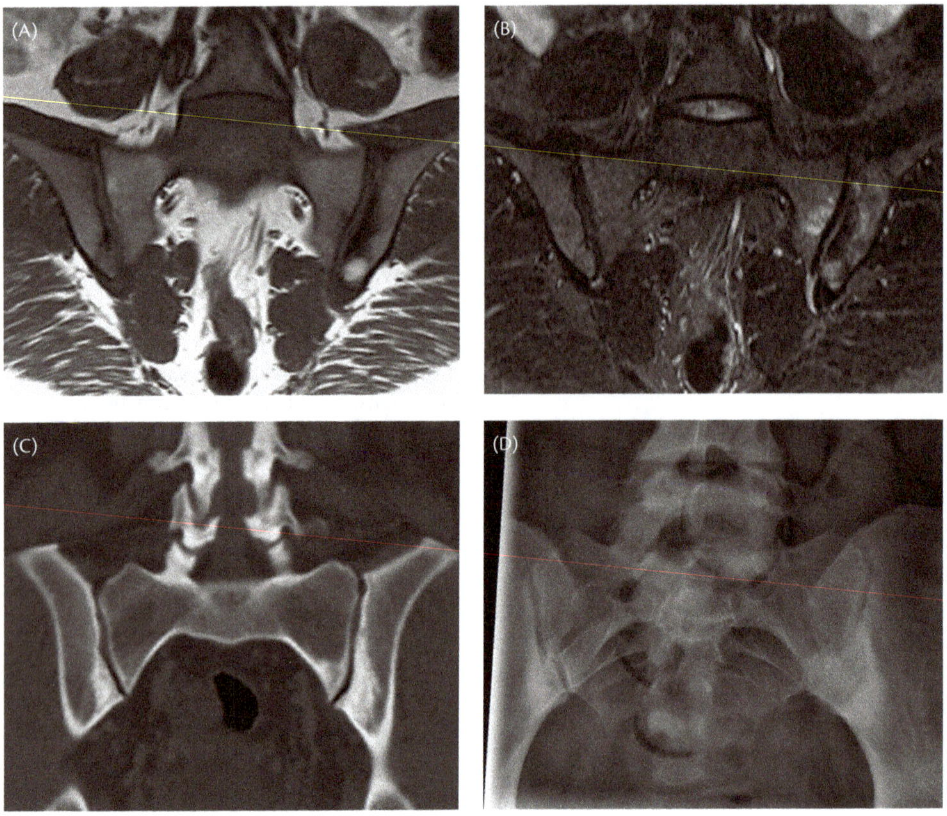

Fig. 13.11 MRI coronal T1W (A) and STIR (B), CT scan (C), and radiograph (D) of SI joints in OCI/osteoarthritis. A 28-year-old female HLA-B27-positive patient with inflammatory-type buttock pain was clinically followed for 10 years. MRI scan was performed at age 28, and because aetiology of SI joint findings was unproven, she was given a trial of biologic therapy without response. On follow-up, CT scan and radiograph 5 years after MRI (after a second pregnancy) confirmed OCI on both studies and osteoarthritis on CT scan. All modalities show subchondral sclerosis of the left ilium, with right iliac sclerosis more visible on later studies (C, D). Definite BME is visible on both sides of the left SI joint on MRI (B) and was present on 11 slices, although it was mild on most images. The MRI was suspicious for possible erosion, but follow-up CT showed no erosion. The CT scan (C) confirms bilateral hyaline cartilage thinning and intra-articular gas typical for osteoarthritis.

profound, with osteomyelitis and intraosseous abscess formation extending further from the joint surface than is usual in SpA.

BME is a common feature of stress fractures, which may be seen in overuse injuries and in osteoporotic patients with insufficiency fractures. These are invariably confined to either the sacrum or the ilium and are not associated with articular erosion. Prominent BME may be seen in the SI joint in female patients immediately post-partum and usually settles with conservative management. Other arthropathies may rarely affect the SI joints, such as gout and RA, but SI joint involvement is very rare at initial presentation.

MRI-based semiquantitative scoring of spondyloarthritis lesions in the sacroiliac joint

Formal scoring methods for quantifying disease activity in the SI joints on MRI have been proposed that can be generally categorized as being primarily based on either a global scheme that focuses on overall assessment of the SI joints or a more detailed method that scores several consecutive semicoronal images that depict the cartilaginous portion of the SI joint. The presence and extent of BME in the cartilaginous portion of the joint is the primary MRI feature that is scored, although one method also scores inflammation in the joint space and the ligamentous portion of the joint by assessing semiaxial slices through the joint (Aarhus method (15)).

In the Berlin method, each SI joint is divided into quadrants and each quadrant is graded 0–3 according to the estimated percentage volume of the quadrant with BME, leading to a scoring range of 0–24 (44). The Leeds method similarly grades the extent of BME per SI joint quadrant but incorporates intensity of BME in the assessment of severity (45). A major limitation of scoring methods based on percentage of SI joint quadrant or subcortical bone affected with BME is that inflammation occurs concomitantly with structural lesions such as erosion and fat metaplasia and these methods do not elaborate how this impacts scoring.

In the SPARCC method, each SI joint is divided into quadrants, and the presence of marrow oedema in each quadrant is scored dichotomously (present/absent) on consecutive semicoronal slices assessed from anterior to posterior, with additional weighting for intensity and depth (Fig. 13.12) (46). Methodological details are provided in an online training module (http://www.carearthritis.com/MRI_scoring_modules.php). The SPARCC method has been shown to be highly discriminatory in placebo-controlled clinical trials of both AS and nr-axSpA (47, 48). The ASAS conducted a multi-reader exercise evaluating the different scoring methods for reliability and sensitivity to change according to the requirements of the OMERACT filter (49). Agreement between readers and sensitivity to change was better for the more detailed SPARCC scoring method.

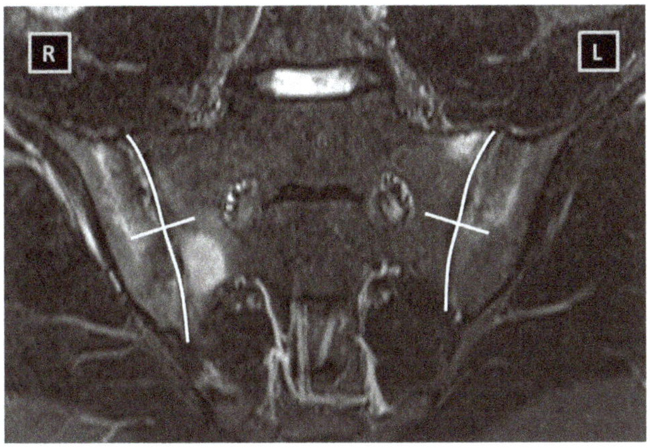

Fig. 13.12 MRI SI joints—coronal STIR—quantitative assessment of inflammation. In the SPARCC method, each SI joint is divided into quadrants, and presence of BME in each quadrant is scored dichotomously (present/absent) on six consecutive semicoronal slices assessed from anterior to posterior, with additional weighting for intensity and depth. On this image, SPARCC BME score would be 6, with BME positive in three upper quadrants (right ilium, left sacrum, left ilium) and two lower quadrants (right ilium and sacrum). The right lower sacral quadrant is also positive for 'depth' as BME is continuously present for a depth of over 1 cm from the articular surface. Score for intensity is 0—the same quadrant is very bright at the perimeter of the lesion but the centre is just below threshold for 'intensity' score. Heterogeneous signals in the right upper sacrum and left lower ilium are below threshold for scoring BME.

Several scoring methods have been developed for quantification of structural lesions in the SI joints on T1W scans. One method scores fat lesions dichotomously (present/absent) according to SI joint quadrants and a 0–8 scoring range based on a global evaluation of the SI joints (50). A second method scores fat metaplasia in both cartilaginous and ligamentous compartments using a grading scheme based on the extent of subcortical bone affected (51). Erosion in the SI joints has also been quantified according to a grading scheme based on the number of erosions per SI joint (1 = 1–2, 2 = 3–5, 3 = > 5 erosions per SI joint) (50). In a second method, erosion is graded in both cartilaginous and ligamentous compartments and severity is graded based on the extent of subcortical bone affected (51).

A scoring method that quantifies fat metaplasia, erosion, backfill, and ankylosis has also been developed. The SPARCC Sacroiliac Joint Structural Score (SSS) is based on assessment of five consecutive slices through the SI joints starting from the transitional slice, division of each SI joint into quadrants, and dichotomous (present/absent) scoring of lesions in each quadrant (52). Methodological details are provided at http://www.carearthritis.com/MRI_scoring_modules.php.

Conclusion

Although radiography of the SI joints remains the cornerstone of evaluation of SpA by imaging, recent advances have firmly established a role for MRI. Moreover, MRI has contributed to our understanding of the pathogenesis and progression of SpA, particularly through the identification of subchondral BME as an early feature and fat metaplasia as an intermediary tissue in the pathway to ankylosis. Finally, MRI has now been shown to provide tools for the quantitative assessment of both active and structural lesions, thereby facilitating the endeavours of basic and clinical researchers.

References

1. Schichikawa K, Tsyimoto M, Nishioka J, Nishibayashi Y, Matsumoto K. Histopathology of early sacroiliitis and enthesitis in ankylosing spondylitis. In: Ziff M, Cohen SB (eds) Advances in Inflammation Research, Volume 9: The Spondyloarthropathies. New York, Raven Press, 1985, pp. 15–24.
2. van den Berg R, Lenczner G, Feydy A, et al. Agreement between clinical practice and trained central reading in reading of sacroiliac joints on plain pelvic radiographs. Results from the DESIR cohort. Arthritis Rheumatol 2014;66:2403–11.
3. Ryan LM, Carrera GF, Lightfoot RW Jr, Hoffman RG, Kozin F. The radiographic diagnosis of sacroiliitis: a comparison of different views with computed tomograms of the sacroiliac joint. Arthritis Rheum 1983;26:760–3.
4. Battistone MJ, Manaster BJ, Reda DJ, Clegg DO. Radiographic diagnosis of sacroiliitis—are sacroiliac views really better? J Rheumatol 1998;25:2395–401.
5. Mau W, Zeidler H, Mau R, Majewski A, Freyschmidt J, Deicher H. Outcome of possible ankylosing spondylitis in a 10 years' follow-up study. Clin Rheumatol 1987;6(Suppl 2):60–6.
6. Sampaio-Barros PD, Bertolo MB, Kraemer MH, Marques-Neto JF, Samara AM. Undifferentiated spondyloarthropathies: a 2-year follow-up study. Clin Rheumatol 2001;20:201–6.
7. Poddubnyy D, Rudwaleit M, Haibel H, et al. Rates and predictors of radiographic sacroiliitis progression over 2 years in patients with axial spondyloarthritis. Ann Rheum Dis 2011;70:1369–74.
8. Oostveen J, Prevo R, den Boer J, van de Laar M. Early detection of sacroiliitis on magnetic resonance imaging and subsequent development of sacroiliitis on plain radiography. A prospective, longitudinal study. J Rheumatol 1999;26:1953–8.
9. Bennett AN, McGonagle D, O'Connor P, et al. Severity of baseline magnetic resonance imaging-evident sacroiliitis and HLA-B27 status in early inflammatory back pain predict radiographically evident ankylosing spondylitis at eight years. Arthritis Rheum 2008;58:3413–18.
10. Van der Linden S.M., Valkenburg H.A., Cats A. Evaluation of diagnostic criteria for ankylosing spondylitis: a proposal for modification of the New York criteria. Arthritis Rheum 1984;27:361–8.
11. Jaremko JL, Liu L, Winn NJ, Ellsworth JE, Lambert RG. Diagnostic utility of magnetic resonance imaging and radiography in juvenile spondyloarthritis: evaluation of the sacroiliac joints in controls and affected subjects. J Rheumatol 2014;41:963–70.
12. O'Shea FD, Boyle E, Salonen DC, et al. Inflammatory and degenerative sacroiliac joint disease in a primary back pain cohort. Arthritis Care Res 2010;62:447–54.
13. Geijer M, Gothlin GG, Gothlin JH. The clinical utility of computed tomography compared to conventional radiography in diagnosing sacroiliitis. A retrospective study on 910 patients and literature review. J Rheumatol 2007;34:1561–5.
14. Devauchelle-Pensec V, D'Agostino MA, Marion J, et al. Computed tomography scanning facilitates the diagnosis of sacroiliitis in patients with suspected spondylarthritis: results of a prospective multicenter French cohort study. Arthritis Rheum 2012;64:1412–19.
15. Puhakka KB, Jurik AG, Egund N, et al. Imaging of sacroiliitis in early seronegative spondylarthropathy. Assessment of abnormalities by MR in comparison with radiography and CT. Acta Radiol 2003;44:218–29.
16. Yu W, Feng F, Dion E, Yang H, Jiang M, Genant HK. Comparison of radiography, computed tomography and magnetic resonance imaging in the detection of sacroiliitis accompanying ankylosing spondylitis. Skeletal Radiol 1998;27:311–20.
17. Blum U, Buitrago-Tellez C, Mundinger A, et al. Magnetic resonance imaging (MRI) for detection of active sacroiliitis—a prospective study comparing conventional radiography, scintigraphy, and contrast enhanced MRI. J Rheumatol 1996;23:2107–15.
18. Song IH, Carrasco-Fernandez J, Rudwaleit M, Sieper J. The diagnostic value of scintigraphy in assessing sacroiliitis in ankylosing spondylitis: a systematic literature search. Ann Rheum Dis 2008;67:1535–40.

19. Unlu E, Pamuk ON, Cakir N. Color and duplex Doppler sonography to detect sacroiliitis and spinal inflammation in ankylosing spondylitis: can this method reveal response to antitumor necrosis factor therapy? J Rheumatol 2007;34:110–16.
20. Klauser A, Halpern EJ, Frauscher F, et al. Inflammatory low back pain: high negative predictive value of contrast-enhanced color Doppler ultrasound in the detection of inflamed sacroiliac joints. Arthritis Rheum 2005;53:440–4.
21. Klauser AS, De Zordo T, Bellmann-Weiler R, et al. Feasibility of second-generation ultrasound contrast media in the detection of active sacroiliitis. Arthritis Rheum 2009;61:909–16.
22. Muche B, Bollow M, Francois RJ, Sieper J, Hamm B, Braun J. Anatomic structures involved in early- and late-stage sacroiliitis in spondylarthritis. Arthritis Rheum 2003;48:1374–84.
23. Puhakka KB, Jurik AG, Schiottz-Christensen B, et al. Magnetic resonance imaging of sacroiliitis in early seronegative spondylarthropathy. Abnormalities correlated to clinical and laboratory findings. Rheumatology (Oxford) 2004;43:234–7.
24. Ahlstrom H, Feltelius N, Nyman R, Hallgren R. Magnetic resonance imaging of sacroiliac joint inflammation. Arthritis Rheum 1990;33:1763–9.
25. Braun J, Bollow M, Eggens U, Konig H, Distler A, Sieper J. Use of dynamic magnetic resonance imaging with fast imaging in the detection of early and advanced sacroiliitis in spondyloarthropathy patients. Arthritis Rheum 1994;37:1039–45.
26. Braun J, Bollow M, Seyrekbasan F, et al. Computed tomography guided corticosteroid injection of the sacroiliac joint in patients with spondyloarthropathy with sacroiliitis: clinical outcome and followup by dynamic magnetic resonance imaging. J Rheumatol 1996;23:659–64.
27. Bollow M, Fischer T, Reisshauer H, et al. Quantitative analyses of sacroiliac biopsies in spondylarthropathies: T cells and macrophages predominate in early and active sacroiliitis—cellularity correlates with the degree of enhancement detected by magnetic resonance imaging. Ann Rheum Dis 2000;59:135–40.
28. Maksymowych WP, Wichuk S, Chiowchanwisawakit P, Lambert RG, Pedersen SJ. Fat metaplasia and backfill are key intermediaries in the development of sacroiliac joint ankylosis in patients with ankylosing spondylitis. Arthritis Rheumatol 2014;66:2958–67.
29. Weber U, Pedersen SJ, Ostergaard M, Rufibach K, Lambert R, Maksymowych WP. Can erosions on MRI of the sacroiliac joints be reliably detected in patients with ankylosing spondylitis? A cross-sectional study. Arthritis Res Ther 2012;14:R124.
30. Bollow M, Hermann KG, Biedermann T, Sieper J, Schontube M, Braun J. Very early spondyloarthritis: where the inflammation in the sacroiliac joints starts. Ann Rheum Dis 2005;64:1644–6.
31. Bollow M, Braun J, Hamm B, et al. Early sacroiliitis in patients with spondyloarthropathy: evaluation with dynamic gadolinium-enhanced MR imaging. Radiology 1995;194:529–36.
32. Heuft-Dorenbosch L, Landewe R, Weijers R, et al. Combining information obtained from magnetic resonance imaging and conventional radiographs to detect sacroiliitis in patients with recent onset inflammatory back pain. Ann Rheum Dis 2006;65:804–8.
33. Weber U, Lambert RG, Østergaard M, Hodler J, Pedersen SJ, Maksymowych WP. The diagnostic utility of magnetic resonance imaging in spondylarthritis: an international multicenter evaluation of one hundred eighty-seven subjects. Arthritis Rheum 2010;62:3048–58.
34. Weber U, Østergaard M, Lambert RGW, et al. Candidate lesion-based criteria for defining a positive sacroiliac joint MRI in two cohorts of patients with axial spondyloarthritis. Ann Rheum Dis 2015;74(11):1976–82.
35. Aydin SZ, Maksymowych WP, Bennett AN, McGonagle D, Emery P, Marzo-Ortega H. Validation of the ASAS criteria and definition of a positive MRI of the sacroiliac joint in an inception cohort of axial spondyloarthritis followed up for 8 years. Ann Rheum Dis 2012;71:56–60.
36. Gong Y, Zheng N, Chen SB, et al. Ten years' experience with needle biopsy in the early diagnosis of sacroiliitis. Arthritis Rheum 2012;64:1399–406.
37. Mandl P, Navarro-Compán V, Terslev L, et al. EULAR recommendations for the use of imaging in the diagnosis and management of spondyloarthritis in clinical practice. Ann Rheum Dis 2015;74(7):1327–39
38. Rudwaleit M, Jurik AG, Hermann KGA, et al. Defining active sacroiliitis on magnetic resonance imaging (MRI) for classification of axial spondyloarthritis: a consensual approach by the ASAS/OMERACT MRI Group. Ann Rheum Dis 2009;68:1520–7.
39. Marzo-Ortega H, McGonagle D, O'Connor P, et al. Baseline and 1-year magnetic resonance imaging of the sacroiliac joint and lumbar spine in very early inflammatory back pain. Relationship between symptoms, HLAB27, and disease extent and persistence. Ann Rheum Dis 2009;68:1721–7.
40. Weber U, Lambert RGW, Pedersen SJ, Hodler J, Østergaard M, Maksymowych WP. Assessment of structural lesions in sacroiliac joints enhances diagnostic utility of magnetic resonance imaging in early spondylarthritis. Arthritis Care Res 2012;62:1763–71.
41. Madsen KB, Egund N, Jurik AG. Grading of inflammatory disease activity in the sacroiliac joints with magnetic resonance imaging: comparison between short-tau inversion recovery and gadolinium contrast-enhanced sequences. J Rheumatol 2010;37:393–400.
42. De Hooge M, van den Berg R, Navarro-Compan V, et al. Magnetic resonance imaging of the sacroiliac joints in the early detection of spondyloarthritis: no added value of gadolinium compared with short tau inversion recovery sequence. Rheumatology (Oxford) 2013;52(7):1220–4.
43. Weiss PF, Xiao R, Biko DM, Johnson AM, Chauvin NA. Detection of inflammatory sacroiliitis in children with magnetic resonance imaging: is gadolinium-contrast enhancement necessary? Arthritis Rheumatol 2015;67(8):2250–6.
44. Hermann KGA, Braun J, Fischer T, Reisshauer H, Bollow M. [Magnetic resonance tomography of sacroiliitis: anatomy, histological pathology, MR-morphology, and grading.] Radiologe 2004;44:217–28.
45. Barkham N, Keen HI, Coates LC, et al. Clinical and imaging efficacy of infliximab in HLA-B27-positive patients with magnetic resonance imaging-determined early sacroiliitis. Arthritis Rheum 2009;60:946–54.
46. Maksymowych WP, Inman RD, Salonen D, et al. Spondyloarthritis Research Consortium of Canada magnetic resonance imaging index for assessment of sacroiliac joint inflammation in ankylosing spondylitis. Arthritis Rheum 2005;53:703–9.
47. Lambert RGW, Salonen D, Rahman P, et al. Adalimumab significantly reduces both spinal and sacroiliac joint inflammation in patients with ankylosing spondylitis. Arthritis Rheum 2007;56:4005–14.
48. Dougados M, van der Heijde D, Sieper J, et al. Symptomatic efficacy of etanercept and its effect on objective signs of inflammation in early nonradiographic axial spondyloarthritis: a multicenter, randomized, double-blind, placebo-controlled trial. Arthritis Rheumatol 2014;66:2091–102.
49. Landewe RB, Hermann KG, van der Heijde DM, et al. Scoring sacroiliac joints by magnetic resonance imaging. A multiple-reader reliability experiment. J Rheumatol 2005;32:2050–5
50. Song, I-H. Hermann KG. Haibel H, et al. Relationship between active inflammatory lesions in the spine and sacroiliac joints and new development of chronic lesions on whole-body MRI in early axial spondyloarthritis: results of the ESTHER trial at week 48. Ann Rheum Dis 2011;70:1257–63.
51. Madsen KB, Jurik AG. Magnetic resonance imaging grading system for active and chronic spondylarthritis changes in the sacroiliac joint. Arthritis Care Res 2010;62:11–18.
52. Maksymowych WP, Wichuk S, Chiowchanwisawakit P, Lambert RG, Pedersen SJ. Development and preliminary validation of the Spondyloarthritis Research Consortium of Canada Magnetic Resonance Imaging Sacroiliac Joint Structural Score. J Rheumatol 2015;42:79–86.

CHAPTER 14

Imaging: spine

Xenofon Baraliakos and Kay-Geert A. Hermann

Introduction to imaging the spine

The pathognomonic findings in the spine of patients with axSpA are, similar to those of the SI joints, mainly inflammatory, osteodestructive, and osteoproliferative in nature, many being located at the entheseal junction to the bone. Clinically, these pathologies are associated with chronic back pain, in the majority of cases with IBP, while spinal stiffness can also occur without pain (1, 2).

In the spine, spondylitis, SpA, and (non-infectious) spondylodiscitis are the main inflammatory manifestations (3), followed by post-inflammatory changes such as fat metaplasia (4), and later on by new bone formation resulting in syndesmophytes and ankylosis (5). The so-called bamboo spine, which has been described in many books in the past, can occur in up to 15% of patients with established AS (6).

Although these characteristic changes can occur during the course of the disease in the majority of patients, their prevalence and the velocity of disease progression and severity can show great variations between individual patients and during different time periods (7). The pathogenesis and the relatively complex pathogenic process between inflammation and formation of structural changes in the spine of axSpA patients are still incompletely understood. This is of special interest since the axial involvement in axSpA is not only characterized by inflammatory and osteoproliferative changes but also by erosive changes which occur during the process of osteoproliferation (8).

The capacity of the available imaging techniques to detect the variety of relevant pathologies in axSpA shows large differences. For assessment of structural changes in the axial skeleton, conventional radiographs are still considered the standard of reference (3, 6). CT is used mainly for assessment of structural changes in the SI joints, but its use is limited to special diagnostic situations due to its radiation exposure. For detection of inflammatory changes, MRI is currently the standard of reference (9).

For classification of axSpA according to the current classification criteria, only changes in the SI joints are considered relevant (10). Nevertheless, some patients may well show spinal involvement in the absence of pathology in the SI joints (3), which still allows for diagnosis of axSpA, both AS- and nr-axSpA. For study purposes, different scoring systems have been proposed for assessment of both the inflammatory and the structural changes in axSpA (11–13).

Finally, structural changes (presence of syndesmophytes, shown by X-ray) and the degree of inflammatory changes in the SI joints (shown by MRI, in combination with HLA-B27) have been found to have prognostic value for the future course of the disease (6, 14).

Imaging of the spine in axial spondyloarthritis

Although spinal changes are known to occur in more advanced stages of the disease and should thus be considered more clinically relevant for diagnosing axSpA, they have not been part of the classification criteria for AS or axSpA, since only 3–5% of patients with AS will show any changes in the spine prior to the SI joints (15). Furthermore, a caveat when interpreting new bone formation in the context of axSpA is also the difficulty to differentiate syndesmophytes (thin bone growth along the course of the anterior longitudinal ligament) from spondylophytes (thicker new bone growing more horizontally, as a sign of degenerative changes) (Fig. 14.1), especially in patients with longer disease duration (16). Nevertheless, syndesmophytes have significant predictive value for further spinal radiographic progression, since the presence of one syndesmophyte is associated with increased risk for development of more syndesmophytes (6). How much time is needed until structural lesions of the spine develop is not entirely clear yet. However, within the first 16 years of AS, bony changes have been reported to be present in more than 50% of patients (17). Overall, both, inflammatory and structural spinal changes play an important role in the evaluation of spinal imaging and also affect treatment decision regarding anti inflammatory agents such as NSAIDs and TNF blockers, which are known to significantly decrease vertebral osteitis (which is considered to represent spinal inflammation) but may also have a positive effect in the retardation of new bone formation (syndesmophytes) (18, 19). However, currently, clinical symptoms such as pain, stiffness, and loss of function are considered to be most important for any decision on treatment in axSpA.

Conventional radiographs

As with conventional radiography of the SI joints, conventional radiographs of the spine are not able to detect spinal inflammatory lesions such as spondylitis and SpA (20). Nevertheless, X-rays are the gold standard for the assessment of structural spinal changes. The visualization of osteoproliferative or erosive processes in the vertebrae represents the spinal damage that has already occurred and is useful in documentation of the disease progression. In general, spinal changes related to axSpA can be osteodestructive (erosions) or hyperproliferative (vertebral squaring, bony sclerosis, disc calcifications, syndesmophytes, bony bridging, vertebral ankylosis) (Figs 14.1 and 14.2). Syndesmophytes are characterized by vertical growth along the course of the annulus fibrosus, which may end with bridging between two adjacent vertebral bodies (Fig. 14.3) (20–23).

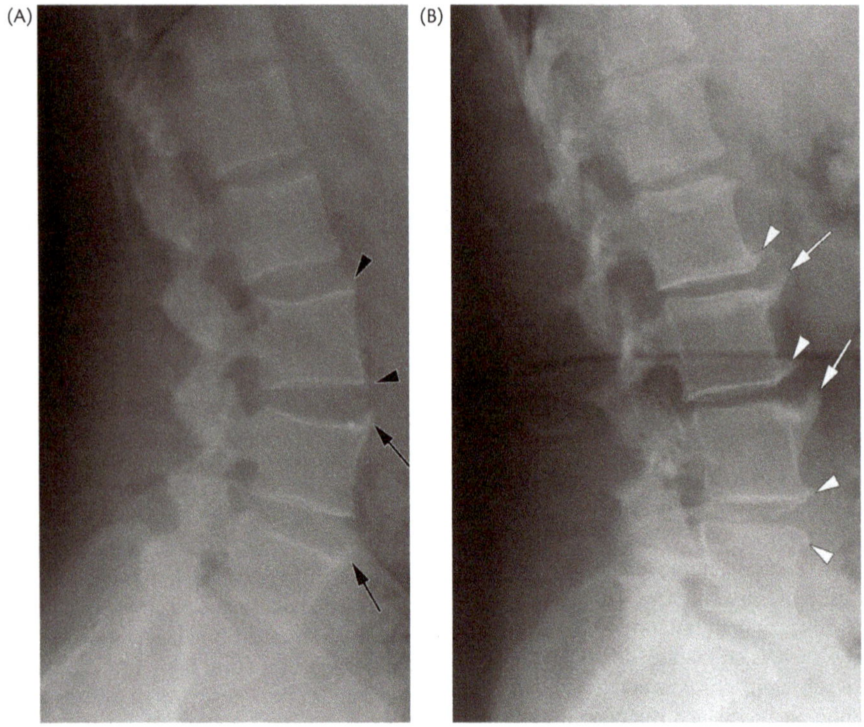

Fig. 14.1 (A) A 43-year-old man with axSpA. Evidence of large syndesmophytes (black arrows) at the anterior edges of the upper endplates of L4 and L5. Note also early syndesmophytes growing at L3 (black arrowheads). (B) A 59-year-old woman with degenerative disc disease. Large spondylophytes (osteophytes) are seen at L3 and L4 (white arrows) as well as smaller spondylophytes at L2 to L5 (white arrowheads). While syndesmophytes are usually thinner than spondylophytes, their identifying feature is the vertical growth direction alongside the annulus fibrosus fibres. In contrast, spondylophytes (osteophytes) are rather bulgy and growth starts primarily horizontal in direction (best seen at white arrowheads), with secondary vertical (or round) growth as spondylophytes are getting larger (white arrows).

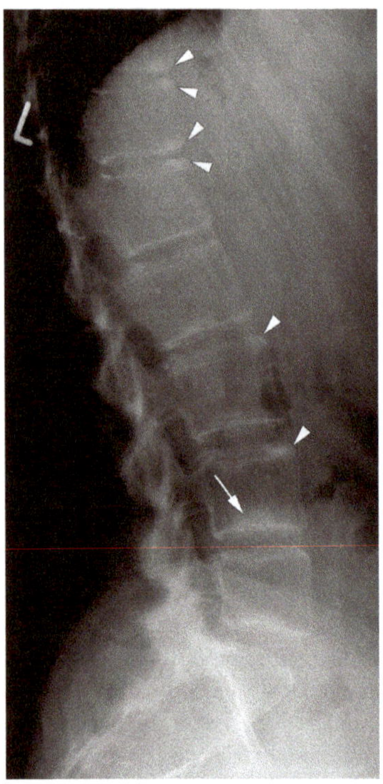

Fig. 14.2 A 47-year-old man with axSpA. There are multiple 'shiny corners' (arrowheads) as signs of vertebral new bone formation at the annulus fibrosus attachments. Note also hemicircular bone sclerosis at L4 (arrow) as a sign of disc involvement.

Furthermore, also the lateral parts of the vertebral bodies, the facet joint (Fig. 14.4) and costovertebral joints, are frequently affected in AS. Nevertheless, since these areas are difficult to assess by most imaging procedures and especially by X-ray, involvement of these joints is frequently underdiagnosed. Also, in some patients, involvement (ankylosis) of the facet joints may be present in those who might not show any presence of osteoproliferation of the vertebral bodies (24), suggesting that these joints may be affected also in earlier courses of the disease.

Magnetic resonance imaging

Technical aspects

In comparison to conventional X-rays, imaging with CT and MRI has an advantage because they can provide multidimensional images by digital image processing. Pathologies can be visualized in different orientations and planes. The spine is most frequently imaged in sagittal orientation, although coronal as well as transverse slices do provide additional information and may highlight the anatomy better. However, only the sagittal plane is included in the definition of the minimum requirement for imaging (25). The AP view used by conventional radiographs is also frequently used in order to capture syndesmophytes. When using CT and MRI, the slices should cover the entire vertebra, including the vertebral body but also the posterior (spinous processes) and the lateral (facet joints, costovertebral joints) elements.

The assessment of active lesions can be performed by so-called water-sensitive MRI techniques, where (hyper)-vascularized areas such as vessels, cerebrospinal fluid, but also BME can be visualized.

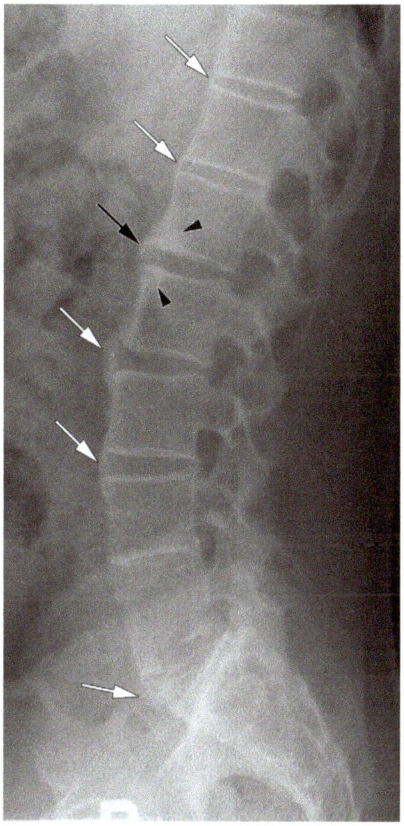

Fig. 14.3 A 53-year-old man with axSpA, demonstrating multiple bridging syndesmophytes (white arrows) leading to bony ankylosis of vertebral segments. Note the vertical alignment and thin appearance of most bridging syndesmophytes. There is one segment unaffected and another one features a large syndesmophyte at the lower endplate of L1 (black arrow) that has not yet fused with L2. Severe vertebral bone sclerosis (designated as 'shiny corners') is also seen (black arrowheads).

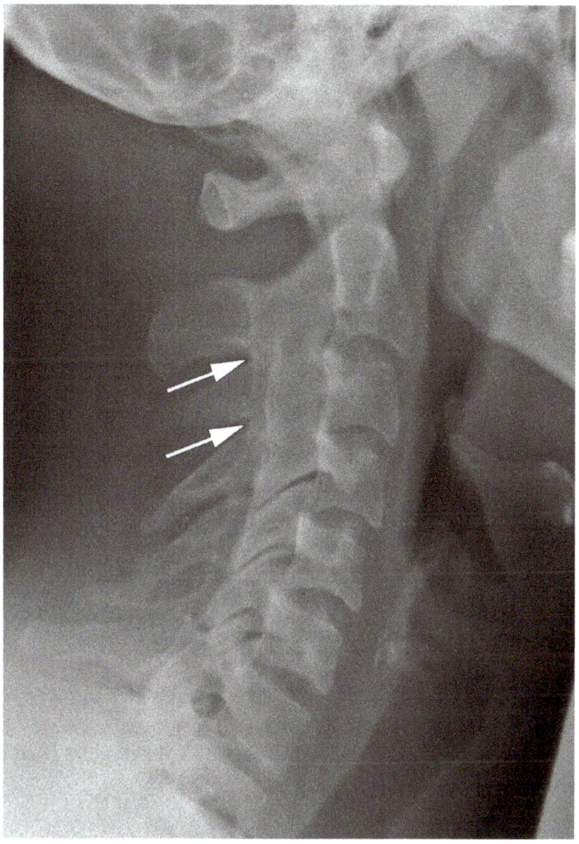

Fig. 14.4 A 26-year-old man with axSpA. Facet joints at C2/3 and C3/4 demonstrate bony ankylosis (arrows).

Such techniques are the T2W gradient-echo sequence with fat saturation (T2FS), the STIR technique, and the T1W turbo spin-echo sequence after application of a contrast agent (Gd) with fat suppression (T1/Gd) (26, 27). The T2FS and the STIR technique are able to assess inflammation by depiction of BME. Both techniques work without the use of contrast agents and apply different types of fat suppression, but the resulting images are similar; thus the term T2FS is used to cover both in this chapter. The T1/Gd sequence detects inflammation by visualization of the enhancement of contrast agents in the hypervascularized areas. As a general rule, use of these contrast agents can be omitted, especially in the setting of clinical trials (28, 29). However, detection of enthesitis may benefit from Gd-enhanced MRI sequences (30). An overview of typical MRI techniques and the signal intensity of different lesions is shown in Table 14.1.

For the assessment of chronic/structural lesions, the currently most frequently used MRI sequence is the T1W turbo spin-echo sequence (usually performed without the application of contrast material), and also gradient echo (GE) techniques (31).

Whole-body MRI is a technique to image most joints and entheses of the body and is capable of showing the extent of disease in both early and late axSpA (32–35). However, the additional effort reveals lesions at the appendicular skeleton in only about 15–20% of cases and thus imaging of the SI joints and spine is usually regarded as sufficient for the routine diagnostic workup of patients with suspected SpA.

Characterization of spinal lesions in axial spondyloarthritis by using magnetic resonance imaging

MRI of the spine is considered the most sensitive method for the assessment of inflammatory lesions related to axSpA (36, 37), being also used as an indicator of disease activity, for measuring response to biologic treatment, and as a possible predictor of response to treatment (38). MRI has also been successfully used to assess structural changes (37).

The characteristic findings when using spinal MRI for assessment of disease activity in patients with axSpA are spondylitis, inflammation of the facet and costovertebral joints, and (abacterial) spondylodiscitis, while fat metaplasia, especially at the vertebral edges, is considered to be a typical sign of post-inflammatory lesions.

Spondylitis is pathognomonic for BME related to axSpA and can be considered as an early sign of the disease. It represents active osteitis and enthesitis at the junction of the annulus fibrosus and the vertebral body (Fig. 14.5). Spondylitis is typically seen as a hyperintense signal in T2FS or T1/Gd sequences, with a corresponding hypointense signal in T1W sequences. Lesions most frequently occur at the anterior vertebral edges (spondylitis anterior) but can also be present at the posterior edges (spondylitis posterior) (Fig. 14.6); however, some controversy still exists about the frequency of involvement of spinal structures in early and late axSpA (39). When turning into a post-inflammatory change, the

Table 14.1 Overview of typical MRI techniques and the signal intensity of different lesions

	Sequence	Cerebrospinal fluid	Intervertebral disc	Subcutaneous fat tissue	Inflammatory lesion	Post-inflammatory lesion (fat metaplasia)
Fat-sensitive	T1W	Hypointense	Hypointense	Hyperintense	Hypointense	Hyperintense
Water-sensitive	T2-regular	Hyperintense	Hyperintense	Hyperintense	Hyperintense	Hyperintense
	STIR	Hyperintense	Hyperintense	Hypointense	Hyperintense	Hypointense
	T2FS	Hyperintense	Hyperintense	Hypointense	Hyperintense	Hypointense
	T1/Gd (fat suppressed)	Hypointense	Hypointense	Hypointense	Hyperintense	Hypointense

pathological signal is altered, and usually of low signal intensity in STIR sequences and high signal intensity in T1W sequences (Fig. 14.7) (5). This process is not completely understood to date, but some kind of healing and development of fibrous tissue (with a vast proportion of fatty tissue) does occur (4, 40).

Facet joint and costovertebral joint involvement is similarly characterized by hyperintense signal in T2FS and T1/Gd MRI sequences and hypointense signals in T1W MRI (Fig. 14.8). Active and structural changes of facet and especially of costosternal and costovertebral joints may also be found relatively frequently in young patients with AS, and can be associated with a reduced chest expansion. Since age does not have an influence on thoracic expansion, a clearly pathological chest expansion may even be used as a diagnostic sign in AS (41).

Abacterial spondylodiscitis is characterized by a hemispherical erosive lesion surrounded by an area of BME in one of two adjacent vertebral bodies. MRI is able to detect such changes already in early phases of the disease, in contrast to conventional X-ray where only the consequences of spondylodiscitis are visible as areas with sclerosis (42, 43). Furthermore, normal findings on conventional radiographs can be accompanied by positive inflammatory findings on MRI indicative of spondylodiscitis (42, 43). Overall, asymptomatic spondylodiscitis may occur even in multiple spinal segments in approximately 8–15% of AS patients (20, 44), while such findings were reported to occur in up to 31% of patients with enteropathic SpA (45).

An overview of the typical MRI lesions found in patients with axSpA is shown in Table 14.2.

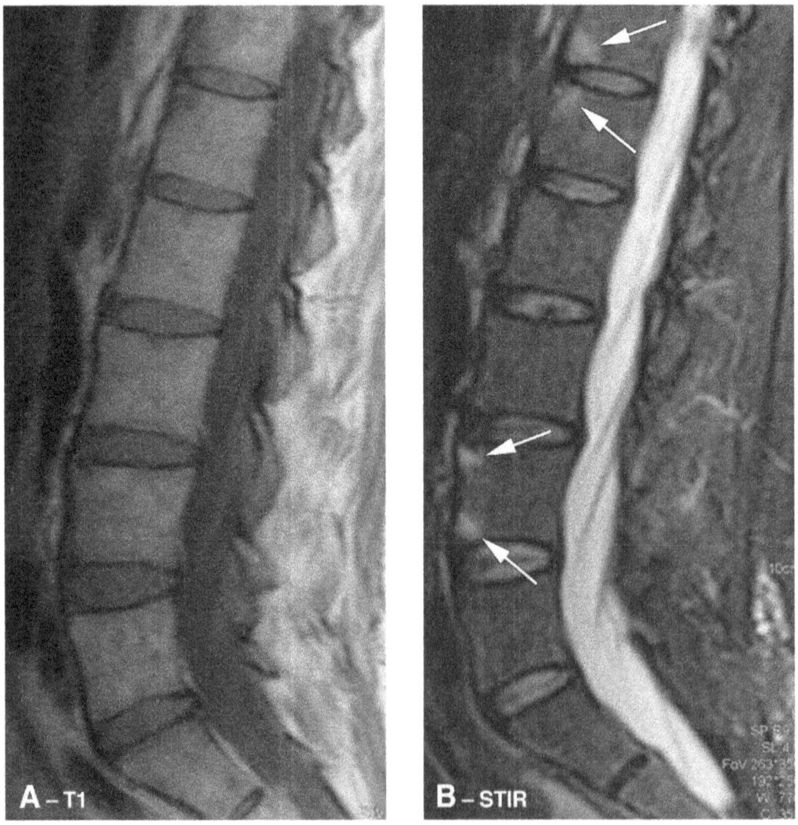

Fig. 14.5 A 51-year-old woman with axSpA. (A) T1W MRI sequence in sagittal orientation. (B) Sagittal STIR sequence. There is active anterior spondylitis at the T12 lower endplate, L1 upper endplate, and L4 both endplates (arrows), characterized by increased signal intensity on STIR at the edges of the vertebral bodies. Note the corresponding slight decrease of signal intensity on T1 in the same areas.

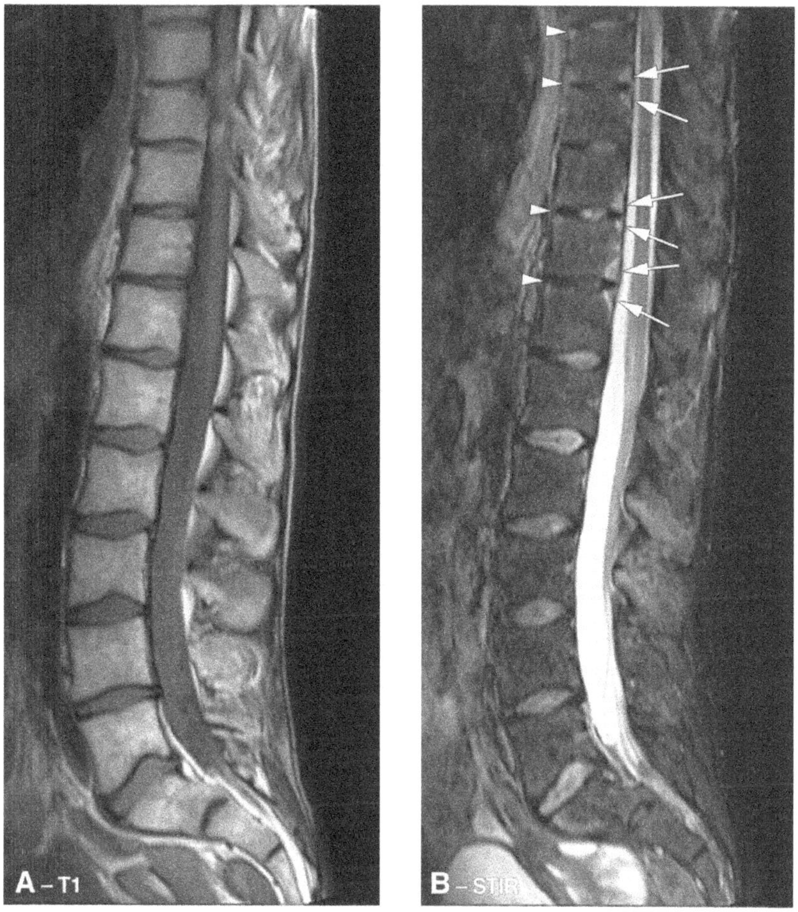

Fig. 14.6 A 37-year-old man with axSpA. (A) T1W MRI sequence in sagittal orientation. (B) Sagittal STIR sequence. There is active posterior spondylitis at T8 to T12 (arrows), characterized by triangular hyperintense lesions at posterior edges of vertebral corners. Corresponding slight loss of signal intensity is seen on T1. There are also several slight manifestations of anterior spondylitis (arrowheads) evident. Note the central slice position, as myelon and cauda equina are well seen!

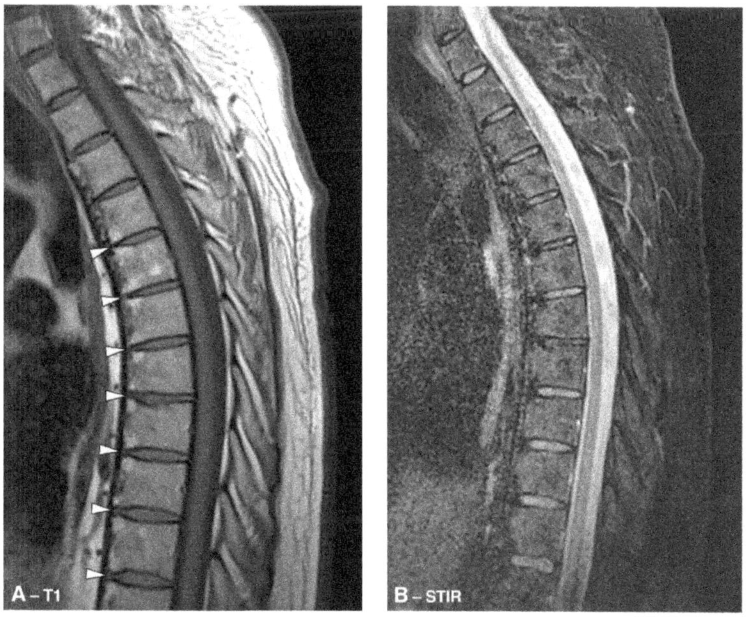

Fig. 14.7 A 44-year-old man with axSpA. (A) T1W MRI sequence in sagittal orientation. (B) Sagittal STIR sequence. There is fat metaplasia of vertebral edges from T4/5 down to T10/11 (arrowheads), characterized by increased signal intensity in T1. The corresponding STIR does not show any sign of inflammation; in fact an even lower signal intensity compared to the normal bone marrow is seen at the involved vertebral edges.

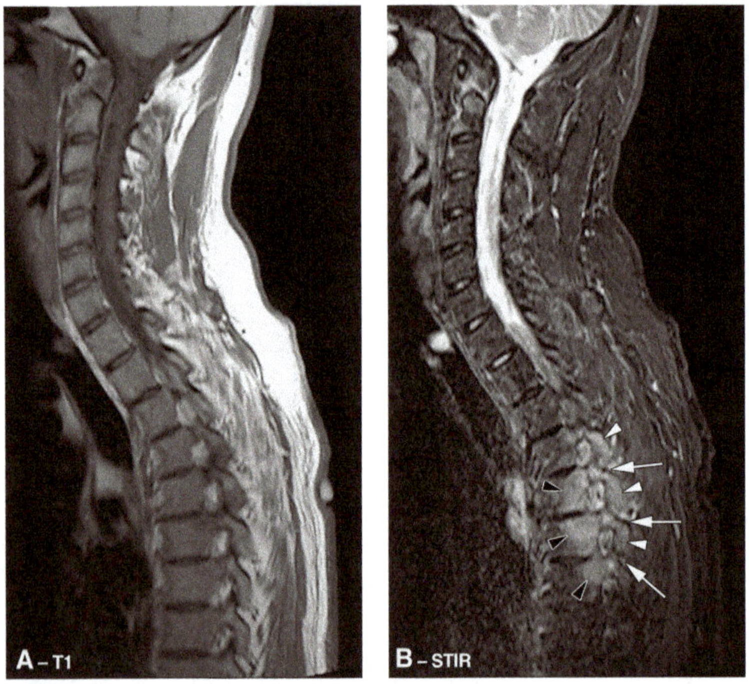

Fig. 14.8 Same patient as in Fig. 14.6. (A) T1W MRI sequence in sagittal orientation. (B) Sagittal STIR sequence. Inflammatory changes are affecting the thoracic facet joints (white arrows), which demonstrate osteitis within adjacent pedicles (white arrowheads), as well as the costovertebral joints, whose involvement is indicated by osteitis of the posterior aspect of thoracic vertebrae (black arrowheads). Corresponding signal loss in T1 is minimal due to the small structures involved. Note the lateral slice position (as opposed to Fig. 14.6) that does not show the spinal cord but depicts costovertebral joints, facet joints, and vertebral pedicles.

Definition of a positive MRI of the spine in axial spondylitis

The definition of a positive MRI of the spine according to ASAS describes osteitis located in the edges of the vertebral bodies (25). Evidence of spondylitis in three or more vertebral edges (independent of whether this is found in anterior or posterior edges) is considered as 'highly suggestive' of axSpA, especially in patients of younger age (<45 years), when degenerative changes are expected to play a minor role for differential diagnosis. For chronic changes, fatty depositions 'at several vertebral corners' may also be indicative of axSpA (25); however, this definition needs further confirmation by more studies conducted in this context.

Table 14.2 Characteristic lesions in the spine of patients with SpA as depicted by MRI

Tissue	Inflammatory changes	Structural changes
Vertebral body	Inflammation (spondylitis) in the bone marrow, most frequently at the corners	Fatty metaplasia Erosion or destruction of the vertebral body (e.g. fracture)—new bone formation (syndesmophytes, ankylosis)
Intervertebral disc	Inflammation (spondylodiscitis)	Ossification of the disc
Facet- and costovertebral joints	Inflammation with or without involvement of the vertebral body	New bone formation and ankylosis in advanced stages
Ligaments	Enthesitis, mainly of the supraspinal and interspinal ligaments	Ligament ossification (in advanced cases)

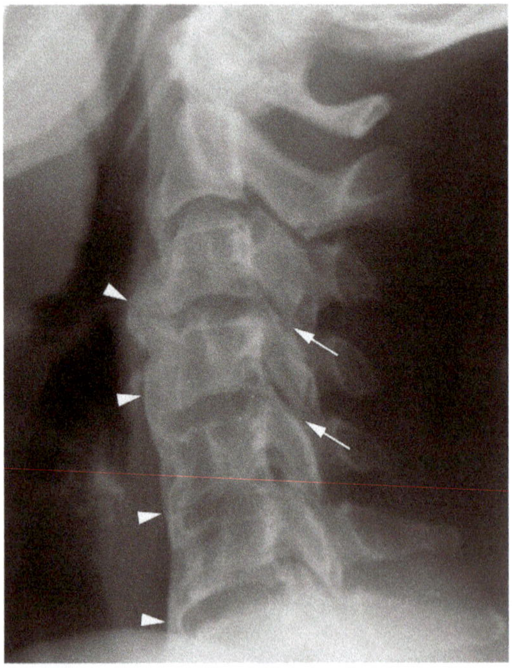

Fig. 14.9 A 53-year-old woman with diffuse idiopathic skeletal hyperostosis. There is bulgy ossification alongside the anterior longitudinal ligament (arrowheads) leading to bony fusion of all cervical vertebral segments. Both intervertebral discs and facet joints (arrows) are not involved, as opposed to end-stage axSpA.

Differential diagnoses for involvement of the spine

Similar to what is known for the SI joints, osteitis (or BME) in the spine cannot be considered specific for axSpA, as it may also be found in other diseases. The most frequent differential diagnoses and pitfalls for interpretation of BME are degenerative changes, fractures, bacterial inflammation, and haemangioma.

Degenerative and proliferative changes can be seen on conventional radiographs as osteophytes which grow in a horizontal direction (spondylophytes) and do not follow the direction of the anterior longitudinal ligament (6). The most typical degenerative changes on MRI are osteochondrosis (segmental degeneration with disc dehydration and erosive changes in the adjacent vertebral endplates) and spondylophytosis (hyperproliferation of the bone in neighbouring vertebral bodies with formation of spondylophytes), which are frequently associated with chronic low back pain in patients of every age. Osteochondrosis is characterized by BME at the vertebral endplate, frequently accompanied by decreased disc height and loss of water content in the adjacent nucleus pulposus. Similarly, Scheuermann's disease starting in childhood is characterized by irregularities of the vertebral endplates and erosive changes on the vertebral surface (46), which are often not recognized before adulthood.

Diffuse idiopathic skeletal hyperostosis (DISH, Forestier's disease) is characterized by chunky osteophytes (Fig. 14.9), often exceeding the length of the anterior longitudinal ligament and causing neurological or other mechanical problems, depending on the spinal site at which they are occurring. Differentiation between AS and DISH regarding the typical ankylosing processes is challenging at times (47). However, a differentiation between AS and DISH on radiographs may be possible since the shape of the spinal bone growth differs. While the typical syndesmophytes are much more frequent in AS, DISH is rather characterized by degenerative spondylophytes and spondylosis (48). CT may be the method of choice to differentiate DISH from AS (49).

A haemangioma represents an accumulation of blood vessels typically located within the vertebral body, mainly in the middle of the vertebra. Although on MRI these findings appear similar to BME, they do represent physiologic abnormalities and do not correlate with any clinical symptoms.

One of the most important inflammatory differential diagnoses of axSpA can be bacterial spondylodiscitis. This finding is characterized by a hyperintense signal which extends from the vertebral body to the surrounding soft tissue, irrespective of anatomical borders (46).

Furthermore, especially in patients with long disease duration and high degree of spinal involvement, spinal fractures may occur in patients with AS due to an underlying osteoporosis in association with a rigid stiffness of the spine, and are a differential diagnosis in

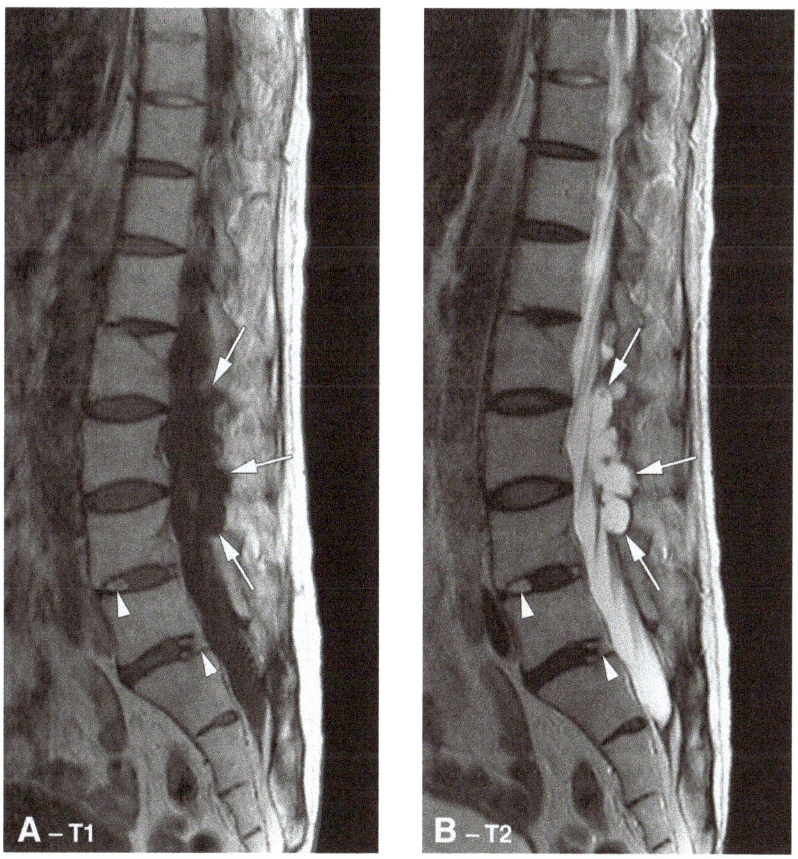

Fig. 14.10 A 53-year-old man with axSpA and cauda equina syndrome. (A) T1W MRI sequence in sagittal orientation. (B) Sagittal T2W sequence (without fat suppression). There are cystic enlargements of the dural sack at L2 to L4 (arrows), leading to atrophy of posterior bony vertebral structures due to its slowly progressing nature. In addition, ankylosis of the intervertebral discs is seen anteriorly at L4/5 and posteriorly at L5/S1 (arrowheads), characterized by hyperintense changes in both T1 and T2, corresponding to yellow (fatty) bone marrow. (Case courtesy of Dr Sandra Hermann, Department of Rheumatology, Charité Medical School, Berlin, Germany.)

those patients (50, 51). Spinal fractures in AS occur most frequently in the cervical (52, 53) but also in the cervicothoracic and the thoracolumbar spine, often due to hyperextension injuries (44, 54). Importantly, due to the decreased bone mineral density and severe ankylosis, non-displaced spinal fractures may not easily be diagnosed by conventional X-ray. The shear forces resulting from spinal movements may lead to dislocation of the injured spinal segment (52). CT examinations of the spine are necessary to detect possible dislocations in patients with persistent or progressive symptoms after injury. Acute fractures show an increased signal intensity on T2FS MRI and variable enhancement in T1/Gd MRI (55), depending on the intensity of hypervascularization, while on T1W MRI a decreased signal intensity can be seen in the same region (54).

Finally, cauda equina syndrome (CES) needs to be mentioned as a relatively rare but typical feature in patients with AS, which may be misdiagnosed, potentially leading to serious clinical symptomatology. CES occurs mainly in patients in advanced stages of AS (56) and is characterized by cysts of the dural sack (Fig. 14.10). The clinical consequence may be compression of nerve structures associated with symptoms such as irradiating pain and limb numbness. It is not well understood why CES can develop in AS, but arachnoiditis due to inflammation of the posterior facet joints leading to adhesions within the thecal sack seems to be a possible explanation (57). Clinically, CES is characterized by slow and progressive sensomotoric loss in the lower limbs, possibly leading to sphincter disturbances and incontinence. The overall prevalence of neurologic symptoms in AS patients is in the range of 2.1% (58), and CES is not an infrequent cause of these (59). The diagnosis of CES is difficult to establish by conventional radiographs alone; therefore CT or MRI need to be performed when it is clinically suspected, both being able to show enlargement of the caudal sack and the dorsal arachnoid diverticula (60).

References

1. Braun J, Sieper J. Ankylosing spondylitis. Lancet 2007;369(9570):1379–90.
2. Braun J, Bollow M, Remlinger G, et al. Prevalence of spondylarthropathies in HLA-B27 positive and negative blood donors. Arthritis Rheum 1998;41(1):58–67.
3. Braun J, Bollow M, Sieper J. Radiologic diagnosis and pathology of the spondyloarthropathies. Rheum Dis Clin North Am 1998;24(4):697–735.
4. Baraliakos X, Heldmann F, Callhoff J, et al. Which spinal lesions are associated with new bone formation in patients with ankylosing spondylitis treated with anti-TNF agents? A long-term observational study using MRI and conventional radiography. Ann Rheum Dise2014;73(10):1819–25.
5. Hermann KG, Althoff CE, Schneider U, et al. Magnetic resonance imaging of spinal changes in patients with spondyloarthritis and correlation with conventional radiography. RadioGraphics2005;25(3):559–70.
6. Baraliakos X, Listing J, Rudwaleit M, et al. Progression of radiographic damage in patients with ankylosing spondylitis: defining the central role of syndesmophytes. Ann Rheum Dis2007;66(7):910–15.
7. Baraliakos X, Listing J, von der Recke A, Braun J. The natural course of radiographic progression in ankylosing spondylitis—evidence for major individual variations in a large proportion of patients. J Rheumatol 2009;36:997–1002.
8. Baraliakos X, Listing J, Haibel H, Sieper J, Braun J. Vertebral erosions associated with spinal inflammation in patients with ankylosing spondylitis identified by magnetic resonance imaging: changes after 2 years of tumor necrosis factor inhibitor therapy. J Rheumatol 2013;40(11):1891–6.
9. Sieper J, Rudwaleit M, Baraliakos X, et al. The Assessment of SpondyloArthritis international Society (ASAS) handbook: a guide to assess spondyloarthritis. Ann Rheum Dis 2009;68(Suppl 2):ii1–44.
10. Rudwaleit M, van der Heijde D, Landewe R, et al. The development of Assessment of SpondyloArthritis international Society classification criteria for axial spondyloarthritis (part II): validation and final selection. Ann Rheum Dis 2009;68(6):777–83.
11. MacKay K, Mack C, Brophy S, Calin A. The Bath Ankylosing Spondylitis Radiology Index (BASRI): a new, validated approach to disease assessment. Arthritis Rheum 1998;41(12):2263–70.
12. Baraliakos X, Listing J, Rudwaleit M, Sieper J, Braun J. Development of a radiographic scoring tool for ankylosing spondylitis only based on bone formation: addition of the thoracic spine improves sensitivity to change. Arthritis Rheum 2009;61(6):764–71.
13. Creemers MC, Franssen MJ, van't Hof MA, Gribnau FW, van de Putte LB, van Riel PL. Assessment of outcome in ankylosing spondylitis: an extended radiographic scoring system. Ann Rheum Dis 2005;64(1):127–9.
14. Bennett AN, McGonagle D, O'Connor P, et al. Severity of baseline magnetic resonance imaging-evident sacroiliitis and HLA-B27 status in early inflammatory back pain predict radiographically evident ankylosing spondylitis at eight years. Arthritis Rheum 2008;58(11):3413–18.
15. Khan MA, van der Linden SM, Kushner I, Valkenburg HA, Cats A. Spondylitic disease without radiologic evidence of sacroiliitis in relatives of HLA-B27 positive ankylosing spondylitis patients. Arthritis Rheum 1985;28(1):40–3.
16. Baraliakos X, Listing J, von der Recke A, Braun J. The natural course of radiographic progression in ankylosing spondylitis—evidence for major individual variations in a large proportion of patients. J Rheumatol 2009;36(5):997–1002.
17. Gran JT, Skomsvoll JF. The outcome of ankylosing spondylitis: a study of 100 patients. Br J Rheumatol 1997;36(7):766–71.
18. Baraliakos X, Haibel H, Listing J, Sieper J, Braun J. Continuous long-term anti-TNF therapy does not lead to an increase in the rate of new bone formation over 8 years in patients with ankylosing spondylitis. Ann Rheum Dis 2014;73(4):710–15.
19. Haroon N, Inman RD, Learch TJ, et al. The impact of tumor necrosis factor alpha inhibitors on radiographic progression in ankylosing spondylitis. Arthritis Rheum 2013;65(10):2645–54.
20. Bollow M. [Magnetic resonance imaging in ankylosing spondylitis (Marie-Struempell-Bechterew disease).] Rofo 2002;174(12):1489–99.
21. Dihlmann W. Current radiodiagnostic concept of ankylosing spondylitis. Skeletal Radiol 1979;4(4):179–88.
22. Calin A. Radiology and spondylarthritis. Baillieres Clin Rheumatol 1996;10(3):455–76.
23. Gaucher AA, Pere PG, Gillet PM. From ankylosing spondylitis to Forestier's disease: ossifying enthesopathy, a unifying concept. J Rheumatol 1990;17(6):854–6.
24. de Vlam K, Mielants H, Veys EM. Involvement of the zygapophyseal joint in ankylosing spondylitis: relation to the bridging syndesmophyte. J Rheumatol 1999;26(8):1738–45.
25. Hermann KG, Baraliakos X, van der Heijde D, et al. Descriptions of spinal magnetic resonance imaging (MRI) lesions and definition of a positive MRI of the spine in axial spondyloarthritis (SpA)—a consensual approach by the ASAS/OMERACT MRI Study Group. Ann Rheum Dis 2012;71(8):1278–88.
26. Braun J, Bollow M, Eggens U, Konig H, Distler A, Sieper J. Use of dynamic magnetic resonance imaging with fast imaging in the detection of early and advanced sacroiliitis in spondylarthropathy patients. Arthritis Rheum 1994;37(7):1039–45.
27. Bollow M, Braun J, Hamm B, et al. Early sacroiliitis in patients with spondyloarthropathy: evaluation with dynamic gadolinium-enhanced MR imaging. Radiology 1995;194(2):529–36.
28. Baraliakos X, Hermann KG, Landewe R, et al. Assessment of acute spinal inflammation in patients with ankylosing spondylitis by magnetic

resonance imaging: a comparison between contrast enhanced T1 and short tau inversion recovery (STIR) sequences. Ann Rheum Dis 2005;64(8):1141–4.

29. Hermann KG, Landewe RB, Braun J, van der Heijde D. Magnetic resonance imaging of inflammatory lesions in the spine in ankylosing spondylitis clinical trials: is paramagnetic contrast medium necessary? J Rheumatol 2005;32(10):2056–60.
30. Klang E, Aharoni D, Hermann KG, et al. Magnetic resonance imaging of pelvic entheses—a systematic comparison between short tau inversion recovery (STIR) and T1-weighted, contrast-enhanced, fat-saturated sequences. Skeletal Radiol 2014;43(4):499–505.
31. Braun J, van der Heijde D. Imaging and scoring in ankylosing spondylitis. Best Pract Res Clin Rheumatol 2002;16(4):573–604.
32. Mager AK, Althoff CE, Sieper J, Hamm B, Hermann KG. Role of whole-body magnetic resonance imaging in diagnosing early spondyloarthritis. Eur J Radiol 2009;71(2):182–8.
33. Althoff CE, Appel H, Rudwaleit M, et al. Whole-body MRI as a new screening tool for detecting axial and peripheral manifestations of spondyloarthritis. Ann Rheum Dis 2007;66(7):983–5.
34. Althoff CE, Sieper J, Song IH, et al. Active inflammation and structural change in early active axial spondyloarthritis as detected by whole-body MRI. Ann Rheum Dis 2013;72(6):967–73.
35. Appel H, Hermann KG, Althoff CE, Rudwaleit M, Sieper J. Whole-body magnetic resonance imaging evaluation of widespread inflammatory lesions in a patient with ankylosing spondylitis before and after 1 year of treatment with infliximab. J Rheumatol 2007;34(12):2497–8.
36. Baraliakos X, Golder W, Brandt J, et al. Analysing acute spinal changes in ankylosing spondylitis—a systematic comparison of conventional X-rays with magnetic resonance imaging (MRI) using established and new scoring systems. Arthritis Rheum 2003;48(9):S177.
37. Braun J, Baraliakos X, Golder W, et al. Analysing chronic spinal changes in ankylosing spondylitis: a systematic comparison of conventional x rays with magnetic resonance imaging using established and new scoring systems. Ann Rheum Dis 2004;63(9):1046–55.
38. Rudwaleit M, Schwarzlose S, Hilgert ES, Listing J, Braun J, Sieper J. MRI in predicting a major clinical response to anti-tumour necrosis factor treatment in ankylosing spondylitis. Ann Rheum Dis 2008;67(9):1276–81.
39. Bochkova AG, Levshakova AV, Bunchuk NV, Braun J. Spinal inflammation lesions as detected by magnetic resonance imaging in patients with early ankylosing spondylitis are more often observed in posterior structures of the spine. Rheumatology (Oxford) 2010;49(4):749–55.
40. Appel H, Sieper J. Spondyloarthritis at the crossroads of imaging, pathology, and structural damage in the era of biologics. Curr Rheumatol Rep 2008;10(5):356–63.
41. van der Linden S, Valkenburg HA, Cats A. Evaluation of diagnostic criteria for ankylosing spondylitis. A proposal for modification of the New York criteria. Arthritis Rheum 1984;27(4):361–8.
42. Rasker JJ, Prevo RL, Lanting PJ. Spondylodiscitis in ankylosing spondylitis, inflammation or trauma? A description of six cases. Scand J Rheumatol 1996;25(1):52–7.
43. Wienands K, Lukas P, Albrecht HJ. [Clinical value of MR tomography of spondylodiscitis in ankylosing spondylitis.] Z Rheumatol 1990;49(6):356–60.
44. Kabasakal Y, Garrett SL, Calin A. The epidemiology of spondylodiscitis in ankylosing spondylitis—a controlled study. Br J Rheumatol 1996;35(7):660–3.
45. Peluso R, Di Minno MN, Bruner V, Soscia E, Castiglione F, Manguso F, et al. Discovertebral Erosions in Patients with Enteropathic Spondyloarthritis. J Rheumatol 2012;39(12):2332–40.
46. Hermann KG, Bollow M. Magnetic resonance imaging of the axial skeleton in rheumatoid disease. Best Pract Res Clin Rheumatol 2004;18(6):881–907.
47. Hermann KG, Bollow M. Rethinking diffuse idiopathic skeletal hyperostosis. Rheumatology (Oxford) 2014;53(11):1917–19.
48. Baraliakos X, Listing J, Buschmann J, von der Recke A, Braun J. A comparison of new bone formation in patients with ankylosing spondylitis and patients with diffuse idiopathic skeletal hyperostosis: a retrospective cohort study over six years. Arthritis Rheum 2012;64(4):1127–33.
49. Yaniv G, Bader S, Lidar M, et al. The natural course of bridging osteophyte formation in diffuse idiopathic skeletal hyperostosis: retrospective analysis of consecutive CT examinations over 10 years. Rheumatology (Oxford) 2014;53(11):1951–7.
50. Fox MW, Onofrio BM, Kilgore JE. Neurological complications of ankylosing spondylitis. J Neurosurg 1993;78(6):871–8.
51. Mitra D, Elvins DM, Speden DJ, Collins AJ. The prevalence of vertebral fractures in mild ankylosing spondylitis and their relationship to bone mineral density. Rheumatology (Oxford) 2000;39(1):85–9.
52. Bernd L, Blasius K, Lukoschek M. [Spinal fractures in ankylosing spondylitis.] Z Orthop Ihre Grenzgeb 1992;130(1):59–63.
53. Broom MJ, Raycroft JF. Complications of fractures of the cervical spine in ankylosing spondylitis. Spine 1988;13(7):763–6.
54. Vinson EN, Major NM. MR imaging of ankylosing spondylitis. Semin Musculoskelet Radiol 2003;7(2):103–13.
55. Shih TT, Chen PQ, Li YW, Hsu CY. Spinal fractures and pseudoarthrosis complicating ankylosing spondylitis: MRI manifestation and clinical significance. J Comput Assist Tomogr 2001;25(2):164–70.
56. Sant SM, O'Connell D. Cauda equina syndrome in ankylosing spondylitis: a case report and review of the literature. Clin Rheumatol 1995;14(2):224–6.
57. Abello R, Rovira M, Sanz MP, et al. MRI and CT of ankylosing spondylitis with vertebral scalloping. Neuroradiology 1988;30(3):272–5.
58. Edgar MA. Letter: nervous system involvement in ankylosing spondylitis. Br Med J 1974;1(904):394.
59. Ahn NU, Ahn UM, Nallamshetty L, et al. Cauda equina syndrome in ankylosing spondylitis (the CES-AS syndrome): meta-analysis of outcomes after medical and surgical treatments. J Spinal Disord 2001;14(5):427–33.
60. Mitchell MJ, Sartoris DJ, Moody D, Resnick D. Cauda equina syndrome complicating ankylosing spondylitis. Radiology 1990;175(2):521–5.

CHAPTER 15

Juvenile-onset spondyloarthritis

Ruben Burgos-Vargas and Shirley M.L. Tse

Current concept and classification

Juvenile-onset spondyloarthritis (JoSpA) refers to the group of HLA-B27-associated paediatric rheumatic diseases that involves the synovium and entheses of peripheral joints in the initial years and, in some patients, the SI and spinal joints several years later (1). Patients with JoSpA may also have anterior uveitis, psoriasis, IBD, and some other EAMs, and represent a disease continuum with adult-onset SpA.

JoSpA might include patients with enthesitis-related arthritis (ERA) and PsA categories of JIA, according to the ILAR classification (2). The opposite does not occur, since ILAR JIA classification does not allow the possibility of clinical overlapping among the different categories, one of the most important features of SpA (3). Thus JoSpA corresponds to the Amor (4) and ESSG criteria (5) application in children (6). The ASAS axial and peripheral classification criteria for SpA in adults (7, 8) have not been validated in children and adolescents, and this should be recognized when referring to JoSpA (9). (Note: in this chapter, we have adopted the acronym JoSpA/ERA to facilitate its comprehension.)

Epidemiological aspects

The prevalence of JoSpA/ERA in the general population is unknown, but its incidence in American and Canadian children has been estimated and varies from 2.1 per 100 000 (10) to 24.0 per 100 000 children in western Canadian Indians (11). The proportion of JoSpA/ERA among children with JIA and adults with AS varies from 10% to 36% (12, 13) and from 8% to 36% (14), respectively, in different populations. Variations may be attributed to study design and probably ethnicity.

Pathogenesis

Similar to adult-onset SpA, the pathogenesis of JoSpA has been linked to genetic susceptibility and triggering factors, such as bacterial infections. In this sense, the origin of the disease relies in part on the HLA-B27 susceptibility hypothesis, but the role of other genes is being explored. On the other hand, the role of mechanical, growth, and developmental factors needs to be investigated.

Genetic factors

The familial occurrence of SpA, especially aggregation of AS in certain families, supports the role of genetic factors in SpA. The HLA-B27 gene is strongly implicated in SpA, particularly as it correlates with AS prevalence in the general population (15, 16). The strongest association of HLA-B27 is with AS, whereas the association with other SpA subsets depends on the clinical phenotype. The prevalence of HLA-B27 in patients with JoSpA/ERA is highly variable; the highest prevalence is seen in patients with AS; the lowest in those with JoPsA and ReA. The risk of radiographic sacroiliitis in HLA-B27-positive JIA children is 85% (17). B*2705 and B*2704 HLA-B27 subtypes are associated with JoSpA in Mexicans (18) and Han Chinese (19), respectively.

Genome-wide screens in adults have implicated a number of other loci, which may include some relevant to childhood disease (20). Of these, ERAP1 in HLA-B27-positive patients and IL-23R, both implicated in antigen presentation to T cells, are associated with AS (20). Interestingly, ERAP2 is linked to both HLA-B27-positive and HLA-B27-negative patients, suggesting a supplementary role of ERAP2 (21). On the other hand, genetic polymorphisms in IFNγ appear to be a predisposing factor to ReA in the Dutch population (22), and solute carrier family 11 member A1 gene polymorphisms in the Chinese population (23). In children and adolescents, association of ERAP1 with JoSpA/ERA in addition to IL-23R to PsA has been demonstrated (24). ERAP1 and IL-23R were not associated with other JIA subtypes.

Several hypotheses concerning the HLA-B27 association with the disease have been postulated. The most popular, but actually the most elusive, is the 'arthritogenic bacteria' theory (25). Most studies' mechanisms correspond to HLA B27 misfolding in the ER and the consequent unfolded protein response, as well as the HLA-B27 free heavy-chain and surface homodimer hypothesis (26, 27), which provokes a proinflammatory cytokine response.

Environmental factors

There is actually little evidence to date that any environmental factors, particularly microbial infections, play a significant role in the pathogenesis of JoSpA/ERA. The exception is ReA, but its definition requires the demonstration of a trigger infectious agent. Weak evidence comes from the demonstration of humoral and cellular responses to various microorganisms (28) or to bacterial components such as peptidoglycan (29) and the outer membrane protein of *Salmonella typhimurium* (30). Only case reports and small series of cases support the role of bacteria in JoSpA/ERA, including detection of bacterial DNA in synovial fluid cells (31) and Toll-like receptors 2 and 4 expression in peripheral blood and synovial fluid cells (32). Interestingly, altered microbiota in the stools of patients with JoSpA/ERA has been recently reported, which opens up a new possibility in defining the relation between bacteria and disease (33).

Histopathology

Very few studies have analysed the histopathology of the synovium, entheses, and other organs in children with JoSpA/ERA. There is hyperplasia of the lining cells, CD68 expression, and CD163+ macrophages in the sublining layer (34). Vascularity is increased and composed of CD146+ endothelial cells, high levels of activated CD8+ cells, TNFβ, IFNγ, IL-2, IL-4, and IL-6 (35). TNFα receptors p55 and p75 are prominently expressed in most cells in tissue inflammation. Immunochemistry and immunofluorescence studies of the tarsal region show scarce inflammatory cells in the synovium, synovial sheaths, and entheses (36). In contrast, there seems to be some differentiation of entheseal cells toward an osteoblastic lineage and the formation of bone islets embedded within the enthesis matrix, suggesting a predominantly mechanical rather than an inflammatory phenomenon. Studies in animal models have identified a role for bone morphogenetic protein signalling (37) and IL-23 on entheseal resident TCR (38).

The clinical picture

JoSpA categories are recognized by clinical features, laboratory tests and imaging characteristics. While some characteristics correspond to inflammatory, potentially reversible changes, others result from structural damage. Throughout the course of the disease, overlaps between one clinical condition and another may occur and the diagnostic category may change.

Presenting features and differential diagnosis

Children and adolescents with JoSpA/ERA may present to the clinic with a short history of isolated monoarthritis, oligoarthritis, or enthesitis. More rarely they complain of polyarthritis or SI/gluteal pain as presenting symptoms. Differential diagnoses include joint infection, pigmented villonodular synovitis, trauma, sport and overuse injuries, osteochondrosis, hypermobility syndromes, mechanical as well as other causes of back pain, and disorders of growth and development. Interestingly, at least one-third of patients with JoSpA recall doing strenuous sport activities several weeks before the onset of their arthritis or enthesitis. Differential diagnosis is less difficult when the combination of arthritis and enthesitis occur simultaneously or contiguously. Likewise, the concomitant presentation of isolated peripheral and axial symptoms, although rare, may be easier to recognize. In these patients, HLA-B27 might be helpful in establishing the diagnosis.

The clinical manifestations of JoSpA/ERA differ in some aspects from those of adult-onset SpA, particularly AS. Children and adolescents with AS typically have peripheral arthritis and enthesitis in the initial years, with axial symptoms emerging 5–10 years later, whereas most adults with AS have IBP at onset (39–48). Early lower limb involvement may be associated with a greater need for hip replacement than in those with adult onset AS (41, 46). This may be the consequence of more serious hip involvement or longer disease duration. In general, more JoSpA/ERA cases result in functional classes III and IV (42), and their mean BASFI is higher (45). The contrary has been also found, with better scores of BASFI, Health Assessment Questionnaire (HAQ), and HRQoL, and less fatigue than patients with adult-onset AS (47). Nevertheless, the clinical course of JoSpA/ERA is often more severe as a consequence of peripheral involvement.

General aspects

Lower limb arthritis and/or enthesitis occur in nearly all patients, and their patterns differ very little among specific diagnostic entities. Arthritis and enthesitis may not parallel each other in regard to date of onset and throughout the disease course. Likewise, they might differ in relative severity, duration, and consequences. On the other hand, the distinction between arthritis and enthesitis as the cause of pain may be difficult at some sites, for example, the SI joints and the feet.

Peripheral arthritis and enthesitis

The most common finding in patients with JoSpA/ERA at onset is unilateral or asymmetric monoarthritis or oligoarthritis involving the knee, ankle, or mid-tarsus (Fig. 15.1) (1). Less frequently, the disease starts in the metatarsophalangeal (MTP), and interphalangeal (IP) joints of the feet, the hips, and rarely the upper extremity joints. Hip involvement at disease onset should raise the suspicion for a diagnosis of JoSpA/ERA, as it is uncommon amongst the other JIA subtypes. Usually, the course of arthritis consists of recurring episodes of monoarthritis or oligoarthritis lasting from weeks to months, followed by a period of remission or low disease activity. However, there are cases with persistent arthritis and increasing number of joints involved, including the hips.

Enthesitis might not parallel arthritis at onset or during the disease course, but in most cases inflammation at peripheral sites determines the disease severity and ultimately can affect the physical function and quality of life of patients. The attachments of plantar fascia, Achilles tendon, and patellar ligaments are the entheses most frequently involved, followed by the ligament and tendon insertions at the talonavicular joint and base of the fifth metatarsal bone (1, 49). Upper limb entheses, such as those on the shoulder and epicondyles, as well as those at the iliac crest, may also be found.

The involvement of the feet is certainly complex. Besides ankle swelling and enthesitis at the plantar fascia and Achilles tendon, tenosynovitis involving the peroneal and tibial tendons, leading to massive swelling extending to the mid tarsus, is often found. The resulting inflammation causes the characteristic tarsitis, which is seen in up to one-third of JoSpA/ERA patients at disease onset. Severe cases of swelling of the retrocalcaneal bursa have also been seen.

Axial involvement

Up to 80% of children with JoSpA/ERA will not have clinical evidence of sacroiliitis or spondylitis at disease onset or during the initial years of disease (50–52). However, some children may have isolated episodes of gluteal or back pain or a clinical pattern that includes neck, back, and gluteal pain, reduced spinal mobility, and radiographic sacroiliitis fulfilling the diagnosis of AS, accompanied by severe polyarthritis and enthesitis in less than 3 years (53). Overall, most children and adolescents who develop axial symptoms are recognized 5–10 years after disease onset, yet sacroiliitis may still occur up to 20 years after clinical onset. This evolution is more likely in boys (17, 54), particularly those who are HLA-B27-positive (17, 50, 51), age at onset ≥ 8 years, with early hip involvement (17, 54, 56) and back pain (52), polyarthritis (53, 55), enthesitis (52), polyenthesitis (55), tarsitis (52), and elevated ESR for at least 6 months (54). Radiographic sacroiliitis (Fig. 15.2) and MRI sacroiliitis and spondylitis (Fig. 15.3) may be found in patients without back pain or in patients complaining of back symptoms that seldom fulfill IBP criteria. Specifically, the

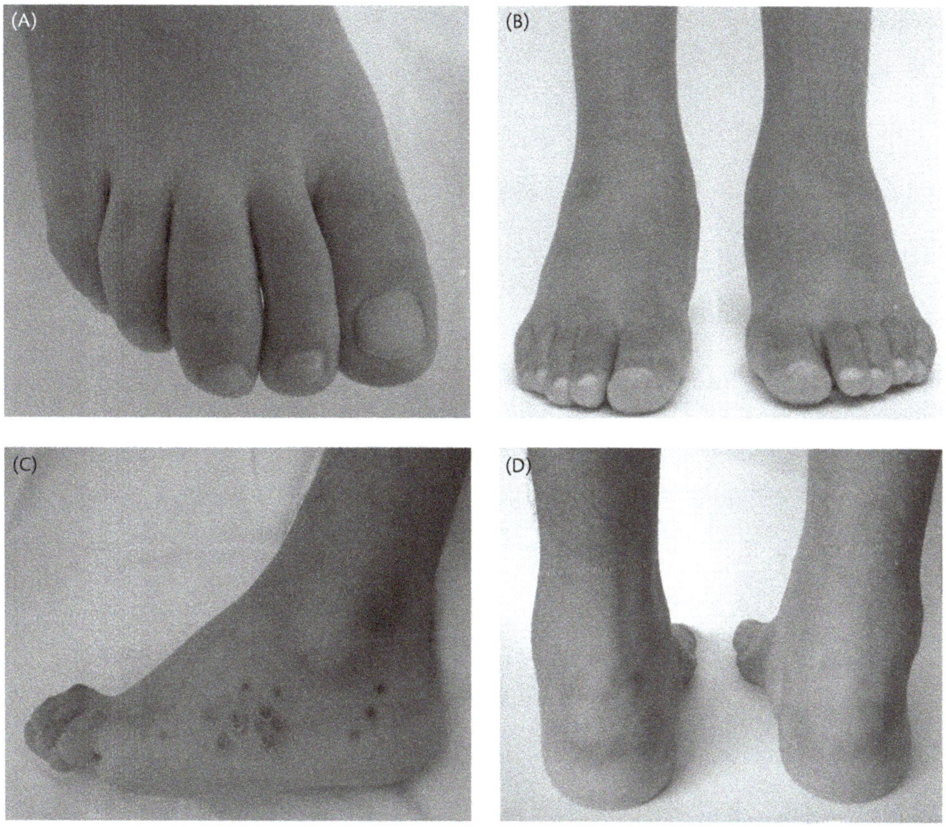

Fig. 15.1 (See colour plate section). Involvement of the feet in patients with JoSpA. (A) Dactylitis of third digit in a 12-year-old boy with uSpA. (B) Diffuse swelling of tarsal region of an 11-year-old boy with JoAS. (C) Tarsal swelling, hyperextension of digits, and keratoderma blennorrhagica in a 16-year-old boy with chronic ReA. (D) Diffuse swelling of posterior aspect of feet including ankles, Achilles, and peroneal and tibial posterior tendons in a 12-year-old-boy with uSpA.

Modified from Burgos-Vargas R, Vázquez-Mellado J. Reactive arthritides. In: Cassidy JT, Petty RE, eds. Textbook of pediatric rheumatology, 5th ed. Philadelphia: Elsevier Saunders, 2005:604–612 and Reprinted from Rheumatic Disease Clinics of North America, 28, Burgos-Vargas R, The juvenile-onset spondyloarthritides, Copyright (2002) with permission from Elsevier. In: Weisman MH, van der Heijde D, Reveille JD, eds. Ankylosing spondylitis and the spondyloarthropathies. St Louis: Elsevier Mosby, 2006:94–106.

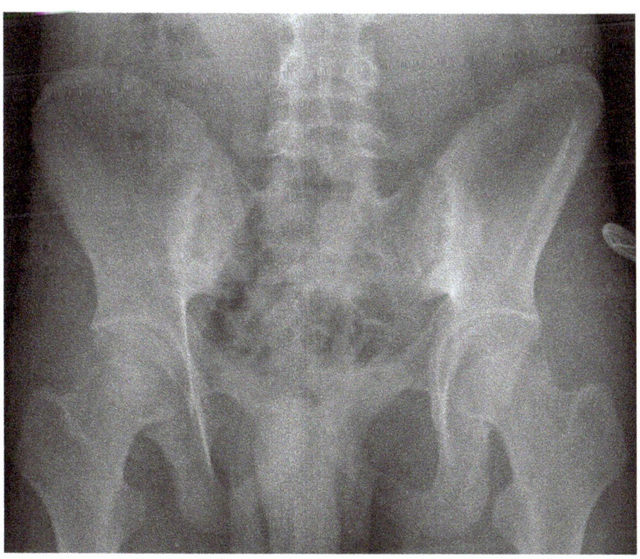

Fig. 15.2 Grade 3 bilateral sacroiliitis in a 14-year-old boy with 6 years' disease duration. There is subchondral sclerosis of iliac bone, joint surface irregularities, which include erosions on both sides, and joint space narrowing of hips.

Weisman MH, van der Heijde D, Reveille JD, eds. Ankylosing spondylitis and the spondyloarthropathies. St. Louis: Elsevier Mosby, 2006:94–106.

combination of insidious onset, alternating gluteal pain, improvement with exercise but not with rest, and nocturnal pain are rarely reported in JoSpA/ERA. In most cases, the relevance of axial symptoms increases with duration and progression of the disease course in patients with AS (52).

From inflammatory symptoms to structural changes

At a certain point during the course of the disease, there is osteocartilaginous proliferation at the tendon and ligament attachments to bone (57). The mechanisms involved in this phenomenon are not well characterized. In adults, syndesmophytes may emerge from inflamed (58–60) but also non-inflamed areas of the entheses in the spine (61). Inflammatory mediators and bone lineage proteins seem responsible for such a process (57). While the former are important in the early stages of the disease, the latter become prominent as the disease progresses. Since enthesophytes and syndesmophytes may also be found in sites not previously infiltrated by inflammatory cells, there is a strong suggestion that a mechanical stress may be responsible for generating bone proliferation in studies of adult SpA (62). There are no similar studies in patients with JoSpA/ERA. However, studies involving the feet in patients with tarsitis in both the early inflammatory and chronic ankylosing

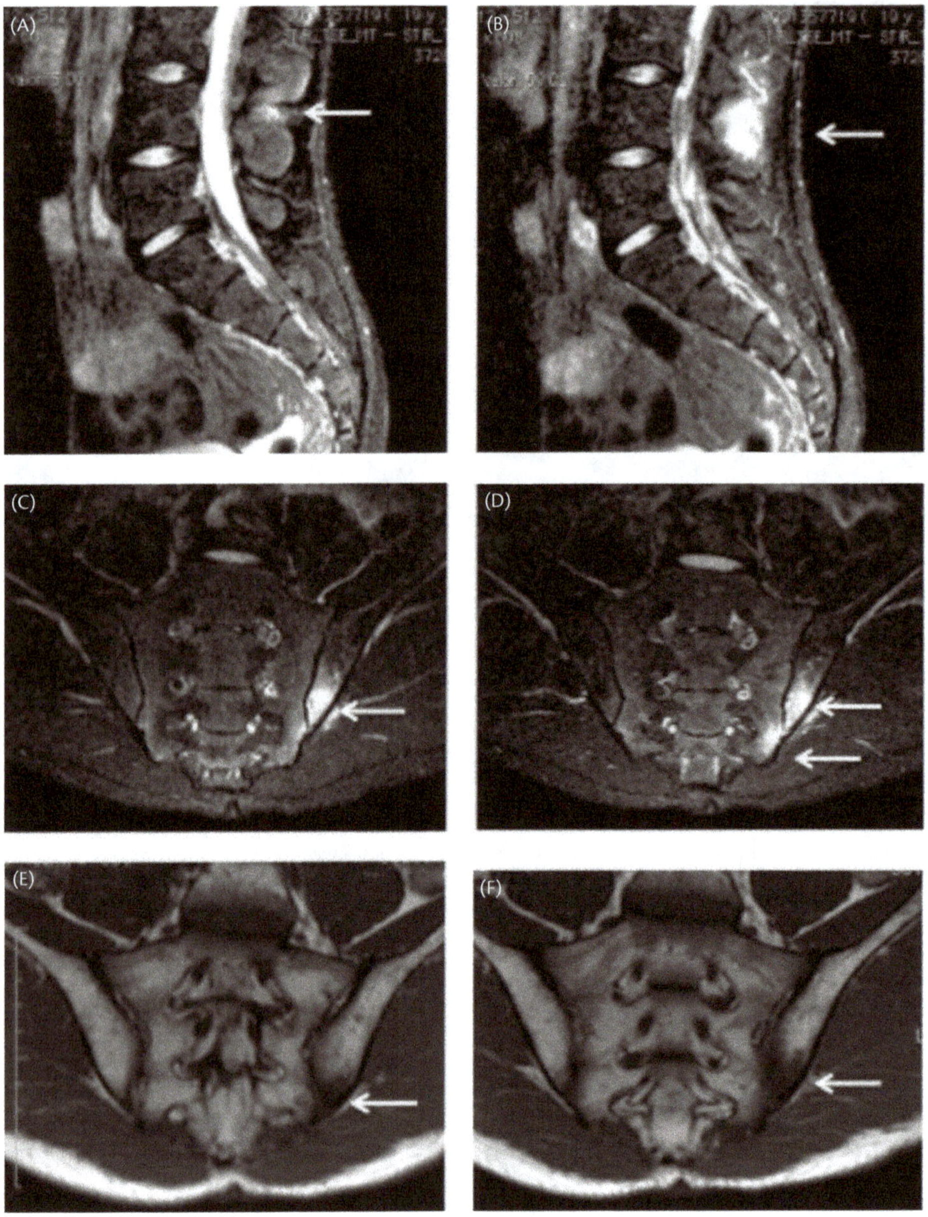

Fig. 15.3 STIR and T1 MR image sequences of SI and spinal joints of an HLA-B27-positive 18-year-old boy with recurrent peripheral arthritis and enthesitis for 7 years and intermittent gluteal and back pain during the last 12 months. (A, B) STIR sequence shows oedema of sacrum and iliac bones. (B, C) T1 sequence showing erosions and fat loss in the area corresponding to the oedema found in STIR sequence. (D–F) There is bone oedema corresponding to L4–L5 zygapophyseal joints.

stages of the disease suggest that the peripheral disease mirrors axial involvement (Fig. 15.4) (36, 63).

Health-related quality of life and functioning

Before the era of TNFi, only 17% (64) and less than 50% (65) of patients with JoSpA/ERA were in remission by 5–10 years after disease onset, respectively. About 50% of patients still have active disease 17 years after onset (66), and 60% have functional limitations after 10 years, particularly those with active disease for more than 5 years (65). Compared with other JIA categories, patients with JoSpA/ERA have more pain, higher childhood HAQ scores, poorer physical health, lower physical functioning, and lower HRQoL (54, 67, 68). Prognostic factors associated with a failure to achieve remission include the presence of AS in a first-degree relative, HLA-DRB1*08, ankle or hip arthritis within the first 6 months of disease, development of sacroiliitis, and persistently elevated ESR within the first 6 months of onset (54).

Imaging studies

Radiographic, MRI, and US with power Doppler studies provide information about diagnosis and classification, disease progression, and therapeutic efficacy. Radiographic findings include osteopenia, joint space narrowing, and, in some cases, ankylosis; these changes

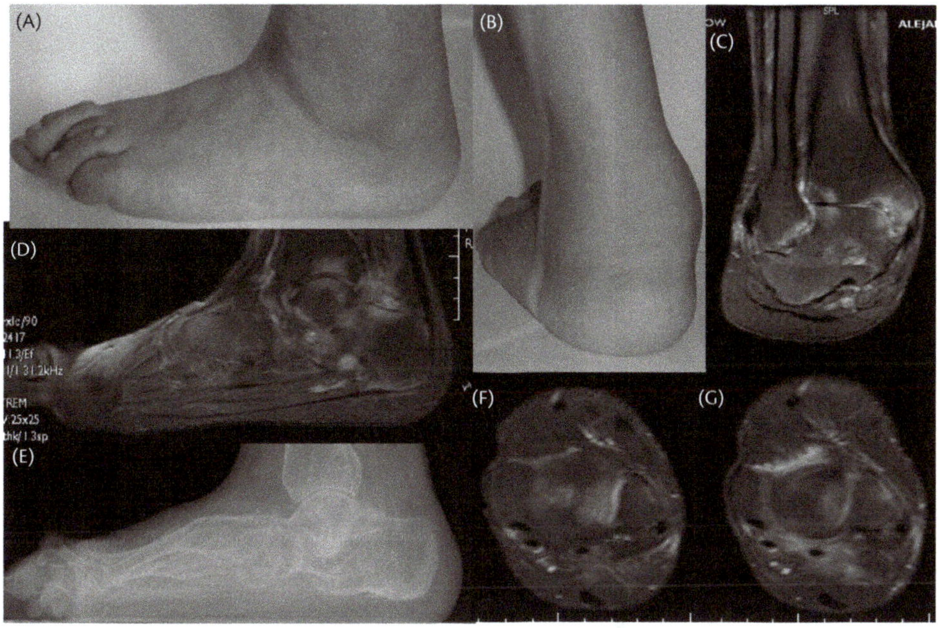

Fig. 15.4 Composite images of ankylosing tarsitis in a 16-year-old boy with AS of 9 years' duration and complete ankylosis of tarsal bones and grade 2 bilateral sacroiliitis. (A, B) Flat-foot and swelling around ankle. (C–F) STIR MR images showing oedema in various tarsal bones, joint spaces (C, D), and soft tissues (E, F) surrounding tendons of posterior aspect of foot on coronal view (arrows). (G) Complete ankylosis of tarsal bones and an enthesophyte at plantar fascia attachment.
Modified from Burgos-Vargas R. A case of childhood-onset ankylosing spondylitis: diagnosis and treatment. Nat Clin Pract Rheumatol 2009;5:52–57.

are more characteristic in the hip and mid-foot. Despite the development of enthesophytes in the calcaneus and base of the fifth metatarsal bone, it generally does not seem to occur in the spine or pelvis until after many years of disease activity. With the exception of the small joints of the feet and hands, hips, and SI joints, erosive and destructive changes are rarely seen.

MRI studies have been useful in detecting areas of active inflammation and structural abnormalities. Compared to radiographs, MRI is more sensitive in the detection of acute and chronic changes in the SI joint. There is a trend to identify subclinical sacroiliitis on MRI in patients with JoSpA/ERA (69, 70), but further studies are needed to determine its value as a diagnostic tool, and particularly if subclinical sacroiliitis on MRI is to be able to inform any specific treatment. T1 and STIR sequences are usually enough to evaluate the involvement of the joints, entheses, and tendons (71). However, the use of Gd might be recommended for small joints, but probably not for the SI and spinal joints. As the majority of JoSpA/ERA patients have peripheral involvement, whole-body MRI protocols may be a potentially valuable tool for early detection and monitoring of both peripheral and axial disease activity in this population (Fig. 15.5) (72).

US with power Doppler of the joints and particularly the entheses, including tendons and bursae, is highly sensitive to detect inflammatory changes, including active synovitis and bursitis. US may also detect tendon thickening as well as chronic lesions such as enthesophytes, erosions, and cortical irregularities (73–75). However, US lacks specificity and might not correlate with clinical examination. In fact, some findings in US studies of JoSpA/ERA patients are similar to those found in healthy children (74).

Clinical presentation

Before the 1980s, most clinical descriptions referred to JoAS and Reiter's syndrome; undifferentiated forms became clearly recognized in the early 1980s (76, 77). Currently, the recognition of early JoSpA/ERA forms may result in the introduction of effective treatment in the inflammatory stage of the disease.

Undifferentiated spondyloarthritis

Undifferentiated SpA is the most common type of SpA in children and, in a variable proportion of cases, may be the earliest form of AS. Previously, this group was named HLA-B27-associated SpA and enthesopathy in childhood (76) or seronegative enthesopathy and arthropathy syndrome (77), but now it is currently recognized and referred to as ERA (2). While an unknown proportion of patients achieve disease remission, up to 70% and 90% of Mexican (50) and Canadian (51) children, respectively, but fewer Italian children (78) fulfill AS criteria approximately 10 years after onset. The frequency of polyarthritis, enthesopathy, and IBP is increased in HLA-B27-positive children. MRI may show subclinical sacroiliitis in a few cases (64, 66).

Juvenile-onset ankylosing spondylitis

This term refers to AS starting before the age of 16 years. The diagnosis, according to mNY criteria (79), is usually made 5–10 years after onset (52, 80). This situation makes AS a rare diagnosis before the age of 16. As mentioned in the section 'Axial involvement', back complaints in the paediatric population are uncommon and often do not resemble IBP. On the other hand, most patients with adult-onset AS have back pain at onset. Radiographic sacroiliitis is commonly found in symptomatic patients (Fig. 15.2). MRI may show acute sacroiliitis in symptomatic patients, but may also be found in asymptomatic patients (Fig. 15.3). Around 5–10% of patients may have high-grade fever, weight loss, muscle weakness, fatigue, lymph node enlargement, leukocytosis, or anaemia in the active inflammatory phase of the disease (52, 80). Up to 27% have

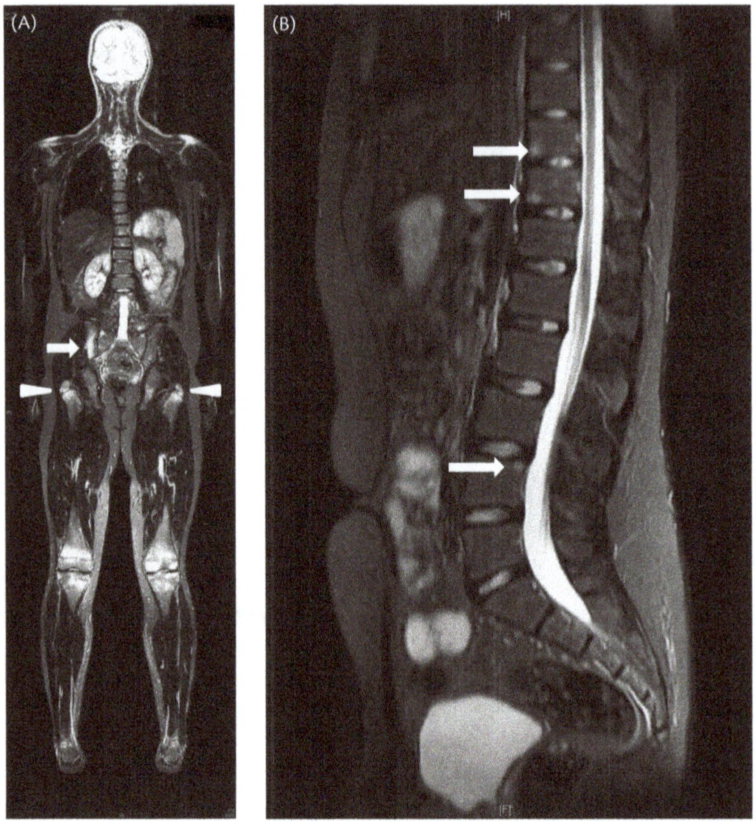

Fig. 15.5 Whole-body STIR MRI in a 15-year-old HLA-B27-positive adolescent boy with ERA. (A) Abnormal signal within SI joints, especially on the right, with high intra-articular signal extending into iliac bone (arrow). Right SI joint also demonstrates irregularity and sclerosis, suggestive of erosive changes. High signal is noted at bilateral proximal femoral metaphyses at region of greater trochanter (arrowheads). High signal is also noted in left ischium, in addition to bilateral involvement of metaphysis and epiphyses of distal femur, and proximal and distal tibia. (B) Corner inflammatory lesions within vertebral bodies (arrows).

acute anterior uveitis and around 80% have non-specific GI manifestations. Cardiovascular manifestations are rare in children (81), and amyloidosis seldom occurs in the modern era. Although adult patients with AS might have better BASFI, HAQ, and QoL scores as well as less fatigue, the course of JoAS seems to be more severe in regard to disease activity, disability, and hip involvement than in adult-onset disease, because of the frequency of peripheral arthritis and enthesitis.

Reactive arthritis

The term reactive arthritis is restricted to HLA-B27-associated arthritis triggered by *Salmonella, Yersinia, Campylobacter*, and *Shigella*. Since viable *Chlamydia* have been found within the joints, the possibility of *Chlamydia* induced ReA may represent an infectious arthritis and be more appropriately referred to as 'an infectious non-suppurative arthritis', which challenges the concept of ReA as a non-septic arthritis (82, 83). Reiter's syndrome (an eponym which has been abandoned) refers to ReA with associated conjunctivitis and urethritis or cervicitis.

Infection typically occurs 2–4 weeks before the onset of arthritis, but many patients might not report any symptom of infection. ReA has occurred in up to 10% of children with yersiniosis (84), 8% with salmonellosis (85), and, in particular, 12% with *Salmonella typhimurium* phage type 135a infection (86). Joint involvement in ReA predominates in the lower extremities (87, 88), but some patients with *Salmonella* and *Yersinia* ReA often have involvement of the hand joints (89, 90). ReA is usually mild and sporadic in HLA-B27-negative children or those triggered by *Yersinia* or *Campylobacter* infection. In contrast, HLA-B27-positive children may evolve into AS. A confident diagnosis normally requires identification of a triggering infection, but in individual cases this seldom occurs. EAMs include aphthous stomatitis, conjunctivitis, erythema nodosum, circinate balanitis, keratoderma blennorrhagica (Fig. 15.1), uveitis, and urethritis/cervicitis. More rarely seen features include aortic insufficiency, myocarditis, and pericarditis (84–90).

Juvenile-onset psoriatic arthritis

The condition of JoPsA is defined by the concomitant occurrence of arthritis and psoriasis in individuals younger than 16 years of age (91). JoPsA includes two main patient subpopulations: the first one, which is not related to SpA, is mainly composed of young girls with polyarthritis involving the hands, dactylitis, and antinuclear antibodies, while the second subpopulation includes more frequently HLA-B27 boys with persistent oligoarthritis, enthesitis, and axial symptoms (81–94). In JoPsA, arthritis occurs before psoriasis in 50% of cases, psoriasis as the initial manifestation in 40%, and simultaneous occurrence of psoriasis and arthritis in 10%. Seventy percent of children have oligoarthritis at onset and polyarthritis develops shortly after in most patients (74, 91, 92). Small joints and wrist arthritis differentiates oligo-PsA from oligo-JIA (95). Radiographic changes include osteopenia and joint space narrowing, periostitis, erosions, destructive changes, and ankylosis in joints of the hand, cervical spine, and hips. MRI can demonstrate inflammatory changes in the SI and spinal joints, as well as in peripheral sites (96).

The age of disease onset is usually between 7 and 13 years of age. Most children have slight or mild skin and nail lesions; 80% may have psoriasis vulgaris (91, 92). Chronic iridocyclitis occurs in 15%, whereas fever, pericarditis, IBD, and amyloidosis are rarely seen (89, 90). Predictors of PsA in children with JIA in the initial 6 months include psoriasis in a first-degree relative, age at onset more than 6 years, HLA-DRB1*11/12, dactylitis, and ankle or toe arthritis (74).

ILAR criteria (2) may also include patients with arthritis or psoriasis and dactylitis, nail pitting, or a family history of psoriasis. Yet, a patient fulfilling such criteria might be classified with undifferentiated arthritis if he is a HLA-B27-positive boy older than 16 years of age at onset or if he has a first-degree relative with SpA features, including anterior uveitis and IBD. In contrast to such criteria (2), the clinical picture of such groups of patients (91, 92) is akin to the SpA concept and PsA classification. Moreover, around 25% of patients with JoPsA according to the Vancouver criteria (92) may not fulfill the ILAR criteria (94).

Crohn's disease and ulcerative colitis

Eighteen to thirty percent of patients with CD and 15% of those with UC have their first symptoms before the age of 20 (97). Peripheral arthritis occurs in 9% and 10–20% of patients with CD and UC, respectively; 1.7% have onset of arthritis 1 year after the onset of their IBD and 4.2% by 10 years (98). Most patients have peripheral arthritis with or without axial symptoms. Around 50% of children with arthritis associated with IBD have single or recurrent attacks of lower limb monoarthritis or oligoarthritis for less than 4 weeks (99); half of such children have simultaneous episodes of arthritis and gut exacerbations (98, 99). This type of arthritis does not resemble that of JoSpA/ERA, and permanent functional limitations or joint damage do not develop in most patients. In contrast, spondylitis and radiographic sacroiliitis in IBD patients generally have no relationship with the gut exacerbations and are seen more frequently in older boys who are HLA-B27 positive.

Ankylosing tarsitis

Ankylosing tarsitis refers to a distinct set of clinical and radiographic findings, including inflammatory changes, which were originally described in HLA-B27-associated JoSpA/ERA (63). Some of these findings resemble those of the spine and SI joints in AS. Patients with ankylosing tarsitis have midfoot swelling associated with perimalleolar and Achilles tendon swelling; decreased mobility of the tarsal, ankle, and MTP joints; pes planus; and hyperextension of the MTP joints (Fig. 15.4). Radiographic, MRI, and US features have been described above. Histopathologic findings include slight inflammatory changes along with the formation of bone islets embedded within the enthesis matrix (36). Ankylosing tarsitis may occur in patients with undifferentiated JoSpA/ERA and with axSpA before the appearance of radiographic sacroiliitis.

Therapeutic recommendations

The purpose of treatment is to reduce the signs and symptoms of disease activity and to improve the quality of life of children and adolescents with JoSpA/ERA (100). The disease waxes and wanes and often has a chronic course extending into adulthood. Until recently, there has been no evidence that any treatment might halt disease progression (101). However, biologic therapies seem to have changed the outlook for these children.

NSAIDs provide symptomatic relief for most patients with mild symptoms, but may be ineffective in patients with severe disease. Nearly all patients receive SSZ at some time, but its efficacy is limited (102). MTX is also used in JoSpA/ERA, but there is no clear evidence of efficacy in these patients and its application is extrapolated from its efficacy in treating peripheral arthritis in JIA patients. These drugs may have some efficacy in psoriasis, anterior uveitis, and keratoderma blennorrhagica. Oral and intra-articular glucocorticoids—including injection of the SI joints (103)—may be beneficial in patients with moderate to severe disease activity that does not respond to NSAIDs.

The use of TNFi represents the most significant advance in therapy for JoSpA/ERA, including AS and PsA (104–113). Despite the lack of specific recommendations for the treatment of JoSpA/ERA, TNFi are commonly prescribed in patients with peripheral arthritis and enthesitis not responding to NSAIDs, SSZ, MTX, or glucocorticoid intra-articular injections. TNFi are also used as initial treatment in those patients with predominantly axial involvement of the SI joints or spine. The anti-inflammatory effect of etanercept, infliximab, and adalimumab is often seen within the first few weeks of treatment, and long-term administration of these drugs provides sustained relief. Efficacy is seen in clinical outcome measures including active joint counts, enthesitis counts, inflammatory markers (CRP and ESR), physical function, quality of life, and SpA disease activity instruments. MRI of peripheral and SI joints may also show significant reduction of inflammation with TNFi (Figs 15.6 and 15.7). However, retrospective studies of JoSpA/ERA suggest that fewer patients actually achieve inactive disease, sustained remission, or successful discontinuation of TNFi compared to other JIA subgroups (108, 111–113). One study showed continued progression of radiographic sacroiliitis in some patients treated with TNFi for more than 5 years (101). In general, TNFα blockers have been considered safe and well tolerated. However, the US Food and Drug Administration (FDA) issued a boxed warning highlighting some side-effects of TNFi therapy (114). The selection of TNFi should be made based on patient preference. In the presence of certain EAMs such as uveitis and IBD, the monoclonal TNFi are preferable.

Peripheral involvement may affect walking, climbing stairs, and standing. Patients with axial disease may have a significant reduction in spinal mobility and chest expansion. Therefore patients should be enrolled in physical and occupational therapy programs in which rest, dynamic splints, and exercises for muscle strength and stretching can be implemented on an individual basis. Additionally, foot orthotics, especially cushions under the heel and plantar aspects of the MTP joints, have been useful for the management of peripheral involvement including enthesitis. The use of custom-made foot orthotics can result in improved pain and ambulation and less disability in JIA patients compared to prefabricated inserts and athletic shoes (115). Surgical modalities, such as soft tissue release, synovectomy, tendon repair, arthroplasty, and joint replacement, may be indicated in some patients with certain forms of hip, knee, and MTP disease.

The impact of JoSpA/ERA in children and adolescents on HRQoL can be very significant and often continues as they transition to

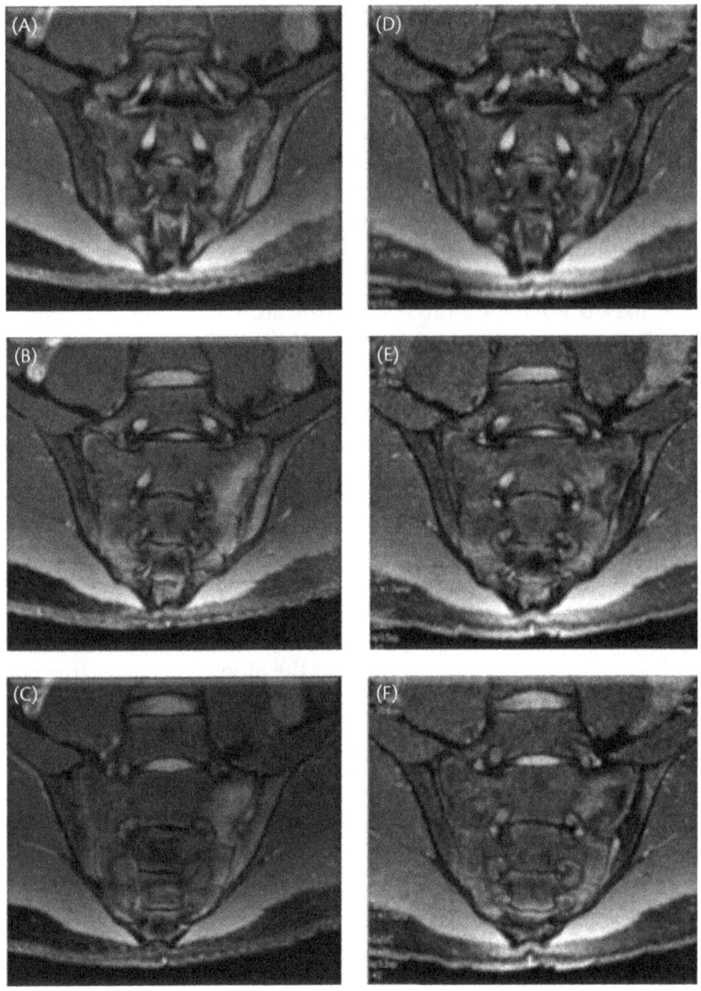

Fig. 15.6 MRI improvement of active sacroiliitis following infusion of infliximab. (A, B) (baseline findings) STIR. (A–C) MRI findings at baseline: there is oedema extending throughout sacrum and iliac bones of left SI joint. There are also clear irregularities (erosions) along mid-portion of sacrum articular surface (arrows). (D–F) MRI changes observed 14 weeks after start of infliximab: while hyperintesive signals (bone oedema) have disapeared, erosions and fat deposition suggest transition to chronic phase.

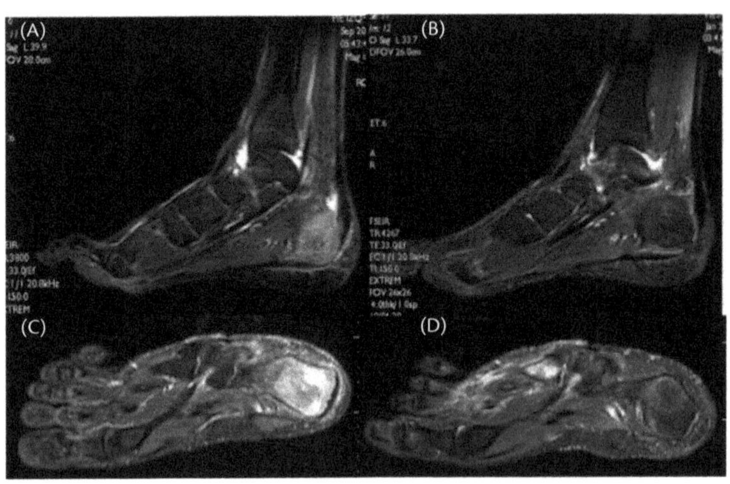

Fig. 15.7 MRI improvement of active arthritis, enthesitis, and bone oedema following infusion of infliximab. (A, B) (baseline findings) STIR MR images of foot of a 15-year-old boy with ankle swelling and painful heel (Achilles tendon and plantar fascia) for 6 months. Sagittal–lateral views showing synovial fluid effusion in posterior and anterior aspect of ankle and retrocalcaneal bursae, and possibly fat as well as bone oedema of calcaneus, including attachments of Achilles tendon and its continuation to plantar fascia. Synovial fluid effusion of ankle joint, oedema around posterior peroneal tendon, and extensive oedema of calcaneus in sagittal–posterior views. Coronal views show extension of oedema in calcaneus. (C, D) STIR MR images obtained 8 weeks after starting infliximab, showing complete resolution of calcaneus oedema and marked reduction of inflammation in ankle joint and retrocalcaneal bursae.

adulthood. Thus it is important to consider the psychological, educational, and socioeconomic aspects of the patient's life in the plan of management. Disease activity and joint damage over time may affect the individual's social life, including personal and family activities, education, and career. Attention to early diagnosis, along with appropriate therapeutic strategies and counselling will lead to improved outcomes in children and adolescents with JoSpA/ERA.

References

1. Burgos-Vargas R. The juvenile-onset spondyloarthritides. Rheum Dis Clin North Am 2002;28:531–60.
2. Petty RE, Southwood TR, Manners P, et al. International League of Associations for Rheumatology classification of juvenile idiopathic arthritis: 2nd revision, Edmonton, 2001. J Rheumatol 2004;31:390–2.
3. Moll JM. 'The Leeds Idea': an historical account of the spondarthritis concept. Reumatismo 2007;59(Suppl 1):13–18.
4. Amor B, Dougados M, Mijiyawa M. [Critères des classification des spondylartropaties.] Rev Rhum Mal Osteoartic 1990;57:85–9.
5. Dougados M, van der Linden S, Juhlin R, et al. The European Spondylarthropathy Study Group preliminary criteria for the classification of spondylarthropathy. Arthritis Rheum 1991;34:1218–27.
6. Prieur AM, Listrat V, Dougados M. [Criteres de classification des spondyloarthropathies chez les enfants.] Arch Franc Ped 1993;50:379–85.
7. Rudwaleit M, van der Heijde D, Landewe R, et al. The development of Assessment of SpondyloArthritis international Society classification criteria for axial spondyloarthritis (part II): validation and final selection. Ann Rheum Dis 2009;68:777–83.
8. Rudwaleit M, van der Heijde D, Landewe R, et al. The Assessment of SpondyloArthritis International Society classification criteria for peripheral spondyloarthritis and for spondyloarthritis in general. Ann Rheum Dis 2011;70:25–31.
9. Burgos-Vargas R. The Assessment of the Spondyloarthritis International Society concept and criteria for the classification of axial spondyloarthritis and peripheral spondyloarthritis: a critical appraisal for the pediatric rheumatologist. Pediatr Rheumatol Online J 2012;10:14.
10. Malleson PN, Fung MY, Rosenberg AM, for the Canadian Pediatric Rheumatology Association. The incidence of pediatric rheumatic diseases: results from the Canadian Pediatric Rheumatology Association Disease Registry. J Rheumatol 1996;23:1981–7.
11. Boyer GS, Lanier AT, Templin DW. Prevalence rates of spondyloarthropathies, rheumatoid arthritis, and other rheumatic disorders in an Alaskan Inupiat Eskimo population. J Rheumatol 1998;15:678–83.
12. Yilmaz M, Kendirli SG, Altintas DU, et al. Juvenile idiopathic arthritis profile in Turkish children. Pediatr Int 2008;50:154–8.
13. Kunjir V, Venugopalan A, Chopra A. Profile of Indian patients with juvenile onset chronic inflammatory joint disease using the ILAR classification criteria for JIA: a community-based cohort study. J Rheumatol 2010;37:1756–62.
14. Lau CS, Burgos-Vargas R, Louthrenoo W, et al. Features of spondyloarthropathies around the world. Rheum Dis Clin North Am 1998;24:753–70.
15. Brown MA. Breakthroughs in genetic studies of ankylosing spondylitis. Rheumatology (Oxford) 2008;47:132–7.
16. Reveille JD. An update on the contribution of the MHC to AS susceptibility. Clin Rheumatol 2014;33:749–57.
17. Flato B, Smerdel A, Johnston V, et al. The influence of patient characteristics, disease variables, and HLA alleles on the development of radiographically evident sacroiliitis in juvenile idiopathic arthritis. Arthritis Rheum 2002;46:986–94.
18. López-Larrea C, Gonzalez-Roces S, Peña M, et al. Characterization of B27 haplotypes by oligotyping and genomic sequencing in the Mexican Mestizo population with ankylosing spondylitis: juvenile and adult onset. Hum Immunol 1995;43:174–80.
19. Mou Y, Wu Z, Gu J, et al. HLA-B27 polymorphism in patients with juvenile and adult-onset ankylosing spondylitis in southern China. Tissue Antigens 2010;75:56–60.
20. International Genetics of Ankylosing Spondylitis Consortium, Cortes A, Hadler J, et al. Identification of multiple risk variants for ankylosing spondylitis through high-density genotyping of immune-related loci. Nat Genet 2013;45:730–8.
21. Robinson PC, Costello ME, Leo P, et al. ERAP2 is associated with ankylosing spondylitis in HLA-B27-positive and HLA-B27-negative patients. Ann Rheum Dis 2015;74(8):1627–9.
22. Doorduyn Y, Van Pelt W, Siezen CL, et al. Novel insight in the association between salmonellosis or campylobacteriosis and chronic illness, and the role of host genetics in susceptibility to these diseases. Epidemiol Infect 2008;136:1225–34.
23. Chen YJ, Lin CH, Ou TT, et al. Solute carrier family 11 member A1 gene polymorphisms in reactive arthritis. J Clin Immunol 2007;27:46–52.
24. Hinks A, Martin P, Flynn E, et al. Subtype specific genetic associations for juvenile idiopathic arthritis: ERAP1 with the enthesitis related arthritis subtype and IL23R with juvenile psoriatic arthritis. Arthritis Res Ther 2011;13:R12.
25. Schittenhelm RB, Sian TC, Wilmann PG, Dudek NL, Purcell AW. Revisiting the arthritogenic peptide theory: quantitative not qualitative changes in the peptide repertoire of HLA-B27 allotypes. Arthritis Rheumatol 2015;67:702–13.
26. Alvarez-Navarro C, López de Castro JA. ERAP1 structure, function and pathogenetic role in ankylosing spondylitis and other MHC-associated diseases. Mol Immunol 2014;57(1):12–21.
27. Colbert RA, Tran TM, Layh-Schmitt G. HLA-B27 misfolding and ankylosing spondylitis. Mol Immunol 2014;57:44–51.
28. Life P, Hassell A, Williams K, et al. Responses to gram negative enteric bacterial antigens by synovial T cells from patients with juvenile chronic arthritis: recognition of heat shock protein HSP60. J Rheumatol 1993;20:1388–96.
29. Burgos-Vargas R, Howard A, Ansell BM. Antibodies to peptidoglycan in juvenile onset ankylosing spondylitis and pauciarticular onset juvenile arthritis associated with chronic iridocyclitis. J Rheumatol 1986;13:760–5.
30. Singh YP, Singh AK, Aggarwal A, et al. Evidence of cellular immune response to outer membrane protein of *Salmonella typhimurium* in patients with enthesitis-related arthritis subtype of juvenile idiopathic arthritis. J Rheumatol 2011;38:161–6.
31. Pacheco-Tena C, Alvarado de la Barrera C, López-Vidal Y, et al. Bacterial DNA in synovial fluid cells of patients with juvenile onset spondyloarthropathies. Rheumatology (Oxford) 2001;40:920–7.
32. Myles A, Aggarwal A. Expression of Toll-like receptors 2 and 4 is increased in peripheral blood and synovial fluid monocytes of patients with enthesitis-related arthritis subtype of juvenile idiopathic arthritis. Rheumatology (Oxford) 2011;50:481–8.
33. Stoll ML, Kumar R, Morrow CD, et al. Altered microbiota associated with abnormal humoral immune responses to comensal organisms in enthesitis-related arthritis. Arthritis Res Ther 2014; 16(6):486.
34. Kruithof E, Van den Bossche V, De Rycke L, et al. Distinct synovial immunopathologic characteristics of juvenile-onset spondylarthritis and other forms of juvenile idiopathic arthritis. Arthritis Rheum 2006;54:2594–604.
35. Grom AA, Murray KJ, Luyrink L, et al. Patterns of expression of tumor necrosis factor alpha, tumor necrosis factor beta, and their receptors in synovia of patients with juvenile rheumatoid arthritis and juvenile spondylarthropathy. Arthritis Rheum 1996;39:1703–10.
36. Pacheco-Tena C, Pérez-Tamayo R, Pineda C, et al. Bone lineage proteins in the entheses of the midfoot in patients with spondyloarthritis. J Rheumatol 2015;42:630–7.
37. Lories RJ, Derese I, Luyten FP. Modulation of bone morphogenetic protein signaling inhibits the onset and progression of ankylosing enthesitis. J Clin Invest 2005;115:1571–9.

38. Sherlock JP, Joyce-Shaikh B, Turner SP, et al. IL-23 induces spondyloarthropathy by acting on ROR-γt+CD3+CD4−CD8−entheseal resident T cells. Nat Med 2012;18:1069–76.
39. Riley MJ, Ansell BM, Bywaters EG. Radiological manifestations of ankylosing spondylitis according to age at onset. Ann Rheum Dis 1971;30:138–48.
40. Marks SH, Barnett M, Calin A. A case-control study of juvenile- and adult-onset ankylosing spondylitis. J Rheumatol 1982;9:739–41.
41. Calin A, Elswood J. The natural history of juvenile-onset ankylosing spondylitis: a 24-year retrospective case-control study. Br J Rheumatol 1988;27:91–3.
42. Garcia-Morteo O, Maldonado-Cocco JA, Suarez-Almazor ME, Garay E. Ankylosing spondylitis of juvenile onset: comparison with adult onset disease. Scand J Rheumatol 1983;12:246–8.
43. Burgos-Vargas R, Naranjo A, Castillo J, Katona G. Ankylosing spondylitis in the Mexican mestizo: patterns of disease according to age at onset. J Rheumatol 1989;16:186–91.
44. Baek HJ, Shin KC, Lee YJ, Kang SW, Lee EB, Yoo CD. Juvenile onset ankylosing spondylitis (JAS) has less severe spinal disease course tan adult onset ankylosing spondylitis (AAS): clinical comparison between JAS and AAS in Korea. J Rheumatol 2002; 29:1780–5.
45. Stone M, Warren RW, Bruckel J, Cooper D, Cortinovis D, Inman RD. Juvenile onset ankylosing spondylitis is associated with worse functional outcomes than adult-onset ankylosing spondylitis. Arthritis Rheum 2005;53:445–51.
46. Gensler LS, Ward MM, Reveille JD, Learch TJ, Weisman MH, Davis JC Jr. Clinical, radiographic and functional differences between juvenile-onset and adult-onset ankylosing spondylitis: results from the PSOAS cohort. Ann Rheum Dis 2008;67:233–7.
47. O'Shea FD, Boyle E, Riarh R, Tse SM, Laxer RM, Inman RD. Comparison of clinical and radiographic severity of juvenile-onset versus adult-onset ankylosing spondylitis. Ann Rheum Dis 2009;68:1407–12.
48. Ozgocmen S, Ardicoglu O, Kamanli A, Kaya A, Durmus B, Yildirim K. Pattern of disease onset, diagnostic delay, and clinical features in juvenile onset and adult onset ankylosing spondylitis. J Rheumatol 2009;36:2830–3.
49. Weiss PF, Klink AJ, Behrens EM, et al. Enthesitis in an inception cohort of enthesitis-related arthritis. Arthritis Care Res (Hoboken) 2011;63:1307–12.
50. Burgos-Vargas R, Clark P. Axial involvement in the seronegative enthesopathy and arthropathy syndrome and its progression to ankylosing spondylitis. J Rheumatol 1989;16:192–7.
51. Cabral DA, Oen KG, Petty RE. SEA syndrome revisited: a long-term followup of children with a syndrome of seronegative enthesopathy and arthropathy. J Rheumatol 1992;19:1282–5.
52. Burgos-Vargas R, Vázquez-Mellado J. The early clinical recognition of juvenile-onset ankylosing spondylitis and its differentiation from juvenile rheumatoid arthritis. Arthritis Rheum 1995;38:835–44.
53. Burgos-Vargas R, Vázquez-Mellado J, Cassis N, et al. Genuine ankylosing spondylitis in children: a case-control study of patients with early definite disease according to adult onset criteria. J Rheumatol 1996;23:2140–7.
54. Flatø B, Hoffmann-Vold AM, Reiff A, et al. Long-term outcome and prognostic factors in enthesitis-related arthritis: a case-control study. Arthritis Rheum 2006;54:3573–82.
55. Pagnini I, Savelli S, Matucci-Cerinic M, et al. Early predictors of juvenile sacroiliitis in enthesitis-related arthritis. J Rheumatol 2010;37:2395–401.
56. Stoll ML, Bhore R, Dempsey-Robertson M, et al. Spondyloarthritis in a pediatric population: risk factors for sacroiliitis. J Rheumatol 2010;37:2402–8.
57. Hreggvidsdottir HS, Noordenbos T, Baeten DL. Inflammatory pathways in spondyloarthritis. Mol Immunol 2014;57:28–37.
58. Baraliakos X, Listing J, Rudwaleit M, et al. The relationship between inflammation and new bone formation in patients with ankylosing spondylitis. Arthritis Res Ther 2008;10(5):R104.
59. Maksymowych WP, Chiowchanwisawakit P, Clare T, et al. Inflammatory lesions of the spine on magnetic resonance imaging predict the development of new syndesmophytes in ankylosing spondylitis: evidence of a relationship between inflammation and new bone formation. Arthritis Rheum 2009;60:93–102.
60. van der Heijde D, Machado P, Braun J, et al. MRI inflammation at the vertebral unit only marginally predicts new syndesmophyte formation: a multilevel analysis in patients with ankylosing spondylitis. Ann Rheum Dis 2012;71:369–73.
61. Chiowchanwisawakit P, Lambert RG, Conner-Spady B, et al. Focal fat lesions at vertebral corners on magnetic resonance imaging predict the development of new syndesmophytes in ankylosing spondylitis. Arthritis Rheum 2011;63:2215–25.
62. Masi AT. Might axial myofascial properties and biomechanical mechanisms be relevant to ankylosing spondylitis and axial spondyloarthritis? Arthritis Res Ther 2014;16(2):107.
63. Burgos-Vargas R, Granados-Arriola J. Ankylosing spondylitis and related diseases in the Mexican Mestizo. In: Khan MA (ed) Spine: State of the Art Reviews. Vol 4. Ankylosing Spondylitis and Related Spondyloarthropathies. Philadelphia, Hanley & Belfus, 1990, p. 665.
64. Minden K, Kiessling U, Listing J, et al. Prognosis of patients with juvenile chronic arthritis and juvenile spondyloarthropathy. J Rheumatol 2000;27:2256–63.
65. Flato B, Aasland A, Vinje O, et al. Outcome and predictive factors in juvenile rheumatoid arthritis and juvenile spondyloarthropathy. J Rheumatol 1988;25:366–75.
66. Minden K, Niewerth M, Listing J, et al. Long-term outcome in patients with juvenile idiopathic arthritis. Arthritis Rheum 2002;46:2392–401.
67. Flatø B, Lien G, Smerdel-Ramoya A, et al. Juvenile psoriatic arthritis: long-term outcome and differentiation from other subtypes of juvenile idiopathic arthritis. J Rheumatol 2009;36:642–50.
68. Weiss PF, Beukelman T, Schanberg LE, et al. Enthesitis-related arthritis is associated with higher pain intensity and poorer health status in comparison with other categories of juvenile idiopathic arthritis: the Childhood Arthritis and Rheumatology Research Alliance Registry. J Rheumatol 2012;39:2341–51.
69. Bollow M, Biedermann T, Kannenberg J, et al. Use of dynamic magnetic resonance imaging to detect sacroiliitis in HLA-B27 positive and negative children with juvenile arthritides. J Rheumatol 1998;25:556–64.
70. Weiss PF, Colbert RA. Radiography versus magnetic resonance imaging (MRI) in juvenile spondyloarthritis: is the MR image everything? J Rheumatol 2014;41:832–3.
71. Weiss PF, Xiao R, Biko DM, Johnson AM, Chauvin NA. Detection of inflammatory sacroiliitis in children with magnetic resonance imaging: is gadolinium-contrast enhancement necessary? Arthritis Rheumatol 2015;67(8):2250–6.
72. Aquino MR, Tse SM, Gupta S, et al. Whole-body MRI of juvenile spondyloarthritis: protocols and pictorial review of characteristic patterns. Pediatr Radiol 2015;45:754–62.
73. Jousse-Joulin S, Breton S, Cangemi C, et al. Ultrasonography for detecting enthesitis in juvenile idiopathic arthritis. Arthritis Care Res (Hoboken) 2011;63:849–55.
74. Aydin SZ, Tan AL, Hodsgon R, et al. Comparison of ultrasonography and magnetic resonance imaging for the assessment of clinically defined knee enthesitis in spondyloarthritis. Clin Exp Rheumatol 2013;31:933–6.
75. Weiss PF, Chauvin NA, Klink AJ, et al. Detection of enthesitis in children with enthesitis-related arthritis: dolorimetry compared to ultrasonography. Arthritis Rheumatol 2014;66(1):218–27.
76. Jacobs JC, Johnston AD, Berdon WE. HLA-B27 associated spondyloarthritis and enthesopathy in childhood: clinical, pathologic and radiographic observations in 58 patients. J Pediatr 1982;100:521–8.
77. Rosenberg AM, Petty RE. A syndrome of seronegative enthesopathy and arthropathy in children. Arthritis Rheum 1982;25:1041–7.
78. Olivieri I, Cutro MS, D'Angelo S, et al. Low frequency of axial involvement in southern Italian Caucasian children with HLA-B27 positive

juvenile onset undifferentiated spondyloarthritis. Clin Exp Rheumatol 2012;30:290–6.
79. van der Linden S, Valkenburg HA, Cats A. Evaluation of diagnostic criteria for ankylosing spondylitis. A proposal for modification of the New York criteria. Arthritis Rheum 1984;27:361–8.
80. Schaller JG, Bitnum S, Wedgwood RJ. Ankylosing spondylitis with childhood onset. J Pediatr 1969;74:505–16.
81. Stamato T, Laxer RM, de Freitas C, et al. Prevalence of cardiac manifestations of juvenile ankylosing spondylitis. Am J Cardiol 1995;75:744–6.
82. Hannu T, Inman R, Granfors K, Leirisalo-Repo M. Reactive arthritis or post-infectious arthritis? Best Pract Res Clin Rheumatol 2006;20:419–33.
83. Gracey E, Inman RD. *Chlamydia*-induced ReA: immune imbalances and persistent pathogens. Nat Rev Rheumatol 2011;8:55–9.
84. Hoogkamp-Korstanje JA, Stolk-Engelaar VM. *Yersinia enterocolitica* infection in children. Pediatr Infect Dis J 1995;14:771–5.
85. Mattila L, Leirisalo-Repo M, Pelkonen P, et al. Reactive arthritis following an outbreak of *Salmonella bovis morbificans* infection. J Infect 1998;36:289–95.
86. Lee AT, Hall RG, Pile KD. Reactive joint symptoms following an outbreak of *Salmonella typhimurium* phage type 135a. J Rheumatol 2005;32:524–7.
87. Burgos-Vargas R, Vázquez-Mellado J. Reactive arthritides. In: Cassidy JT, Petty RE (eds) Textbook of Pediatric Rheumatology, 5th edn. Philadelphia, Elsevier Saunders, 2005, pp. 604–12.
88. Rosenberg AM, Petty RE. Reiter's disease in children. Am J Dis Child 1979;133:394–8.
89. Kanakoudi-Tsakalidou F, Pardalos G, Prastidou-Gertsi P, et al. Persistent or severe course of reactive arthritis following *Salmonella enteritidis* infection. Scand J Rheumatol 1998;27:431–6.
90. Tacceti G, Trappani S, Ermini M, et al. Reactive arthritis triggered by *Yersinia enterocolitica*: a review of 18 pediatric cases. Clin Exp Rheumatol 1994;12:681–5.
91. Shore A, Ansell BM. Juvenile psoriatic arthritis—an analysis of 60 cases. J Pediatr 1982;100:529–35.
92. Southwood TR, Petty RE, Malleson PN, et al. Psoriatic arthritis in children. Arthritis Rheum 1989;32:1014–21.
93. Hamilton ML, Gladman DD, Shore A, et al. Juvenile psoriatic arthritis and HLA antigens. Ann Rheum Dis 1990;49:694–7.
94. Stoll ML, Zurakowski D, Nigrovic LE, et al. Patients with juvenile psoriatic arthritis comprise two distinct populations. Arthritis Rheum 2006;54:3564–72.
95. Huemer C, Malleson PN, Cabral DA, et al. Patterns of joint involvement at onset differentiate oligoarticular juvenile psoriatic arthritis from pauciarticular juvenile rheumatoid arthritis. J Rheumatol 2002;29:1531–5.
96. Lee EY, Sundel RP, Kim S, et al. MRI findings of juvenile psoriatic arthritis. Skeletal Radiol 2008;37:987–96.
97. Burbige EJ, Huang SH, Bayless TM. Clinical manifestations of Crohn's disease in children and adolescents. Pediatrics 1975;55:866–71.
98. Jose FA, Garnett EA, Vittinghoff E, et al. Development of extraintestinal manifestations in pediatric patients with inflammatory bowel disease. Inflamm Bowel Dis 2009;15:63–8.
99. Lindsley C, Schaller JG. Arthritis associated with inflammatory bowel disease in children. J Pediatr 1974;84:16–20.
100. Tse SM, Burgos-Vargas R, Colbert RA. Juvenile spondyloarthritis treatment recommendations. Am J Med Sci 2012;343:367–70.
101. Hugle B, Burgos-Vargas R, Inman RD, et al. Long-term outcome of anti-tumor necrosis factor alpha blockade in the treatment of juvenile spondyloarthritis. Clin Exp Rheumatol 2014;32:424–31.
102. Burgos-Vargas R, Vázquez-Mellado J, Pacheco-Tena C, et al. A 26-week randomised, double-blind, placebo-controlled exploratory study of sulfasalazine in juvenile onset spondyloarthropathies. Ann Rheum Dis 2002;61:941–2.
103. Fritz J, Tzaribachev N, Thomas C, et al. Evaluation of MR imaging guided steroid injection of the sacroiliac joints for the treatment of children with refractory enthesitis-related arthritis. Eur Radiol. 2011;21:1050–7.
104. Henrickson M, Reiff A. Prolonged efficacy of etanercept in refractory enthesitis-related arthritis. J Rheumatol 2004;31:2055–61.
105. Tse SM, Burgos-Vargas R, Laxer RM. Anti-tumor necrosis factor alpha blockade in the treatment of juvenile spondylarthropathy. Arthritis Rheum 2005;52:2103–8.
106. Sulpice M, Deslandre CJ, Quartier P. Efficacy and safety of TNF-alpha antagonist therapy in patients with juvenile spondyloarthropathies. Joint Bone Spine 2009;76:24–7.
107. Otten MH, Prince FH, Ten Cate R, et al. Tumour necrosis factor (TNF)-blocking agents in juvenile psoriatic arthritis: are they effective? Ann Rheum Dis 2011;70:337–40.
108. Otten MH, Prince FH, Twilt M, et al. Tumor necrosis factor–blocking agents for children with enthesitis-related arthritis—data from the Dutch Arthritis and Biologicals in Children Register, 1999–2010. J Rheumatol 2011;38:2258–63.
109. Horneff G, Fitter S, Foeldvari I, et al. Double-blind, placebo-controlled randomized trial with adalimumab for treatment of juvenile onset ankylosing spondylitis (JoAS): significant short term improvement. Arthritis Res Ther 2012;14:R230.
110. Horneff G, Burgos-Vargas R, Constantin T, et al. Efficacy and safety of open-label etanercept on extended oligoarticular juvenile idiopathic arthritis, enthesitis-related arthritis and psoriatic arthritis: part 1 (week 12) of the CLIPPER study. Ann Rheum Dis 2014;73:1114–22.
111. Donnithorne KJ, Cron RQ, Beukelman T. Attainment of inactive disease status following initiation of TNF-α inhibitor therapy for juvenile idiopathic arthritis: enthesitis-related arthritis predicts persistent active disease. J Rheumatol 2011;38:2675–81.
112. Boiu S, Marniga E, Bader-Meunier B, et al. Functional status in severe juvenile idiopathic arthritis in the biologic treatment era: an assessment in a French paediatric rheumatology referral centre. Rheumatology (Oxford) 2012;51:1285–92.
113. Oen K, Tucker L, Huber AM, et al. Predictors of early inactive disease in a juvenile idiopathic arthritis cohort: results of a Canadian multicenter, prospective inception cohort study. Arthritis Rheum 2009;61:1077–86.
114. Beukelman T, Haynes K, Curtis JR, et al. Safety Assessment of Biological Therapeutics Collaboration. Rates of malignancy associated with juvenile idiopathic arthritis and its treatment. Arthritis Rheum 2012;64:1263–71.
115. Powell M, Seid M, Szer IS. Efficacy of custom foot orthotics in improving pain and functional status in children with juvenile idiopathic arthritis: a randomized trial. J Rheumatol 2005;32:943–50.

CHAPTER 16

Extra-articular manifestations: uveitis

James T. Rosenbaum

Introduction to uveitis

Definition

Uvea is the Latin word for grape. The Roman anatomists thought that the middle section of the eye was a grape-like structure. The uvea lies between the sclera and the retina. The anterior uvea is the iris. The posterior uveal tract is the choroid, a vascular tissue that helps to oxygenate the retina. Uveitis is the term that describes inflammation of any part of the uveal tract. Uveitis is subdivided into anatomic subsets, such as anterior uveitis (which includes either iritis or iridocyclitis), panuveitis, or choroiditis. Uveitis is generally diagnosed by an examination with a slit lamp and an indirect ophthalmoscope. If leukocytes are detected in the anterior chamber of the eye or in the vitreous humor and no infection is present, a diagnosis of uveitis is made. Since neither the anterior chamber nor the vitreous humor is technically part of the uveal tract, some experts prefer the term intraocular inflammation to uveitis. Inflammation of the uvea is often associated with inflammation of adjacent structures. Thus retinochoroiditis and chorioretinitis are both subsets of uveitis. A panuveitis refers to inflammation occurring in the anterior chamber, vitreous humor, and retina and/or choroid. A group called the Standardization of Uveitis Nomenclature (SUN) has recommended the term intermediate uveitis when inflammation is primarily in the vitreous humor, and posterior uveitis for inflammation that affects the retina or choroid (1).

Epidemiology

A study based on patients receiving care from the Northern California Kaiser system concluded that uveitis has a point prevalence of 115.3 per 100 000 and an incidence of 52.4 per 100 000 (2). Although these numbers are modest, uveitis accounts for about 10% of the acquired blindness in the USA (3). In terms of years of visual morbidity, uveitis is comparable to either diabetes or macular degeneration. Both diabetic retinopathy and macular degeneration tend to affect patients near the end of life. In contrast, uveitis frequently affects individuals during young adulthood or even childhood, so that a relatively uncommon problem nonetheless accounts for many years of morbidity (4).

Differential diagnosis of a red eye

Not all patients with uveitis present with a red eye. For example, children with JIA and anterior uveitis have disease that begins so insidiously that the eye is typically not red. Patients who have solely an intermediate or posterior uveitis also do not characteristically develop a red eye. The AAU typical of AS should be associated with eye redness with few exceptions.

The differential diagnosis of eye redness includes conjunctivitis and episcleritis. Both of these conditions do not typically cause pain and neither should be associated with leukocytes in the anterior chamber. A scleritis, on the other hand, is painful. When it affects just one sector of the eye, it is relatively easy to distinguish redness from scleritis versus redness from anterior uveitis (Fig. 16.1). A diffuse scleritis might be more of a challenge since some patients with scleritis do have an anterior uveitis in association with it. Patients with scleritis have a tender globe which is not typical of iritis. AAU also tends to cause a smaller pupil because of spasm of the ciliary muscles. The redness tends to be at the limbus, the junction between the cornea and the sclera (Fig. 16.2). Acute closed-angle glaucoma also causes eye redness and is identified by the marked elevation of intraocular pressure and usually a pupil in mid-position. A slit lamp examination combined with measurement of the intraocular pressure can generally distinguish among these causes of ocular redness.

Rheumatologists should refer patients to an ophthalmologist if the patient is experiencing pain as opposed to discomfort, if there is sensitivity to light (photophobia), if there is any change in visual acuity, or if the problem is simply persistent.

Differential diagnosis of uveitis

Just as arthritis is not a single disease, the term uveitis describes multiple different diseases. The differential diagnosis is aided greatly by characterizing the uveitis. Does it affect one eye or both eyes? Did it start suddenly or insidiously? Does it follow a continuous course or is it episodic? Is it associated with complications such as glaucoma, cataract, macular oedema, posterior synechiae (adherence of the

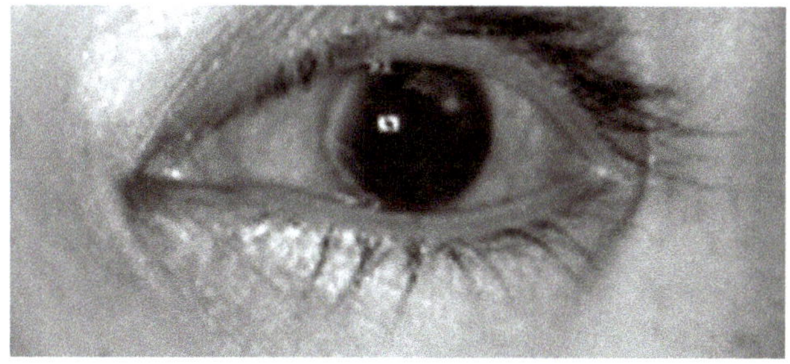

Fig. 16.1 (See colour plate section). Scleritis. Although the surface of this eye is diffusely red, the eye is redder nasally. A sector of redness suggests a scleritis or episcleritis.

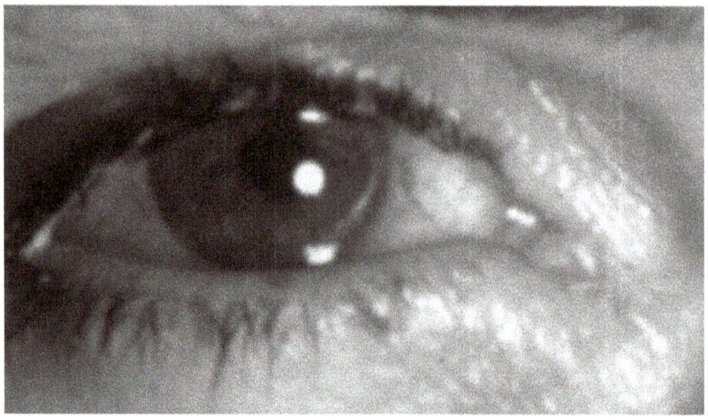

Fig. 16.2 (See colour plate section). AAU or iritis. The redness is especially prominent at the junction between the cornea and sclera. Slit lamp examination should reveal leukocytes in the anterior chamber.

iris to the anterior lens capsule), band keratopathy (deposition of calcium in the corneal epithelium), or retinal detachment? What is the size and location of any leukocytes which have attached to the corneal endothelium? And what anatomic portion of the eye is predominantly affected? Just as characteristics like this would narrow the differential diagnosis among RA, osteoarthritis, and gout, these types of features aid an experienced ophthalmologist a great deal in determining the likely cause of a uveitis.

Uveitis is also classified on the basis of aetiology (Box 16.1). By convention, various infections are considered as causes of uveitis, just as tuberculosis and gonorrhoea enter into the differential diagnosis of arthritis. Many forms of uveitis are presumed to be immune-mediated, but the inflammation is usually confined to the eye. Other forms of uveitis are immune-mediated, but the illness is systemic, with inflammation also occurring in other organ systems (Box 16.2). A variety of medications are known to have the potential to induce uveitis (5). Some diseases will mimic uveitis by causing cells to appear in the anterior chamber or the vitreous humor. These so-called masquerades include leukaemia, lymphoma, retinoblastoma, retinal detachment, and retinal degeneration. About 30% of patients with uveitis have a disease that does not fit readily into a diagnostic niche. They are generally labelled as having idiopathic uveitis. Since the aetiology is presumably immunologic, some suggest that a better term is primary uveitis to distinguish this disease from that secondary to an illness like AS. Undifferentiated uveitis is another term that has been proposed (6).

Box 16.1 Broad categories of disease that cause uveitis

Infections (examples include herpes simplex, herpes zoster, syphilis, and tuberculosis)

Immune processes mostly confined to the eye (examples include birdshot retinochoroidopathy, sympathetic ophthalmia, multifocal choroiditis, serpiginous choroiditis)

Masquerade syndromes (examples include leukaemia and lymphoma)

Systemic immune diseases (see Box 16.2)

Drug reactions (TNFi, rifampicin, bisphosphonates)

Trauma (ophthalmic surgery)

Idiopathic

Box 16.2 Systemic, immune-mediated diseases associated with uveitis. (Diseases are listed in approximate order of frequency (most common to least common) as seen in the author's referral-based clinic in Portland, Oregon, USA.)

AS

Sarcoidosis

JIA

PsA

IBD

ReA/enthesitis

Tubulo-interstitial nephritis with uveitis (TINU)

Multiple sclerosis

Behçet's disease

Vogt–Koyanagi–Harada disease

Relapsing polychondritis

Cogan's syndrome, Kawasaki's disease, and other forms of vasculitis

Autoinflammatory diseases such as Blau syndrome and neonatal-onset multisystem inflammatory disease (NOMID)

Sweet's syndrome

SLE

Rheumatic fever

Relationship of HLA-B27 to uveitis

B27 and uveitis: general

About 85% of all uveitis is predominantly anterior uveitis (2). Usually anterior uveitis responds to topical corticosteroid therapy (see section 'Treating active disease'). Centres that specialize in the care of patients with uveitis tend to evaluate a disproportionate share of intermediate and posterior uveitis which is less responsive to topical therapy. Shortly after a group from London reported an association between HLA-B27 and AS (7), the same group discovered that about 50% of patients with anterior uveitis were HLA-B27 positive (8). HLA-B27-associated uveitis is easily the most common identifiable form of uveitis in Europe and North America.

Characteristics of B27-associated uveitis

The uveitis associated with HLA-B27 tends to have a sudden onset that can follow a prodrome of discomfort in the eye for a day or two (9, 10). It is rare for both eyes to be affected simultaneously. The uveitis can be severe, but it generally completely resolves after no more than 2 months of inflammation. Males develop B27-associated iritis more commonly than females by about a ratio of 3:2. While both eyes are not simultaneously inflamed, recurrences are the rule and these recurrences sometimes flip-flop to affect the eye opposite the first attack. The uveitis associated with HLA-B27 results in hypopyon (a cellular response that is intense such that cells produce a visible meniscus in the anterior chamber) about one attack in seven (11). Posterior synechiae are common with HLA-B27-associated uveitis, and fibrin is sometimes visible in the anterior chamber.

Herpes simplex also causes a unilateral anterior uveitis that is recurrent. Herpes simplex can usually be identified because it may cause corneal scarring or atrophy of pigment in the iris. It also tends not to resolve simply by treatment with topical corticosteroids.

Herpes simplex keratouveitis usually causes an elevation of the intraocular pressure, while HLA-B27-associated anterior uveitis tends to lower the intraocular pressure.

Many of the same genes that predispose to AS including HLA-B27 and IL-23 receptor also influence susceptibility to anterior uveitis (12). However, there appear to be genetic factors that contribute to the likelihood to develop anterior uveitis independently of the risk of developing SpA (12).

Likelihood of spondyloarthritis if a patient has B27-associated uveitis

Studies have reached variable conclusions about the likelihood that a patient has spondyloarthropathy if he or she is B27 positive and has a uveitis. A large study from Paris published in 2004 concluded that about 80% of patients with B27-associated anterior uveitis have a spondyloarthropathy (13). This percentage included patients with definite AS, possible AS, uSpA, PsA, and IBD. This study was conducted prior to the publication of diagnostic criteria for axSpA that have been proposed by the ASAS group. By ASAS criteria, a patient has axSpA if he or she is HLA-B27 positive, has inflammatory low back pain by history, and has an episode of uveitis. By ASAS criteria, radiographic sacroiliitis is not required to diagnoses SpA. Using these criteria, closer to 90% of patients with B27-associated iritis might have SpA. The majority of patients who are seen by an ophthalmologist with B27-associated uveitis and inflammatory low back pain are unaware that their back discomfort is causally related to their eye disease (9).

A group from Dublin has proposed an algorithm to evaluate patients with anterior uveitis in an emergency department for SpA (14). Using this algorithm, the authors studied only patients who were not already known to have spondyloarthropathy. The authors concluded that 40% of patients seen in an emergency department for anterior uveitis had an associated SpA which had not been previously diagnosed. Another study used US to identify 'occult' SpA among patients with AAU. This report noted US evidence for enthesitis in 55.6% of patients with HLA-B27-associated AAU. Controls with other forms of uveitis had enthesitis much less frequently.

Studies also vary a great deal in estimating the frequency of AAU among patients with AS. An important variable is how long the study followed patients, since younger patients may eventually develop AAU but not have had an episode early in the course of disease. In studies with a long duration of follow-up, as many as 50% of all patients with AS provide a history of at least one episode of iritis.

Uveitis and inflammatory bowel disease or psoriatic arthritis

Arthritis in association with CD, UC, and psoriasis can take on several different patterns, including one that is predominantly axial and one that is predominantly peripheral. In parallel to this, some patients with IBD or PsA develop sudden onset, unilateral, episodic anterior uveitis that is indistinguishable from the uveitis associated with AS. About half of those with uveitis in association with IBD (10) or PsA (15) will have uveitis that is bilateral, insidious in onset, chronic in duration, and/or predominating in the vitreous humor. About half of the patients with uveitis in association with IBD and PsA are HLA-B27 positive. The frequency of uveitis as a complication of IBD and PsA is lower than the frequency of uveitis in association with AS. Although studies vary, the frequency of uveitis is roughly 5% for either disease.

Uveitis and juvenile ankylosing spondylitis

Children who are HLA-B27 positive with AS also tend to develop uveitis (16). While the uveitis most characteristic of JIA is bilateral, insidious in onset, and chronic in duration, the uveitis associated with juvenile AS is sudden in onset, unilateral, and usually brief in duration (16). The JIA subset that develops bilateral, insidious-onset anterior uveitis is usually female between the ages of 2 and 6. The juvenile AS subset is usually older and tends to be male.

Laboratory testing for B27-associated uveitis

HLA-B27 testing can be informative in patients with sudden-onset, unilateral anterior uveitis. For example, it helps establish a diagnosis of axSpA by the ASAS criteria, as discussed in the section 'Likelihood of spondyloarthritis if a patient has B27-associated uveitis'. In addition, HLA-B27-positive patients are at greater risk for recurrent attacks of uveitis.

The association of HLA-B27 with a bilateral anterior uveitis or a vitritis is weak. Typing patients for HLA-B27 in the setting of a bilateral or intermediate uveitis will produce positive results that frequently represent a coincidence rather than a cause and effect relationship.

Treatment of uveitis in association with axial spondyloarthritis

Prevention

Several medications have been studied in well-designed trials for prevention of uveitis. SSZ is clearly effective (17, 18) as are TNFi (19–21). In general, antibodies to TNF are more active than ETN for treating uveitis (22). For example, a retrospective study from the Cleveland Clinic of patients with many different forms of uveitis found that 100% of those treated with infliximab had improvement of uveitis, compared to 33% treated with ETN (22). Evidence does, however, support ETN as effective in reducing the frequency of uveitis attacks (19). Patients who have an established pattern of several attacks of B27-associated AAU per year are good candidates for SSZ therapy. A risk-benefit analysis to justify a TNFi for this indication is more problematic because of the greater cost and risk with biologic therapy. It is easier to justify the biologic therapy if both joint and eye disease are poorly controlled. Just as TNFi are a paradoxical cause of psoriasis, TNFi are likewise a rare cause of uveitis (23). In this regard, ETN is also a more likely cause than a monoclonal antibody.

Retrospective data support the contention that NSAIDs prevent attacks of uveitis (24), and MTX is also probably active in this regard (25), but the randomized controlled data in support of SSZ make it the drug of first choice to prevent iritis flares in the rare patient who has very frequent attacks of uveitis.

Treating active disease

Most patients with B27-associated AAU can be adequately treated with topical corticosteroids. Prednisolone acetate is the most common selection. A dilating drop is also often added because this helps to prevent posterior synechiae. In addition, some pain is due to spasm of the muscle controlling the pupil size. Cycloplegia can relieve this pain. Difluprednate is a form of topical corticosteroid that is more potent than prednisolone acetate. Complications of topical corticosteroids include cataractogenesis and elevated intraocular pressure. Difluprednate is more efficacious than prednisolone acetate, but also more likely to induce these complications.

A minority of patients do not respond to topical therapy alone. Options for these patients include a short course of oral prednisone or a periocular injection of a corticosteroid such as triamcinolone.

Episodes of iritis should be monitored by an ophthalmologist so that the intraocular pressure is controlled and so that excessive therapy leading to a cataract is not prescribed. However, patients who experience multiple attacks learn to recognize the prodrome that marks the onset of an attack. It is very appropriate for these individuals to self-medicate at the start of the prodrome, with the proviso that an ophthalmologist will be consulted at the earliest possible convenient time.

Why uveitis and spondyloarthritis coexist

Arthritis and uveitis coexist in multiple diseases in addition to SpA. Other examples include JIA, Blau syndrome, sarcoidosis, Kawasaki's disease, and infections like Lyme disease and Whipple's disease. The explanation for this coexistence is unclear, and indeed multiple factors might contribute, including genes, as discussed in the section 'Characteristics of B27-associated uveitis'. Some potential auto-antigens such as type II collagen and aggrecan are common to both the eye and joint. It is also possible that similarities between the eye and joint might allow immune complexes to deposit. Similarities could also allow a foreign antigen such as a bacterial cell wall to deposit (26).

In at least three animal models, uveitis and arthritis coexist. Arthritis can be induced in BALB/c mice by immunization with the proteoglycan aggrecan (27). Susceptible animals develop sacroiliitis reminiscent of SpA. These same mice often develop an anterior uveitis. Intriguingly, inhibiting gamma interferon will ameliorate the joint disease while exacerbating the eye inflammation (28).

Adjuvant arthritis was described more than 50 years ago. Immunization of selected rat strains with killed mycobacteria in mineral oil produces an asymmetric arthritis with new bone formation and some spinal involvement. Some of these rats also develop a chronic, granulomatous uveitis (29).

Finally, the SKG mouse described by Sakaguchi and colleagues has a defect in ZAP-70, a transmembrane molecule involved in T cell signalling (30, 31). If these mice are challenged, as with curdlan from yeast cell wall, an arthritis develops. Some investigators have called attention to the similarity of this disease to SpA (30). Both bowel involvement reminiscent of CD and uveitis have been reported.

Conclusion

In summary, AAU is the most common, clinically apparent EAM of AS. In many patients, the uveitis is a clue to the existence of the associated joint disease, and, in some patients, the uveitis is the dominant manifestation of the entire clinical spectrum. Understanding this relationship from both a clinical perspective and a research perspective promises to improve the management of this troubling aspect of AS.

References

1. Jabs DA, Nussenblatt RB, Rosenbaum JT. Standardization of uveitis nomenclature for reporting clinical data. Results of the First International Workshop. Am J Ophthalmol 2005;140:509–16.
2. Gritz DC, Wong IG. Incidence and prevalence of uveitis in northern California; the Northern California Epidemiology of Uveitis Study. Ophthalmology 2004;111:491–500; discussion 500.
3. Nussenblatt RB. The natural history of uveitis. Int Ophthalmol 1990;14:303–8.
4. Suttorp-Schulten MSA, Rothova A. The possible impact of uveitis in blindness, a literature survey. Br J Ophthalmol 1996;80:844–8.
5. Fraunfelder R, Rosenbaum JT. Drug induced uveitis: prevention and management. Drug Safety 1997;17:197–207.
6. Jabs DA, Busingye J. Approach to the diagnosis of the uveitides. Am J Ophthalmol 2013;156:228–36.
7. Brewerton DA, Hart FD, Nicholls A, Caffrey M, James DC, Sturrock RD. Ankylosing spondylitis and HL-A 27. Lancet 1973;1:904–7.
8. Brewerton DA, Caffrey M, Nicholls A, Walters D, James DC. Acute anterior uveitis and HL-A 27. Lancet 1973;302:994–6.
9. Rosenbaum JT. Characterization of uveitis associated with spondyloarthritis. J Rheumatol 1989;16:792–6.
10. Lyons JL, Rosenbaum JT. Uveitis associated with inflammatory bowel disease compared with uveitis associated with spondyloarthropathy. Arch Ophthalmol 1997;115:61–4.
11. D'Alessandro LP, Forster DJ, Rao NA. Anterior uveitis and hypopyon. Am J Ophthalmol 1991;112:317–21.
12. Martin TM, Rosenbaum JT. An update on the genetics of HLA B27-associated acute anterior uveitis. Ocul Immunol Inflamm 2011;19:108–14.
13. Monnet D, Breban M, Hudry C, Dougados M, Brezin AP. Ophthalmic findings and frequency of extraocular manifestations in patients with HLA-B27 uveitis: a study of 175 cases. Ophthalmology 2004;111:802–9.
14. Haroon M, O'Rourke M, Ramasamy P, Murphy CC, FitzGerald O. A novel evidence-based detection of undiagnosed spondyloarthritis in patients presenting with acute anterior uveitis: the DUET (Dublin Uveitis Evaluation Tool). Ann Rheum Dis 2015;74(11):1990–5.
15. Paiva ES, Macaluso DC, Edwards A, Rosenbaum JT. Characterisation of uveitis in patients with psoriatic arthritis. Ann Rheum Dis 2000;59:67–70.
16. Burgos-Vargas R, Vazquez-Mellado J, Gomez-Gordillo M, Katona G. Uveitis of juvenile ankylosing spondylitis. J Rheumatol 1989;15(6):1039.
17. Munoz-Fernandez S, Hidalgo V, Fernandez-Melon J, et al. Sulfasalazine reduces the number of flares of acute anterior uveitis over a one-year period. J Rheumatol 2003;30:1277–9.
18. Dougados M, Berenbaum F, Maetzel A, Amor B. Prevention of acute anterior uveitis associated with spondyloarthropathy induced by salazosulfapyridine. Rev Rhum 1993;60:81–3.
19. Braun J, Baraliakos X, Listing J, Sieper J. Decreased incidence of anterior uveitis in patients with ankylosing spondylitis treated with the anti-tumor necrosis factor agents infliximab and etanercept. Arthritis Rheum 2005;52:2447–51.
20. Wendling D, Paccou J, Berthelot JM, et al. New onset of uveitis during anti-tumor necrosis factor treatment for rheumatic diseases. Semin Arthritis Rheum 2011;41:503–10.
21. Rudwaleit M, Rodevand E, Holck P, et al. Adalimumab effectively reduces the rate of anterior uveitis flares in patients with active ankylosing spondylitis: results of a prospective open-label study. Ann Rheum Dis 2009;68:696–701.
22. Galor A, Perez V, Hammel J, Lowder C. Differential effectiveness of etanercept and infliximab in the treatment of ocular inflammation. Ophthalmology 2006;113:2317–23.
23. Lim LL, Fraunfelder FW, Rosenbaum JT. Do tumor necrosis factor inhibitors cause uveitis? A registry-based study. Arthritis Rheum 2007;56:3248–52.

24. Levinson RD, Rosenbaum JT. Nonsteroidal anti-inflammatory drugs for prophylaxis of acute anterior uveitis. Ocul Immunol Inflamm 2010;18:69–71.
25. Munoz-Fernandez S, Garcia-Aparicio AM, Hidalgo MV, et al. Methotrexate: an option for preventing the recurrence of acute anterior uveitis. Eye (Lond) 2009;23:1130–3.
26. Rosenbaum JT, Cousins S. Uveitis and arthritis: experimental models and clinical correlates. Semin Arthritis Rheum 1982;11:383–9.
27. Kezic JM, Glant TT, Rosenbaum JT, Rosenzweig HL. Neutralization of IL-17 ameliorates uveitis but damages photoreceptors in a murine model of spondyloarthritis. Arthritis Res Ther 2012;14:R18.
28. Kezic JM, Davey MP, Glant TT, Rosenbaum JT, Rosenzweig HL. Interferon-gamma regulates discordant mechanisms of uveitis versus joint and axial disease in a murine model resembling spondylarthritis. Arthritis Rheum 2012;64:762–71.
29. Petty RE, Johnston W, McCormick AQ, Hunt DWC, Rootman J, Rollins DF. Uveitis and arthritis induced by adjuvant: clinical, immunologic and histologic characteristics. J Rheumatol 1989;16:499–505.
30. Rehaume LM, Mondot S, Aguirre de Carcer D, et al. ZAP-70 genotype disrupts the relationship between microbiota and host, leading to spondyloarthritis and ileitis in SKG mice. Arthritis Rheumatol 2014;66:2780–92.
31. Ruutu M, Thomas G, Steck R, et al. Beta-glucan triggers spondylarthritis and Crohn's disease-like ileitis in SKG mice. Arthritis Rheum 2012;64:2211–22.

CHAPTER 17

Extra-articular manifestations: inflammatory bowel disease

Dirk Elewaut, Heleen Cypers, Matthew L. Stoll, and Charles O. Elson

Introduction to inflammatory bowel disease

SpA and IBD are entities that share common genetic and pathogenic mechanisms. A significant and reciprocal overlap exists between IBD and SpA, as evident from clinical observations and the tendency for familial aggregation. A significant number of SpA patients develop IBD, in particular CD, with a prevalence around 5–10%. Conversely, up to 30% of IBD patients develop articular disease similar to SpA (1–3). Data from a number of human and animal studies suggest that this clinical overlap stems—at least in part—from an overlap in immune-mediated pathways and that gut infection or inflammation may act as a trigger for arthritis in SpA. The first clue for a pathogenic link between the bowel and joint in SpA came from the observation that patients with certain gastrointestinal infections (*Campylobacter* spp, *Yersinia* spp, *Salmonella* spp, and *Shigella* spp) could develop an ReA, with a pattern of joint involvement typical for SpA. Up to 20% of these patients eventually develop AS (1). Moreover, in the 1980s, Cuvelier et al. showed that up to half of all SpA (axial and peripheral) patients display microscopic signs of bowel inflammation, commonly without associated gastro-intestinal symptoms (4). This has since been confirmed by several other investigators (5–10).

Bowel inflammation in SpA can affect the ileum as well as the colon, but is most prominent in the terminal ileum. Two types of inflammation can be distinguished based on histopathological characteristics: an acute type resembling infectious enterocolitis with infiltration of the epithelium with granulocytes but normal mucosal architecture, and a chronic type showing a chronic lymphoplasmacytic cellular infiltrate in the lamina propria and disturbance of mucosal architecture (Fig. 17.1). The latter type of inflammation bears particular resemblance to early CD (4). Patients with this type of inflammation also have a higher risk of evolution to full-blown CD (up to 20%), suggesting that chronic bowel inflammation in SpA could represent a preclinical form of CD. Follow-up studies showed a clear clinical relationship between gut and joint inflammation, with remission of joint inflammation being associated with disappearance of gut inflammation, and vice versa. Importantly, microscopic bowel inflammation has also been shown to be associated with a more severe SpA disease phenotype and a higher risk of developing structural damage(i.e. evolution to AS), further indicating a role for intestinal inflammation in the pathogenesis of SpA (11, 12).

The current working hypothesis of the pathogenesis of IBD is that these diseases are due to a dysregulated immune response, particularly a pathogenic CD4 T cell response, to the intestinal microbiota in a genetically susceptible host. Two lines of evidence support this hypothesis. The first is a large amount of data on experimental colitis in gene-targeted mice, which found that the intestinal microbiota was required for colitis to occur in most colitis models, and that CD4 effector T cells were the major mediators of colon inflammation (13). The second is the genetic data coming from GWAS in humans with CD and UC, which has identified many gene variants involved in host interactions with microbes (14). These independent lines of inquiry are complementary and both support the hypothesis above. That being said, in humans with IBD there is also a large environmental component that is as yet poorly defined. For example, there

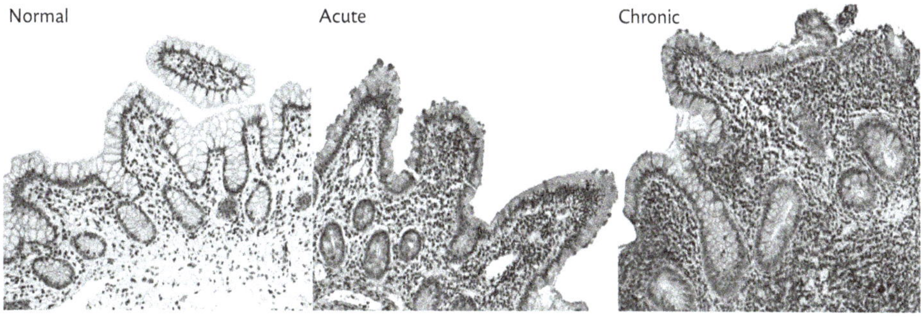

Fig. 17.1 (See colour plate section). Histological subtypes of microscopic bowel inflammation in SpA.

are large differences in IBD prevalence in the same genetically susceptible populations living in different countries. Moreover, the children of migrants from third world to first world countries develop IBD at a much higher frequency than in their native countries. This is also true of allergy and other immune-mediated diseases.

The sections that follow discuss various components of the pathogenesis of IBD and overlaps with SpA.

Intestinal microbiota

The human intestinal microbiota consists of approximately 100 trillion organisms per person, which, among them, contain about 3 million genes (the *microbiome*), one hundred times the number of unique genes in the human body (15). Despite being of microbial origin, many of these genes encode for proteins performing functions that are of direct relevance to human physiology, such as absorption of nutrients, drug metabolism, and vitamin synthesis. The last decade has witnessed significant advances in the ability to interrogate the microbiome, using techniques such as sequencing of the 16S ribosomal DNA and next generation sequencing of all microbial DNA (the *metagenome*). Although both 16S sequencing and metagenomics can provide taxonomic information on the microbiota in a sample, the metagenome data also permit direct assessment of the functional potential of the sample (16).

Numerous studies have evaluated the intestinal microbiota of subjects with IBD. One consistent finding has been decreased alpha diversity (i.e. alterations in the richness and evenness of the intestinal microbiota) (17). Richness refers to the variety of unique organisms present in the sample, while evenness, in effect, speaks to the likelihood that two sequences picked at random will represent the same species. Both appear to be altered in subjects with IBD. For example, one study found 266 unique species in the faeces of paediatric subjects with UC, compared to 758 among healthy control subjects, and UC subjects refractory to corticosteroid treatment demonstrated even lower species counts (142 vs 338) compared to steroid-responsive subjects (18). Similarly, a study of newly diagnosed children with CD and UC demonstrated decreased diversity, as measured by the Shannon and Simpson indexes, among CD (but not UC) patients compared to healthy controls, with both of these indexes being markers of evenness (19). At the taxonomic level, substantial alterations in the contents of the microbiota are generally reported in these studies. Although individual studies vary, common themes have been increases in the Proteobacteria phylum and decreased abundance of Firmicutes, including a specific organism called *Faecalibacterium prausnitzii* (20), which has been found to have anti-inflammatory properties. Functional consequences of these alterations include decreased production of short-chain fatty acids such as butyrate and proprionate, which are essential for enterocyte health and also appear to have a direct anti-inflammatory potential (21).

That the microbiota is altered in IBD does not directly prove that the alterations are responsible for the inflammatory phenotype, as it is plausible that alterations could result from the inflammatory process itself as well as from its therapy. Although some of the medications used to treat IBD, particularly antibiotics, are likely to alter the contents of the microbiota, alterations have been reported in newly diagnosed subjects naïve to immunosuppressive therapy (19). A role for altered microbiota in the pathogenesis of the disease is also supported by therapeutic responses to alterations of the microbiota. A meta-analysis of 35 studies of subjects with CD or UC concluded that addition of probiotics to standard therapy in patients with UC, although not CD, resulted in improved remission rates (22). Conversely, antibiotics can improve remission rates in CD, although their role in UC is less clear (23).

Recent studies have focused as well on faecal microbial transplants. Initial studies were limited to subjects with chronic *Clostridium difficile* infection in the context of IBD, some of whom responded to treatment (24); more recently, a prospective study of faecal microbial transplantation (FMT) in children with IBD likewise showed improvements in markers of active IBD in nine paediatric subjects, seven of whom went into remission (25). However, not all investigators are equally enthusiastic (26). Finally, another therapeutic approach for IBD is exclusive enteral nutrition (EEN), which several studies have shown to be equivalent to corticosteroids in the induction of remission (27, 28). Although its mechanism has not yet been defined, microbial alterations have been reported (29).

Given the reciprocity between bowel and joint inflammation in SpA and the overlap with IBD, intestinal microbiota could play a role in SpA as well. This could be either through a direct mechanism, whereby microorganisms or fragments thereof traffic to the joints, causing inflammation, or indirectly whereby bacteria trigger an autoimmune reaction against self-antigens by molecular mimicry. Alternatively, intestinal bacteria could skew the immune system toward a proinflammatory state, ultimately leading to joint inflammation. A proposed mechanism for linking gut and joint inflammation is recirculation of lymphocytes and macrophages primed in the intestinal mucosa and reactivated in the joint. In ReA, there is some evidence for the first mechanism: specific proliferation of synovial fluid T cells to antigens of ReA-triggering microbes has been seen (30, 31). Also, identical T cell expansions in the colon and synovium of a patient with enterogenic ReA have been shown (32). Bacterial antigens, DNA, and RNA from ReA-associated microorganisms have been detected in synovial fluid and synovial tissue from ReA patients in multiple studies (33–36). However, nucleic acids from many other bacteria, mainly commensals from skin and gut, have also been found in synovial fluid of ReA patients (37, 38). Bacterial nucleic acids can be detected in various forms of arthritis, such as RA, and neither necessarily reflect the presence of the complete bacterial genome nor indicate pathogenic significance (39–42). Moreover, long-term antibiotics have shown no benefit in ReA and peripheral SpA (43, 44).

Klebsiella has for a long time been hypothesized to be implicated in SpA pathogenesis, mainly based on elevated IgA antibodies in serum of SpA patients (45, 46). However, at this moment, a causal role for *Klebsiella* in SpA pathogenesis is still controversial and results supporting this hypothesis have not consistently been reproduced (47). The most compelling evidence for a role of microbiota in development of arthritis has come from animal models: HLA-B27-tg rats as well as SKG mice, representing animal models for SpA and IBD (as discussed in the section 'Lessons learned from experimental models'), do not develop disease when they are held in germ-free conditions (48). Moreover, an altered gut microbiome in HLA-B27 tg rats was recently revealed, with an increase in *Prevotella* spp and *Bacteroides vulgatus* and a decrease in Rikenellaceae compared to wild-type animals (49). The administration of prebiotics reduced colitis and prevented arthritis in these rats, and this effect was associated with alterations to the intestinal

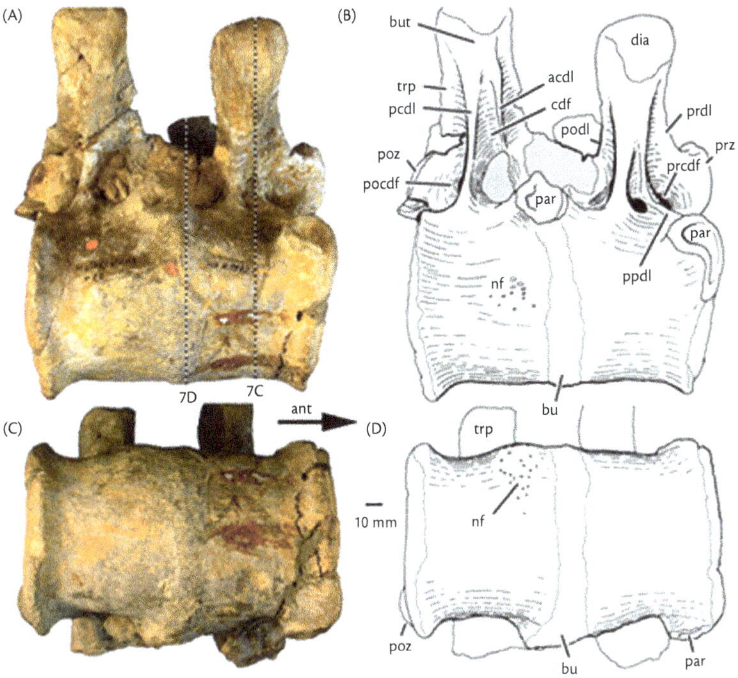

Fig. 1.1 Fused thoracic segment of *Phytosauria indet* from the Late Triassic of Halberstadt. (A, B) Right lateral view; (C, D) ventral view.
Witzmann F, Schwarz-Wings D, Hampe O, Fritsch G, Asbach P 2014: Evidence of Spondyloarthropathy in the Spine of a Phytosaur (Reptilia: Archosauriformes) from the Late Triassic of Halberstadt, Germany. Plos One 9:e85511.

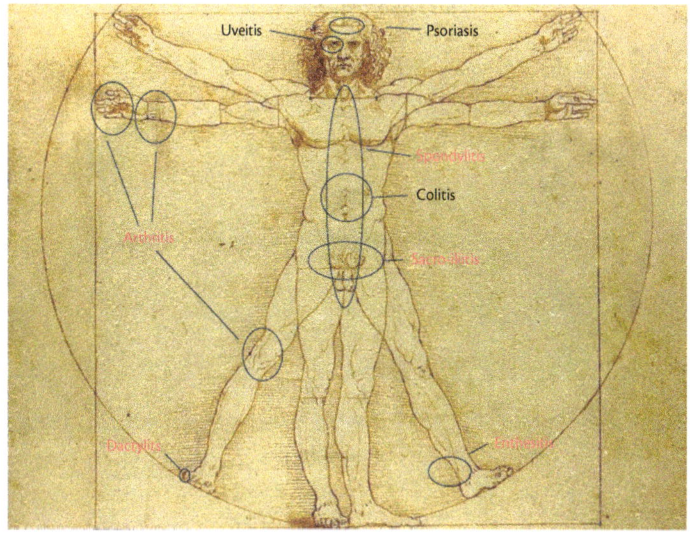

Fig. 3.3 Multiorgan involvement in SpA indicated on Leonardo da Vinci's Vitruvian Man.

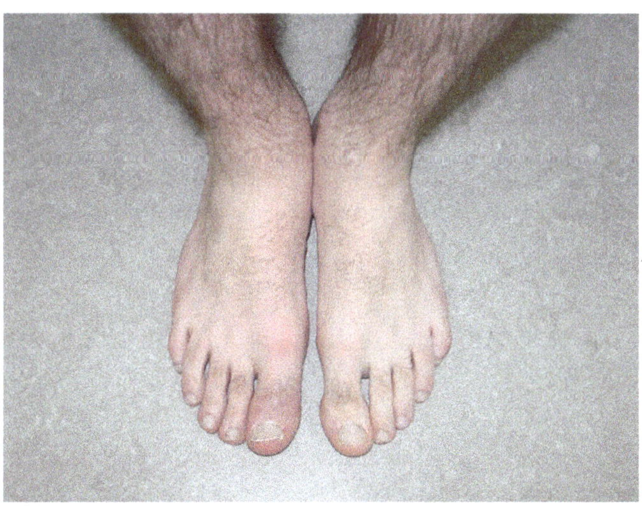

Fig. 4.1 A 25-year-old man, HLA-B27 positive, presenting with arthritis of the right toe and right ankle. This pattern of arthritis is typical of SpA.
Courtesy of M. Rudwaleit.

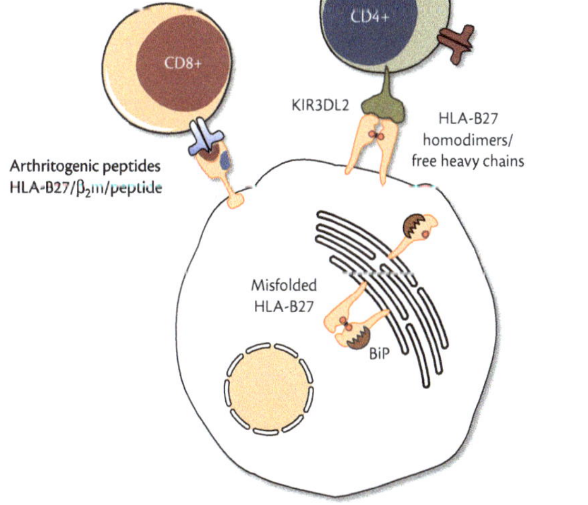

Fig. 6.1 Proposed mechanisms linking HLA-B27 to disease pathogenesis. HLA-B27 displays foreign peptides to CD8+ T cells during an infection. The T cells cross-react with self-peptides presented by HLA-B27 and thus become 'autoreactive'. Self-peptides that are specifically responsible for arthritis would be considered 'arthritogenic peptides'. HLA-B27 can form dimers on the cell surface that are capable of interacting with KIRs such as KIR3DL2, and then triggering CD4+ T cells to produce proinflammatory cytokines. HLA-B27, because of its tendency to misfold, can accumulate inside the cell where it can cause ER stress. The response to ER stress can promote proinflammatory cytokine production.

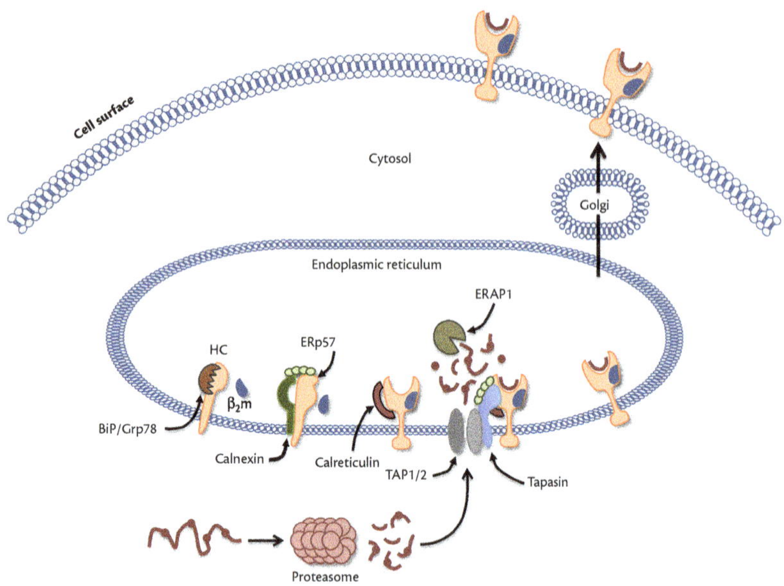

Fig. 6.2 HLA class I assembly pathway. HLA class I heavy chains are synthesized in the ER, where they interact transiently with several chaperones (binding immunoglobulin protein (BiP), calnexin, calreticulin) to facilitate folding. ERp57 is an oxidoreductase that facilitates disulphide bond formation. Folded heavy chains can bind β_2m, but remain in the ER tethered to tapasin and the peptide loading complex until optimal peptides can bind. Peptides are produced in the cytosol and transported into the ER via peptide transporters (transporter associated with antigen processing (TAP1/2), where they are further trimmed by the aminopeptidase ERAP1 (and ERAP2; not shown). Optimized HLA class I complexes are transported to the cell surface through the Golgi.

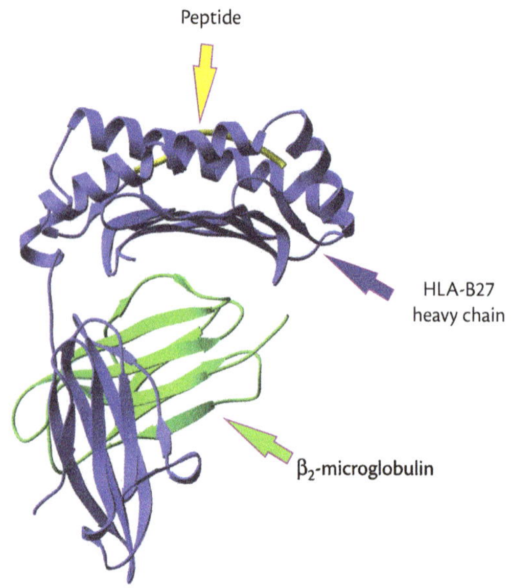

Fig. 6.3 Ribbon diagram of HLA-B27 modelled from its crystal structure. The HLA-B27 heavy chain and non-covalently attached to β_2m are arrowed. The folded heavy chain forms a peptide-binding groove, which contains a peptide, whose backbone only is shown here (arrowed). Many of the amino acids that differ between HLA-B alleles line the peptide binding groove. TCRs interact with bound peptide as regions of the HLA class I heavy chain. Only the membrane distal portion of the HLA class I molecule is shown.

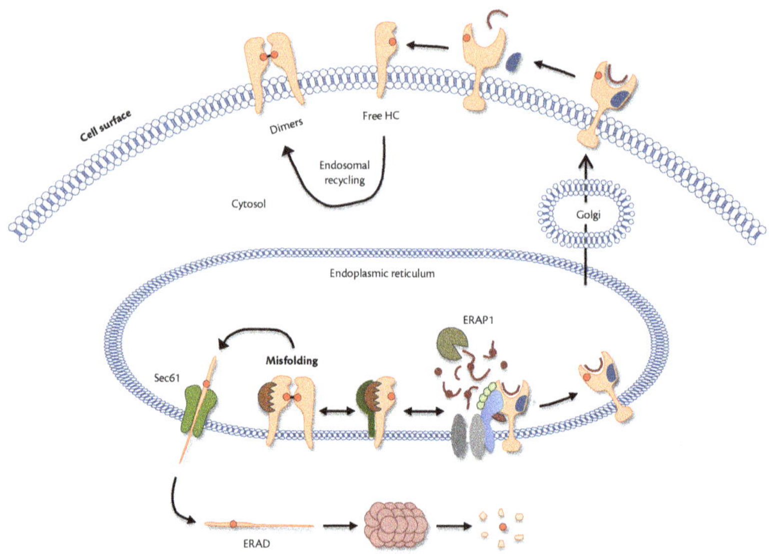

Fig. 6.4 Aberrant features of HLA-B27 cell biology. Cell surface HLA-B27 complexes can lose β_2m (and peptide) and remain as free heavy chains on the cell surface, or form disulphide-linked dimers during endosomal recycling. Newly synthesized heavy chains are slow to fold and bind β_2m in the ER, and exhibit a prolonged association with BiP. They have a tendency to dimerize due to the oxidizing environment. Accumulation of misfolded and BiP-bound heavy chains can cause ER stress.

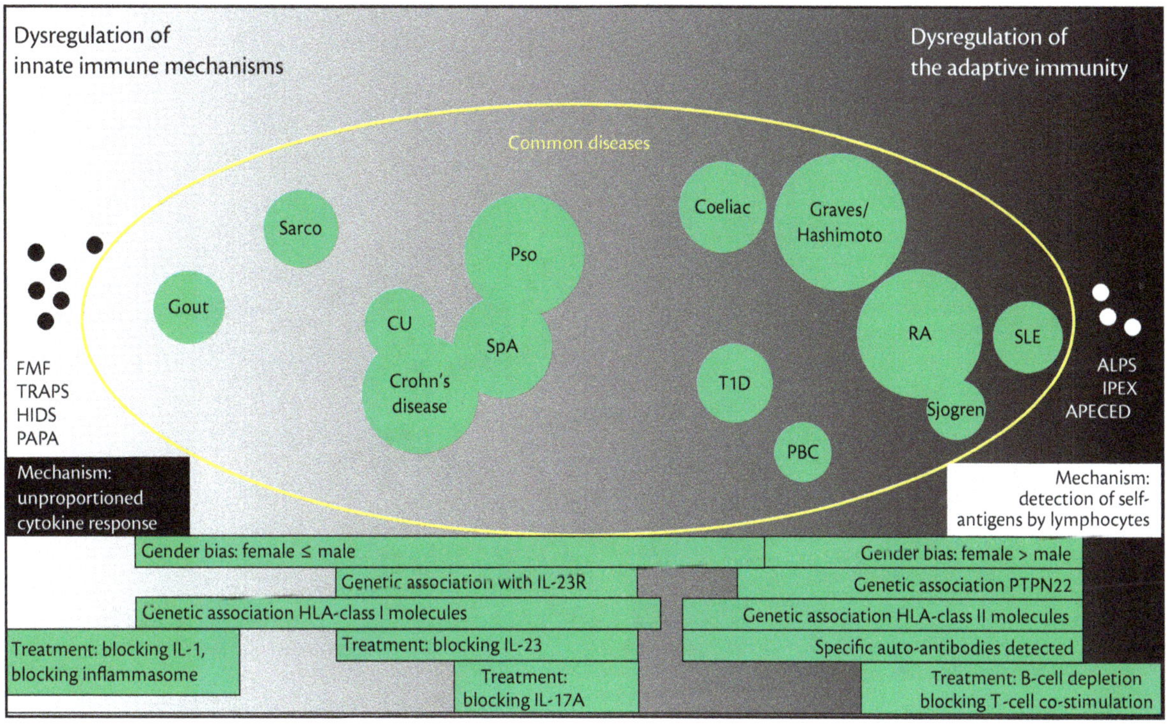

Fig. 7.1 Clustering of immune-mediated diseases based on acquired versus innate immune mechanisms. Rare monogenic diseases define the extremes of a spectrum between disease phenotypes that are caused by, on the one hand, problems in specific recognition of self-antigens by the adaptive immune system and, on the other hand, uncontrolled or inappropriate activation of innate cytokine pathways. A selection of common diseases is placed in the spectrum, based upon gender bias, genetic associations, and response to treatments. FMF, Familial Mediterranean fever; TRAPS, TNF receptor-associated periodic syndrome; HIDS, hyperimmunoglobinaemia D with periodic fever syndrome; PAPA, pyogenic arthritis pyoderma gangrenosum and severe cystic acne; ALPS, autoimmune lymphoproliferative syndrome; IPEX, immune dysregulation polyendrocrinopathy enteropathy X-linked; APECED, autoimmune polyendocrinopathy–candidiasis–ectodermal dystrophy syndrome; Sarco, sarcoidosis; CU, colitis ulcerosa; Pso, psoriasis; T1D, type I diabetes; RA, rheumatoid arthritis; PBC, primary biliary cirrhosis; SLE, systemic lupus erythematosus.

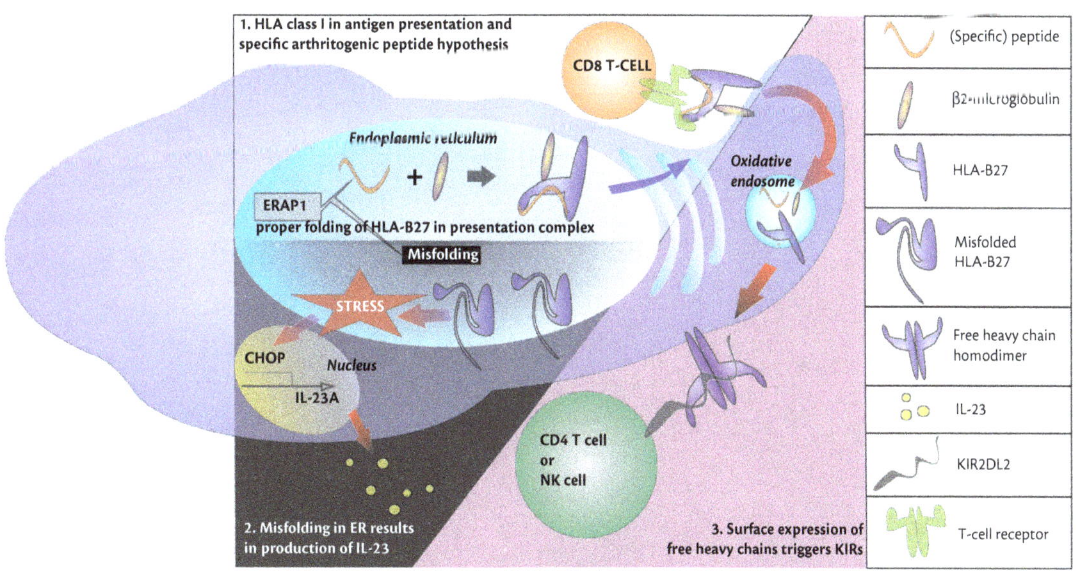

Fig. 7.2 Three theories on the contribution of HLA-B27 to SpA pathophysiology. HLA-B27 forms a heterotrimeric complex with peptide and β_2m, known as the presentation complex. The arthritogenic peptide hypothesis proposes that HLA-B27 binds a restricted peptide that is recognized by autoreactive CD8 T cells. The second theory states that misfolding of HLA-B27 occurs during formation of the presentation complex. A stress reaction is induced that is known as the unfolded protein response. This response includes upregulation of the transcription factor CHOP, which leads to expression of IL-23A. The third theory describes that the presentation complex can be internalized and that free forms of HLA-B27, including a homodimer, can be re-expressed on the cell surface. KIRs expressed on CD4+ T cells or NK cells can be triggered upon recognition of free heavy chain forms of HLA-B27. The recently discovered interaction of HLA-B27 with ERAP1, can be important for the creation of a restricted specific peptide described in the arthritogenic peptide hypothesis. Alternatively, ERAP1 is known to influence peptide availability, thus influencing the folding kinetics in the ER, which can lead to misfolding. ERAP1, Endoplasmic reticulum-associated aminopeptidase 1; CHOP, C/EBP homologous protein; IL-23, interleukin 23; KIR3DL2, killer immunoglobulin receptor 3DL2.

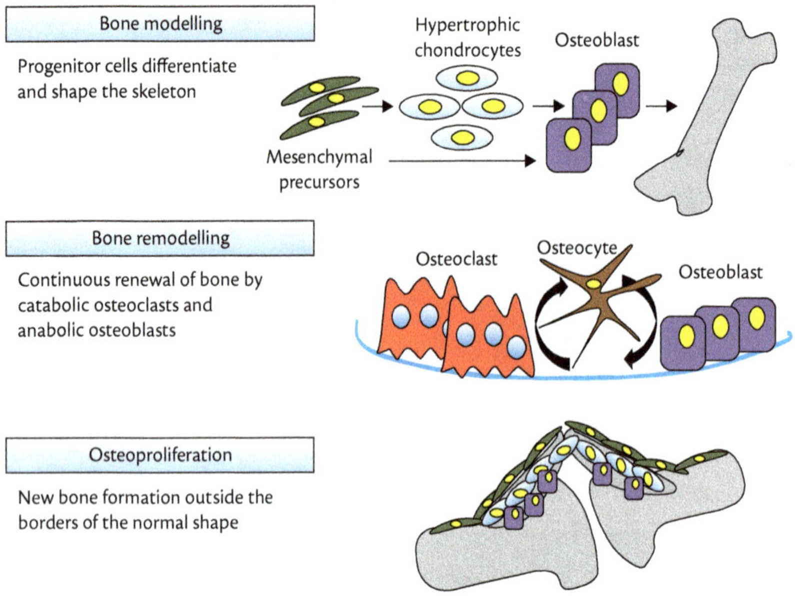

Fig. 10.1 Concepts of bone formation. Bone modelling is a developmental process that determines the shape and structure of the skeleton. In this well-orchestrated process, progenitors differentiate by endochondral or direct bone formation. Bone remodelling refers to the continuous renewal of the skeleton by bone-resorbing osteoclasts (multinucleated cells) and bone-forming osteoblasts. The osteocytes are mechanosensitive cells and orchestrate the bone remodelling cycle. Bone modelling in SpA is a disease-associated process, in which new bone formation occurs outside the original borders of the skeleton.

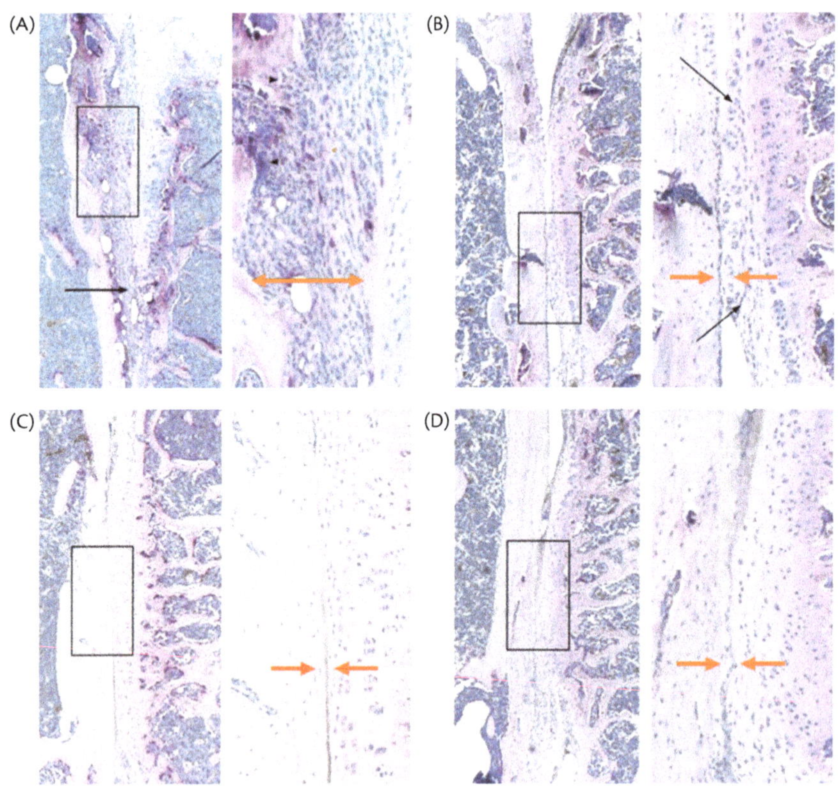

Fig. 10.4 Blockade of Dickkopf (DKK)-1 leads to ankylosis of SI joints. Microphotographs of tartrate-resistant acid phosphatase (TRAP)-stained sections counterstained with haematoxylin of SI joints of TNF tg mice. Framed inserts within left pictures show regions depicted in close-up pictures on the right. (A) Vehicle-treated TNF tg mouse with marked synovial inflammation in the SI joint (arrow) and multiple osteoclasts (arrowheads) and bone erosion (star). (B–D) Various degrees of bony proliferations and joint ankylosis after treatment with anti-DKK antibody: (B) localized chondro-osteophyte leading to narrowing of the joint gap (arrows); (C) bone and hypertrophic cartilage filling the entire joint gap; (D) bony ankylosis. Original magnification 5× (left), 20× (right). Purple dots represent osteoclasts and orange arrows mark the joint gap.

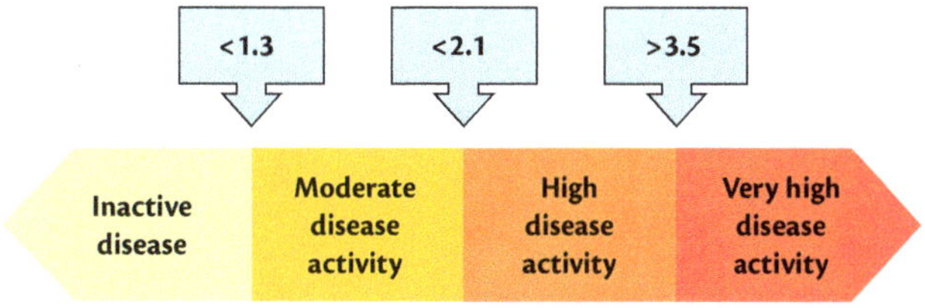

Fig. 12.2 ASDAS cut-offs for status scores.
Reproduced from Ann Rheum Dis, Machado P, Landewe R, Lie E, Kvien TK, Braun J, Baker D, et al. 70, 47–53, 2011 with permission from BMJ Publishing Group Ltd.

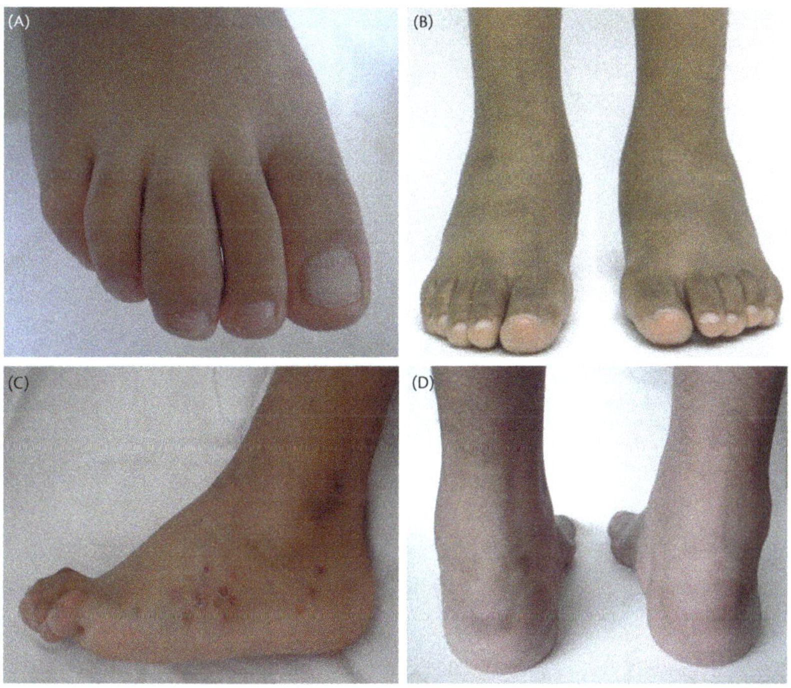

Fig. 15.1 Involvement of the feet in patients with JoSpA. (A) Dactylitis of third digit in a 12-year-old boy with uSpA. (B) Diffuse swelling of tarsal region of an 11-year-old boy with JoAS. (C) Tarsal swelling, hyperextension of digits, and keratoderma blennorrhagica in a 16-year-old boy with chronic ReA. (D) Diffuse swelling of posterior aspect of feet including ankles, Achilles, and peroneal and tibial posterior tendons in a 12-year-old-boy with uSpA.
Modified from Burgos-Vargas R, Vázquez-Mellado J. Reactive arthritides. In: Cassidy JT, Petty RE, eds. Textbook of pediatric rheumatology, 5th ed. Philadelphia: Elsevier Saunders, 2005:604–612 and Reprinted from Rheumatic Disease Clinics of North America, 28, Burgos-Vargas R, The juvenile-onset spondyloarthritides, Copyright (2002) with permission from Elsevier. In: Weisman MH, van der Heijde D, Reveille JD, eds. Ankylosing spondylitis and the spondyloarthropathies. St Louis: Elsevier Mosby, 2006:94–106.

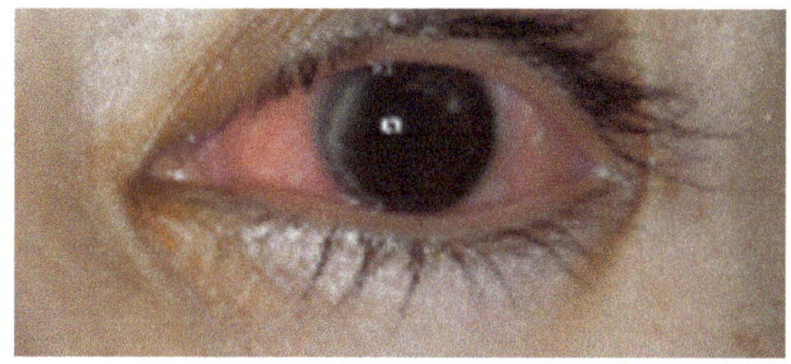

Fig. 16.1 Scleritis. Although the surface of this eye is diffusely red, the eye is redder nasally. A sector of redness suggests a scleritis or episcleritis.

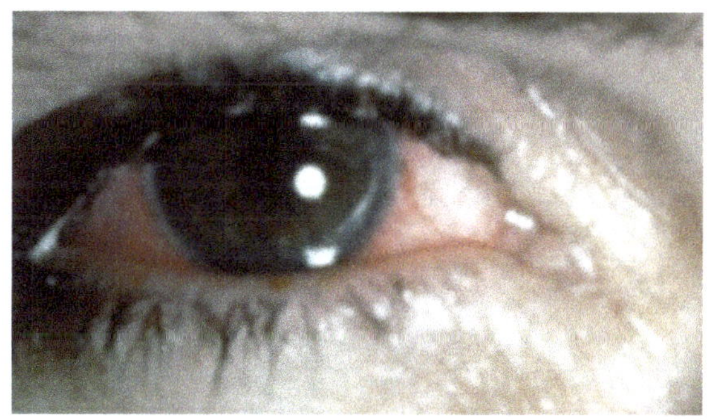

Fig. 16.2 AAU or iritis. The redness is especially prominent at the junction between the cornea and sclera. Slit lamp examination should reveal leukocytes in the anterior chamber.

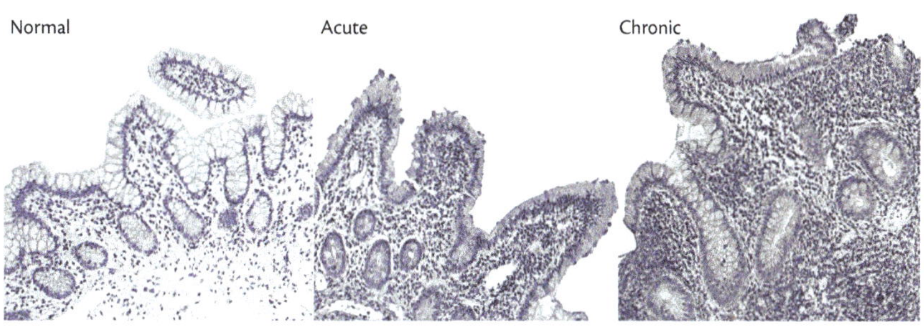

Fig. 17.1 Histological subtypes of microscopic bowel inflammation in SpA.

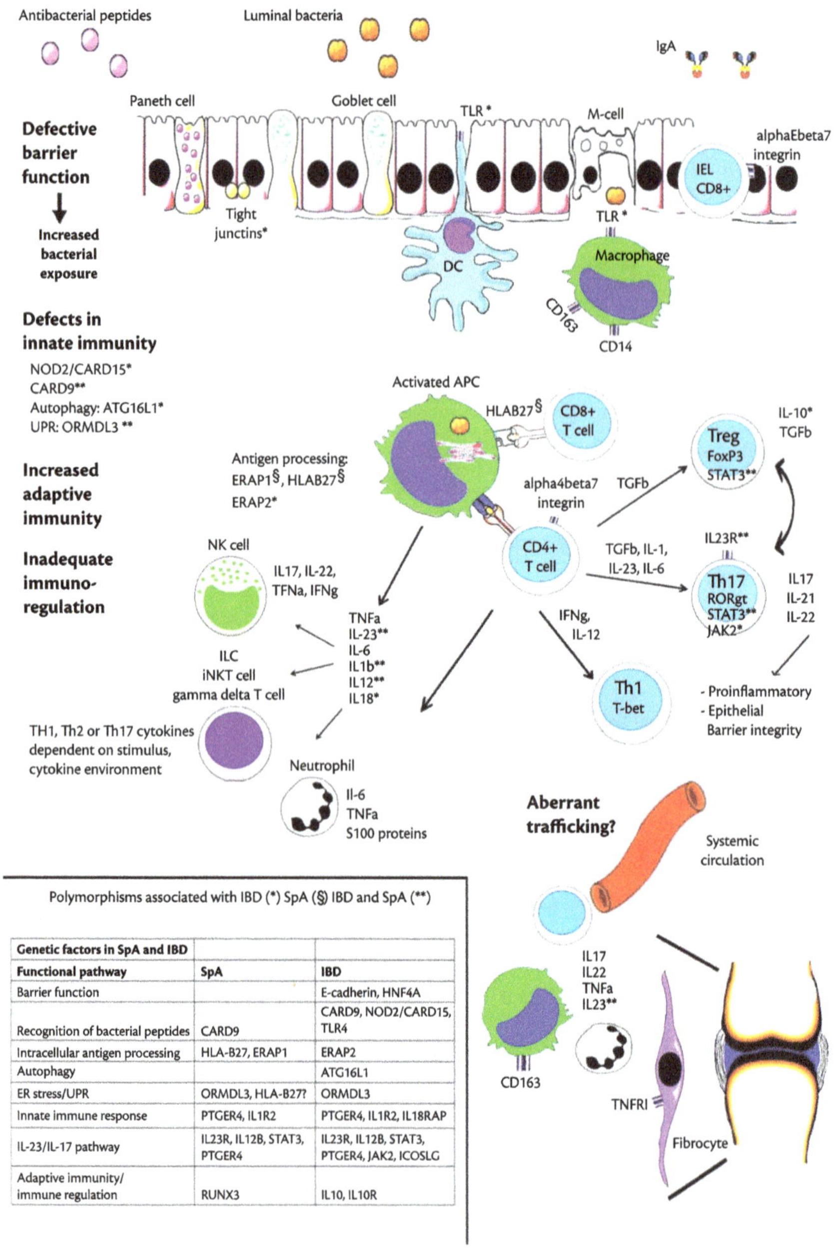

Polymorphisms associated with IBD (*) SpA (§) IBD and SpA (**)

Genetic factors in SpA and IBD		
Functional pathway	**SpA**	**IBD**
Barrier function		E-cadherin, HNF4A
Recognition of bacterial peptides	CARD9	CARD9, NOD2/CARD15, TLR4
Intracellular antigen processing	HLA-B27, ERAP1	ERAP2
Autophagy		ATG16L1
ER stress/UPR	ORMDL3, HLA-B27?	ORMDL3
Innate immune response	PTGER4, IL1R2	PTGER4, IL1R2, IL18RAP
IL-23/IL-17 pathway	IL23R, IL12B, STAT3, PTGER4	IL23R, IL12B, STAT3, PTGER4, JAK2, ICOSLG
Adaptive immunity/ immune regulation	RUNX3	IL10, IL10R

Fig. 17.2 Genetic factors in IBD and SpA and the link with pathogenesis.

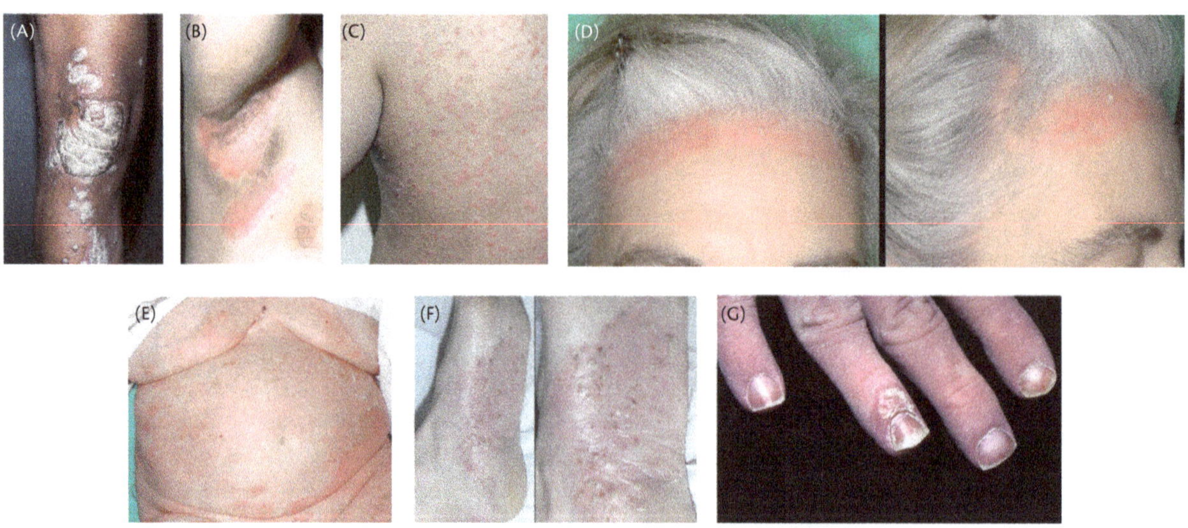

Fig. 18.1 Clinical manifestations of psoriasis. (A) Typical erythematosquamous plaques on the knee; (B) inverse psoriasis in the axilla, lacking the typical scaling but with well-demarked margins; (C) guttate psoriasis with an exanthematous distribution of hyperkeratotic papule 'sand' small plaques on the trunk; (D) scalp psoriasis affecting a small zone of the forehead; (E) generalized pustular psoriasis; (F) localized pustular psoriasis in plantar location; (G) nail psoriasis, featuring distal onycholysis (ring finger) and an 'oil drop' (index finger).

The photos from patients and histologies have been prepared by Dr E. Laffite and Prof. G. Kaya, Dpt. of Dermatology, Geneva University Hospital. They are part of the GRAPPA slide library and reproduced here with permission.

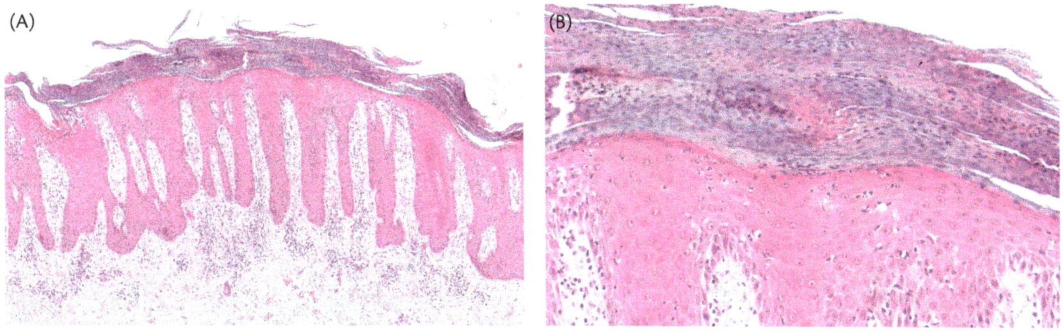

Fig. 18.2 Histological characteristics of plaque-type psoriasis. The typical epidermal features of akanthosis and papillomatosis, along with a dense mononuclear inflammatory infiltrate, are readily visible at low magnification (A), while the detail (B) shows pronounced parakeratosis.
The photos from patients and histologies have been prepared by Dr E. Laffite and Prof. G. Kaya, Dpt. of Dermatology, Geneva University Hospital. They are part of the GRAPPA slide library and reproduced here with permission.

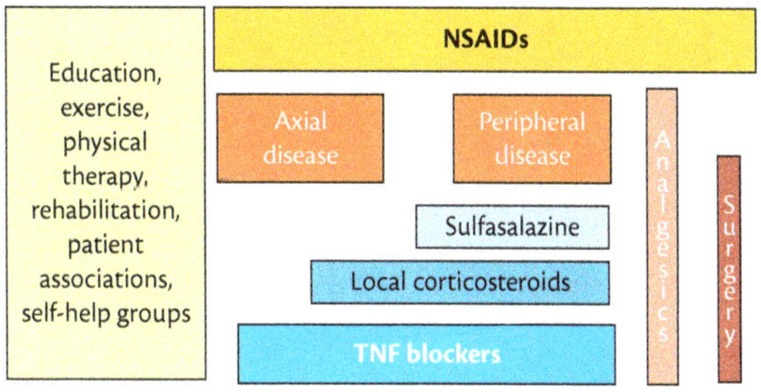

Fig. 22.1 ASAS/EULAR recommendations for the management of AS.
Reproduced from Ann Rhuem Dis, Zochling, J et al., 65, 442–52, 2006 with permission from BMJ Publishing Group Ltd. Reproduced from Ann Rhuem Dis, Braun et al., 70, 896–904, 2011 with permission from BMJ Publishing Group Ltd.

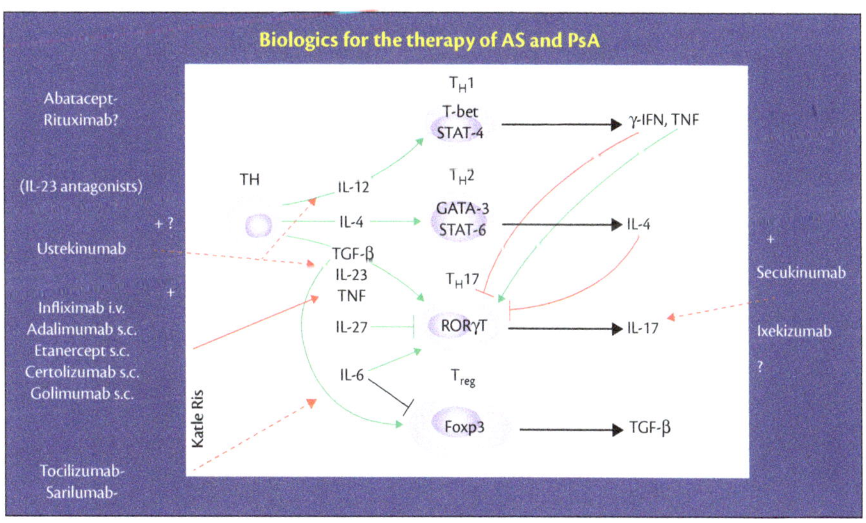

Fig. 22.3 Biologics for the therapy of AS and PsA. + Efficacy proven; – no efficacy in clinical trials; ?, not tested or results not unequivocal.
Adapted from Steinman L, Nat Med 13:144 (2007), IV ANOV I, (2006), Tato CM Nature 44 1:166 (2006).

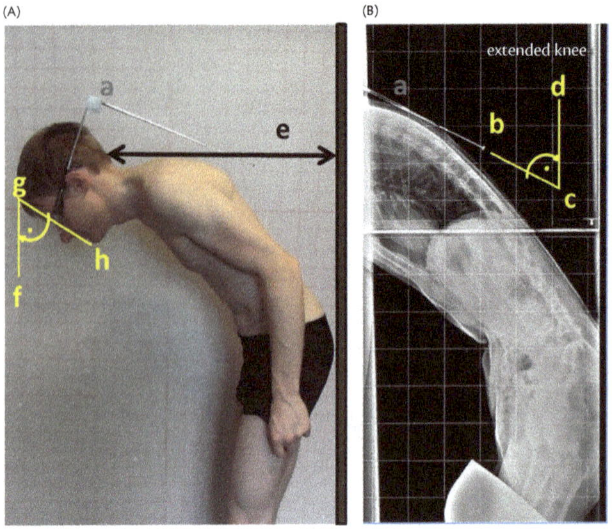

Fig. 23.3 Documentation of deranged posture clinically on standing photograph (A) and lateral X-ray (B). 'AS-spectacles', angulated and telescoping extensions on a spectacles frame, (a) allow documentation and measurement of visual axis without X-ray exposure of the head. On standing X-ray, the angle bcd between extension of the frame and the plumb-line indicates how many degrees are lost from horizontal vision. If performed standing with knees and hips extended maximally, one lateral X-ray of the trunk stores all information on global sagittal imbalance. In the case discussed, there is no thoracic hyperkyphosis and deformity derives exclusively from loss of lumbar lordosis and hip joints fused in flexion. Occiput–wall distance (e) is a measure of sagittal trunk imbalance. Chin–brow-angle fgh similar to the AS-spectacles indicates position of head and visual axis, respectively.

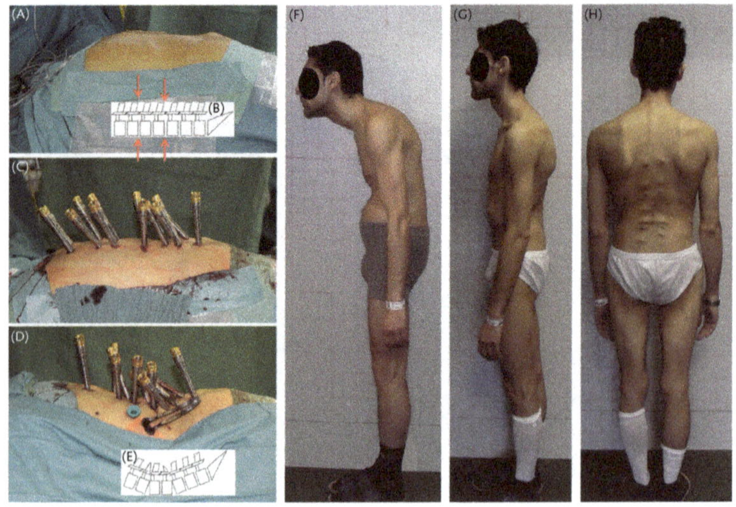

Fig. 23.8 MiDVO-R. (A) Patient positioned prone on the operative table after sterile draping. (B) Schematic of the posterior and anterior sites of osteotomies (arrows). (C) After percutaneous implantation of fixation screws and before osteotomies. (D) Change from C-shape to S-shape of the spine: microscope-assisted posterior and thoracoscopic/retroperitoneal anterior osteotomies performed, allowing correction. (E) Schematic of correction to Th12/L1 and L2/L3. (F) The same patient preoperatively in maximum extension. (G) Postoperative situation viewed from the side. (H) Directly postoperative, viewed from the back: stab incisions from screw implantation, two small incisions from posterior osteotomies, and laterally at the left side the thoracoscopic entry and at the right side the retroperitoneoscopic entry can be seen.

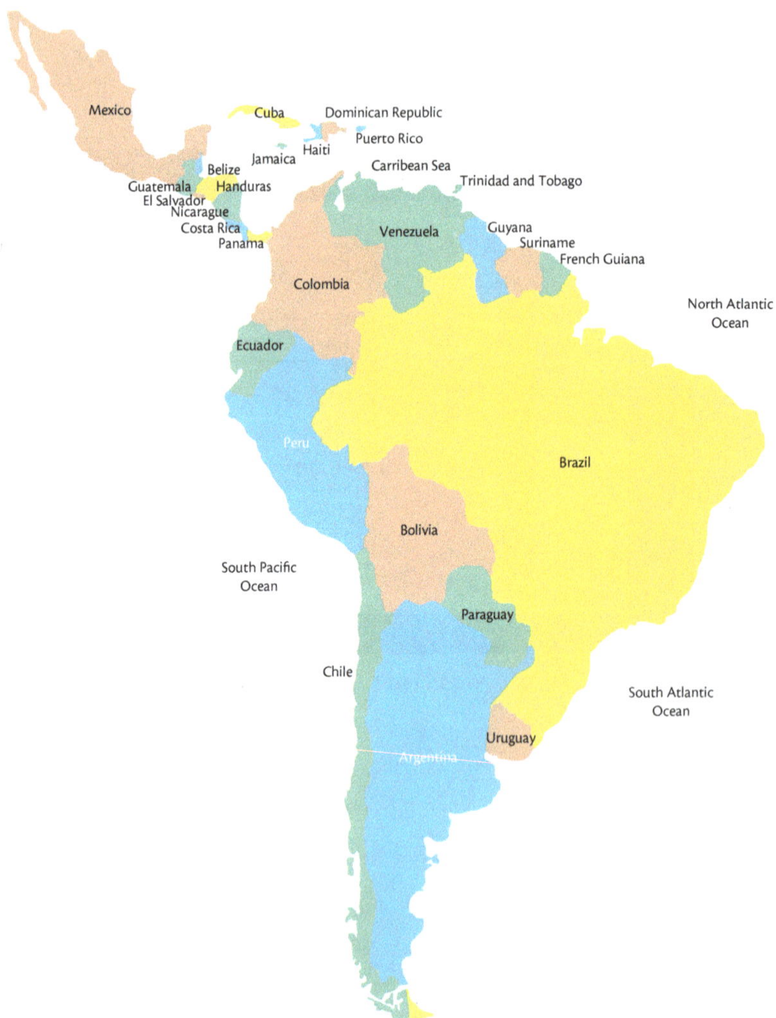

Fig. 29.1 Map of Latin America.

microbiota, decreased tissue proinflammatory cytokines, and increased immunomodulatory molecules (50).

A 2002 study evaluated the composition of the faecal microflora of 15 AS patients and 15 matched controls by denaturing gradient gel electrophoresis. No specific differences in colonization profiles were discernible between patients and controls, but there was a higher prevalence of sulphate-reducing bacteria in patients with AS (51). More recently, microbiome analyses in SpA patients have been conducted using high-throughput 16S rRNA gene sequencing, demonstrating a relatively lower diversity of intestinal microbiota in PsA characterized by a reduction in *Akkermansia* and *Ruminococcus* spp, which have also been shown to be reduced in IBD (52). A higher abundance of Lachnospiraceae, Veillonellaceae, Prevotellaceae, Porphyromonadaceae, and Bacteroidaceae was found in the terminal ileum of AS patients compared to healthy controls (53), and decreased *F. prausnitzii* has been reported in the stool of children with SpA (54). One 2010 RCT in 63 active SpA patients, however, did not show a beneficial effect of probiotics on disease activity, fatigue, quality of life, or intestinal symptoms, but it is possible that such therapies still need fine-tuning to be effective (55).

Genetics in inflammatory bowel disease and overlap with SpA

GWAS performed in subjects with CD and UC have detected upwards of 160 polymorphisms associated with IBD. Some are unique to either UC or CD, but the majority are associated with both UC and CD (14). Many of the polymorphisms associated with IBD are in genes involved with one of a limited number of functional pathways, including innate and adaptive immunity, processing of intracellular bacteria, and barrier function (14). The common theme of many of these polymorphisms is that they impact the handling of commensal organisms.

SpA is to a significant extent a genetically determined disease. A review of genetics in SpA is beyond the scope of this chapter and the focus here is on the overlap with IBD. There is indeed a remarkable genetic overlap between SpA and IBD. An Iceland genealogy database showed a three-fold increased risk of developing IBD in first-degree relatives of patients with AS, and vice versa (56). The same group also showed increased faecal calprotectin concentrations (a marker for intestinal inflammation) in patients with AS as well as in their first-degree relatives (57). Elevated faecal calprotectin levels were also reported in a study of paediatric SpA patients (58). A 2013 genotyping analysis on a cohort of European, East Asian, and Latin American patients displayed considerable concordant overlap of AS susceptibility loci with CD (12 loci), UC (11 loci), and coeliac disease (six loci) (59). Shared genetic factors have been mostly found in the IL-23/IL-17 pathway: these include polymorphisms in the IL-23 receptor gene, the IL-12B gene, signal transducer and activator of transcription 3 (STAT3), and prostaglandin E receptor 4 (PTGER4). Others have a role in innate immunity (caspase recruitment domain-containing protein 9, CARD9) or ER stress and autophagy (ORMDL Sphingolipid Biosynthesis Regulator 3, ORMDL3) (60), as shown in Fig. 17.2.

Epithelial cells and barrier

Defective barrier function can promote IBD by permitting direct access of commensal enteric organisms to the systemic immune system. While bacteria present in typically sterile locations generally result in a robust inflammatory response, we live in a state of immunologic detente with our gut microbiota. Homeostasis with the microbiota is mediated in part by lack of exposure of the systemic immune system to the microbes. So long as the commensal organisms are maintained within the intestinal lumen, periodic sampling of the lumen by intestinal dendritic cells generally results in a tolerogenic IgA response (61). This occurs largely through secretory IgA, which binds to commensal organisms, then crosses into the mucosa by binding to IgA receptors on microfold (M) cells (62). This results in the presentation of the bacterial components to tolerogenic CD11c+ CD11b+ CD103+ dendritic cells, which produce IL-10 and induce IgA class-switching of antigen-reactive B cells (63, 64). However, damage to the intestinal barrier can result in translocation of the commensal organisms or their products into the lamina propria, resulting in priming of innate immune responses and adaptive immunity.

Beyond the tight junctions of the epithelial cells, there are several components of a barrier within the lumen that minimize access of the luminal bacteria to the intestinal wall. One such component is the secretory IgA function, which by binding to commensal organisms prevents them from gaining access to the epithelium and subepithelium (65, 66). Another important component of the barrier consists of intestinal mucin, produced by goblet cells. The critical role played by intestinal mucins was demonstrated by mice deficient in the muc2 gene, which develop colitis and colon cancer (67). Not unexpectedly, they have bacteria present in normally sterile areas (68).

Antimicrobial peptides, such as RegIIIγ and cryptidins, that are produced by epithelial cells maintain a sterile zone above the intestinal epithelium (69). Interestingly, production of these peptides is dependent upon myeloid differentiation factor (MyD88), indicating that TLR signalling is likely to play a role in induction of these peptides (69, 70). Mice deficient in RegIIIγ have increased T cell immunity to the microbiota, as evidenced by increased numbers of CD4+ IFNγ cells and intestinal IgA (69).

Several polymorphisms associated with IBD can result in impaired barrier function. For example, a GWAS in UC identified the CDH1 locus on 16q22 (71). This locus codes for E-cadherin, a glycoprotein that is responsible for tight junctions between colonic epithelial cells, and is also responsible for enterocyte repair in the context of mucosal injury (71). This same study also identified the hepatocyte nuclear factor 4 alpha (HNF4A) locus on 20q13. This gene codes for the transcription factor HNF4A, which is also critical for epithelial organization and barrier formation. Mice deficient in HNF4A developed a severe colitis following colonic injury by dextran sulfate (72). Likewise, an epithelial cell conditional knockout of the CDH1 gene in mice resulted in damage to the intestinal wall, bloody diarrhoea, and death (73).

Innate immunity

Defects in innate immune responses conferring susceptibility to IBD seem to involve diminished bacterial sensing or impaired handling of commensal bacteria (e.g. through perturbed autophagy or ER stress responses). The innate immune response to bacterial antigens is mediated through germline-encoded receptors called pattern recognition receptors (PRRs) such as TLRs and nucleotide oligomerization domains (NODs). One of the earliest and most important polymorphisms identified in IBD is in the NOD2 (74).

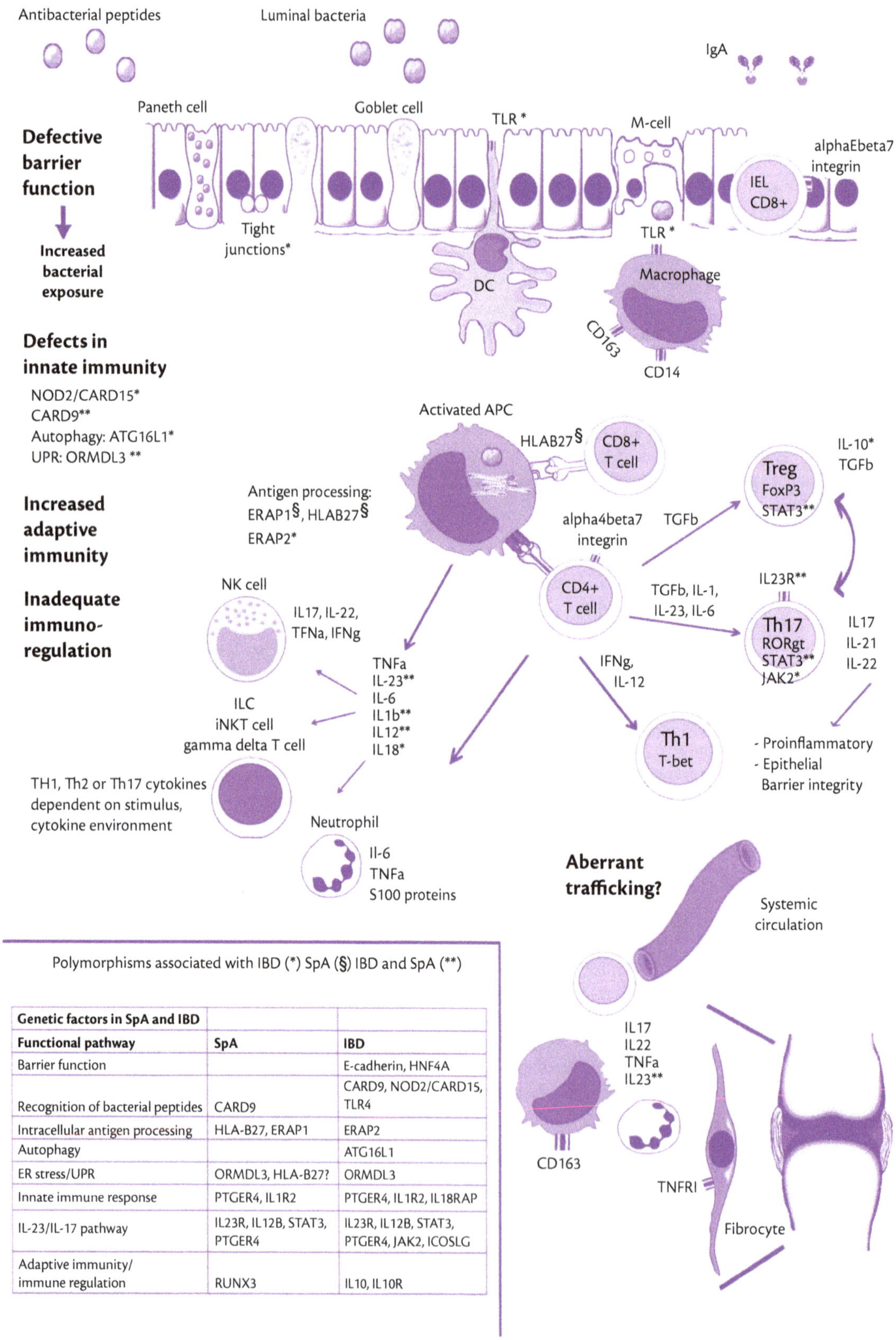

Genetic factors in SpA and IBD		
Functional pathway	**SpA**	**IBD**
Barrier function		E-cadherin, HNF4A
Recognition of bacterial peptides	CARD9	CARD9, NOD2/CARD15, TLR4
Intracellular antigen processing	HLA-B27, ERAP1	ERAP2
Autophagy		ATG16L1
ER stress/UPR	ORMDL3, HLA-B27?	ORMDL3
Innate immune response	PTGER4, IL1R2	PTGER4, IL1R2, IL18RAP
IL-23/IL-17 pathway	IL23R, IL12B, STAT3, PTGER4	IL23R, IL12B, STAT3, PTGER4, JAK2, ICOSLG
Adaptive immunity/ immune regulation	RUNX3	IL10, IL10R

Fig. 17.2 (See colour plate section). Genetic factors in IBD and SpA and the link with pathogenesis.

NOD2 recognizes muramyl dipeptide (MDP), a component of peptidoglycan that is present on most Gram-positive as well as Gram-negative bacteria (75). Thus NOD2 is a critical pattern recognition molecule, which by definition recognizes widely conserved microbial motifs and triggers rapid immunologic activation through the innate immune system (76). The NOD2 mutation associated with CD results in decreased innate immune signalling following binding of MDP (61). While this failure to initiate innate immune responses to commensal organisms can result in improper bacterial handling and may contribute to dysbiosis in IBD (77), it can also result in increased adaptive immunity to commensal organisms. Specifically, CD patients with at least one NOD2 polymorphism, compared to those with the wild-type allele, have elevated IgG anti-flagellin antibodies (78). In SpA patients, the overall prevalence of these NOD2 polymorphisms is not altered compared to healthy controls. However, they were shown to be associated with a higher risk of chronic gut inflammation (79, 80).

TLR4 binds with LPS, a component of Gram-negative bacteria. This leads to activation of the NFκB signalling pathway and a pro-inflammatory response. An association between two TLR4 mutations (Asp299Gly and Thr399Ile), causing a diminished response to LPS, was found in IBD. However, the frequency of these TLR4 mutations did not differ between patients with AS and HLA-B27-positive healthy controls (81).

A shared association between IBD and SpA involves the CARD9 gene (14, 59). CARD9 mediates signalling from dectin-1 and dectin-2 receptors, which recognize β-glucan, a component of bacterial and fungal cell walls. CARD9-deficient mice exhibit impaired intestinal epithelial repair (82). On the contrary, β-glucan administration to SKG mice (discussed in the section 'Lessons learned from experimental models') leads to an SpA/IBD-like disease (83).

Recent studies have identified defective autophagy as a critical mechanism by which the NOD2 polymorphism is associated with IBD. Autophagy is the process by which cytoplasmic materials are targeted to the lysosome for degradation. The canonical function of autophagy has been considered to be the maintenance of cellular homeostasis (84). However, recent studies have shown that it is also a process by which intracellular pathogens are degraded (84). This process, which takes place within intestinal epithelial cells and is dependent upon MyD88, is triggered by binding of NOD2 to invasive organisms, followed by recruitment of autophagy related 16-like 1, polymorphisms which are also associated with CD, to the cell membrane of the intestinal epithelial cell (84). That facilitates uptake and degradation of the organism. Mice unable to perform this function have dissemination of pathogenic as well as commensal organisms to extra-intestinal sites (84). The ATG16L1 polymorphisms associated with CD have as yet not been found to be associated with AS.

Another mechanism important for maintenance of cellular homeostasis is the UPR in response to ER stress, occurring when unfolded or misfolded proteins accumulate in the ER lumen. Polymorphisms in ORMDL3, overexpression of which facilitates the activation of the UPR, were found to be associated with CD as well as with AS, suggesting a role for ER stress in both diseases (85).

Adaptive immunity

Several GWAS polymorphisms are associated with altered adaptive immunologic responses. One such polymorphism is in the IL-23R gene and is also associated with AS and psoriasis (14). IL-23R is a heterodimer consisting of an α chain, IL-23R, and a β chain, the IL-12β1, which is shared with the IL-12 receptor (86). It binds IL-23, a cytokine produced by activated macrophages, dendritic cells, and Paneth cells (87), which supports the survival of effector Th17 cells thought to be critical to IBD and related conditions (86). The polymorphism associated with IBD results in production of a splice variant that is solubilized and thus serves as a decoy receptor for IL-23, resulting in decreased signalling of IL-23 through its membrane-bound receptor (88). This protective IL-23R polymorphism associated with IBD is predicted to result in less CD4 T effector function, because IL-23 is a major survival factor for T effector cells, particularly CD4 Th17 cells (86). IL-23R polymorphisms have also been shown to be associated with AS (89). A histopathological study showed an increased expression of IL-23 in the bowel of CD as well as of AS patients (87). Moreover, IL-23 and IL-17 are increased in synovial fluid and facet joints of SpA patients, reinforcing the role for this pathway in pathogenesis (90).

It is important to note that IL-23R is also found on many other IL-17-producing cells besides Th17 cells, such as γδ T cells, innate lymphoid cells type 3 (ILC3s), and mucosal-associated invariant T (MAIT) cells (91, 92).

Immune regulation is also impaired in IBD. CD4+CD25+ as well as CD4+FoxP3+ T cells in the intestine induce class-switching of B cells to produce IgA antibodies against commensal organisms (93, 94), in that depletion of regulatory T (Treg) cells results in substantially decreased intestinal IgA levels (94). Ablation of STAT3 in regulatory T cells in mice resulted in fatal intestinal inflammation, due to unconstrained T effector function (95). In humans with IBD, regulatory T cells are present in the lesions and function normally in in vitro assays. There may not be enough of them or they may not function properly in an inflammatory setting. Importantly, STAT3 polymorphisms are associated with IBD (14), suggesting that altered regulatory function may be responsible for some of the manifestations of the disease. Data on Treg cells in SpA are conflicting, with some investigators describing increased numbers of Treg cells in peripheral blood of AS patients, while others have not found this. Frequencies in synovial fluid were found to be increased in peripheral SpA patients compared to AS and RA patients (96). Expansion of IL-10-producing Treg cells was seen in the ileum of AS patients with chronic inflammation (97).

Several other polymorphisms in IBD are in genes coding for cytokines that influence IL-23 production and regulatory T cell function. Polymorphisms in IL-10 or its receptor are associated with both UC and CD, and loss-of-function mutations in this gene result in infantile enterocolitis that is poorly responsive to standard therapies and instead requires bone marrow transplantation (98). Recently, an association with IL-10 SNPs was also described in AS (99), and there is some evidence for a dysregulation of the IL-10 pathway in SpA from in vitro and animal studies (100). Polymorphisms in STAT3, important for Th17/Treg differentiation, are associated with both IBD and AS (14, 95, 101). Additional polymorphisms involved in Th17 differentiation include janus kinase 2 (JAK2) and inducible T-cell co-stimulator ligand (ICOSLG) (20).

The most important genetic factor in SpA is HLA-B27, most prominently in AS, with 75–95% of AS patients being HLA-B27 positive (102). In IBD the overall prevalence of HLA-B27 is comparable to that of a healthy control population; however, in patients with spondylitis and sacroiliitis, the prevalence has been reported to be between 25 and 78% (103–105). The physiological role of HLA-B27 is antigen presentation to CD8+ T cells, so initial hypotheses linking HLA-B27 with SpA involved HLA-B27 binding-specific (Gram-negative) bacterial peptides, presenting them to cytotoxic T cells, which then crossreact with endogenous peptides, leading to chronic inflammation. Anti-HLA-B27 monoclonal antibodies were found to bind *Klebsiella, Shigella*, and *Yersinia* antigens, indeed suggesting shared or crossreactive antigens. HLA-B27 has also been shown to share amino acid sequences that are identical to those found in Gram-negative bacterial proteins (106–108). However, no arthritogenic auto-antigen has yet been identified in AS. Also, the HLA-B27-tg rat model is not dependent on CD8+ T cells. On the other hand, SNPs in the runt-related transcription factor 3 (RUNX3) gene, involved in CD8+ T cell differentiation, were shown to be associated with AS (59, 109). The discovery of polymorphisms in ERAP-1 (which encodes an ER aminopeptidase involved in peptide trimming before HLA class I presentation) associated with HLA-B27-positive SpA patients, suggests that aberrant intracellular peptide processing leading to altered antigenic peptide presentation (rather than presentation of a pathogenic peptide) could be a mechanism by which HLA-B27 might predispose to disease (60, 110). Alternatively, it has been postulated that ERAP-SNPs might influence HLA-B27 misfolding leading to ER stress. However, a recent study did not find a difference in ER stress gene expression in AS patients stratified according to HLA-B27 and ERAP-SNPs expression, suggesting that other mechanisms are involved (111).

HLA-B27 might also be involved in increased translocation of certain enteric bacteria, leading to increased adaptive immunity, through defective clearing of intracellular bacteria in macrophages, analogous to mechanisms suggested in IBD pathogenesis (112). Alternatively, or additionally, HLA-B27 may contribute to SpA pathogenesis through triggering of innate immunity leading to a local proinflammatory environment in the bowel and the joint. Two hypotheses have been proposed for this, although results from animal models and functional studies do not consistently support these: HLA-B27 may form heavy chain dimers, which in turn are recognized by NK-type receptors on NK cells, monocytes, B cells, and T cells. A second hypothesis is based on the fact that HLA-B27 has a tendency to misfold in the ER, activating the UPR. A chronically activated UPR leads to a proinflammatory state, which includes upregulation of IL-23. Thus the latter hypothesis links HLA-B27 with IL-23R polymorphisms in SpA (113, 114).

Immune response against commensal organisms

Adaptive immunity

Studies in colitic mice led to the identification of microbiota flagellins as immunodominant antigens (115), antibodies against which were subsequently found to be present in about 50% of humans with CD (116). When present in patients with CD, they are associated with a complicated course (116). Specifically, patients positive for CBir1 flagellin antibodies have increased incidence of small-bowel internal-penetrating and fibrostenosing disease in adults (2005), as well as a more aggressive phenotype in children (117). The source of the flagellin antigens is *Clostridium* subphylum XIVa, mostly from the Lachnospiracaea family (118). In vitro studies are also suggestive of an immunodominant role for flagellin antigens in CD. Peripheral blood monocytes obtained from CD patients produced elevated IL-6 when exposed to flagellins, compared to monocytes obtained from either UC subjects or healthy controls (119). Likewise, lamina propria monocytes obtained from CD patients produced increased IFNγ when exposed to flagellin antigens, compared to mononuclear cells obtained from UC patients or from controls (119). Whether the antibodies against flagellins themselves are pathogenic or are markers of a T-cell-directed process awaits further exploration; however, adoptive transfer of TCR transgenic CD4 T cells specific for flagellin results in colitis, implicating the cellular response as being pathogenic (115).

Multiple other antigenic targets have been identified in subsets of individuals with CD, apparently in mutually exclusive subsets of patients. These antigens include serum IgA and IgG antibodies against oligomannan, generally known as anti-*Saccharomyces cerevisiae* antibodies; IgA antibodies against I2, derived from *Pseudomonas fluorescens*; and IgA antibodies against *E. coli* outer membrane protein (Omp) C (120). Additionally, peripheral anti-neutrophil cytoplasmic antibodies (pANCA) are associated with UC (120). Many of these antibodies have also been reported in most but not all studies of adults with SpA (121–124).

The conclusion of a 2012 systematic review, however, was that none of the current IBD-related antibodies, individually or in combination, has sufficient sensitivity to replace conventional tools in diagnosis of IBD. They may be predictive of a complicated disease course and may be useful in the differentiation between CD and UC (125).

Innate immunity

Macrophages appear to have altered function in IBD. In health, intestinal macrophages are characterized by absent CD14 expression and are generally refractory to inflammatory stimulation, despite retaining phagocytic capacity (126). Consistent with these observations, they produce the anti-inflammatory cytokine IL-10 and contribute to the differentiation of Treg rather than Th17 cells (127). In contrast, in CD lesions, intestinal macrophages do express CD14 and produce high levels of inflammatory cytokines, such as IL-23, TNFα, and IL-6 (128). Conversely, peripheral blood myeloid cells appear to have impaired function, demonstrating diminished neutrophil infiltration and clearance of killed *E. coli* injected into the forearm of human volunteers (129). Along those lines, peripheral blood mononuclear cells exposed to a variety of TLR ligands had impaired TNF production by macrophages derived from CD patients compared to healthy control subjects (130). The genetic underpinnings of this impaired macrophage function are unclear, as no links between known IBD-associated polymorphisms and macrophage function were identified (130). However, polymorphisms in IL18RAP, which is associated with IBD, resulted in diminished signalling via IL-18 and IL-1, resulting in impaired production of TNF and other proinflammatory cytokines (131).

In SpA there is some evidence for a preferred polarization to M2-type macrophages, as CD163+ macrophages, but not CD68+ macrophages, were found to be increased in SpA versus RA synovium. Moreover, the number of CD163+ macrophages correlated with global inflammation as well as with impaired lymphocyte activation. Interestingly, CD163+ macrophages were also found to be increased in colon mucosa of SpA and CD (but not UC) patients (132, 133). On the other hand, peripheral blood macrophages in AS show higher IL-23 production in response to LPS when compared to healthy controls (without signs of UPR induction) (134).

Another innate cell with altered function in IBD are ILCs present in the gut and additional tissues. ILCs are recently recognized cells that have a lymphoid origin and morphology without any capacity to rearrange antigen-specific receptors (135). ILCs have been categorized into three groups (ILC1–3), corresponding roughly to Th1, Th2, and Th17 T cells, all of which express CD127 (135). Of particular interest in IBD are the ILC3, characterized by expression of the Th17-associated transcription factor ROR-γt. A subset of these ILCs express MHC class II and present microbiota-related antigens in vivo to T cells (136, 137). Presentation of microbiota antigens to CD4 T cells by ILCs does not result in proliferative responses; instead, they delete microbiota-specific CD4 T effector cells (136, 137), and selective depletion of MHC II molecules in ILCs resulted in increased IgG levels against a variety of commensal bacteria and spontaneous colitis. ILCs were found in increased numbers in the inflamed colon of CD compared to UC patients, but the role of ILCs in human IBD awaits further clarification.

The role of ILC in the gut in SpA has not been extensively investigated. Innate-like resident lymphoid cells have been described in a murine collagen antibody-induced model of SpA. These IL-23R+, ROR-γt+CD3+CD4–CD8–, entheseal resident T cells were shown to respond to raised systemic levels of IL-23 by making IL-17A and IL-22 (138). Recently, one study reported an increase of ILC3-like cells (e.g. Lyn-RORc-Tbet+ NKp44+ cells) in the gut, synovial fluid, and bone marrow of patients with AS, which had the capacity to produce IL-17 and IL-22 and expressed α4β7 (139).

Two innate-like T cell populations with possible significance for SpA and IBD are iNKT cells and γδ T cells. Natural killer T (NKT) cells are innate-like T cells which also express NK cell-associated receptors and have important immunoregulatory properties. The most abundant and best characterized subset has an invariant TCR alpha chain with a typical Vα14-Jα18 (murine) or Vα24-Jα18 (human) rearrangement and a restricted TCR Vβ repertoire, and is referred to as invariant natural killer T (iNKT) cells. They recognize glycolipids bound to the MHC class I-like molecule CD1d, and quickly respond through the production of large amounts of Th1, Th2, and Th17 cytokines, the balance of which depends on the microenvironment as well as on the type of ligand by which the NKT cells are activated. Through this capacity, they may modulate various autoimmune diseases, although they have been shown to be able to promote as well as ameliorate certain diseases (140). In the TNFΔ^{ARE} model, a mouse model for SpA with combined ileal Crohn's-like disease and SpA due to enhanced TNF mRNA stability, disease was aggravated in NKT-deficient (Jα18–/–) mice. The chronic TNFα exposure in this model led to increased cross-talk between DCs and iNKT cells by increased CD1d expression, something that has also been shown in DCs of SpA patients. The inflammatory DCs from these mice stimulated iNKT cells to produce immunomodulatory cytokines by CD1d-mediated presentation of endogenous glycolipids. iNKT cells may therefore represent a naturally occurring counter-regulatory mechanism to attenuate TNF-driven inflammation (141).

γδ T cells are a minor population of peripheral blood, but are abundant in epithelial layers such as the skin and intestine, where they have a role in epithelial homeostasis and repair. They express a TCR comprised of γ and δ chains, which bind to an antigen independent of MHC/peptide complexes. They recognize microbiota-derived phosphoantigens, non-classic MHC class I molecules, and heat shock protein-derived peptides. Dependent on the microenvironment, γδ T cells show phenotypic and functional plasticity with Th1-, Th2-, Th17-, and Treg-like phenotypes (142). An increased number of IL-23R-positive γδ cells was found in peripheral blood of AS patients, compared to PsA, RA, and healthy controls. Moreover, these cells appeared to be a more important source of IL-17 than conventional Th17 cells (143). Both expansion and reduction of circulating or mucosal γδ cells have been reported in IBD (144). One study examining biopsies of SpA patients with gut inflammation showed an increased number of αβ intraepithelial lymphocytes, whereas γδ T cells showed no changes. This was the case as well for biopsies of CD patients in this study (145).

Lessons learned from experimental models

Many animal models of IBD have been developed, and they can be categorized according to mechanism into the following categories: spontaneous (genetic models), microbial-induced, chemical (dextran sulfate), and immune (transfer of colitogenic T cells) (13). In most of the spontaneous models, the CD4 T cell is the effector cell. Another feature of several of these models is the dependence upon an intact microbiota. For example, mice deficient in T-bet and RAG2 develop a severe form of UC (TRUC model) (146). Two lines of evidence in this model show that the microbiota are themselves at least partly responsible for the disease: (1) absence of disease when anaerobic organisms were depleted with the antibiotic metronidazole; and (2) horizontal transfer of the phenotype when T-bet–/– but RAG-sufficient mice were caged together (146). Subsequent studies identified two specific organisms, *Klebsiella pneumoniae* and *Proteus mirabella*, as being implicated in the colitis (147). Similarly, IL-10-deficient mice develop a chronic enterocolitis due to absence of the regulatory function provided by the cytokine; this condition is less severe in specific pathogen-free conditions compared to the typical housing conditions, and does not occur in germ-free IL-10-deficient mice (148).

Animal studies have also given insight as to how the intestinal microbiome shapes the mucosal immune system. For instance, segmented filamentous bacteria (SFB) have been shown to modulate the host immune system in mice through induction of IgA and Th17 cells (149). Mice lacking secondary lymphoid organs spontaneously develop specific antinuclear antibodies; this is dependent on ROR-γt and IL-17R and it is also associated with increased SFB colonization of the gut, further strengthening the role of these bacteria in generating Th17 responses (150). Colonization of mice with *Clostridia* species induces Treg cell development by stimulation of TGFβ production (151). Butyrate, a fermentation product of certain commensal bacteria, has been shown to induce the differentiation of colonic Treg cells in mice, and a reduction in butyrate-producing bacteria has been shown in IBD and juvenile SpA patients (20, 152, 153).

Three animal models combining gut and SpA-like joint inflammation are the HLA-B27-tg rat model, the TNFΔ^{ARE} murine model, and SKG mice treated with β-glucan. These models illustrate different mechanisms by which SpA-like disease can occur. For instance, both gut and joint disease in SKG mice and HLA-B27-tg rats is CD4 T cell-dependent, whereas arthritis was found to be T cell-independent in TNFΔ^{ARE} mice. Given the polygenic nature of human SpA, it is also very likely that multiple pathways would be involved in disease pathogenesis depending on the genetic background of a certain patient and environmental influences.

HLA-B27-tg rats develop enterocolitis, peripheral arthritis, sacroiliitis, and sometimes spondylitis of tail vertebrae (154). Although the canonical function of HLA-B27 is to present antigen to CD8 T cells, the latter are actually dispensable in this disease (109). However, the requirement for CD4 T cells is evidenced by the absence of disease development in thymectomized rats. As mentioned in the section 'Intestinal microbiota', these animals do not develop disease if they are held in a germ-free environment, which supports the hypothesis that the gut microbiome is a factor in the pathogenesis of both IBD and SpA (48). Also, in this model the relation between HLA-B27 upregulation, accumulation of its misfolded heavy chains, followed by the unfolded protein response and arthritis was shown for the first time (155, 156). However, although as expected, additional human β2-microglobulin reduced HLA-B27 misfolding and triggering of unfolded protein responses, surprisingly the frequency and severity of arthritis was increased, whereas no evidence of colitis was seen. Moreover, the clinical and histopathological features of this arthropathy resembled human SpA more than did the original B27-tg rats. This also implies that in this model, gut inflammation seems not to be a necessary prerequisite for the development of SpA-like articular disease (157).

The SKG mouse strain is characterized by mutation in ZAP-70, which leads to an increase of IL-17-skewed autoreactive T cells due to deficient thymic negative selection. These mice spontaneously develop an RA-like autoimmune arthritis. However, when treated with β-1,3-glucan (curdlan), a major component of bacterial and fungal cell walls, they develop a disease very similar to human SpA, with enthesitis, sacroiliitis, peripheral arthritis, dactylitis, plantar fasciitis, vertebral inflammation, ileitis resembling CD, and unilateral uveitis, illustrating the importance of interactions between the immune system and microbiota in the development of a specific disease phenotype (83). This model is T cell- and IL-23-dependent and is dependent on the microbial environment, as untreated SKG mice housed in germ-free conditions remain healthy (158). Moreover, in this model, the differential impact of genetic background and microbiota on specific disease characteristics was clearly shown: development of ileitis (and concurrent ileal IL-23 expression, ER stress, and IL-17 production) after curdlan injection was dependent on microbiota and TLR-4 signalling (i.e. absent in curdlan-treated germ-free SKG mice and significantly attenuated in TLR4-/- mice). Also, wild-type mice injected with curdlan developed arthritis, but not ileitis. Arthritis and spondylitis still developed in germ-free SKG mice, but with a low incidence, indicating that the microbiome still influenced the severity of the arthritis. Arthritis histological scores did not differ between TLR-4+/+ and TLR4-/- mice (159). Interestingly, inoculation of SKG mice with *Chlamydia muridarum* leads to a TNF-dependent ReA-like disease with arthritis, spondylitis, and dermatitis, but not colitis (160).

TNFα has emerged as a key cytokine in both IBD and SpA, which is illustrated by the beneficial effect of TNFα inhibitors in both conditions. Increased TNFα in synovial tissues and SI joints of SpA patients has been shown (161). A model particularly useful to examine TNF-driven gut and joint inflammation is the $TNF\Delta^{ARE}$ murine model. By deletion of the AU-rich elements in the regulatory sequences of the murine TNF genome, a chronic and dysregulated TNF production occurs, leading to a phenotype dominated by IBD-like intestinal inflammation and SpA-like joint disease with synovitis and sacroiliitis (162). Signalling through TNFRI was shown to be essential for the development of both bowel inflammation and arthritis. (note: gene polymorphisms linked to TNFRI are associated with SpA). Moreover, TNFRI expression limited to the stromal compartment (i.e. synovial fibroblasts and intestinal myofibroblasts) appeared to provide a sufficient target for TNF in the development of both gut and joint inflammation (163).

Mechanistic insights gleaned from therapeutic trials

The development of targeted biologic therapies has enabled new insights into the underlying mechanisms of disease based upon response to therapy. Several biologics have been trialed in IBD, with varying success (Table 17.1). Many of these trials have also been conducted in SpA. Whereas some biologic therapies were effective in both conditions, others showed clearly different effects.

TNF inhibitors

The rationale for use of TNFi in IBD and SpA is that TNF is a proximal member of an important inflammatory cytokine cascade. There are currently five TNFi on the market, of which four are monoclonal antibodies directed against TNF, with the fifth (ETN) being a soluble receptor comprised of the TNF p75 receptor fused to human IgG1 (153).

TNFi are the most widely studied of all the biologics in the management of both CD and UC. A detailed review of all of the therapeutic trials is beyond the scope of this chapter, so the reader is referred elsewhere (164). A meta-analysis of studies published to date in UC identified nine trials enrolling 1226 subjects, reporting improved short-term and long-term response rates (165). Likewise, a systematic review of adalimumab in CD identified six studies demonstrating good short-term and long-term responses, as well as mucosal healing (166). A separate meta-analysis identified three randomized trials of infliximab in CD and four of golimumab, also showing improved efficacy of inducing remission and maintaining healing (167). Interestingly, despite its effectiveness in the related conditions of psoriasis (168) and SpA (169), ETN was ineffective in CD (170). The reason for the differential responsivity to ETN compared to the monoclonal antibodies in CD is unclear. Hypotheses that have been put forward to explain this discrepancy include differences in bioavailability and pharmacodynamics, as well as biological effects at the cellular level: ETN seems less potent in inducing apoptosis of T cells and inhibiting IFNγ production, which might be a more important factor in IBD (171–173). However, certolizumab does not induce apoptosis, yet is effective in CD patients (174). An alternative explanation might be that ETN predominantly binds soluble TNF, whereas monoclonal antibodies bind both soluble and membrane-bound TNF. Inhibition of the latter may be crucial for the treatment of IBD (175). The effect of the different TNFi on microscopic gut inflammation in SpA, and the possible evolution to overt IBD, has not been investigated yet.

Anti-integrin (natalizumab, vedolizumab)

Migration of lymphocytes from the vasculature into the intestinal wall requires binding of the α4β7 integrin on the surface of the leukocyte to vascular cell adhesion molecule (VCAM) or mucosal addressin cell adhesion molecule 1 (MADCAM-1), the latter specifically present in the gut (176). The α4 integrin is targeted by natalizumab, an IgG4 monoclonal antibody directed against integrins (176). Two trials of natalizumab have been conducted in IBD.

Table 17.1 Effectiveness of different biologic therapies in SpA and IBD

		AS	PsA	IBD
TNFα inhibitors				
	Infliximab	Effective	Effective	Effective
	Adalimumab	Effective	Effective	Effective
	ETN	Effective	Effective	Ineffective
	Golimumab	Effective	Effective	Effective in UC, no trials in CD
	Certolizumab	Effective	Effective	Effective, but not approved in the EU
Anti-IL-17	Secukinumab	Effective in two phase III RCTs in both TNFi-naive patients and TNFi-non-responders (MEASURE 1 and 2)	Effective in two phase III RCTs in both TNFi-naive patients and TNFi-non-responders (FUTURE 1 and 2)	Ineffective
Anti-IL-12/IL-23	Ustekinumab	Effective in phase II open-label study (TOPAS)	Effective in phase III RCT in both TNFi-naive patients and TNFi-non-responders (PSUMMIT 1 and 2)	Effective in phase II RCT in TNFi-resistant CD patients versus placebo Phase III trials ongoing in CD and UC
JAK3 inhibition	Tofacitinib	Dose-ranging phase I trial ongoing	Phase III trial ongoing	No significant difference versus placebo in phase II trial in CD. Extension study ongoing. Effective in phase II trial in UC versus placebo. Phase III trials ongoing
Anti-integrin	Vedolizumab (α4β7 integrin)	No trials	No trials	Effective in UC (TNFi-naïve > TNFi-non responders) CD: not more effective than placebo in inducing clinical remission at week 6 in TNFi-non responders. Higher remission rates seen in TNFi-naive patients. Higher remission rates at week 52 in responders to induction. Other phase III trials in CD and UC ongoing
	Natalizumab (α4 integrin)	No trials	No trials	Effective but serious adverse events (PML). Reintroduced in 2006 in the USA using a surveillance programme and only in patients on no other immunosuppressive therapy
T cell co-stimulation blockade	Abatacept	Ineffective in two small open-label studies in AS and axSpA	Modest effect in phase II trial	Ineffective
B cell depletion	Rituximab	Modest effect in small open-label study in TNFi-naïve patients, but not in TNFi-non-responders	Modest effect in two small open-label trials	Ineffective in small RCT in UC; no other trials
For ongoing trials see https://Clinicaltrials.gov				

PML, Progressive multifocal leukoencephalopathy.

The first trial enrolled 905 subjects with CD to receive induction with natalizumab or placebo. At week 10, there was a small but statistically significant difference in the percentage of subjects with a 70-point drop in the Crohn's Disease Activity Index (CDAI) (56% vs 49%, $p = 0.05$), favouring natalizumab (177). Responders were permitted entry into the maintenance phase, in which subjects were randomized to receive the same dose of natalizumab or placebo until week 52, the outcome in this case being the proportion who sustained their response to induction therapy. This maintenance of response was observed in 103 of 168 (61%) of subjects treated with natalizumab, compared to only 48 of 170 (28%) of patients exposed to placebo ($p < 0.001$). The second study enrolled 509 subjects with CD to receive natalizumab, with outcome assessed at weeks 8–12 (178). In this study, the primary endpoint of a 70-point drop in the CDAI maintained through weeks 8–12 was seen in 48% of subjects treated with natalizumab, compared to 32% of controls. These studies led to approval of this drug, but enthusiasm for its use was dampened by reports of progressive multifocal leukoencephalopathy (176).

A different anti-integrin agent, vedolizumab, was developed to target more specifically the α4β7 integrin that is responsible for gut homing, and was evaluated in a study of 315 CD patients with prior exposure to TNFi (179). Subjects received vedolizumab 300 mg intravenously or placebo at weeks 0, 2, and 6, with the primary outcome being remission at week 6. The results indicated that the likelihood of remission was similar among the drug and placebo arms (15.2% vs 12.1%, respectively, $p = 0.433$), although there were significant differences in the secondary outcomes of remission at week 10 and CDAI response at week 6, both favouring vedolizumab. Additionally, a second arm of the study evaluated 101 subjects who were naïve to TNFi, reporting higher remission rates at week 6 (31.4% vs 12%, $p = 0.012$), as well as remission at week 10 and CDAI response at week 6, among subjects treated with vedolizumab. It is known that after infection, effector CD4 T cells have a limited lifespan, and that is likely true as well during chronic IBD. The success of these agents is compatible with the need for replenishment of pathogenic CD4 T cells from a circulating memory pool (180, 181).

Vedolizumab has also been studied in subjects with UC. The first trial was a dose-ranging study, in which subjects received placebo or 2 mg/kg, 6 mg/kg, or 10 mg/kg at 0, 2, 4, and 12 weeks (182). This was primarily a pharmacokinetics and safety study involving only 46 subjects, although effectiveness outcomes were evaluated as well. No serious adverse events attributed to the drug or serious infectious events were identified. With respect to effectiveness, drug-treated patients were more likely to demonstrate a partial Mayo score response (e.g. 60–80% at day 113) compared to placebo-treated patients (33% at day 113.) A subsequent phase 3 study exposed 374 subjects to vedolizumab (300 mg) or placebo at weeks 0 and 2, in addition to another 521 subjects who received the drug open-label (183). Responders at week 6 were subsequently randomized to receive vedolizumab every 4 weeks, every 8 weeks, or placebo as maintenance therapy for up to 52 weeks. The primary outcome at week 6 was a clinical response using the Mayo clinical scale, and the primary outcome for maintenance therapy was clinical remission at week 52. At week 6, response was seen in 47.1% of the drug arm, compared to 25.5% of placebo-treated patients. Likewise, remission at 52 weeks was observed in 44.8% of subjects receiving the drug every 4 weeks, 41.8% receiving the drug every 8 weeks, and only 15.9% of the placebo arm.

An increase in T cells carrying αEβ7 integrin (an adhesion molecule expressed on leukocytes at mucosal sites) has been described in intestinal mucosa of SpA patients, even in the absence of histological signs of gut inflammation (184). Its ligand E-cadherin was also shown to be upregulated in inflamed bowel mucosa of IBD as well as SpA patients (185). Moreover, increased expression of β7 integrins (αEβ7 and α4β7) was noted on synovial T cell lines from SpA, although this might also be the result of T cell activation, so it does not provide direct evidence for their intestinal origin (186, 187). There is no information on the effect of anti-integrin medications on arthritis in patients with IBD and concomitant joint disease.

JAK3 inhibition (tofacitinib)

The JAK family of receptors is associated with multiple cytokine receptors, including those for IL-2, IL-6, and IL-12. Upon ligation of the receptor, JAKs become activated and phosphorylate themselves, and then phosphorylate STAT3 and other downstream proteins. STAT3 dimerizes and then translocates into the nucleus, leading to activation of a variety of proinflammatory genes (188). The importance of the JAK-STAT signalling pathway to immunologic functioning is illustrated by severe combined immunodeficiency syndromes resulting from mutations in JAK3 (189). Tofacitinib is a selective oral inhibitor of the JAK family of kinases and is the only oral biologic currently available. This was studied in UC at doses of 0.5, 3, 10, and 15 mg twice daily for 8 weeks, the endpoint being a clinical response. The highest dose resulted in a statistically significant incidence of a clinical response (38/49 vs 20/48 in the placebo arm), while all three of the higher doses resulted in an increased likelihood of attaining clinical remission (190).

A dose-ranging study on tofacitinib in AS as well as a phase 3 trial in PsA are currently ongoing (https://Clinicaltrials.gov).

Anti-IL-23/-IL-12 (p40)

The role of Th17 cells in IBD has been discussed in 'Genetics in inflammatory bowel disease and overlap with SpA: Adaptive immunity'; thus the IL-17 pathway became an obvious therapeutic target. The first medication to target the pathway was ustekinumab, which is a humanized monoclonal antibody directed against the shared p40 subunit of IL-23 and IL-12. In a crossover study, 104 individuals with CD were given ustekinumab (either 90 mg subcutaneously for 4 consecutive weeks), a single intravenous dose of 4.5 mg/kg, or placebo (191). A clinical response, defined as a reduction of at least 25% and 70 points in the CDAI, was seen in slightly more ustekinumab-treated patients at weeks 4 and 6 (53% vs 30%, $p = 0.02$), which was not sustained at week 8 (49% vs 40%, $p = 0.34$). In a second study, 526 patients were randomly assigned to receive induction with intravenous ustekinumab at doses of 1, 3, or 6 mg/kg, or placebo. In the maintenance phase of the study, responders and non-responders were both re-recruited and randomized to receive either placebo or subcutaneous ustekinumab 90 mg at weeks 8 and 16, with outcome assessed at week 22. The primary endpoint of a 100-point reduction in the CDAI at week 6 was observed in 39.7% at the highest dose, compared to 23.5% in the placebo-treated patients; subjects who received lower doses had non-significant differences compared to placebo (192). Likewise, in the maintenance phase, a clinical response was seen in 69.4% versus 42.5% ($p < 0.001$), although improvement was only seen in the patients who responded to induction therapy.

A phase 3 double-blind, placebo-controlled, randomized trial in PsA (PSUMMIT 2) showed that ustekinumab (at 45/90 mg q12 weeks) led to significant and sustained (at 1 year) clinical improvement in both skin and joint symptoms (including in TNFi-experienced patients) (193). A prospective phase 2 open-label trial with ustekinumab (90 mg subcutaneously at baseline, week 4, and week 16) was also performed in AS, showing ASAS40 response in 65% of patients at week 24 (194).

Anti-IL-17A

In the context of these findings, secukinumab, a monoclonal antibody directed against IL-17A, was tested in CD (195). Fifty-nine subjects were assigned to secukinumab 10 mg/kg versus placebo intravenous × 2 doses 3 weeks apart, with outcome assessed at week 6. The investigators used a novel Bayesian analysis that incorporated historical controls, ultimately concluding that the likelihood of secukinumab being superior to placebo was only 4.4%, and the reduction in CDAI was actually higher in the controls (63.1 vs 29.2). This difference favouring placebo was most pronounced among patients with baseline markers of inflammation (elevated CRP or faecal calprotectin).

On the contrary, secukinumab has shown very rapid and high clinical response rates in moderate to severe plaque psoriasis (196). In a phase 2 placebo-controlled trial in 42 patients with PsA, however, the primary endpoint of ACR20 response at week 6 was not met. However, clinical responses, acute-phase reactant, and quality of life improvements were greater with secukinumab versus placebo (197). Moreover, results from two phase 3 trials (FUTURE 1 and 2) in PsA showed positive results of secukinumab (75/150/300 mg per 4 weeks after an intravenous or subcutaneous loading dose the first 4 weeks) versus placebo with regards to disease activity and structural damage, regardless of prior TNFi exposure (198, 199). In AS, a phase 2 trial with secukinumab showed very good and rapid results in patients with inadequate response to NSAIDs: more than 60% of patients reached the primary endpoint of ASAS20 response at week 6 (compared to 17% in the placebo group) (200). Two placebo-controlled phase 3 trials in AS were also recently reported (MEASURE 1 and 2: secukinumab 75/150 mg subcutaneously administered every 4 weeks after, respectively, an intravenous or subcutaneous loading dose for the first 4 weeks), showing positive responses regardless of prior TNFi exposure (201). The unexpected difference in response to IL-17 blockade in SpA and IBD has not yet been explained. Possibly this could be attributable to the assumed physiological role of IL-17 and IL-22 in gut homeostasis and the maintaining of epithelial barrier integrity versus a more pathological role of these cytokines in the joint (202).

T cell co-stimulation blockade (abatacept)

T cell activation of B cells requires co-stimulation with surface molecules such as CD28 (present on T cells) and CD80 and CD86 (present on B cells) (203). Cytotoxic T lymphocyte antigen 4 (CTLA-4) is expressed on activated T cells and binds to CD80/86, serving as a decoy receptor by preventing binding to CD28 (203). Abatacept is a solubilized CTLA-4 molecule fused to human IgG, which is approved for RA and JIA (204). Sandborn et al. (2012) studied abatacept in subjects with both UC and CD in a single trial, recruiting a total of 451 CD patients and 591 UC patients (205). Subjects were dosed with abatacept at 30 mg/kg, 10 mg/kg, 3 mg/kg, or placebo intravenously at weeks 0, 2, 4, and 8. Responders were assigned randomly to receive abatacept 10 mg/kg or placebo intravenously every 4 weeks through week 52. In the induction phase, CDAI response was observed in 14.5% of placebo-treated CD subjects, compared to only 15.5%, 10.2%, and 17.2% of subjects treated with the increasing doses of abatacept, all of which differences were not statistically significant. Among the responders, remission at week 52 was observed in 23.8% (10 of 42) of subjects receiving abatacept, compared to 11.1% (5 of 45) of placebo subjects. The results in the UC patients were not any more promising. Induction phase response was seen in 29.5% of placebo-treated subjects, which was actually higher than any of the three drug arms. Among the responders, remission in the maintenance phase was seen in an equal number (17.2%) of drug-treated versus placebo-treated patients.

There are several possible explanations for these findings, which are compatible with the evidence discussed in the section 'Immune response against commensal organisms', supporting roles for activated T cells in IBD. These include involvement of CD28-independent pathways in co-stimulation, diminished requirement for co-stimulation in the activation of T effector-memory cells compared to naïve T cells, and inhibition by abatacept of the activation of regulatory T cells (206). In a prospective open-label pilot study in 15 TNFi-naive AS patients and 15 TNFi- non responders, abatacept (10 mg/kg) failed to demonstrate efficacy (207). In PsA, however, an ACR20 response of 48% was seen in the abatacept (10 mg/kg) group, which was significantly higher than what was seen in the placebo group (208).

B cell depletion (rituximab)

The final class of biologics to be tested in human subjects with IBD is rituximab, which binds to the CD20 receptor present on mature B cells and depletes them (209). This was a small trial, limited to 24 subjects with UC, of whom 16 received rituximab 1 g × two infusions, the standard dosing in RA (210). Although depletion was effective, no significant difference was reported in response rate at week 4 (9/16 rituximab vs 3/8 placebo) or week 12 (5/16 rituximab vs 1/8 placebo) (211). Since the data from RA indicate that longer follow-up times are required to observe a maximal therapeutic effect (210), it is unclear what the outcome may have been if a larger sample size and more optimal study design had been employed.

Rituximab has been tested in small trials in SpA: in a phase II clinical trial in 20 patients with active AS rituximab 2–1 g was modestly efficacious in TNFi-naïve patients (50% achieved an ASAS20 response, 40% an ASAS40 response, 30% achieved ASAS partial remission, and 50% achieved a BASDAI50 response), but not in patients with inadequate response to TNFi (212). In an open-label study of nine PsA patients, rituximab showed some efficacy (213). Another open-label study in 21 patients with PsA showed modest improvement in arthritis and psoriasis, especially in TNFi-naïve patients (214).

References

1. Leirisalo-Repo M. Prognosis, course of disease, and treatment of the spondyloarthropathies. Rheum Dis Clin North Am 1998;24(4):737–51, viii.
2. Palm O, Moum B, Ongre A, Gran JT. Prevalence of ankylosing spondylitis and other spondyloarthropathies among patients with inflammatory bowel disease: a population study (the IBSEN study). J Rheumatol 2002;29(3):511–15.
3. Shivashankar R, Loftus EV Jr, Tremaine WJ, et al. Incidence of spondyloarthropathy in patients with Crohn's disease: a population-based study. J Rheumatol 2012;39(11):2148–52.
4. Cuvelier C, Barbatis C, Mielants H, De Vos M, Roels H, Veys E. Histopathology of intestinal inflammation related to reactive arthritis. Gut 1987;28(4):394–401.
5. Grillet B, de Clerck L, Dequeker J, Rutgeerts P, Geboes K. Systematic ileocolonoscopy and bowel biopsy study in spondylarthropathy. Br J Rheumatol 1987;26(5):338–40.
6. Lee YH, Ji JD, Kim JS, et al. Ileocolonoscopic and histologic studies of Korean patients with ankylosing spondylitis. Scand J Rheumatol 1997;26(6):473–6.
7. Leirisalo-Repo M, Turunen U, Stenman S, Helenius P, Seppala K. High frequency of silent inflammatory bowel disease in spondylarthropathy. Arthritis Rheum 1994;37(1):23–31.
8. Porzio V, Biasi G, Corrado A, et al. Intestinal histological and ultrastructural inflammatory changes in spondyloarthropathy and rheumatoid arthritis. Scand J Rheumatol 1997;26(2):92–8.
9. Simenon G, Van Gossum A, Adler M, Rickaert F, Appelboom T. Macroscopic and microscopic gut lesions in seronegative spondyloarthropathies. J Rheumatol 1990;17(11):1491–4.
10. Van Praet L, Van den Bosch FE, Jacques P, et al. Microscopic gut inflammation in axial spondyloarthritis: a multiparametric predictive model. Ann Rheum Dis 2013;72(3):414–17.
11. De Vos M, Mielants H, Cuvelier C, Elewaut A, Veys E. Long-term evolution of gut inflammation in patients with spondyloarthropathy. Gastroenterology 1996;110(6):1696–703.
12. Van Praet L, Jans L, Carron P, et al. Degree of bone marrow oedema in sacroiliac joints of patients with axial spondyloarthritis is linked to

gut inflammation and male sex: results from the GIANT cohort. Ann Rheum Dis 2014;73(6):1186–9.
13. Saleh M, Elson CO. Experimental inflammatory bowel disease: insights into the host–microbiota dialog. Immunity 2011;34(3):293–302.
14. Lees CW, Barrett JC, Parkes M, Satsangi J. New IBD genetics: common pathways with other diseases. Gut 2011;60(12):1739–53.
15. Qin J, Li R, Raes J, et al. A human gut microbial gene catalogue established by metagenomic sequencing. Nature 2010;464(7285):59–65.
16. Human Microbiome Project Consortium. Structure, function and diversity of the healthy human microbiome. Nature 2012;486(7402):207–14.
17. Nagalingam NA, Lynch SV. Role of the microbiota in inflammatory bowel diseases. Inflamm Bowel Dis 2012;18(5):968–84.
18. Michail S, Durbin M, Turner D, et al. Alterations in the gut microbiome of children with severe ulcerative colitis. Inflamm Bowel Dis 2012;18(10):1799–808.
19. Hansen R, Russell RK, Reiff C, et al. Microbiota of de-novo pediatric IBD: increased *Faecalibacterium prausnitzii* and reduced bacterial diversity in Crohn's but not in ulcerative colitis. Am J Gastroenterol 2012;107(12):1913–22.
20. Huttenhower C, Kostic AD, Xavier RJ. Inflammatory bowel disease as a model for translating the microbiome. Immunity 2014;40(6):843–54.
21. Segain JP, Raingeard de la Bletiere D, Bourreille A, et al. Butyrate inhibits inflammatory responses through NFkappaB inhibition: implications for Crohn's disease. Gut 2000;47(3):397–403.
22. Ghouri YA, Richards DM, Rahimi EF, Krill JT, Jelinek KA, DuPont AW. Systematic review of randomized controlled trials of probiotics, prebiotics, and synbiotics in inflammatory bowel disease. Clin Exp Gastroenterol 2014;7:473–87.
23. Kerman DH, Deshpande AR. Gut microbiota and inflammatory bowel disease: the role of antibiotics in disease management. Postgrad Med. 2014;126(4):7–19.
24. Austin M, Mellow M, Tierney WM. Fecal microbiota transplantation in the treatment of *Clostridium difficile* infections. Am J Med 2014;127(6):479–83.
25. Suskind DL, Brittnacher MJ, Wahbeh G, et al. Fecal microbial transplant effect on clinical outcomes and fecal microbiome in active Crohn's disease. Inflamm Bowel Dis 2015;21(3):556–63.
26. Ianiro G, Bibbo S, Scaldaferri F, Gasbarrini A, Cammarota G. Fecal microbiota transplantation in inflammatory bowel disease: beyond the excitement. Medicine (Baltimore) 2014;93(19):e97.
27. Soo J, Malik BA, Turner JM, et al. Use of exclusive enteral nutrition is just as effective as corticosteroids in newly diagnosed pediatric Crohn's disease. Dig Dis Sci 2013;58(12):3584–91.
28. Cameron FL, Gerasimidis K, Papangelou A, et al. Clinical progress in the two years following a course of exclusive enteral nutrition in 109 paediatric patients with Crohn's disease. Aliment Pharmacol Ther 2013;37(6):622–9.
29. Leach ST, Mitchell HM, Eng WR, Zhang L, Day AS. Sustained modulation of intestinal bacteria by exclusive enteral nutrition used to treat children with Crohn's disease. Aliment Pharmacol Ther 2008;28(6):724–33.
30. Gaston JS, Life PF, Granfors K, et al. Synovial T lymphocyte recognition of organisms that trigger reactive arthritis. Clin Exp Immunol 1989;76(3):348–53.
31. Sieper J, Braun J, Wu P, Kingsley G. T cells are responsible for the enhanced synovial cellular immune response to triggering antigen in reactive arthritis. Clin Exp Immunol 1993;91(1):96–102.
32. May E, Marker-Hermann E, Wittig BM, Zeitz M, Meyer zum Buschenfelde KH, Duchmann R. Identical T-cell expansions in the colon mucosa and the synovium of a patient with enterogenic spondyloarthropathy. Gastroenterology 2000;119(6):1745–55.
33. Gaston JS, Cox C, Granfors K. Clinical and experimental evidence for persistent *Yersinia* infection in reactive arthritis. Arthritis Rheum 1999;42(10):2239–42.
34. Gerard HC, Branigan PJ, Schumacher HR Jr, Hudson AP. Synovial *Chlamydia trachomatis* in patients with reactive arthritis/Reiter's syndrome are viable but show aberrant gene expression. J Rheumatol 1998;25(4):734–42.
35. Granfors K, Jalkanen S, Lindberg AA, et al. *Salmonella* lipopolysaccharide in synovial cells from patients with reactive arthritis. Lancet 1990;335(8691):685–8.
36. Granfors K, Jalkanen S, von Essen R, et al. *Yersinia* antigens in synovial-fluid cells from patients with reactive arthritis. N Engl J Med 1989;320(4):216–21.
37. Cox CJ, Kempsell KE, Gaston JS. Investigation of infectious agents associated with arthritis by reverse transcription PCR of bacterial rRNA. Arthritis Res Ther 2003;5(1):R1–8.
38. Siala M, Jaulhac B, Gdoura R, et al. Analysis of bacterial DNA in synovial tissue of Tunisian patients with reactive and undifferentiated arthritis by broad-range PCR, cloning and sequencing. Arthritis Res Ther 2008;10(2):R40.
39. Gerard HC, Wang Z, Wang GF, et al. Chromosomal DNA from a variety of bacterial species is present in synovial tissue from patients with various forms of arthritis. Arthritis Rheum 2001;44(7):1689–97.
40. Olmez N, Wang GF, Li Y, Zhang H, Schumacher HR. Chlamydial nucleic acids in synovium in osteoarthritis: what are the implications? J Rheumatol 2001;28(8):1874–80.
41. Pacheco-Tena C, Alvarado De La Barrera C, Lopez-Vidal Y, et al. Bacterial DNA in synovial fluid cells of patients with juvenile onset spondyloarthropathies. Rheumatology (Oxford) 2001;40(8):920–7.
42. van der Heijden IM, Wilbrink B, Tchetverikov I, et al. Presence of bacterial DNA and bacterial peptidoglycans in joints of patients with rheumatoid arthritis and other arthritides. Arthritis Rheum 2000;43(3):593–8.
43. Sieper J, Fendler C, Laitko S, et al. No benefit of long-term ciprofloxacin treatment in patients with reactive arthritis and undifferentiated oligoarthritis: a three-month, multicenter, double-blind, randomized, placebo-controlled study. Arthritis Rheum 1999;42(7):1386–96.
44. Smieja M, MacPherson DW, Kean W, et al. Randomised, blinded, placebo controlled trial of doxycycline for chronic seronegative arthritis. Ann Rheum Dis 2001;60(12):1088–94.
45. Ahmadi K, Wilson C, Tiwana H, Binder A, Ebringer A. Antibodies to *Klebsiella pneumoniae* lipopolysaccharide in patients with ankylosing spondylitis. Br J Rheumatol 1998;37(12):1330–33.
46. Maki-Ikola O, Lehtinen K, Nissila M, Granfors K. IgM, IgA and IgG class serum antibodies against *Klebsiella pneumoniae* and *Escherichia coli* lipopolysaccharides in patients with ankylosing spondylitis. Br J Rheumatol 1994;33(11):1025–29.
47. Stone MA, Payne U, Schentag C, Rahman P, Pacheco-Tena C, Inman RD. Comparative immune responses to candidate arthritogenic bacteria do not confirm a dominant role for *Klebsiella pneumonia* in the pathogenesis of familial ankylosing spondylitis. Rheumatology (Oxford) 2004;43(2):148–55.
48. Taurog JD, Richardson JA, Croft JT, et al. The germfree state prevents development of gut and joint inflammatory disease in HLA-B27 transgenic rats. J Exp Med 1994;180(6):2359–64.
49. Lin P, Bach M, Asquith M, et al. HLA-B27 and human beta2-microglobulin affect the gut microbiota of transgenic rats. PLoS One 2014;9(8):e105684.
50. Hoentjen F, Welling GW, Harmsen HJ, et al. Reduction of colitis by prebiotics in HLA-B27 transgenic rats is associated with microflora changes and immunomodulation. Inflamm Bowel Dis 2005;11(11):977–85.
51. Stebbings S, Munro K, Simon MA, et al. Comparison of the faecal microflora of patients with ankylosing spondylitis and controls using molecular methods of analysis. Rheumatology (Oxford) 2002;41(12):1395–401.
52. Scher JU, Ubeda C, Artacho A, et al. Decreased bacterial diversity characterizes the altered gut microbiota in patients with psoriatic arthritis, resembling dysbiosis in inflammatory bowel disease. Arthritis Rheumatol 2015;67(1):128–39.
53. Costello ME, Ciccia F, Willner D, et al. Intestinal dysbiosis in ankylosing spondylitis. Arthritis Rheumatol 2014 Nov 21; doi 10.1002/art.38967.

54. Stoll ML, Kumar R, Morrow CD, et al. Altered microbiota associated with abnormal humoral immune responses to commensal organisms in enthesitis-related arthritis. Arthritis Res Ther 2014;16(6):486.
55. Jenks K, Stebbings S, Burton J, Schultz M, Herbison P, Highton J. Probiotic therapy for the treatment of spondyloarthritis: a randomized controlled trial. J Rheumatol 2010;37(10):2118–25.
56. Thjodleifsson B, Geirsson AJ, Bjornsson S, Bjarnason I. A common genetic background for inflammatory bowel disease and ankylosing spondylitis: a genealogic study in Iceland. Arthritis Rheum 2007;56(8):2633–39.
57. Bjarnason I, Helgason KO, Geirsson AJ, et al. Subclinical intestinal inflammation and sacroiliac changes in relatives of patients with ankylosing spondylitis. Gastroenterology 2003;125(6):1598–605.
58. Stoll ML, Punaro M, Patel AS. Fecal calprotectin in children with the enthesitis-related arthritis subtype of juvenile idiopathic arthritis. J Rheumatol 2011;38(10):2274–75.
59. Cortes A, Hadler J, Pointon JP, et al. Identification of multiple risk variants for ankylosing spondylitis through high-density genotyping of immune-related loci. Nat Genet 2013;45(7):730–8.
60. Reveille JD. Genetics of spondyloarthritis--beyond the MHC. Nat Rev Rheumatol 2012;8(5):296–304.
61. Alexander KL, Targan SR, Elson CO 3rd. Microbiota activation and regulation of innate and adaptive immunity. Immunol Rev 2014;260(1):206–20.
62. Mantis NJ, Cheung MC, Chintalacharuvu KR, Rey J, Corthesy B, Neutra MR. Selective adherence of IgA to murine Peyer's patch M cells: evidence for a novel IgA receptor. J Immunol 2002;169(4):1844–51.
63. Iwasaki A, Kelsall BL. Unique functions of CD11b+, CD8 alpha+, and double-negative Peyer's patch dendritic cells. J Immunol 2001;166(8):4884–90.
64. Cerutti A. Location, location, location: B-cell differentiation in the gut lamina propria. Mucosal Immunol 2008;1(1):8–10.
65. Kaetzel CS. The polymeric immunoglobulin receptor: bridging innate and adaptive immune responses at mucosal surfaces. Immunol Rev 2005;206:83–99.
66. Corthesy B. Multi-faceted functions of secretory IgA at mucosal surfaces. Front Immunol 2013;4:185.
67. Johansson ME, Phillipson M, Petersson J, Velcich A, Holm L, Hansson GC. The inner of the two Muc2 mucin-dependent mucus layers in colon is devoid of bacteria. Proc Natl Acad Sci USA 2008;105(39):15064–9.
68. Johansson ME, Gustafsson JK, Holmen-Larsson J, et al. Bacteria penetrate the normally impenetrable inner colon mucus layer in both murine colitis models and patients with ulcerative colitis. Gut 2014;63(2):281–91.
69. Vaishnava S, Yamamoto M, Severson KM, et al. The antibacterial lectin RegIIIgamma promotes the spatial segregation of microbiota and host in the intestine. Science 2011;334(6053):255–8.
70. Cash HL, Whitham CV, Behrendt CL, Hooper LV. Symbiotic bacteria direct expression of an intestinal bactericidal lectin. Science 2006;313(5790):1126–30.
71. UK IBD Genetics Consortium, Barrett JC, Lee JC, et al. Genome-wide association study of ulcerative colitis identifies three new susceptibility loci, including the HNF4A region. Nat Genet 2009;41(12):1330–4.
72. Ahn SH, Shah YM, Inoue J, et al. Hepatocyte nuclear factor 4alpha in the intestinal epithelial cells protects against inflammatory bowel disease. Inflamm Bowel Dis 2008;14(7):908–20.
73. Schneider MR, Dahlhoff M, Horst D, et al. A key role for E-cadherin in intestinal homeostasis and Paneth cell maturation. PLoS One 2010;5(12):e14325.
74. Hugot JP, Chamaillard M, Zouali H, et al. Association of NOD2 leucine-rich repeat variants with susceptibility to Crohn's disease. Nature 2001;411(6837):599–603.
75. Girardin SE, Boneca IG, Viala J, et al. Nod2 is a general sensor of peptidoglycan through muramyl dipeptide (MDP) detection. J Biol Chem 2003;278(11):8869–72.
76. Biswas A, Petnicki-Ocwieja T, Kobayashi KS. Nod2: a key regulator linking microbiota to intestinal mucosal immunity. J Mol Med (Berl) 2012;90(1):15–24.
77. Strober W, Asano N, Fuss I, Kitani A, Watanabe T. Cellular and molecular mechanisms underlying NOD2 risk-associated polymorphisms in Crohn's disease. Immunol Rev 2014;260(1):249–60.
78. Papadakis KA, Yang H, Ippoliti A, et al. Anti-flagellin (CBir1) phenotypic and genetic Crohn's disease associations. Inflamm Bowel Dis 2007;13(5):524–30.
79. Crane AM, Bradbury L, van Heel DA, et al. Role of NOD2 variants in spondylarthritis. Arthritis Rheum 2002;46(6):1629–33.
80. Laukens D, Peeters H, Marichal D, et al. CARD15 gene polymorphisms in patients with spondyloarthropathies identify a specific phenotype previously related to Crohn's disease. Ann Rheum Dis 2005;64(6):930–5.
81. Adam R, Sturrock RD, Gracie JA. TLR4 mutations (Asp299Gly and Thr399Ile) are not associated with ankylosing spondylitis. Ann Rheum Dis 2006;65(8):1099–101.
82. Sokol H, Conway KL, Zhang M, et al. Card9 mediates intestinal epithelial cell restitution, T-helper 17 responses, and control of bacterial infection in mice. Gastroenterology 2013;145(3):591–601.e3.
83. Ruutu M, Thomas G, Steck R, et al. β-Glucan triggers spondylarthritis and Crohn's disease-like ileitis in SKG mice. Arthritis Rheum 2012;64(7):2211–22.
84. Benjamin JL, Sumpter R Jr, Levine B, Hooper LV. Intestinal epithelial autophagy is essential for host defense against invasive bacteria. Cell Host Microbe 2013;13(6):723–34.
85. Laukens D, Georges M, Libioulle C, et al. Evidence for significant overlap between common risk variants for Crohn's disease and ankylosing spondylitis. PLoS One 2010;5(11):e13795.
86. Di Cesare A, Di Meglio P, Nestle FO. The IL-23/Th17 axis in the immunopathogenesis of psoriasis. J Invest Dermatol 2009;129(6):1339–50.
87. Ciccia F, Bombardieri M, Principato A, et al. Overexpression of interleukin-23, but not interleukin-17, as an immunologic signature of subclinical intestinal inflammation in ankylosing spondylitis. Arthritis Rheum 2009;60(4):955–65.
88. Langrish CL, McKenzie BS, Wilson NJ, de Waal Malefyt R, Kastelein RA, Cua DJ. IL-12 and IL-23: master regulators of innate and adaptive immunity. Immunol Rev 2004;202:96–105.
89. Rahman P, Inman RD, Gladman DD, Reeve JP, Peddle L, Maksymowych WP. Association of interleukin-23 receptor variants with ankylosing spondylitis. Arthritis Rheum 2008;58(4):1020–5.
90. Appel H, Maier R, Bleil J, et al. In situ analysis of interleukin-23- and interleukin-12-positive cells in the spine of patients with ankylosing spondylitis. Arthritis Rheum 2013;65(6):1522–9.
91. Sutton CE, Mielke LA, Mills KH. IL-17-producing gammadelta T cells and innate lymphoid cells. Eur J Immunol 2012;42(9):2221–31.
92. Treiner E. Mucosal-associated invariant T cells in inflammatory bowel diseases: bystanders, defenders, or offenders? Front Immunol 2015;6:27.
93. Cerutti A, Rescigno M. The biology of intestinal immunoglobulin A responses. Immunity 2008;28(6):740–50.
94. Cong Y, Feng T, Fujihashi K, Schoeb TR, Elson CO. A dominant, coordinated T regulatory cell-IgA response to the intestinal microbiota. Proc Natl Acad Sci USA 2009;106(46):19256–61.
95. Chaudhry A, Rudra D, Treuting P, et al. CD4+ regulatory T cells control TH17 responses in a Stat3-dependent manner. Science 2009;326(5955):986–91.
96. Appel H, Wu P, Scheer R, et al. Synovial and peripheral blood CD4+FoxP3+ T cells in spondyloarthritis. J Rheumatol 2011;38(11):2445–51.
97. Ciccia F, Accardo-Palumbo A, Giardina A, et al. Expansion of intestinal CD4+CD25(high) Treg cells in patients with ankylosing spondylitis: a putative role for interleukin-10 in preventing intestinal Th17 response. Arthritis Rheum 2010;62(12):3625–34.
98. Engelhardt KR, Grimbacher B. IL-10 in humans: lessons from the gut, IL-10/IL-10 receptor deficiencies, and IL-10 polymorphisms. Curr Top Microbiol Immunol 2014;380:1–18.

99. Robinson PC, Claushuis TA, Cortes A, et al. Genetic dissection of acute anterior uveitis reveals similarities and differences in associations observed with ankylosing spondylitis. Arthritis Rheumatol 2015;67(1):140–51.
100. Stebbings SM, Taylor C, Tannock GW, Baird MA, Highton J. The immune response to autologous bacteroides in ankylosing spondylitis is characterized by reduced interleukin 10 production. J Rheumatol 2009;36(4):797–800.
101. Danoy P, Pryce K, Hadler J, et al. Association of variants at 1q32 and STAT3 with ankylosing spondylitis suggests genetic overlap with Crohn's disease. PLoS Genet 2010;6(12):e1001195.
102. Brewerton DA, Hart FD, Nicholls A, Caffrey M, James DC, Sturrock RD. Ankylosing spondylitis and HL-A 27. Lancet 1973;1(7809):904–7.
103. de Vlam K, Mielants H, Cuvelier C, De Keyser F, Veys EM, De Vos M. Spondyloarthropathy is underestimated in inflammatory bowel disease: prevalence and HLA association. J Rheumatol 2000;27(12):2860-65.
104. Purrmann J, Zeidler H, Bertrams J, et al. HLA antigens in ankylosing spondylitis associated with Crohn's disease. Increased frequency of the HLA phenotype B27,B44. J Rheumatol 1988;15(11):1658–61.
105. Steer S, Jones H, Hibbert J, et al. Low back pain, sacroiliitis, and the relationship with HLA-B27 in Crohn's disease. J Rheumatol 2003;30(3):518–22.
106. Alvarez-Navarro C, Cragnolini JJ, Dos Santos HG, et al. Novel HLA-B27-restricted epitopes from *Chlamydia trachomatis* generated upon endogenous processing of bacterial proteins suggest a role of molecular mimicry in reactive arthritis. J Biol Chem 2013;288(36):25810–25.
107. Frauendorf E, von Goessel H, May E, Marker-Hermann E. HLA-B27-restricted T cells from patients with ankylosing spondylitis recognize peptides from B*2705 that are similar to bacteria-derived peptides. Clin Exp Immunol 2003;134(2):351–9.
108. Scofield RH, Warren WL, Koelsch G, Harley JB. A hypothesis for the HLA-B27 immune dysregulation in spondyloarthropathy: contributions from enteric organisms, B27 structure, peptides bound by B27, and convergent evolution. Proc Natl Acad Sci USA 1993;90(20):9330–4.
109. May E, Dorris ML, Satumtira N, et al. CD8 alpha beta T cells are not essential to the pathogenesis of arthritis or colitis in HLA-B27 transgenic rats. J Immunol 2003;170(2):1099–105.
110. Evans DM, Spencer CC, Pointon JJ, et al. Interaction between ERAP1 and HLA-B27 in ankylosing spondylitis implicates peptide handling in the mechanism for HLA-B27 in disease susceptibility. Nat Genet 2011;43(8):761–7.
111. Kenna TJ, Lau MC, Keith P, et al. Disease-associated polymorphisms in ERAP1 do not alter endoplasmic reticulum stress in patients with ankylosing spondylitis. Genes Immun 2015;16(1):35–42.
112. Qian BF, Tonkonogy SL, Sartor RB. Aberrant innate immune responses in TLR-ligand activated HLA-B27 transgenic rat cells. Inflamm Bowel Dis 2008;14(10):1358–65.
113. Colbert RA, Tran TM, Layh-Schmitt G. HLA-B27 misfolding and ankylosing spondylitis. Mol Immunol 2014;57(1):44–51.
114. Braem K, Lories RJ. Insights into the pathophysiology of ankylosing spondylitis: contributions from animal models. Joint Bone Spine 2012;79(3):243–8.
115. Lodes MJ, Cong Y, Elson CO, et al. Bacterial flagellin is a dominant antigen in Crohn disease. J Clin Invest 2004;113(9):1296–306.
116. Targan SR, Landers CJ, Yang H, et al. Antibodies to CBir1 flagellin define a unique response that is associated independently with complicated Crohn's disease. Gastroenterology 2005;128(7):2020–8.
117. Dubinsky MC, Lin YC, Dutridge D, et al. Serum immune responses predict rapid disease progression among children with Crohn's disease: immune responses predict disease progression. Am J Gastroenterol 2006;101(2):360–7.
118. Duck LW, Walter MR, Novak J, et al. Isolation of flagellated bacteria implicated in Crohn's disease. Inflamm Bowel Dis 2007;13(10):1191–201.
119. Shen C, Landers CJ, Derkowski C, Elson CO, Targan SR. Enhanced CBir1-specific innate and adaptive immune responses in Crohn's disease. Inflamm Bowel Dis 2008;14(12):1641–51.
120. Landers CJ, Cohavy O, Misra R, et al. Selected loss of tolerance evidenced by Crohn's disease-associated immune responses to auto- and microbial antigens. Gastroenterology 2002;123(3):689–99.
121. Stoll ML. Gut microbes, immunty, and spondyloarthritis. Clin Immunol 2015;159(2):134–42.
122. Matzkies FG, Targan SR, Berel D, et al. Markers of intestinal inflammation in patients with ankylosing spondylitis: a pilot study. Arthritis Res Ther 2012;14(6):R261.
123. Mundwiler ML, Mei L, Landers CJ, Reveille JD, Targan S, Weisman MH. Inflammatory bowel disease serologies in ankylosing spondylitis patients: a pilot study. Arthritis Res Ther 2009;11(6):R177.
124. Wallis D, Asaduzzaman A, Weisman M, et al. Elevated serum anti-flagellin antibodies implicate subclinical bowel inflammation in ankylosing spondylitis: an observational study. Arthritis Res Ther 2013;15(5):R166.
125. Prideaux L, De Cruz P, Ng SC, Kamm MA. Serological antibodies in inflammatory bowel disease: a systematic review. Inflamm Bowel Dis 2012;18(7):1340–55.
126. Smythies LE, Sellers M, Clements RH, et al. Human intestinal macrophages display profound inflammatory anergy despite avid phagocytic and bacteriocidal activity. J Clin Invest 2005;115(1):66–75.
127. Denning TL, Wang YC, Patel SR, Williams IR, Pulendran B. Lamina propria macrophages and dendritic cells differentially induce regulatory and interleukin 17-producing T cell responses. Nat Immunol 2007;8(10):1086–94.
128. Kamada N, Hisamatsu T, Okamoto S, et al. Unique CD14 intestinal macrophages contribute to the pathogenesis of Crohn disease via IL-23/IFN-gamma axis. J Clin Invest 2008;118(6):2269–80.
129. Smith AM, Rahman FZ, Hayee B, et al. Disordered macrophage cytokine secretion underlies impaired acute inflammation and bacterial clearance in Crohn's disease. J Exp Med 2009;206(9):1883–97.
130. Sewell GW, Rahman FZ, Levine AP, et al. Defective tumor necrosis factor release from Crohn's disease macrophages in response to Toll-like receptor activation: relationship to phenotype and genome-wide association susceptibility loci. Inflamm Bowel Dis 2012;18(11):2120–7.
131. Hedl M, Zheng S, Abraham C. The IL18RAP region disease polymorphism decreases IL-18RAP/IL-18R1/IL-1R1 expression and signaling through innate receptor-initiated pathways. J Immunol 2014;192(12):5924–32.
132. Baeten D, Demetter P, Cuvelier CA, et al. Macrophages expressing the scavenger receptor CD163: a link between immune alterations of the gut and synovial inflammation in spondyloarthropathy. J Pathol 2002;196(3):343–50.
133. Baeten D, Moller HJ, Delanghe J, Veys EM, Moestrup SK, De Keyser F. Association of CD163+ macrophages and local production of soluble CD163 with decreased lymphocyte activation in spondylarthropathy synovitis. Arthritis Rheum 2004;50(5):1611–23.
134. Zeng L, Lindstrom MJ, Smith JA. Ankylosing spondylitis macrophage production of higher levels of interleukin-23 in response to lipopolysaccharide without induction of a significant unfolded protein response. Arthritis Rheum 2011;63(12):3807–17.
135. Hazenberg MD, Spits H. Human innate lymphoid cells. Blood 2014;124(5):700–9.
136. Hepworth MR, Monticelli LA, Fung TC, et al. Innate lymphoid cells regulate CD4+ T-cell responses to intestinal commensal bacteria. Nature 2013;498(7452):113–17.
137. Hepworth MA, Fung TC, Masur SH, et al. Immune tolerance. Group 3 innate lymphoid cells mediate intestinal selection of commensal bacteria-specific CD4+ T cells. Science 2015;348(6238):1031–5.
138. Sherlock JP, Joyce-Shaikh B, Turner SP, et al. IL-23 induces spondyloarthropathy by acting on ROR-γt+ CD3+CD4–CD8– entheseal resident T cells. Nat Med 2012;18(7):1069–76.
139. Ciccia F, Guggino G, Rizzo A, et al. Type 3 innate lymphoid cells producing IL-17 and IL-22 are expanded in the gut, in the peripheral

blood, synovial fluid and bone marrow of patients with ankylosing spondylitis. Ann Rheum Dis 2015;74(9):1739–47.
140. Drennan MB, Aspeslagh S, Elewaut D. Invariant natural killer T cells in rheumatic disease: a joint dilemma. Nat Rev Rheumatol 2010;6(2):90–8.
141. Jacques P, Venken K, Van Beneden K, et al. Invariant natural killer T cells are natural regulators of murine spondylarthritis. Arthritis Rheum 2010;62(4):988–99.
142. Paul S, Shilpi, Lal G. Role of gamma-delta (gammadelta) T cells in autoimmunity. J Leukoc Biol 2015;97(2):259–71.
143. Kenna TJ, Davidson SI, Duan R, et al. Enrichment of circulating interleukin-17-secreting interleukin-23 receptor-positive gamma/delta T cells in patients with active ankylosing spondylitis. Arthritis Rheum 2012;64(5):1420–9.
144. Al-Mossawi MH, Ridley A, Kiedel S, Bowness P. The role of natural killer cells, gamma delta T-cells and other innate immune cells in spondyloarthritis. Curr Opin Rheumatol 2013;25(4):434–9.
145. Cuvelier CA, De Wever N, Mielants H, De Vos M, Veys EM, Roels H. Expression of T cell receptors alpha beta and gamma delta in the ileal mucosa of patients with Crohn's disease and with spondylarthropathy. Clin Exp Immunol 1992;90(2):275–9.
146. Garrett WS, Lord GM, Punit S, et al. Communicable ulcerative colitis induced by T-bet deficiency in the innate immune system. Cell 2007;131(1):33–45.
147. Garrett WS, Gallini CA, Yatsunenko T, et al. Enterobacteriaceae act in concert with the gut microbiota to induce spontaneous and maternally transmitted colitis. Cell Host Microbe 2010;8(3):292–300.
148. Kuhn R, Lohler J, Rennick D, Rajewsky K, Muller W. Interleukin-10-deficient mice develop chronic enterocolitis. Cell 1993;75(2):263–74.
149. Ivanov, II, Atarashi K, Manel N, et al. Induction of intestinal Th17 cells by segmented filamentous bacteria. Cell 2009;139(3):485–98.
150. Van Praet JT, Donovan E, Vanassche I, et al. Commensal microbiota influence systemic autoimmune responses. Embo j 2015;34(4):466–74.
151. Atarashi K, Tanoue T, Shima T, et al. Induction of colonic regulatory T cells by indigenous *Clostridium species*. Science 2011;331(6015):337–41.
152. Furusawa Y, Obata Y, Fukuda S, et al. Commensal microbe-derived butyrate induces the differentiation of colonic regulatory T cells. Nature 2013;504(7480):446–50.
153. Stoll ML, Cron RQ. Treatment of juvenile idiopathic arthritis: a revolution in care. Pediatr Rheumatol Online J 2014;12:13.
154. Hammer RE, Maika SD, Richardson JA, Tang JP, Taurog JD. Spontaneous inflammatory disease in transgenic rats expressing HLA-B27 and human beta 2m: an animal model of HLA-B27-associated human disorders. Cell 1990;63(5):1099–112.
155. Turner MJ, Delay ML, Bai S, Klenk E, Colbert RA. HLA-B27 up-regulation causes accumulation of misfolded heavy chains and correlates with the magnitude of the unfolded protein response in transgenic rats: implications for the pathogenesis of spondylarthritis-like disease. Arthritis Rheum 2007;56(1):215–23.
156. Turner MJ, Sowders DP, DeLay ML, et al. HLA-B27 misfolding in transgenic rats is associated with activation of the unfolded protein response. J Immunol 2005;175(4):2438–48.
157. Tran TM, Dorris ML, Satumtira N, et al. Additional human beta2-microglobulin curbs HLA-B27 misfolding and promotes arthritis and spondylitis without colitis in male HLA-B27-transgenic rats. Arthritis Rheum 2006;54(4):1317–27.
158. Benham H, Rehaume LM, Hasnain SZ, et al. Interleukin-23 mediates the intestinal response to microbial beta-1,3-glucan and the development of spondyloarthritis pathology in SKG mice. Arthritis Rheumatol 2014;66(7):1755–67.
159. Rehaume LM, Mondot S, Aguirre de Carcer D, et al. ZAP-70 genotype disrupts the relationship between microbiota and host, leading to spondyloarthritis and ileitis in SKG mice. Arthritis Rheumatol 2014;66(10):2780–92.
160. Baillet AC, Rehaume LM, Benham H, et al. High *Chlamydia* burden promotes tumor necrosis factor-dependent reactive arthritis in SKG mice. Arthritis Rheumatol 2015;67(6):1535–47.
161. Braun J, Bollow M, Neure L, et al. Use of immunohistologic and in situ hybridization techniques in the examination of sacroiliac joint biopsy specimens from patients with ankylosing spondylitis. Arthritis Rheum 1995;38(4):499–505.
162. Kontoyiannis D, Pasparakis M, Pizarro TT, Cominelli F, Kollias G. Impaired on/off regulation of TNF biosynthesis in mice lacking TNF AU-rich elements: implications for joint and gut-associated immunopathologies. Immunity 1999;10(3):387–98.
163. Armaka M, Apostolaki M, Jacques P, Kontoyiannis DL, Elewaut D, Kollias G. Mesenchymal cell targeting by TNF as a common pathogenic principle in chronic inflammatory joint and intestinal diseases. J Exp Med 2008;205(2):331–7.
164. Billiet T, Rutgeerts P, Ferrante M, Van Assche G, Vermeire S. Targeting TNF-alpha for the treatment of inflammatory bowel disease. Expert Opin Biol Ther 2014;14(1):75–101.
165. Huang X, Lv B, Jin HF, Zhang S. A meta-analysis of the therapeutic effects of tumor necrosis factor-alpha blockers on ulcerative colitis. Eur J Clin Pharmacol 2011;67(8):759–66.
166. Song YN, Zheng P, Xiao JH, Lu ZJ. Efficacy and safety of adalimumab for the Crohn's disease: a systematic review and meta-analysis of published randomized placebo-controlled trials. Eur J Clin Pharmacol 2014;70(8):907–14.
167. Ford AC, Sandborn WJ, Khan KJ, Hanauer SB, Talley NJ, Moayyedi P. Efficacy of biological therapies in inflammatory bowel disease: systematic review and meta-analysis. Am J Gastroenterol 2011;106(4):644–59, quiz 60.
168. Strohal R, Chimenti S, Vena GA, Girolomoni G. Etanercept provides an effective, safe and flexible short- and long-term treatment regimen for moderate-to-severe psoriasis: a systematic review of current evidence. J Dermatolog Treat 2013;24(3):199–208.
169. Dougados M, van der Heijde D, Sieper J, et al. Symptomatic efficacy of etanercept and its effects on objective signs of inflammation in early nonradiographic axial spondyloarthritis: a multicenter, randomized, double-blind, placebo-controlled trial. Arthritis Rheumatol 2014;66(8):2091–102.
170. Sandborn WJ, Hanauer SB, Katz S, et al. Etanercept for active Crohn's disease: a randomized, double-blind, placebo-controlled trial. Gastroenterology 2001;121(5):1088–94.
171. Furst DE, Wallis R, Broder M, Beenhouwer DO. Tumor necrosis factor antagonists: different kinetics and/or mechanisms of action may explain differences in the risk for developing granulomatous infection. Semin Arthritis Rheum 2006;36(3):159–67.
172. Zou J, Rudwaleit M, Brandt J, Thiel A, Braun J, Sieper J. Up regulation of the production of tumour necrosis factor alpha and interferon gamma by T cells in ankylosing spondylitis during treatment with etanercept. Ann Rheum Dis 2003;62(6):561–4.
173. Zou J, Rudwaleit M, Brandt J, Thiel A, Braun J, Sieper J. Down-regulation of the nonspecific and antigen-specific T cell cytokine response in ankylosing spondylitis during treatment with infliximab. Arthritis Rheum 2003;48(3):780–90.
174. Bourne T, Fossati G, Nesbitt A. A PEGylated Fab' fragment against tumor necrosis factor for the treatment of Crohn disease: exploring a new mechanism of action. BioDrugs 2008;22(5):331–7.
175. Perrier C, de Hertogh G, Cremer J, et al. Neutralization of membrane TNF, but not soluble TNF, is crucial for the treatment of experimental colitis. Inflamm Bowel Dis 2013;19(2):246–53.
176. Danese S, Panes J. Development of drugs to target interactions between leukocytes and endothelial cells and treatment algorithms for inflammatory bowel diseases. Gastroenterology 2014;147(5):981–9.
177. Sandborn WJ, Colombel JF, Enns R, et al. Natalizumab induction and maintenance therapy for Crohn's disease. N Engl J Med 2005;353(18):1912–25.

178. Targan SR, Feagan BG, Fedorak RN, et al. Natalizumab for the treatment of active Crohn's disease: results of the ENCORE Trial. Gastroenterology 2007;132(5):1672–83.
179. Sands BE, Feagan BG, Rutgeerts P, et al. Effects of vedolizumab induction therapy for patients with Crohn's disease in whom tumor necrosis factor antagonist treatment failed. Gastroenterology 2014;147(3):618–27 e3.
180. Hand TW, Dos Santos LM, Bouladoux N, et al. Acute gastrointestinal infection induces long-lived microbiota-specific T cell responses. Science 2012;337(6101):1553–6.
181. Kanai T, Nemoto Y, Tomita T, Totsuka T, Watanabe M, Hibi T. Persistent retention of colitogenic CD4+ memory T cells causes inflammatory bowel diseases to become intractable. Inflamm Bowel Dis 2009;15(6):926–34.
182. Parikh A, Leach T, Wyant T, et al. Vedolizumab for the treatment of active ulcerative colitis: a randomized controlled phase 2 dose-ranging study. Inflamm Bowel Dis 2012;18(8):1470–9.
183. Feagan BG, Rutgeerts P, Sands BE, et al. Vedolizumab as induction and maintenance therapy for ulcerative colitis. N Engl J Med 2013;369(8):699–710.
184. Demetter P, Van Huysse JA, De Keyser F, et al. Increase in lymphoid follicles and leukocyte adhesion molecules emphasizes a role for the gut in spondyloarthropathy pathogenesis. J Pathol 2002;198(4):517–22.
185. Demetter P, Baeten D, De Keyser F, et al. Subclinical gut inflammation in spondyloarthropathy patients is associated with upregulation of the E-cadherin/catenin complex. Ann Rheum Dis 2000;59(3):211–16.
186. Elewaut D, De Keyser F, Van Den Bosch F, et al. Enrichment of T cells carrying beta7 integrins in inflamed synovial tissue from patients with early spondyloarthropathy, compared to rheumatoid arthritis. J Rheumatol 1998;25(10):1932–7.
187. Van Damme N, Elewaut D, Baeten D, et al. Gut mucosal T cell lines from ankylosing spondylitis patients are enriched with alphaEbeta7 integrin. Clin Exp Rheumatol 2001;19(6):681–7.
188. Villarino AV, Kanno Y, Ferdinand JR, O'Shea JJ. Mechanisms of Jak/STAT signaling in immunity and disease. J Immunol 2015;194(1):21–7.
189. Noguchi M, Yi H, Rosenblatt HM, et al. Interleukin-2 receptor gamma chain mutation results in X-linked severe combined immunodeficiency in humans. Cell 1993;73(1):147–57.
190. Sandborn WJ, Ghosh S, Panes J, et al. Tofacitinib, an oral Janus kinase inhibitor, in active ulcerative colitis. N Engl J Med 2012;367(7):616–24.
191. Sandborn WJ, Feagan BG, Fedorak RN, et al. A randomized trial of Ustekinumab, a human interleukin-12/23 monoclonal antibody, in patients with moderate-to-severe Crohn's disease. Gastroenterology 2008;135(4):1130–41.
192. Sandborn WJ, Gasink C, Gao LL, et al. Ustekinumab induction and maintenance therapy in refractory Crohn's disease. N Engl J Med 2012;367(16):1519–28.
193. Ritchlin C, Rahman P, Kavanaugh A, et al. Efficacy and safety of the anti-IL-12/23 p40 monoclonal antibody, ustekinumab, in patients with active psoriatic arthritis despite conventional non-biological and biological anti-tumour necrosis factor therapy: 6-month and 1-year results of the phase 3, multicentre, double-blind, placebo-controlled, randomised PSUMMIT 2 trial. Ann Rheum Dis 2014;73(6):990–9.
194. Poddubnyy D, Hermann KG, Callhoff J, Listing J, Sieper J. Ustekinumab for the treatment of patients with active ankylosing spondylitis: results of a 28-week, prospective, open-label, proof-of-concept study (TOPAS). Ann Rheum Dis 2014;73(5):817–23.
195. Hueber W, Sands BE, Lewitzky S, et al. Secukinumab, a human anti-IL-17A monoclonal antibody, for moderate to severe Crohn's disease: unexpected results of a randomised, double-blind placebo-controlled trial. Gut 2012;61(12):1693–700.
196. Rich P, Sigurgeirsson B, Thaci D, et al. Secukinumab induction and maintenance therapy in moderate-to-severe plaque psoriasis: a randomized, double-blind, placebo-controlled, phase II regimen-finding study. Br J Dermatol 2013;168(2):402–11.
197. McInnes IB, Sieper J, Braun J, et al. Efficacy and safety of secukinumab, a fully human anti-interleukin-17A monoclonal antibody, in patients with moderate-to-severe psoriatic arthritis: a 24-week, randomised, double-blind, placebo-controlled, phase II proof-of-concept trial. Ann Rheum Dis 2014;73(2):349–56.
198. McInnes IB, Mease PJ, Kirkham B, et al. Secukinumab, a human anti-interleukin-17A monoclonal antibody, in patients with psoriatic arthritis (FUTURE 2): a randomised, double-blind, placebo-controlled, phase 3 trial. Lancet 2015;386(9999):1137–46.
199. Mease PJ, McInnes IB, Kirkham B, et al. Secukinumab inhibition of interleukin-17A in patients with psoriatic arthritis. N Engl J Med 2015;373(14):1329–39.
200. Baeten D, Baraliakos X, Braun J, et al. Anti-interleukin-17A monoclonal antibody secukinumab in treatment of ankylosing spondylitis: a randomised, double-blind, placebo-controlled trial. Lancet 2013;382(9906):1705–13.
201. Baeten D, Sieper J, Braun J, et al. Secukinumab, an interleukin-17A inhibitor, in ankylosing spondylitis. N Engl J Med 2015;373(26):2534–48.
202. De Wilde K, Debusschere K, Beeckman S, Jacques P, Elewaut D. Integrating the pathogenesis of spondyloarthritis: gut and joint united? Curr Opin Rheumatol 2015;27(2):189–96.
203. Cron RQ. A signal achievement in the treatment of arthritis. Arthritis Rheum 2005;52(8):2229–32.
204. Stoll ML, Cron RQ. Treatment of juvenile idiopathic arthritis in the biologic age. Rheum Dis Clin North Am 2013;39(4):751–66.
205. Sandborn WJ, Colombel JF, Sands BE, et al. Abatacept for Crohn's disease and ulcerative colitis. Gastroenterology 2012;143(1):62–9 e4.
206. Mayer L, Kaser A, Blumberg RS. Dead on arrival: understanding the failure of CTLA4-immunoglobulin therapy in inflammatory bowel disease. Gastroenterology 2012;143(1):13–17.
207. Song IH, Heldmann F, Rudwaleit M, et al. Treatment of active ankylosing spondylitis with abatacept: an open-label, 24-week pilot study. Ann Rheum Dis 2011;70(6):1108–10.
208. Mease P, Genovese MC, Gladstein G, et al. Abatacept in the treatment of patients with psoriatic arthritis: results of a six-month, multicenter, randomized, double-blind, placebo-controlled, phase II trial. Arthritis Rheum 2011;63(4):939–48.
209. Grillo-Lopez AJ, White CA, Varns C, et al. Overview of the clinical development of rituximab: first monoclonal antibody approved for the treatment of lymphoma. Semin Oncol 1999;26(5Suppl 14):66–73.
210. Emery P, Deodhar A, Rigby WF, et al. Efficacy and safety of different doses and retreatment of rituximab: a randomised, placebo-controlled trial in patients who are biological naive with active rheumatoid arthritis and an inadequate response to methotrexate (Study Evaluating Rituximab's Efficacy in MTX iNadequate rEsponders (SERENE)). Ann Rheum Dis 2010;69(9):1629–35.
211. Leiper K, Martin K, Ellis A, et al. Randomised placebo-controlled trial of rituximab (anti-CD20) in active ulcerative colitis. Gut 2011;60(11):1520–6.
212. Song IH, Heldmann F, Rudwaleit M, et al. Different response to rituximab in tumor necrosis factor blocker-naive patients with active ankylosing spondylitis and in patients in whom tumor necrosis factor blockers have failed: a twenty-four-week clinical trial. Arthritis Rheum 2010;62(5):1290–7.
213. Jimenez-Boj E, Stamm TA, Sadlonova M, et al. Rituximab in psoriatic arthritis: an exploratory evaluation. Ann Rheum Dis 2012;71(11):1868–71.
214. Mease P, Kavanaugh A, Genovese M, Ritchlin C, Rosengren S, Quistberg A. Rituximab in psoriatic arthritis provides modest clinical improvement and reduces expression of inflammatory biomarkers in skin lesions. Arthritis Rheum 2010;62(Suppl 10):S818.

CHAPTER 18

Extra-articular manifestations: psoriasis

Wolf-Henning Boehncke and Dafna D. Gladman

Introduction to psoriasis

Psoriasis is a chronic-recurrent inflammatory skin disease, affecting about 2% of the world's population (1). In 2014, the WHO's member states adopted a resolution on psoriasis, recognizing it as 'a chronic, non-communicable, painful, disfiguring, and disabling disease for which there is no cure'. The resolution also acknowledges the psychosocial burden of the disease and that many people with psoriasis suffer due to lack of awareness and access to sufficient treatment. This resolution echoes the readily measurable psychological burden of the disease, which in comparative studies is ranked second only to depression (2). Much of this is due to the visible disfiguration of psoriasis patients that often triggers reactions ranging from irritation to disgust among others. It also takes into account the high physical burden of the disease, which is at least comparable to other major diseases such as cancer (2). This result becomes readily understandable when looking at symptoms such as pain, itch, and bleeding, which are regularly reported by patients (3). The burden of disease is further increased by a number of comorbid conditions, including metabolic syndrome and resulting CVDs (4). Finally, joint involvement in the form of PsA is present in around 30% of psoriasis patients seen by dermatologists in Europe and North America (5).

Psoriasis is a multifaceted disease with a variety of skin lesions as well as joint manifestations. The latter might be considered to be part of the psoriatic disease itself or associated with it, according to different points of view. This chapter focuses on the clinical features of psoriasis of the skin and its underlying pathogenesis, taking into account the current status of genetic research in the field. It also describes PsA, and the association of psoriasis with SpA.

Classification

The classification of psoriasis has long been based on clinical signs and symptoms. This approach also underlies the ICD-10 coding system. More recently, genetics have shed a different light on what was previously regarded as a rather monolithic entity. This section briefly summarizes classifications based on both approaches (Table 18.1). A different level of complexity is introduced by the term 'psoriasis vulgaris', which has previously only rarely been used in the Anglo-American literature but has now been adopted by geneticists.

The commonest clinical manifestation of psoriasis is multiple plaques, which develop over weeks or months. This manifestation is called chronic plaque-type psoriasis and can be differentiated

Table 18.1 Classification of psoriasis based on clinical and genetic criteria

Clinical criteria	Composite definition	Genetic markers
L40* Psoriasis L40.0* psoriasis vulgaris ◆ Chronic plaque-type ◆ Inverse ◆ Erythroderma L40.1* generalized pustular psoriasis L40.2* acrodermatitis continua suppurativa L40.3* psoriasis pustulosa palmoplantaris L40.4* psoriasis guttata	Type 1 ◆ Association with HLA-Cw6 ◆ Positive family history ◆ Manifestation <30 years Type 2 ◆ No association with HLA-Cw6 ◆ Sporadic ◆ Manifestation >40 years	Psoriasis vulgaris ◆ >30 PSORSs Guttate psoriasis ◆ PSORS1 DITRA (minority of cases with generalized pustular psoriasis) ◆ Mutations in the IL36RN gene ◆ Lack of association with PSORS1

*ICD-10 coding; PSORS, psoriasis susceptibility locus; DITRA, deficiency of interleukin thirty-six receptor antagonist.

from psoriasis developing in an acute exanthematic manner, which is called guttate psoriasis. Often, nails and scalp are involved. Psoriasis affecting skin folds is referred to as inverse psoriasis. Psoriasis is among those skin diseases that can result in the clinical state of erythroderma, with no or almost no normal skin being visible any more, as the whole organ is affected by the disease. All of these manifestations, with the exception of guttate psoriasis (L40.4), are summarized as 'psoriasis vulgaris' based on the current ICD-10 classification (L40.0). These manifestations can be separated clinically from pustular forms of psoriasis, comprising generalized pustular psoriasis (L40.1), as well as two types of localized pustular psoriasis, namely acrodermatitis continua suppurative (L40.2) and psoriasis pustulosa palmoplantaris (L40.3).

Early genetic studies previously identified a locus on chromosome 6 comprising MHC genes as the most important genetic locus associated with chronic plaque-type psoriasis. This locus has been termed psoriasis susceptibility locus 1 (PSORS1); it accounts for around 50% of the heritability of psoriasis (6). The risk allele is most likely HLA-C*06. Based on this finding, two types of chronic plaque-type psoriasis have been differentiated: type 1 psoriasis was defined as cases being associated with HLA-C*06, a positive family history of psoriasis, and an early disease onset (<30 years), while type 2 psoriasis includes sporadic cases lacking a positive family history, not showing an association with HLA-C*06, and a manifestation after the age of 40 (7). More recently, GWAS helped to identify around 40 more genes associated with different clinical manifestations of psoriasis, allowing for a refined genetic classification. As these are crucial to better understand the underlying pathogenesis, they are reviewed in the respective sections of this chapter.

Clinical features

Non-pustular psoriasis

The classical appearance of plaque-type psoriasis comprises multiple monomorphic, well-demarked, infiltrated, red, scaly plaques (Fig. 18.1A). Depending on the chronicity of the lesion, the colour of the plaque may resemble any shade between a light salmon-red and a deep burgundy red to purple. The more pronounced the infiltration, the more profound is the formation of a rim along the demarcation of the lesional skin. Scales are coarse, with a silvery to asbestos-like colour. Predilection sites for these plaques comprise elbows, knees, the umbilical and sacral regions. As psoriasis can principally manifest at any site of the body, the status of erythroderma can arise if the whole skin organ is affected. The typical scaling can be absent in cases of so-called inverse psoriasis, affecting intertriginous sites such as axillae and groin (Fig. 18.1B).

Actually, the primary lesions of non-pustular psoriasis are not plaques but rather hyperkeratotic papules. This can readily be observed in guttate psoriasis (Fig. 18.1C). Here, psoriasis takes a more acute exanthematic course, and multiple droplet-like lesions appear simultaneously, covering a large portion of the body surface area. This manifestation is often seen in children in association with an upper respiratory tract infection.

Psoriasis of scalp and nails

Scalp psoriasis is common, affecting around 80% of the patients (8). This manifestation is often long-standing and may cover a huge portion of the head (9). Sites commonly affected comprise the forehead, where the lesions typically extend several centimetres beyond the scalp, the retro-auricular region, and the external auditory canal (Fig. 18.1D). While non-scarring alopecia is readily observed in the case of scalp psoriasis (10), scarring alopecia is seemingly rare and sometimes associated with AIDS (11).

Nail psoriasis, too, is a common feature, observed in around 50% of the patients. It may affect both the nail bed and/or the nail matrix. Fingernails are more often affected than toenails (12). Nail pits are the most frequent manifestation of nail psoriasis, representing superficial punctuate depressions in the nail plate. Other signs and symptoms comprise distal onycholysis, translucent yellow-brownish discoloration in the nail bed ('oil drop') (Fig. 18.1G), as well as thickened and crumbled nail plates which may cause complete dystrophy (13). Nail lesions are more common among patients with PsA than those with psoriasis alone (14). It has been suggested that scalp and nail lesions are risk factors for the development of PsA (15).

Pustular psoriasis

Although less frequent than plaque-type psoriasis, pustular manifestations can readily be observed as well. These can manifest in a generalized or localized manner (Fig. 18.1E and F). More than a decade ago, diagnostic criteria for generalized pustular psoriasis were defined (16): multiple sterile pustules are present on erythematous skin. Patients show systemic symptoms such as fever or nausea as well as at least one out of a list of numerous laboratory anomalies, including signs of inflammation (elevated CRP, leukocytosis), high antistreptolysin O antibody titres, elevated IgG or IgA serum levels, hypoproteinaemia or hypocalcaemia. Localized forms of pustular psoriasis often manifest on hands and feet in the form of palmoplantar pustular psoriasis, while acrodermatitis continua suppurative affects the tips of the fingers and/or toes.

Trigger factors

Psoriasis belongs to those dermatoses exhibiting the so-called Koebner phenomenon, where non-specific trauma provokes the

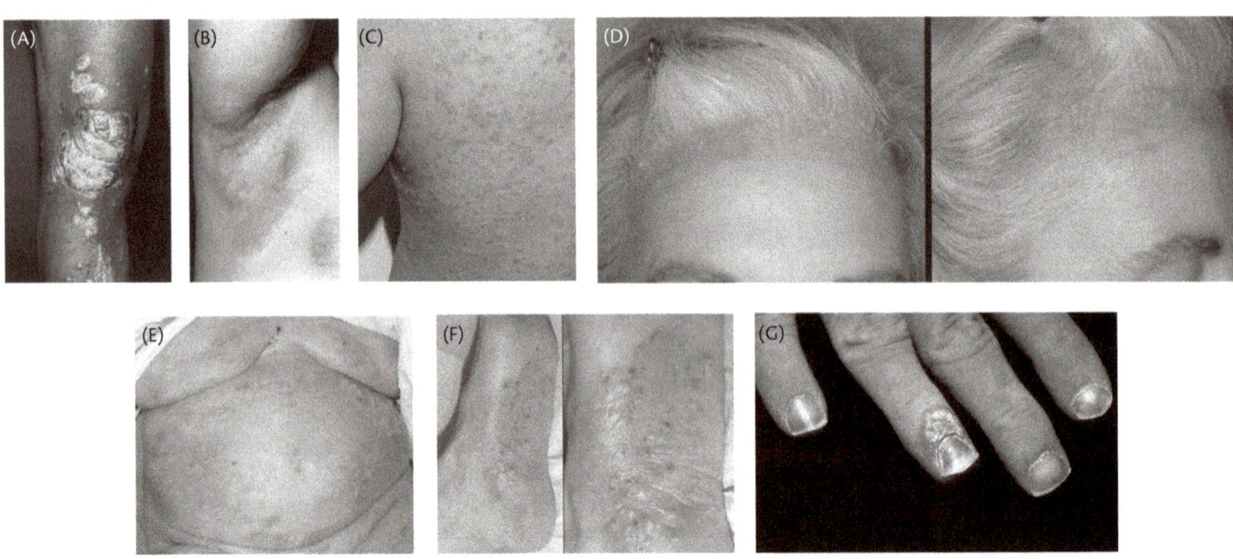

Fig. 18.1 (See colour plate section). Clinical manifestations of psoriasis. (A) Typical erythematosquamous plaques on the knee; (B) inverse psoriasis in the axilla, lacking the typical scaling but with well-demarked margins; (C) guttate psoriasis with an exanthematous distribution of hyperkeratotic papule 'sand' small plaques on the trunk; (D) scalp psoriasis affecting a small zone of the forehead; (E) generalized pustular psoriasis; (F) localized pustular psoriasis in plantar location; (G) nail psoriasis, featuring distal onycholysis (ring finger) and an 'oil drop' (index finger).

The photos from patients and histologies have been prepared by Dr E. Laffite and Prof. G. Kaya, Dpt. of Dermatology, Geneva University Hospital. They are part of the GRAPPA slide library and reproduced here with permission.

manifestation of typical lesions at the site of the irritation. Potential triggers of the Koebner phenomenon include scratching, piercing, tattoos, and surgical interventions. Psoriatic rashes or an exacerbation of psoriasis can be caused by numerous other factors, such as certain drugs (β blockers, lithium, antimalarials, NSAIDs) (17). Moreover, occupational risk factors impairing the skin barrier function are known to negatively influence the course of psoriasis, aggravating palmoplantar psoriasis in particular. Finally, infections play an important role as trigger factors: psoriasis may manifest itself for the first time or worsen after an HIV infection (18). Furthermore, streptococcal pharyngitis in children and adolescents may be observed for a few weeks prior to the manifestation of a psoriatic rash, frequently in the form of guttate psoriasis. This constellation is often reported to be the initial manifestation in the respective patients. It is suggested that similarities between streptococcal superantigens and keratins result in a crossreactivity and subsequent manifestation of a chronic autoimmune response towards the epidermis (19).

Clinical assessment

As stated in the section 'Non-pustular psoriasis', psoriasis commonly presents in the form of infiltrated, red, scaly plaques. Consequently, quantification of these three components in combination with the extent of the lesions represents the standard method of assessing disease severity in clinical trials. The Psoriasis Area and Severity Index (PASI) assesses erythema, induration, and scaling in a semiquantitative manner, scoring each of these from '0' to '4'. Additionally, the percentage of the affected area of the head, trunk, and upper and lower extremities is determined semiquantitatively. The resulting score ranges from '0' to '72'. Moderate-to-severe psoriasis, eligible for a systemic therapy, is usually defined by a score of ≥10. The use of the PASI is hampered by several factors: its range is rather theoretical, and PASI scores beyond 40 are rarely documented. In cases of mild psoriasis, its sensitivity to change is rather limited. Many physicians regard it as labour-intensive and thus would not use the PASI in their daily practice, preferring to determine the body surface area by the number of patient palms that are needed to cover all the psoriasis lesions. Most importantly, the PASI can only be used in patients with plaque-type psoriasis, not taking into account clinically important manifestations such as nail psoriasis and the different impact of lesions depending on the site affected. A lesion on the face might have a substantially higher impact on the patient's well-being than a similar plaque on the trunk.

Physician Global Assessment (PGA) scores are often used instead of the PASI. Numerous such tools exist, including static as well as dynamic scales. A widely used PGA is the five-point static PGA with scores from '0' ('clear') to '4' ('very severe'), each score being defined by descriptions of the type of erythema, induration, and scaling, respectively. Additional scores exist for scalp and nail psoriasis (the Nail Psoriasis Severity Index—NAPSI).

To capture all dimensions of psoriasis, a documentation of patient-reported outcomes is indispensable. One such tool that is widely used for skin disease in general and psoriasis in particular is the Dermatology Life Quality Index (DLQI) (20). This tool comprises ten questions, the answers to which are scored from '0' to '3'. A score ≥ 10 is considered to reflect a very significant burden of disease, while scores <5 indicate a minimally reduced quality of life.

Currently, the 'rule of 10s' is used as an orientation to differentiate between mild versus moderate-to-severe psoriasis. According to this rule, a patient is considered to suffer from moderate-to-severe psoriasis if the PASI or DLQI are >10, or if more than 10% of the body surface is affected. As this rule does not fully capture manifestations other than plaque-type psoriasis, it has been suggested to include additional criteria to define moderate-to-severe psoriasis, such as substantial involvement of two or more of the nails, widespread involvement of the scalp, and psoriasis on visible areas (21). The same document suggests a 50% reduction in the PASI and a DLQI < 5 as treatment goals, achievement of these validating a continuation of the respective therapy, while failure to achieve these criteria should result in considering to adapt the treatment.

An international group is currently developing appropriate outcome measures for psoriasis (22).

Diagnosis and differential diagnosis of psoriasis

The diagnosis of chronic plaque-type psoriasis is usually established clinically, based on the typical appearance of the lesions and possibly a positive personal and family history. Biopsies are rarely needed. The characteristic histology shows epidermal changes such as thickening (akanthosis) and rete ridges reaching deep into the dermis, with the dermal papillae extending far up until close to the skin surface (papillomatosis), along with persisting nuclei in the cornified layer (parakeratosis) (Fig. 18.2). A dense inflammatory infiltrate is present in the dermis, consisting of a mixture of namely T lymphocytes, neutrophilic granulocytes, and macrophages. Some T lymphocytes are also found within the epidermis, where neutrophils might form aggregates, the so-called pustules of Kogoj and Munro's microabscesses. Finally, dilated and elongated capillaries are found within the dermal papillae.

Diagnosing inverse psoriasis clinically might be a challenge. Here, typical manifestations in the form of psoriatic plaques elsewhere, or involvement of the scalp or nails can give important clues. Nail changes as diagnostic features might also be helpful in cases of erythroderma.

Common differential diagnoses of psoriasis comprise tinea capitis and tinea corporis; fungal infections usually exhibit a much finer scaling, which typically is accentuated at the progressing perimeter of the fungal lesions. Seborrheic dermatitis often manifests on the scalp, face, and chest; unlike scalp psoriasis, seborrheic dermatitis of the scalp does not go beyond the hair line. Sometimes a sharp differentiation between these two pathologies is next to impossible, a constellation for which the term 'seborrhiasis' has been coined. Other differential diagnoses include different types of eczema (atopic, irritative, allergic) as well as lichen planus, the latter often exhibiting mucosal involvement, severe itch, and scarring alopecia (in contrast to the usually non-scarring alopecia induced by scalp psoriasis). Finally, pityriasis rosea (self-limiting), pityriasis rubra pilaris, secondary syphilis, and cutaneous lymphomas can sometimes be taken for psoriasis (or vice versa). In case of few lesions, Bowen's disease should also be considered.

Genetics and pathogenesis

The pathogenetic pillars of psoriasis can readily be depicted from the classic clinical appearance of psoriatic plaques, echoed by their histological hallmarks: scaling as well as the histological features of akanthosis, papillomatosis, and parakeratosis highlight epidermal

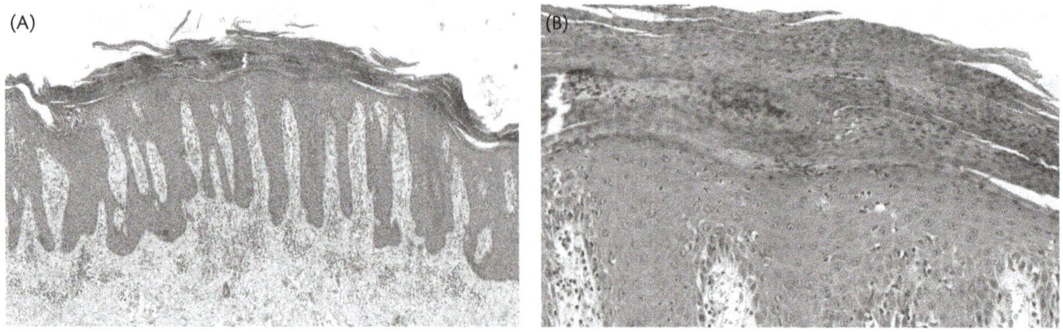

Fig. 18.2 (See colour plate section). Histological characteristics of plaque-type psoriasis. The typical epidermal features of akanthosis and papillomatosis, along with a dense mononuclear inflammatory infiltrate, are readily visible at low magnification (A), while the detail (B) shows pronounced parakeratosis.
The photos from patients and histologies have been prepared by Dr E. Laffite and Prof. G. Kaya, Dpt. of Dermatology, Geneva University Hospital. They are part of the GRAPPA slide library and reproduced here with permission.

hyperproliferation, while erythema and induration reflect the inflammatory nature of these lesions. Admittedly, angioneogenesis as the third cornerstone can only be appreciated at the histological level (in the form of tortuous and elongated capillaries extending into the dermal papillae; see section 'Diagnosis and differential diagnosis of psoriasis').

Genetics have shed more light on the pathogenesis of psoriasis. While it has long been recognized that HLA-C*06 is associated with plaque-type psoriasis, recent GWAS have identified around 40 additional loci. Attempts to group the respective candidate genes point towards several important pathways which are potentially clinically relevant (Table 18.2) (23). These include functions of both the adaptive and the innate immune system. The importance of T lymphocytes in general and Th17 lymphocytes in particular is highlighted by variants in the genes encoding the IL-23R and the untranslated region of IL-12B as indicators of psoriasis risk. Analyses of transcribed genes in lesional psoriatic skin have further suggested a role for T lymphocytes and DCs.

On the other hand, it was also through genetic studies that the concept of psoriasis as a rather 'monolithic' entity has been challenged. This is particularly true for attempts to define generalized pustular psoriasis as a distinct entity. A few years ago, a missense mutation in the IL-36RN gene was identified in Tunisian families and was subsequently confirmed to be present in a considerable percentage of patients with generalized pustular psoriasis in other cohorts around the world (24). This mutation results in the lack of an IL-36R antagonist and hence causes increased signalling of IL-36, resulting in synthesis and secretion of numerous proinflammatory cytokines, including IL-1β, IL-6, and IL-8. The respective disease is currently named DITRA (deficiency of interleukin thirty-six receptor antagonist). The observation that the major psoriasis susceptibility locus, HLA-C*06, is not associated with generalized pustular psoriasis further supports the concept that it is a distinct entity.

Many of the key mechanisms suggested by genetic studies have been further substantiated by experimental work and clinical research on the efficacy of therapies with well-defined modes of action. A widely accepted hypothesis suggests that genetically predisposed individuals respond to environmental factors (stress, microorganisms, drugs, trauma) through an activation of dermal plasmocytoid DCs towards a complex consisting of self-DNA and the antimicrobial peptide LL-37 produced by keratinocytes (25). This activation signal results in the release of IFNα and subsequent activation of more dermal DCs, which in turn secrete, among other mediators, TNFα and IL-23. The former acts on numerous cell types and exhibits multiple proinflammatory effects, such as induction of secondary messengers and adhesion molecules, all of which have important roles in the pathogenesis of psoriasis. The latter is a key factor for the differentiation of Th17 lymphocytes, considered to be important effector cells in the psoriatic inflammation. These lymphocytes secrete IL-17 and IL-22, the latter inducing keratinocyte proliferation. Noteworthy, IL-17 is also produced by numerous cell types other than Th17 lymphocytes, including neutrophils, mast cells, and macrophages. In line with the particular importance of TNFα, on the one hand, and IL-23 and IL-17, on the other hand, biologics blocking specifically either TNFα, IL-23, or IL-17, respectively, have been shown to be highly effective in the treatment of psoriasis (26, 27).

Psoriatic arthritis

PsA, defined as an inflammatory musculoskeletal disease that is usually seronegative for rheumatoid factor, affects some 30% of patients with psoriasis. Although initially thought to be a rare and mild disease, recent data demonstrate that the disease is common and may be quite severe. Since psoriasis occurs in 1–3% of the population and PsA may occur in about a third of people with psoriasis, its prevalence may be as high as 1% of the population (28). Indeed, a prospective study of patients with psoriasis who did not have arthritis at initial visit to the clinic demonstrated that the incidence of PsA was 1.87 per 100 psoriasis cases per year—suggesting an annual incidence of almost 2% (29). This is consistent with the fact that in the studies demonstrating 30% prevalence of PsA among psoriasis patients, the average duration of psoriasis was 15 years (5). PsA affects men and women in an almost equal distribution; however, recent evidence suggests that while men have more severe axial disease and peripheral radiological damage, women tend to demonstrate more functional limitations (30).

Clinical picture of PsA

In their initial description of PsA, Moll and Wright identified five clinical patterns, including distal, oligoarticular, polyarticular, arthritis mutilans, and predominantly axial (31). However, it has become clear that these patterns change over time, such that, most

Table 18.2 Major gene variants associated with psoriasis (adapted from Capon 2012 (23))

Gene	Protein function	Pathway	Comment
TNFA1P3	Inhibitor of TNFα-induced NFκB signalling	NFκB signalling	TNFα inhibitors are clinically effective in treating psoriasis
TNIP1	Inhibitor of TNFα-induced NFκB signalling	NFκB signalling	TNFα inhibitors are clinically effective in treating psoriasis
IL28RA	IL29 receptor subunit	IFN signalling	
IL12B	Shared subunit of IL-12 and IL-23	IL-23 signalling	
IL23R	IL-23 receptor subunit	IL-23 signalling	
IL23A	IL-23 subunit	IL-23 signalling	Ustekinumab (inhibiting IL-12 and IL-23) and specific anti-IL-23 antibodies are clinically effective in treating psoriasis
PSORS1 (HLA-C)	HLA class I antigen	Antigen presentation	
ERAP1	Peptidase processing HLA class I ligands	Antigen presentation	

Italic: genes related to function of the innate immune system; PSORS, psoriasis susceptibility locus; ERAP, endoplasmic reticulum aminopeptidase.

Underlined: genes related to function of the adaptive immune system.

Source: Reprinted with permission of Macmillan Publishers Ltd., J Invest Dermatol, Capon F, Burden AD, Trembath RC, et al., 132, 3 Pt 2, copyright (2012).

recently, only three articular patterns of PsA are recognized, namely peripheral arthritis, axial disease, and axial plus peripheral disease. Indeed, a cluster analysis suggested that peripheral and axial, with or without peripheral, are the important clusters (32). Peripheral arthritis is distinguished from RA because of the involvement of the distal interphalangeal joints, the reddish-purplish discoloration over the inflamed joint, the asymmetry, the presence of dactylitis, enthesitis, and axial involvement, and the presence of flail or fused joints.

Axial disease in PsA

Axial involvement has been reported in 25–70% of patients with PsA, depending on the definition used, and it is usually accompanied by peripheral disease (33). Axial disease alone occurred in only 2–4% of reported series of patients with PsA. Patients with isolated axial disease and psoriasis may be classified as either axSpA with psoriasis or as axial PsA. The definition very much depends on the physician to whom the patients are referred to. Patients with PsA who had axial disease at presentation were more likely to be HLA-B27 positive, have radiographic damage to peripheral joints, and elevated ESR, and less likely to have a family history of PsA (34). It was estimated that after 10 years of follow-up, 15% of the PsA patients would develop axial PsA. Nail dystrophy, number of radiographically damaged joints, periostitis, and elevated ESR increased the risk of developing axial PsA, while swollen joints decreased the risk (34). Over a 10-year period, patients with axial PsA had improvement in neck and back pain, but lateral spinal flexion and cervical mobility deteriorated (35).

Assessment of patients with axial PsA uses the same spinal measurement tools used for AS. The reliability of the measures was demonstrated in the International Spondyloarthritis Inter-Observer Reliability Exercise—the INSPIRE study, which assessed patients with AS and axial PsA (36). Similarly, a Spanish study concluded that patients with axial PsA can be assessed using the same tools used for primary AS (37). Radiographic assessment in patients with axial PsA using the tools developed for AS has also been proven reliable in axial PsA (38).

Axial psoriatic arthritis compared to primary ankylosing spondylitis

Several studies noted that axial PsA differs from primary AS by clinical and radiological features (39–41). Generally axial PsA is not as severe as AS, although disease activity as measured by the BASDAI was not different in the Spanish study (37). These differences support the notion that axial PsA should be maintained as a separate entity. However, although axial disease is diagnosed in about 50% of the patients with PsA, depending on the definition, some 10% of patients diagnosed with AS also have psoriasis. These latter patients may qualify as PsA according to the Classification of Psoriatic Arthritis (CASPAR) criteria (42), as they have inflammatory spinal disease, they would gain two points if they have psoriasis at the current examination, and they would gain another point if their rheumatoid factor is negative, thus gaining three points, which would satisfy the classification criteria. Whether these patients are more severe than their counterparts detected in PsA cohorts is not clear. Patients with AS who have psoriasis appear to be similar to those who do not have psoriasis (43). However, among patients with IBP, the prevalence of psoriasis was 16.6%, much higher than the general population. Patients with IBP and psoriasis had active axial disease as well as enthesitis and dactylitis, both features of PsA (44).

Genetics and pathogenesis of psoriatic arthritis

The pathogenesis of PsA is similar to that of psoriasis in that similar genetic and immunological factors are associated with both. However, patients with PsA differ from those with psoriasis alone in HLA alleles. While HLA-C*06 is a susceptibility allele for PsA compared to the general population, patients with psoriasis who carry the HLA-C*06 allele are less likely to develop PsA, and, if they do, they usually develop it later in the course of their disease (45–47). On the other hand, HLA-B*27, HLA-B*39, and HLA-B*08 are more common among patients with PsA compared to psoriasis without arthritis (45). A recent fine mapping of the MHC region found that the presence of glutamine in position 45 of the HLA-B antigen confers the strongest risk for PsA in patients with psoriasis (48). This polymorphic site is located in the binding groove of HLA-B and can influence the binding of a peptide to the HLA molecule. This finding highlights the role of innate immunity in the pathogenesis of PsA. Moreover, KIR polymorphism has also been associated with PsA (49). The ligands for the receptors are HLA-C molecules. GWAS have not identified genes which differentiate between PsA and psoriasis (50). However, candidate gene studies identified IL-13 in PsA and not in psoriasis without arthritis (51, 52).

Environmental factors are associated with the development of PsA among patients with psoriasis. These include lifting heavy loads, infections, and possibly vaccinations (53). Smoking seems 'protective', although this is due to interaction with HLA-C*06 (54).

Treatment of psoriatic arthritis

The objective of treating patients with PsA is to control both joint and skin manifestations. If the skin disease is mild, initial therapy with non-steroidal anti-inflammatory medications may be sufficient, but if the skin disease is a factor, then systemic medications such as DMARDs would be indicated. It should be noted that topical skin medications do not work for the arthritis. Of the DMARDs, MTX is the one most commonly used, although evidence for its efficacy is lacking. Nonetheless, in clinical practice, MTX seems to control joint inflammation as well as skin psoriasis. Cyclosporin is another medication that can work for both skin and joint manifestations, but it is nephrotoxic and therefore not recommended for prolonged use. LFN has been shown to be effective for PsA, but has only a very mild effect on psoriasis.

Several biologic agents have been proven effective for both psoriasis and PsA (55). All anti-TNF agents, including ETN, adalimumab, cerolizumab, golimumab, and infliximab, work for PsA. The anti-TNF antibodies appear to work better for psoriasis than the anti-TNF receptor, although with the higher dose of ETN, better skin control has been demonstrated. The anti-IL-12/IL-23 ustekinumab has been proven effective for both psoriasis and PsA. While it is highly effective for psoriasis, the effect on the joint disease is not quite as impressive. More recently, anti-IL-17 agents have demonstrated excellent skin responses, and there is emerging evidence for just as impressive joint responses (56). Many of these agents have also been proven effective for axial disease, although there are no specific studies in axial PsA.

Conclusion

Psoriasis is a common comorbidity in patients with axial disease. Whether these patients have PsA or a co-existence of axial SpA and psoriasis is unclear. Patients with axial disease who have peripheral arthritis, enthesitis, and dactylitis can easily be classified as PsA. Either way, there are now several approaches to managing these patients that have been proven effective.

Acknowledgements

The figures in this chapter are taken with permission from the Group for Research and Assessment of Psoriasis and Psoriatic Arthritis (GRAPPA) slide library.

References

1. Christophers E. Psoriasis—epidemiology and clinical spectrum. Clin Exp Dermatol 2001;26:314–20.
2. Rapp SR, Feldman SR, Exum ML, et al. Psoriasis causes as much disability as other major medical diseases. J Am Acad Dermatol 1999;41:401–7.
3. Dubertret L, Mrowietz U, Ranki A, et al. European patient perspectives on the impact of psoriasis:the EUROPSO patient membership survey. Br J Dermatol 2006;155:729–36.
4. Boehncke WH, Boehncke S, Schön MP. Managing comorbid disease in patients with psoriasis. Br Med J 2010;340:b5666.
5. Mease PJ, Gladman DD, Papp KA, et al. Prevalence of rheumatologist-diagnosed psoriatic arthritis in patients with psoriasis in European/North American dermatology clinics. J Am Acad Dermatol 2013;69:729–35.
6. Trembath RC, Clough RL, Rosbotham JL, et al. Identification of a major susceptibility locus on chromosome 6p and evidence for further disease loci revealed by a two stage genome-wide search in psoriasis. Hum Mol Genet 1997;6:813–20.
7. Henseler T, Christophers E. Psoriasis of early and late onset: characterization of two types of psoriasis vulgaris. J Am Acad Dermatol 1985;13:450–6.
8. Papp K, Berth-Jones J, Kragballe K, et al. Scalp psoriasis: a review of current topical treatment options. J Eur Acad Dermatol Venereol 2007;21:1151–60.
9. van de Kerkhof PC, de Hoop D, de Korte J, et al. Scalp psoriasis, clinical presentations and therapeutic management. Dermatology 1998;197:326–34.
10. Runne U. Alopecia psoriatica. Characteristics of an up to now neglected disease picture. Hautarzt 1993;44:691–2.
11. Schön MP, Reifenberger J, Gantke B, et al. Progressive cicatricial psoriatic alopecia in AIDS. Hautarzt 2000;51:935–8.
12. Farber EM, Nall L. Nail psoriasis. Cutis 1992;50:174–8.
13. Tan EST, Chong W-S, Tey HL. Nail psoriasis. Am J Clin Dermatol 2012;13:375–88.
14. Gladman DD, Anhorn KB, Schachter RK, Mervart H. HLA antigens in psoriatic arthritis. J Rheumatol 1986;13:586–92.
15. Wilson FC, Icen M, Crowson CS, et al. Incidence and clinical predictors of psoriatic arthritis in patients with psoriasis: a population-based study. Arthritis Rheum 2009;61:233–9.
16. Umezawa Y, Ozawa A, Kawasima T, et al. Therapeutic guidelines for the treatment of generalized pustular psoriasis (GPP) based on a proposed classification of disease severity. Arch Dermatol Res 2003;295(Suppl 1):S43–54.
17. Basavaraj KH, Ashok NM, Rashmi R, et al. The role of drugs in the induction and/or exacerbation of psoriasis. Int J Dermatol 2010;49:1351–61.
18. Fry L, Baker BS. Triggering psoriasis: the role of infections and medications. Clin Dermatol 2007;25:606–15.
19. Prinz JC. The role of streptococci in psoriasis. Hautarzt 2009;60:109–15.
20. Finlay A, Khan GK. Dermatology Life Quality Index (DLQI)—a simple practical measure for routine clinical use. Clin Exp Dermatol 1994;19:210–16.
21. Mrowietz U, Kragballe K, Reich K, et al. Definition of treatment goals for moderate to severe psoriasis: a European consensus. Arch Dermatol Res 2011;303:1–10.
22. Gottlieb AB, Armstrong AW, Christensen R, et al. The International Dermatology Outcome Measures Initiative as applied to psoriatic disease outcomes: a report from the GRAPPA 2013 Meeting. J Rheumatol 2014;41:1227–9.
23. Capon F, Burden AD, Trembath RC, et al. Psoriasis and other complex trait dermatoses: from loci to functional pathways. J Invest Dermatol 2012;132(3 Pt 2):915–22.
24. Capon F. IL36RN mutations in generalized pustular psoriasis: just the tip of the iceberg? J Invest Dermatol 2013;133:2503–4.
25. Nestle FO, Kaplan DH, Barker J. Psoriasis. N Engl J Med 2009;361:496–509.
26. Langley RG, Elewski BE, Lebwohl M, et al. Secukinumab in plaque psoriasis—results of two phase 3 trials. N Engl J Med 2014;371:326–38.
27. Puig L, López A, Vilarrasa E, García I. Efficacy of biologics in the treatment of moderate-to-severe plaque psoriasis: a systematic review and meta-analysis of randomized controlled trials with different time points. J Eur Acad Dermatol Venereol 2014;28:1633–53.

28. Gladman DD. Early psoriatic arthritis. Rheum Dis Clin North Am 2012;38:373–86.
29. Eder L, Chandran V, Shen H, et al. The incidence of arthritis in a prospective cohort of psoriasis patients. Arthritis Care Res (Hoboken) 2011;63:619–22.
30. Eder L, Thavaneswaran A, Chandran V, et al. Gender difference in disease expression, radiographic damage and disability among patients with psoriatic arthritis. Ann Rheum Dis 2013;72:578–82.
31. Moll JMH, Wright V. Psoriatic arthritis. Semin Arthritis Rheum 1972;3:55–78.
32. Thavaneswaran A, Chandran V, Gladman DD. Cluster analysis of psoriatic arthritis patients at follow-up. Arthritis Rheum 2013;65(Suppl 10):S145.
33. Gladman DD. Axial disease in psoriatic arthritis. Curr Rheumatol Rep 2007;9:455–60.
34. Chandran V, Tolusso DC, Schentag CT, et al. Risk factors for axial inflammatory arthritis in patients with psoriatic arthritis. J Rheumatol 2010;37:809–15.
35. Chandran V, Barrett J, Schentag CT, et al. Axial psoriatic arthritis: update on a longterm prospective study. J Rheumatol 2009;36:2744–50.
36. Gladman DD, Inman R, Cook R, et al. International Spondyloarthritis Inter-Observer Reliability Exercise—the INSPIRE study: I. Assessment of spinal measures. J Rheumatol 2007;34:1733–9.
37. Fernandez-Sueiro JL, Willisch A, Pertega-Diaz S, et al. Evaluation of ankylosing spondylitis spinal mobility measurements in the assessment of spinal involvement in psoriatic arthritis. Arthritis Rheum 2009;15(61):386–92.
38. Biagioni B, Gladman DD, Cook RJ, et al. Reliability of radiographic scoring methods in axial psoriatic arthritis. Arthritis Care Res 2014;66:1417–22.
39. Gladman DD, Brubacher B, Buskila D, et al. Psoriatic spondyloarthropathy in men and women: a clinical, radiographic, and HLA study. Clin Invest Med 1993;15:371–5.
40. Helliwell PS, Hickling P, Wright V. Do the radiological changes of classic ankylosing spondylitis differ from the changes found in the spondylitis associated with inflammatory bowel disease, psoriasis, and reactive arthritis? Ann Rheum Dis 1998;57:135–40.
41. Chandran V, O'Shea FD, Schentag CT, et al. Relationship between spinal mobility and radiographic damage in ankylosing spondylitis and psoriatic spondylitis: a comparative analysis. J Rheumatol 2007;34:2463–5.
42. Taylor W, Gladman D, Helliwell P, et al. Classification criteria for psoriatic arthritis: development of new criteria from a large international study. Arthritis Rheum 2006;54:2665–73.
43. Machado P, Landewé R, Braun J, et al. Ankylosing spondylitis patients with and without psoriasis do not differ in disease phenotype. Ann Rheum Dis 2013;72:1104–5.
44. Richette P, Tubach F, Breban M, Dougados M. Psoriasis and phenotype of patients with early inflammatory back pain. Ann Rheum Dis 2013;72:566–71.
45. Chandran V, Bull SB, Pellett FJ, et al. Human leukocyte antigen alleles and susceptibility to psoriatic arthritis. Hum Immunol 2013;74:1333–8.
46. Eder L, Chandran V, Pellet F, et al. Human leucocyte antigen risk alleles for psoriatic arthritis among patients with psoriasis. Ann Rheum Dis 2012;71:50–5.
47. Winchester R, Minevich G, Steshenko V, et al. HLA associations reveal genetic heterogeneity in psoriatic arthritis and in the psoriasis phenotype. Arthritis Rheum 2012;64:1134–44.
48. Okada Y, Han B, Tsoi LC, et al. Fine mapping major histocompatibility complex associations in psoriasis and its clinical subtypes. Am J Hum Gen 2014;95:162–72.
49. Chandran V, Bull SB, Pellett FJ, et al. Killer immunoglobulin-like receptor gene polymorphism and susceptibility to psoriatic arthritis. Rheumatology 2014;53:233–9.
50. Eder L, Chandran V, Gladman DD. What have we learned about genetic susceptibility in psoriasis and psoriatic arthritis? Curr Opin Rheumatol 2015;27:91–8.
51. Duffin KC, Freeny IC, Schrodi SJ, et al. Association between IL13 polymorphisms and psoriatic arthritis is modified by smoking. J Invest Dermatol 2009;129:2777–83.
52. Eder L, Chandran V, Pellett F, et al. IL13 gene polymorphism is a marker for psoriatic arthritis among psoriasis patients. Ann Rheum Dis 2011;70:1594–8.
53. Eder L, Law T, Chandran V, et al. The association between environmental factors and onset of psoriatic arthritis in patients with psoriasis. Arthritis Care Res 2011;63:1091–7.
54. Eder L, Shanmugarajah S, Thavaneswaran A, et al. The association between smoking and the development of psoriatic arthritis among psoriasis patients. Ann Rheum Dis 2012;71:219–24.
55. Acosta Felquer ML, Coates LC, Soriano ER, et al. Drug therapies for peripheral joint disease in psoriatic arthritis: a systematic review. J Rheumatol 2014;41:2277–85.
56. Mease PJ, Armstrong AW. Managing patients with psoriatic disease: the diagnosis and pharmacologic treatment of psoriatic arthritis in patients with psoriasis. Drugs 2014;74:423–41.

CHAPTER 19

Non-pharmacological management in axial spondyloarthritis

Laura Passalent and Salih Ozgocmen

Introduction to non-pharmacological management

AxSpA is a chronic progressive inflammatory disease characterized by predominant involvement of the axial skeleton (1). The entity of axSpA consists of nr-axSpA (without definitive radiographic sacroiliitis on X-ray examination) and AS (with radiographic sacroiliitis in accordance to the mNY criteria). Patients with axSpA may also present with features of peripheral involvement (2). The presence of inflammatory low back pain is the primary symptom in axSpA, with a significant number of patients presenting with structural or radiographic damage. As a result, axSpA can be debilitating and potentially disabling (2). Disease progression in terms of structural damage may lead to mobility restrictions as a result of spinal fusion and damage to the peripheral joints. Besides this structural damage, several EAMs such as stiffness, pain, fatigue, and organ involvement, in addition to inflammation, may significantly contribute to functional impairment, sleep disturbances, workforce decline, reduced quality of life, and psychological distress (3–5). Due to the fact that axSpA typically presents in early adulthood (i.e. less than 45 years old), the impact of the disease on different aspects of life (career, family, and social life) can be substantial.

In 2010, the ASAS and EULAR updated their management recommendations for AS (6). These recommendations target patients who fulfill the mNY criteria for AS. The experts express that these recommendations are applied to patients with AS; however, they may also apply to patients with early axial SpA who do not yet fulfill the mNY criteria. The ASAS/EULAR panel recommends a multidisciplinary and patient-centred approach that includes a combination of pharmacological and non-pharmacological treatment modalities (6). These updated recommendations describe a number of non-pharmacological interventions as the cornerstone of treatment in patients with AS. The aims of such treatment are to: (1) reduce pain, stiffness, and discomfort; (2) maintain or improve muscle strength, endurance, flexibility, mobility, balance, physical fitness, and social participation; and (3) prevent spinal abnormalities, joint contractures, and deformities (7). This chapter presents the evidence in support of common non-pharmacological interventions for axSpA and provides recommendations regarding the implementation of such treatment strategies.

Physiotherapy

Often, non-pharmacological management comes in the form of physiotherapy (also referred to as physical therapy). The primary objective of physiotherapy is to assist patients to maintain, recover, or improve their physical abilities. Physiotherapy consists of a variety of physical modalities, including exercise, heat, cold, electrotherapy, and manual techniques. Medical rehabilitation (also referred to as physiatry) involves an interdisciplinary approach (which includes physiotherapy expertise) in the prevention, diagnosis, and management of people with disabling medical conditions. The goal of physiotherapy and medical rehabilitation is to maintain or improve patients' independence, social integration, and quality of life.

There exists a wide range of physiotherapy modalities used in the management of patients with axSpA. These include manual therapies ('hands-on' techniques such as massage and joint mobilization), electrophysical agents (diathermy, therapeutic US, low-level laser therapy, infrared or other electrical currents like transcutaneous electrical nerve stimulation (TENS)), thermotherapy (heat or ice packs, paraffin wax, cryotherapy), and exercise therapy. In general, several modalities are combined to provide comprehensive therapy and optimize treatment outcomes. For example, electrophysical agents are often used as an adjunct to manual techniques or exercises. In addition, physiotherapy may be provided in various forms that include individual outpatient treatment or in-patient rehabilitation programmes. Each of these types of physiotherapy are often supplemented by individually prescribed home-based exercise and education programmes. Regulatory rules and standards for rehabilitation professionals, facilities, and reimbursement strategies may change in different countries. An ideal physiotherapy setting may include space for individual therapy, facilities for electrotherapy, hydrotherapy, and special arrangements for testing, education, group communication, and leisure activities.

Physiotherapists are trained healthcare professionals and are experts in the delivery of physiotherapy and rehabilitation programmes. They are well placed to educate patients on regular daily exercises and physical activity; provide instruction on proper posture (Fig. 19.1); and discuss prevention strategies related to sedentary lifestyle and associated comorbidities. Moreover, they are

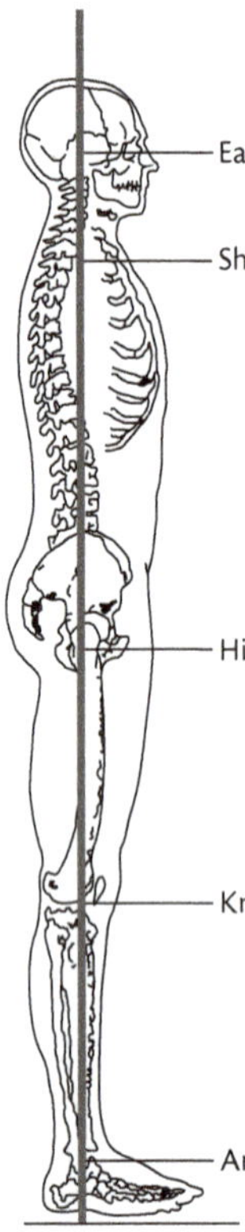

Fig. 19.1 Review of correct posture. (Source: http://www.exercise-ball-exercises.com/images/posture.jpg.)

competent to closely monitor a patient's physical functioning and performance.

For the assessment and monitoring of the physiotherapy interventions, ASAS recommends a core set of domains (8) (Table 19.1). Implementing these specific outcome measures and anthropometric measurements assists in the evaluation of disease activity and physical therapy efficacy. In addition to these ASAS domains, other measurements may be performed for individual patients, such as range-of-motion to monitor peripheral joints with deformities and contractures. Physiotherapy interventions have been shown to be effective for HRQoL and its related components in patients with AS. Therefore validated disease-specific measures like the ASQoL and the newly validated ASAS HI (9, 10) should be considered as key outcome measures.

Table 19.1 Assessment of ASAS core set for physical therapy

Domain	Instrument
Physical function	BASFI
Pain	NRS/VAS (spinal pain/at night due to AS/last week)
Spinal mobility	Chest expansion Modified Schober Occiput to wall Cervical rotation Lateral spinal flexion or BASMI
Spinal stiffness	NRS/VAS (duration of morning stiffness/spine/last week)
Patient global	NRS/VAS (global disease activity/last week)
Fatigue	Fatigue question in BASDAI

NRS/VAS = numeric rating scale/visual analogue scale; BASFI = Bath Ankylosing Spondylitis Functional Index; BASMI = Bath Ankylosing Spondylitis Metrology Index; BASDAI = Bath Ankylosing Spondylitis Disease Activity Index.

Patients with axSpA may develop enthesitis or inflammation of the ligaments, tendons, or periarticular structures, ankylosis of the spinal joints or destruction of the peripheral joints which makes these structures prone to rupture, entrapments, or fractures. Therefore any sudden change in pain or joint malfunction, particularly during stretching or endurance exercises, should alert the practitioner or patients themselves. Furthermore, clinicians should routinely assess other clinical aspects of patients with axSpA who are referred for physiotherapy. This may include cardiopulmonary status and the presence of metallic implants and joint prosthesis which may limit exercises and the application of some physical modalities through this region (i.e. shortwave diathermy). Patients with nr-axSpA, particularly those with short symptom duration, may not have restricted spinal mobility or peripheral joint involvement and may eventually have normal physical functioning. However, patients with nr-axSpA who are smoking and had elevated CRP and active sacroiliitis on MRI are more likely to develop structural damage and are potentially more prone to evolving radiographic sacroiliitis (11, 12). These predictors, in addition to other prognostic indicators, should be evaluated to determine which patients are ideal candidates and would benefit from physiotherapy management.

Exercise

Despite the significant impact of pharmacological therapy on AS outcomes, physical therapy and exercise, regardless of disease stage, remains an essential part of the overall management strategy (Figs 19.2–19.12). The chronic and progressive nature of the disease requires regular, ongoing, and lifelong exercise, despite the fact that non-pharmacological therapies have not been shown to alter disease progression (Table 19.2) (13, 14). Throughout the literature, exercise is the most studied non-pharmacological physical modality in the management of AS. However, there are some difficulties that prevent robust conclusions on the efficacy of exercise (14–17). These are summarized in Box 19.1.

- *This exercise helps to stretch your lower back and buttocks. It's a great exercise to help loosen your muscles and joints first thing in the morning*
- Find a firm surface to lie down on; this can be either the floor or your bed.
- Bend your knees up so that your feet are flat on the surface of the bed.
- Using your hands (or towel looped under your knee), bring one knee in towards your chest.
- Hold for the count of 3.
- Gently lower your knee back down to the bed.
- Now bring your other knee towards your chest.
- Hold for the count of 3.
- Now bring both knees towards your chest.
- Hold for the count of 3.
- Repeat this cycle (right knee, left knee, both knees)
- 10 times.
- * If this exercise causes pain in the knees, hold your legs under the knees when bringing your knees towards your chest.

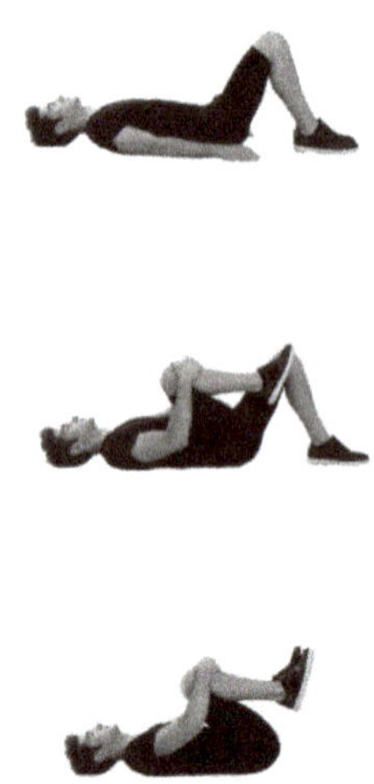

Fig. 19.2 Knees to chest.

- *The pelvic tilt is a strengthening exercise that focuses on your lower abdominals and will help to strengthen your core and promote proper posture.*
- Lie down on your back with your knees bent and your feet flat on the bed.
- Tighten the muscles of your stomach and squeeze your buttocks. At the same time, push your lower back into the bed.
- Hold 5 seconds.
- Gently release.
- Repeat 10–15 times.

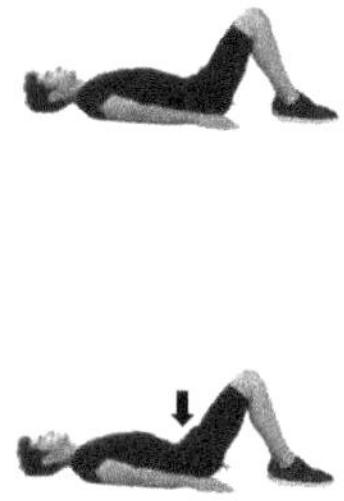

Fig. 19.3 Pelvic tilt.

- *The hamstring muscles are located in the back of the thigh. They connect from the pelvis to the back of the knee joint. Ensuring these muscles are flexible will ensure proper posture.*
- *There are many ways to stretch this muscle; however, the best way to stretch this muscle to avoid undue pressure on the back is to stretch the hamstrings in lying.*
- Lie down on your back with your knees bent and your feet flat on the bed.
- Use a large bath towel or belt and loop the centre of the towel/belt around the ball of your right foot while holding the ends in your hands.
- Gently straighten your knee and flex your ankle (bring your toes towards your nose) and tighten the towel/belt.
- Slowly raise your leg, bringing your toe towards your nose. When you start to feel a discomfort in the back of your thigh, hold this position.
- Hold for 15 seconds.
- Repeat 3–5 times on each leg.
- You may rest your head on a pillow to relax your upper spine during this stretch.

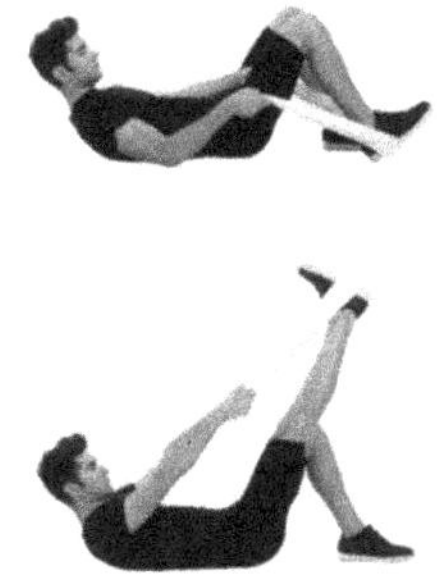

Fig. 19.5 Hamstring stretch.

Several exercise programmes have been described for AS in the literature and include:

- Individualized home-based exercises: these are a series of exercises prescribed to patients according to a predefined protocol of instructions or patients' special needs and that are performed unsupervised and independently.
- Supervised individual exercises: these are individualized exercises that may be performed at home or at a physiotherapy facility under supervision of a qualified instructor such as a physiotherapist. This approach is often chosen in patients early after diagnosis when education is necessary. Supervised exercise regimens can increase motivation, improve self-efficacy, assist in adherence, and ensure that exercise techniques are performed correctly (18).
- Supervised group-based exercises: these are usually offered to patients who may have difficulty adhering to regular independent exercise. Group-based exercises motivate patients to comply with the regimen in an environment where they have social contact with other exercising patients.

Group-based exercise can also be commenced as an in-patient physiotherapy programme. This usually consists of 2–4 weeks of an intensive exercise programme usually focused on posture, flexibility, and strengthening. Other exercise (i.e. respiratory or aerobic exercises), electrotherapy, and hydrotherapy modalities may also be included to relieve symptoms. In many European countries, balneotherapy or spa therapy has a long tradition. This therapy incorporates therapeutic exercises, natural mineral waters, thermal baths, and many other modalities, including mud packs, and massage, and also offers rest and relaxation.

The effect of exercise for AS was examined by a Cochrane review in 2008 (15). The results of this review show that individual home-based and supervised exercise programmes are better than no intervention and improve spinal mobility and physical function. Supervised group physiotherapy is better than home exercise and improves spinal mobility and patient global well-being. A combined in-patient spa-exercise regimen followed by group physiotherapy is better than physiotherapy alone (15). Some new data were added in recent years and substantially confirmed the results of this systematic review.

- *This exercise strengthens your buttocks, abdominals, and lower back. It is a great strengthening exercise to help build and maintain core strength.*
- Lie down on your back with your knees bent and your feet flat on the bed.
- Tighten your stomach muscles and squeeze your buttocks.
- Slowly raise your buttocks off the surface of the bed until your legs form a diagonal with your body.
- Hold 5 seconds.
- Gently release.
- Repeat 10–15 times.
- You may increase the difficulty of this exercise by crossing your hands over your chest or attempting a single leg bridge.

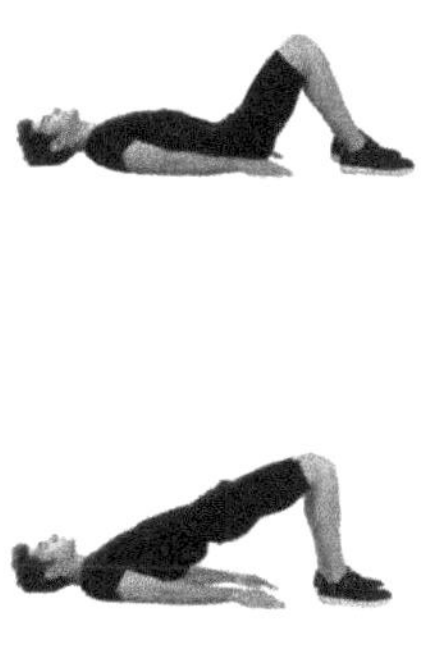

Fig. 19.4 Bridge.

- Lie face down with your hands face down at shoulder level and your elbows bent.
- Relax your back and abdominals.
- Push down with your hands and slowly begin to straighten your elbows. Keep your back and abdominals relaxed.
- Try to straighten your elbows.
- Hold for 3 seconds.
- Slowly return to the face down position.
- Repeat 10 times.
- * Only straighten your elbows within your pain-free range. You should not experience any back pain while attempting this exercise.

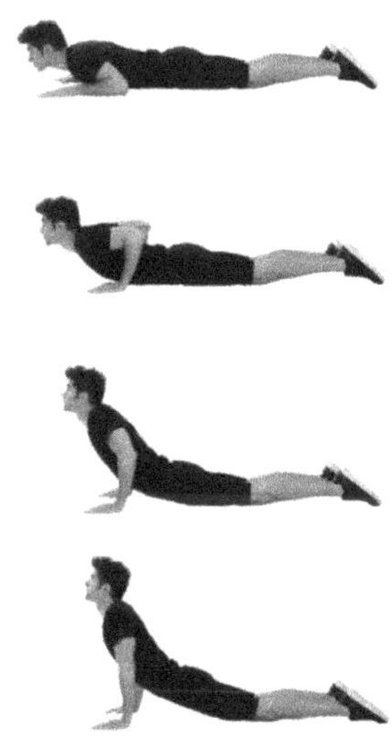

Fig. 19.6 Extension in lying.

- *This is a yoga pose that focuses on stretching the muscles of the torso, buttocks, chest, and arms. It is also a great relaxation position.*
- Start kneeling on your hands and knees.
- Drop your buttocks down towards your heels; as you do this, reach forward as far as you can as your chest drops towards the floor and your abdomen lays against your thighs.
- If you are able, rest your forehead on the ground.
- Hold for 30 seconds.
- Repeat 3–5 times.

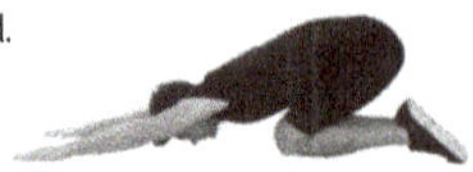

Fig. 19.7 Child's pose.

Home-based exercise programmes

A home-based exercise programme is a key element of a regular lifelong exercise habit. It has the advantage of low cost and is usually preferred by patients who are very active in their worklife and, hence, are unable to dedicate time for group or in-patient physiotherapy programmes. A prospective longitudinal (median follow-up 4.5 years) study consisting of 220 patients with AS examined the effect of unsupervised recreational exercise in addition to specific back exercises on pain severity, stiffness, and functional disability as assessed by the HAQ. Neither duration (minutes per week) nor frequency (times per week) was associated with short-term (6-month) changes in these parameters in the whole group. However, in a subgroup of patients with disease duration of 15 years or less, pain severity and stiffness severity scores improved significantly during periods when exercise was performed more than 200 minutes per week compared with periods when exercise was performed 0–30 minutes per week or less. In the subgroup of patients with long-standing disease, the progression of functional disability over time was lower in those who reported a consistently high frequency of back exercises. The important result from this study is that long-term and consistent back exercises (at least 30 minutes per day and 5 days per week) may help stabilize or decrease the rate of progression in functional disability (19). Another study similarly reported that moderate, consistent exercise can have long-term beneficial effects on both functional capacity and disease activity in patients with AS (18). Recent studies comparing home exercise to standard care or no intervention controls revealed that improvement in physical function, disease activity, chest expansion, and quality of life was in favour of therapeutic exercises (20–22). Improvement has been reported in respiratory muscle strength and pulmonary functions in home-based exercise groups compared to standard care or no intervention (20, 23).

A recently published multicentre Spanish study investigated the feasibility of a structured education and home exercise programme in patients with AS. Patients (n = 381) were randomized to education and exercise or control groups. The intervention group was provided with a 2-hour informative session about AS and instruction on an unsupervised home exercise programme. At 6 months, mean differences (adjusted for BASDAI value, sex, age, and educational level) for BASDAI and BASFI, patient's global, total pain, and ASQoL scores were in favour of education and home exercise group (24). Patients in the education group had significantly increased their knowledge about the disease and its treatments and practised more regular exercise than controls. However, the compliance with the exercise programme was rather low, in accordance with an earlier study reporting that the majority of patients with AS do not participate in exercise on a frequent basis (16).

The efficacy of high-intensity endurance and strength exercise (three times per week) on disease activity and cardiovascular health in patients with active axSpA has been investigated in a pilot study. The results were promising and the exercise group showed significant improvement in ASDAS compared to controls. Also, there were significant improvements in favour of the exercise group in the secondary outcomes, which included disease activity, function, arterial stiffness, peak wave velocity, VO_2 peak, and trunk fat (25). In another study, the effects of a 12-week cardiovascular training (individually monitored Nordic walking, moderate intensity, three units per week) on cardiovascular fitness and perceived disease activity has been investigated in patients with AS. Controls received intervention consisting of monthly 2.5-hour discussion groups on coping strategies and techniques of mindfulness-based stress reduction led by a psychologist. All participants received standard care and attended a weekly 1-hour spinal flexibility exercise group supervised by a physiotherapist. The physical fitness level in the training group was significantly higher than in the control group after 3 months. Also, secondary outcome measures including mean BASDAI and peripheral pain scores were in favour of the training group. Cardiovascular training, in addition to flexibility exercises, increased fitness in patients with AS and reduced their peripheral pain (26).

- *This is a great core strengthening exercise that will strengthen your abdominals, back, and buttock muscles.*
- Start in a kneeling position on your hands and knees. Be sure that your knees are below your hips and your hands are underneath your shoulders.
- Slowly raise your right arm off the bed and hold it straight out in front. Keep your head in a neutral position. Tighten your tummy muscles.
- At the same time, lift your left straight leg off the bed.
- Hold alternate arm and leg for 5 seconds.
- Repeat 10–15 times on each side.

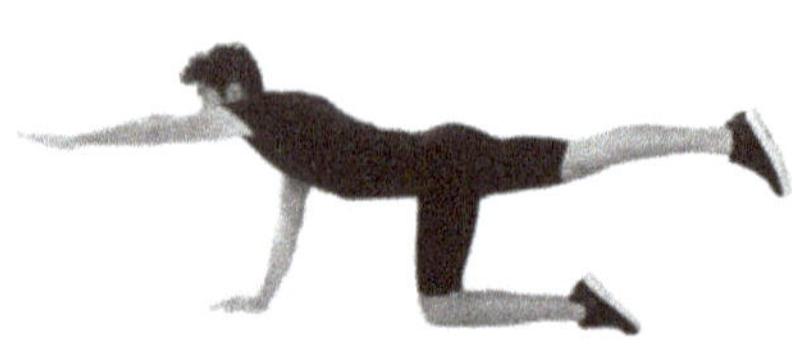

Fig. 19.8 Bird–dog.

- Standing in front of a mirror, if possible loop a towel around your right ankle.
- Bend your right knee and pull the towel while bringing your heel towards your buttocks.
- Bring your heel back enough so that you feel a stretch in the front of your thigh.
- Make sure your knees and thighs remain parallel. Try not to bend forwards at the hips.
- Hold for 15 seconds.
- Repeat 3–5 times on each leg.

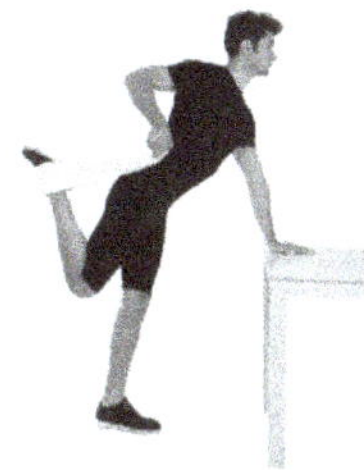

Fig. 19.9 Quadriceps stretch.

Supervised group exercises

Supervised group physiotherapy has been shown to be better than home exercises, according to the last Cochrane review (15). Global posture re-education (GPR) programmes were compared with supervised group exercises. GPR is a physical therapy method focusing on the stretching of antigravitational muscles and strengthening of muscles that are organized on closed kinetic chains to improve postural symmetry (27, 28). Although the level of evidence is moderate to low, this method seems to be comparable or slightly better than supervised group exercises in patients with AS regarding spinal mobility, physical function, and disease activity (20, 27, 29, 30).

Other alternative forms of structured supervised group exercise have been studied to assess their effect in the treatment of AS. For example, the efficacy of Pilates exercises has recently been assessed in patients with AS. Patients were randomized to the Pilates intervention group (1 hour, 3 times per week, for 12 weeks, supervised by a certified trainer) or control group (which received standard care). The Pilates group showed significant improvement in function (BASFI) at week 12 and week 24 compared to controls (31). A more recent study compared the effect of two multimodal home exercises (combination regimen of Pilates, McKenzie, and Heckscher techniques versus stretching, pulmonary exercise, and step-exercise) on pulmonary functions, physical functions, and disease activity in patients with AS. Both groups were provided with education and supervised for 12 weeks and continued individually at home (50 minutes, 3 times per week, for 48 weeks). At the conclusion of the study, improvement in pain, spinal mobility parameters, BASDAI, BASFI, and BASMI was in favour of the combination regimen (combination of Pilates, McKenzie, and Heckscher techniques) (32). The efficacy of Tai Chi has been investigated in a non-randomized controlled study with a small number of patients with AS. Some beneficial effects on disease activity and flexibility have been reported; however, this needs to be further assessed (33).

- *Ball exercises are a great way to strengthen your core. There are numerous exercises that you can do with the ball and at varying degrees of difficulty. Simply sitting on a ball will help improve your core strength. When choosing a ball, make sure it is the right size. Most people will use a 65-cm-diameter ball; however, you can get a smaller or larger ball, depending on your height. When you sit on the ball, keep your feet flat on the floor. Your hips and knees should be at right angles.*
- One simple exercise is to sit on the ball with your feet flat on the floor and your hands on your lap.
- Slowly straighten one knee, while maintaining your balance on the ball.
- Hold 5 seconds.
- Repeat 10–15 times on each leg.

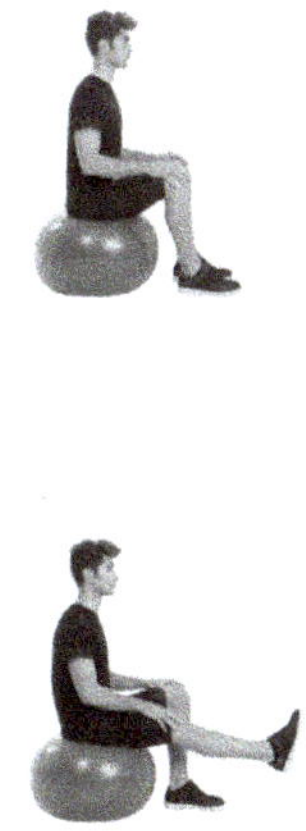

Fig. 19.11 Ball exercises.

In-patient programmes

An in-patient rehabilitation programme makes it possible to provide intensive physiotherapy with multiple sessions per day by using multiple treatment modalities. It also allows for regular supervised exercise and postural training, as well as providing comprehensive patient education. There is evidence that in-patient rehabilitation

- *This stretch focuses on the muscles of the torso and neck.*
- Sit in a straight-back chair, such as a dining room or kitchen chair.
- Sit on the front half of the chair.
- Keeping your posture straight, look over your left shoulder as far as you can, while twisting your torso.
- If you can, hook your left elbow on the back of the chair to help increase the stretch.
- Be sure to keep your buttocks planted on the chair.
- Hold position for 15 seconds.
- Repeat 3–5 times on each side.

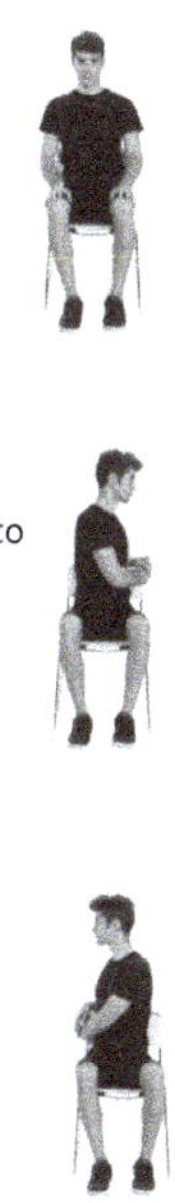

Fig. 19.10 Thoracic rotation.

- *This stretch focuses on the muscles in the front of your chest. Keeping these muscles flexible will assist in maintaining a proper posture.*
- Stand in a corner of a room. Face the corner. Lift both arms to a horizontal position against the walls. Your arms should be at the same height as your shoulders.
- Lean your upper trunk into the corner until you feel the stretch in the front of your chest.
- Hold this position for 15 seconds.
- Repeat 3–5 times.

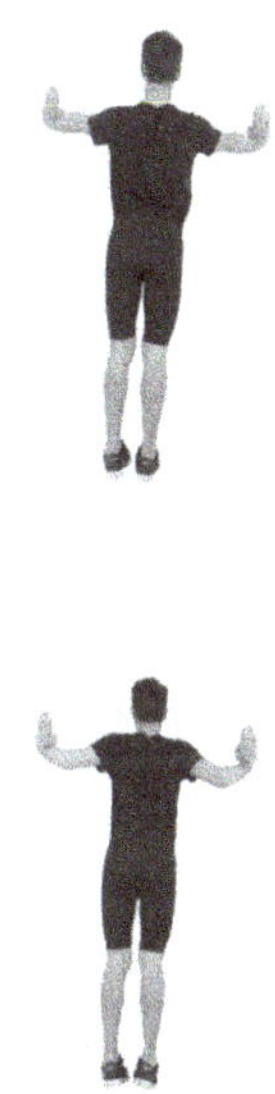

Fig. 19.12 Anterior chest wall stretch.

Table 19.2 Quantity and intensity of exercise prescription (adapted from the American College of Sports Medicine position stand, 2011)

Exercise type	Frequency (days/week)	Intensity	Duration
Cardiorespiratory (aerobic)	3–5	Moderate–vigorous (for most adults) Light–moderate (in deconditioned persons)	20–60 min (150 min/week)
Muscle strength (resistance)	2–3	Resistance equivalent to 60–80% of an individual's one repetition maximal effort; 8–12 repetitions (for most adults) 15–20 repetitions (to improve muscle endurance)	2–4 sets (for most adults)
Flexibility (stretching)	2–3	Stretch to point of slight discomfort	10–30 sec x 4 repetitions (for most adults)

Consensus on evidence-based recommendations for exercise prescription in AS have yet to be established. In the meantime, these guidelines published by the American College of Sports Medicine can be referred to and adapted as indicated when prescribing exercise for patients with axSpA.

Source: Garber CE, Blissmer B, Deschenes MR, Franklin BA, Lamonte MJ, Lee IM, Nieman DC, Swain DP; American College of Sports Medicine. American College of Sports Medicine position stand. Quantity and quality of exercise for developing and maintaining cardiorespiratory, musculoskeletal, and neuromotor fitness in apparently healthy adults: guidance for prescribing exercise. Med Sci Sports Exerc 2011 Jul;43(7):1334–59.

programmes may be more beneficial particularly in young patients (34, 35) and also in patients in the early stages of the disease (36). Previous studies with a small number of patients showed only short-term improvements with in-patient programmes and suggested that efficacy was sustained only if the patients continued with independent home exercises (37, 38). A recently published randomized controlled study revealed that a 3-week in-patient rehabilitation programme had positive effects on disease activity, pain, physical function, and overall well-being, indicating that in-patient rehabilitation programmes can be considered as an important complement to medical treatments in patients with AS (39). Conversely, another study assessing a similar in-patient rehabilitation programme showed that treatment efficacy declined over time, with clinical outcomes (ASAS response criteria) better at 6 weeks than at 12 weeks (34).

Climate may also have a role in treatment efficacy when in-patient rehabilitation is combined with spa or balneotherapy modalities. Four-week in-patient rehabilitation programmes were conducted in Mediterranean and Norwegian settings. While patients in both settings had similar improvement in physical functions, the improvements in the spinal mobility measures and ASAS response criteria were larger and better maintained at least 3 months after rehabilitation in a Mediterranean setting (40).

Box 19.1 Difficulties regarding exercise studies in AS which prevent firm conclusions on the efficacy of exercise

- Heterogeneity of the exercise protocols across studies and outcome measures
- Small sample size, variation in the patient population (axial vs peripheral involvement, disease severity, comorbidities), high rate of withdrawals, absent or short follow-up period, difficulty in blinding patients
- Indefinitely described exercise protocols or exercise modes (frequency, intensity, and duration), underreported physiological response measures, inconformity with the current recommendations (i.e. American College of Sports Medicine's (ACSM) recommendations for developing and maintaining cardiorespiratory fitness, muscular strength, and flexibility in healthy adults)
- Underreported concomitant medications and adherence

Water-based therapies

The efficacy of spa or balneotherapy on clinical outcomes in AS has been investigated in several studies. Balneotherapy was associated with an improvement in most of the outcome measures when compared to conventional exercises and standard care groups (41–48). Swimming and aerobic exercise improves functional capacity, pulmonary functions, and quality of life (49). A recent study showed that water-based exercises improved pain score and quality of life in patients with AS when compared with home-based exercises (50).

Little is known about the physiological effects of spa and exercise on inflammation or inflammatory pathways. In patients with AS, a combined spa and exercise therapy has been shown to increase serum levels of transforming growth factor-beta 1 (TGF-β1), which is an immunomodulating and anti-inflammatory cytokine (51). Further investigation into such phenomenon is warranted.

Tumour necrosis factor alpha inhibitors and rehabilitation in the treatment of patients with axial spondyloarthritis

TNFi have dramatically improved the disease course in patients with AS. Recent studies revealed that the combination of anti-TNF medications with rehabilitation therapies or spa appears to have a synergistic effect in patients with AS (47, 52, 53). The effect of combination therapy with rehabilitation and TNFα blocker (ETN) has been evaluated in a pilot study (52). Nineteen patients with AS underwent a 3-week intensive rehabilitation programme. After 6 months without physiotherapy or home exercises, the patients were reassessed and ETN was initiated (25 mg twice weekly). Three weeks after the initiation of ETN, patients were reintroduced to the same intensive in-patient rehabilitation programme. The primary outcome was the difference in pre- and post-BASFI, and the secondary outcomes were difference in revised Leeds Disability Questionnaire (LDQ), anthropometric measurements, EQ-5D, patient's global health, and 6-minute walking test (6-MWT). Differences between the time points were analysed to assess the efficacy of any rehabilitation arms. Results revealed that a combination treatment improved physical function, disability, and quality of life in patients with active AS.

Another study assessed the efficacy of a 2-week course of combined treatment with rehabilitation and spa versus no intervention in a group of AS patients who were treated with TNFα blockers (ETN and infliximab) for at least 3 months and continued during the study and follow-up period. One group (n = 15) received a combination of rehabilitation (exercises in a thermal pool) and spa (mud packs and thermal bath), and the controls (n = 15) received only TNFα blockers (47). The combined treatment with TNFα blocker, spa, and rehabilitation showed long-term clinical improvement (continued up to 3–6 months), whereas no change in outcome measures was noted in the control group. A recent study also showed that the combination of supervised and home exercises had long-term efficacy, compared to the educational-behavioural programme or no intervention, in terms of anthropometric measurements and disease activity in patients with AS who were under treatment with TNFα blockers (53). A newly published systematic review analysed the efficacy of the combination of TNFα inhibitors and rehabilitation programmes. Inclusion criteria and outcome measurements were comparable across the reviewed studies. The results from these studies showed that combining anti-TNF treatments with rehabilitation programmes enhanced the treatment efficacy in terms of symptom severity, physical functions, daily living activities, quality of life indices, anthropometric measurements, and some exercise parameters (54).

Electrophysical agents and thermotherapies

Electrophysical agents and thermotherapies have a well-established role in physiotherapy practice and are used to reduce pain originating from musculoskeletal structures and prepare the body for exercises and manual techniques. Despite their long tradition in physical therapy, there are little data for their use in patients with SpA. However, experience gained from their use in other rheumatic disorders may promote the use of electrophysical agents and thermotherapies in AS in a similar fashion.

A recent study assessed whole-body hyperthermia using infrared sauna in patients with RA or AS, and failed to show statistically significant improvements in pain, stiffness, and fatigue (55). The efficacy of TENS in AS was evaluated in a small double-blind sham controlled trial, and significant improvement in pain and stiffness in the TENS group was shown (56). A recent randomized double-blind placebo controlled trial showed that magnetic field therapy or magnetotherapy applied to the bilateral hip joints in patients with AS had no superiority in terms of pain, fatigue, morning stiffness, disease activity, functional ability, and quality of life to the placebo (57). In a small study, the effect of whole-body hyperthermy on serum cytokine levels was assessed in patients with AS and in controls. Whole-body hyperthermy caused prolonged decrease in proinflammatory cytokine levels at 24 hours after initiation, mean TNFα levels reduced by 50%, mean IL-1β by 40%, and mean IL-6 by 43% compared to the baseline levels (58).

Self-management and patient education

Successful management of chronic conditions often requires a collaborative effort between the healthcare team and the person living with the chronic condition. In addition to adhering to treatment that has been prescribed by a healthcare provider, patients will often acquire knowledge and skills to actively engage in the self-management of their chronic illness. This may manifest through participation in exercise, altering their diet, and/or lifestyle modifications that are aimed at improving one's overall health and well-being. The success of these self-management strategies is dependent on the effectiveness of the actions individuals take to address their chronic health condition. Support of self-management strategies in the form of patient education is critical in order to ensure effective health behaviour change and positive clinical outcomes. This will help to ensure patients are applying evidence-based strategies in their attempt to self-manage.

Chronic disease self-management strategies typically involve group education provided by an interdisciplinary team of healthcare professionals and/or peers who provide instruction on: symptom management and treatment; physical and psychosocial consequences; and the lifestyle changes that can occur when living with a chronic condition (59). Such self-management patient education has been shown to have beneficial effects on: reduced healthcare utilization; increased disease knowledge, self-efficacy, self-management behaviours (e.g. exercise), medication adherence; improved disease monitoring and better symptom management (60–62).

There is a well-established consensus among AS experts that the treatment of axSpA and AS requires a comprehensive approach that includes patient education (6). In support of this notion is a growing body of evidence illustrating the effectiveness of education programmes for patients with arthritis. A recent Cochrane review of education strategies for patients with RA demonstrated significant benefit with respect to disability, joint counts, patients' global assessment, psychological status, and depression (63). More recently, significant improvement in arthritis self-efficacy, knowledge about arthritis, coping efficacy, and illness intrusiveness were demonstrated following a group-based interdisciplinary education programme for adults with inflammatory arthritis (64). Similar findings have been seen in a variety of self-management programmes aimed at inflammatory arthritis, and have demonstrated positive effects on disability, function, and pain, in addition to self-efficacy (62, 65–68). Despite the evidence supporting patient education programmes for arthritis in general, there has been little investigation into patient education strategies specifically for axSpA. The current evidence suggests that only 40% of patients with AS are being referred for education, even though AS education programmes demonstrate positive effects with respect to mobility, function, self-efficacy, and depression (69–71). AS-specific self-management education strategies that impart knowledge of the disease, in addition to instruction on self-management skills and independent exercise, have shown to be effective with respect to psychological well-being; however, long-term changes are less likely to be sustained longer than 6 months following the initial education session (71).

Informational needs of patients with ankylosing spondylitis

Presumably the development of effective patient education programmes begins with content that is aligned with the informational needs of the patients themselves. A number of studies have examined the informational needs of patients diagnosed with AS and found that patients with AS want to know more about exercise, fatigue, pain, joint dysfunction, and how to improve activities of daily living (72, 73). Furthermore, patients with AS want more information about the latest research and medications, in addition to the standard information pertaining to disease diagnosis, prognosis, and management (73, 74). Table 19.3 outlines the key self-management and patient education topics for patients with axSpA. Despite a comprehensive list of informational needs identified by patients with AS, some patients may decide to refuse disease-related information as it may be considered too overwhelming, or patients may not be in a position to process or accept the information at a particular stage of their diagnosis (72). Moreover, the evidence indicates that the tone in which education information is delivered to patients is important and that patients with AS prefer to have information more positively conveyed, while minimizing any negative connotations associated with the disease (74).

What information are patients with ankylosing spondylitis receiving?

It has been suggested that patients with AS receive significantly more information about diagnosis and medication compared to patients with RA (72). There exists a variety of sources from which patients with AS can obtain information pertaining to their disease, including online and written sources, as well as verbally from their healthcare provider (74). Furthermore, given the almost universal access to online sources of information, it is not surprising that computer-based methods of receiving disease-related information is preferred among patients diagnosed with AS (73, 74). The degree to which patients with AS are seeking online information has yet to be explored in the literature; however, one study examining internet information seeking in RA patients found that 87.5% of patients gathered online medical information prior to their initial consult, versus only 22.8% who sought information from non-computer based sources (75). This figure is higher than similar information-seeking behaviour reported in primary care, where 53.5% of patients used the internet for medical information (76). Evidently the use of computer-based patient education programmes needs to be further examined in AS, as other chronic disease self-management education programmes have proved beneficial with respect to health status (fatigue, pain, shortness of breath) and self-efficacy 1 year after participating in an internet-based chronic disease self-management programme (77).

Table 19.3 Key self-management and patient education topics for patients with axSpA

Disease-related	Diagnosis Prognosis
Management-related	Pharmacological intervention Non-pharmacological intervention
Symptom-related	Fatigue Pain Joint dysfunction
Function-related	Activities of daily living Psychological impact
Social-related	Recreation Community involvement Employment Interpersonal relationships

Clearly there are positive clinical outcomes to be gained through patient education interventions that focus on self-management, as demonstrated in the arthritis literature; however, there remains a significant gap in the scientific literature examining the effectiveness of such strategies as they pertain to AS and axSpA. To begin, further research is required to address the specific educational components that are of most benefit to patients with axSpA. A clear understanding of the factors that influence how patients with axSpA access, integrate, and adhere to education and self-management interventions may assist in the overall function and well-being of this patient population. Second, few studies have examined the long-term outcomes of patient education strategies, suggesting that further investigation into such phenomena is warranted.

Next, application of the most appropriate outcome measures is critical if we are to fully understand the impact of education and self-management interventions in the axSpA population. The ASAS Working Group of OMERACT IV has recommended a number of endpoints for clinical studies for AS that include physical function, pain, spinal mobility, spinal stiffness, and patient global assessment (8). Unfortunately, inclusion of outcomes related to the domains of daily activity and social participation is virtually non-existent in the current literature. These latter domains are found to be restricted in the AS population with respect to recreation, community involvement, employment, and interpersonal relationships (78). Therefore education content and evaluation related to these domains, in addition to the outcomes outlined by the ASAS Working Group of OMERACT IV, will be important in the development, implementation, and evaluation of future education programmes aimed at the AS population. Lastly, exploration of the synergistic effects of patient education strategies with other conventional treatment modalities for AS may reveal new models of treatment that can optimize patient outcomes.

Complementary and alternative medicine (CAM)

CAMs are considered approaches to healthcare that are practiced outside of conventional medicine for specific conditions or well-being (79). The terms 'complementary' and 'alternative' have different connotations. 'Complementary' refers to therapies beyond standard treatment interventions that are applied *in combination* with mainstream medical approaches to a specific condition; whereas 'alternative' refers to therapies outside conventional medicine that are applied *in place of* mainstream medicine (79). Alternative medicine as an approach in and of itself is rare, as the majority of people living in western societies generally use non-mainstream treatment together with conventional management

(79). The interpretation, practice, and convention of CAM may change depending on one's cultural and ethnic origin and where one lives in the world. In general, CAM is a very broad subject and encompasses interventions that involve: *the mind* (e.g. mindful meditation, relaxation therapy); *body practices* (e.g. massage therapy, acupuncture, chiropractic treatment, traditional Chinese medicine); *natural health products* (e.g. herbal remedies, homeopathy, naturopathic interventions); and *dietary supplements* (e.g. vitamins and minerals).

There is very little evidence to support the use of CAM in AS and axSpA; however, its use is common among patients (95%), with the majority of these patients using dietary CAM (72%) or they have consulted with a CAM practitioner (36%) at some point following their diagnosis (80). Other CAM modalities used by patients with AS include massage therapy, acupuncture, naturopathy, and homeopathy (80). Often these alternative forms of therapy are used in conjunction with evidence-based approaches to AS management that include NSAIDs and TNFα inhibitors, as well as conventional exercise and physiotherapy interventions. Unfortunately, a small percentage of patients with AS or axSpA will fail standard treatment, including NSAIDs and/or TNFα inhibitors, with a suboptimal response to conventional management (81, 82). In these unresponsive cases, alternative forms of treatment may represent the only management patients can explore for symptom relief. As the research into the various forms of CAM for axSpA is lacking, evidence as it pertains to low back pain and other types inflammatory arthritis will be considered for the more common practices of CAM, with the understanding that axSpA differs from other forms of inflammatory arthritis and differs from mechanical low back pain.

Massage therapy

There are various forms of massage therapy that can aid in mental relaxation, decrease muscle tension, reduce chronic pain, and improve overall well-being (83). The most recent Cochrane review on massage and low back pain suggests that massage therapy for non-specific low-back pain provides modest benefit with respect to pain relief and return to normal function, when combined with exercise and education (84). Unfortunately, the evidence pertaining to the effect of massage therapy specific to AS is weak and inconclusive, with very few studies found in the literature. One case study reported the effects of short-term Swedish massage on a 47-year-old woman diagnosed with AS and demonstrated improvements in spinal mobility and perceived pain, stiffness, and fatigue (85). Although there exists a small amount of evidence to suggest that massage therapy has some effect on pain reduction and improvement in function in non-specific low back pain, further investigation into the various forms of massage is needed to determine its effect in patients diagnosed with axSpA.

Acupuncture

The popularity of acupuncture as an adjunct to conventional western medical practice has grown since 2005 and the scientific evidence supporting its use has expanded steadily, with evidence supporting its biophysical impact, such as the release of endorphins, serotonin, and cortisol (86–89). The latest Cochrane review for acupuncture and chronic low back pain indicates that acupuncture provides effective immediate short-term pain relief and functional improvement compared to sham treatment, and may be a useful addition to other chronic low back pain interventions (90). Despite evidence suggesting that acupuncture may provide benefit in chronic low back pain, robust evidence for its use in axSpA is lacking. Though the literature shows promise regarding the positive benefits of acupuncture on chronic low back pain, the studies themselves are inconclusive, due to problems associated with small numbers of study subjects, variable acupuncture technique, and the use of non-standardized outcome measures, to name only a few. Further exploration into the clinical and biophysical impact of acupuncture on axSpA using well-designed clinical trials is warranted.

Chiropractic treatment

Chiropractic intervention is often sought by people with low back pain. The most recent Cochrane review examined combined chiropractic treatment, which includes a combination of manual therapies (e.g. spinal manipulation), passive modalities, exercise programmes, and patient education, for non-specific low back pain (91). This review found no clinical evidence to support chiropractic treatment over other treatments to address pain or disability (91). The majority of the literature examining chiropractic treatment for AS consist of case studies and suggest that chiropractic intervention focused on manipulation, mobilization, electrical muscle stimulation, and stretches may result in small improvements in quality of life and spinal flexibility (92, 93). Care must be taken when interpreting the results of case studies, as the data are not sufficient to make conclusions regarding causation. Furthermore, there exist potential problems with secondary data collection, issues of bias, and problems related to external validity. What these case studies offer is a platform for more robust research into the effect of chiropractic management in axSpA.

As chiropractic care is often pursued by patients with chronic back pain, caution should be exercised prior to any patient with AS or suspected AS/axSpA seeking chiropractic management. The Canadian Chiropractic Association's published clinical guidelines advise that: 'inflammatory arthritis such as rheumatoid arthritis, seronegative spondyloarthropathies including acute ankylosing spondylitis characterized by episodes of acute inflammation, demineralization, ligamentous laxity with anatomic subluxation or dislocation, represent an *absolute contraindication* to high-velocity thrust procedures in anatomical regions of involvement' (94). Spinal manipulation in patients with established AS should be avoided due to the risk of osteoporosis and the unknown effects of joint manipulation in actively inflamed joints (95–98). Given the uncertainty of the effect of chiropractic intervention and the potential harm associated with such intervention in AS patients with established syndesmophyte formation and/or osteoporosis, care should be taken prior to undertaking chiropractic treatment, specifically any form of spinal manipulation.

Natural health products and supplements

Natural health products comprise a vast number of products such as herbal remedies, tinctures, and vitamin supplements that may be prescribed by traditional Chinese medicine, naturopathic or homeopathic practitioners. These products may also be obtained by patients, independent of any professional guidance. The use of natural health products in the treatment of AS was reported in a case study of 12 patients with AS who were treated with *Tripterygium wilfordii* (also known as thunder god vine) for 6 weeks (99). The results of this study demonstrated a 60% significant improvement in disease activity and function, with no adverse effects noted (99). Beyond this one case study, there exists a significant gap in the literature examining the effects of natural health products in the AS population. With respect to low back pain and herbal remedies, the Cochrane Collaboration recently published its systematic review of 14 studies examining six herbal medications to address non-specific low back pain. The results indicate that Devil's claw (*Harpagophytum probumbes*), white willow bark (*Salix alba*), cayenne (*Capsicum frutescens*) topical plaster, comfrey (*Symphytum officinale* L.), Brazilian arnica (*Solidago chilensis*) ointments, and lavender essential oil applied by acupressure, were shown to reduce pain more than placebo. Adverse effects in the form of mild, transient GI complaints were described with oral intake of Devil's claw and white willow bark. The quality of the evidence was considered to be low to moderate (100).

Herbal therapy has also been examined in RA. The most recent systematic review looked at 22 studies examining various herbal therapies for RA and showed moderate evidence that oils containing gamma linolenic acid (evening primrose, borage, and blackcurrant seed oil) reduce pain intensity and improve disability for RA. It also found that thunder god vine products may improve some RA symptoms; however, its oral use may be associated with several side-effects (101).

There are a number of considerations that must be addressed when considering natural health product remedies and their various forms. First, the systematic reviews suggest that pooling of data is difficult, given the variation in treatment protocol, such as differences related to dosing, frequency of dosing, and difficulty comparing oral and topical administration. Second, the quality and preparation of such products is not necessarily overseen by a regulatory body, putting the safety of such products into question. Lastly, there is the potential for unknown negative interaction with conventional pharmacological management that could lead to significant adverse events in patients who take natural health products without proper guidance from a trained healthcare provider.

Conclusion

Successful management of AS requires a comprehensive approach that includes a variety of non-pharmacological strategies comprised of physiotherapy and exercise, as well as self-management and patient education. Although axSpA is a relatively new entity, with little data regarding use of non-pharmacological treatments particularly in patients with nr-axSpA, the results in AS could be extrapolated for patients with axSpA. Evidence from the literature reveals that education and exercise continue to be the foundation of non-pharmacological management for patients with axSpA. Conventional exercise protocols consisting of flexibility, stretching, and postural exercises, as well as cardiovascular exercises, have been proven to be beneficial. Aquatic exercises may provide extra benefits. The optimum form of rehabilitation is not yet clear; however, data suggest that an effective rehabilitation strategy should include supervised exercises supported with an educational component. Rehabilitation strategies should be patient-centred and individualized according to the needs and expectations of the patient and also consider clinical status, including the presence of EAMs and comorbidities. Combination of TNFα blockers with a rehabilitation and/or spa programme may have synergistic effects and provide enhanced efficacy regarding numerous outcome parameters, including symptom severity, physical functions, activities of daily living, quality of life indices, and mobility.

Self-management and patient education strategies are also an important component of non-pharmacological management for people with AS. Improved self-efficacy, treatment adherence, disease monitoring, and symptom management can result from appropriate patient education strategies. Education topics should be identified by the patients themselves and include information pertaining to diagnosis, prognosis, management, and how best to mitigate the physical and psychosocial impact of the disease on patients' daily lives.

In general, the value of CAM as an evidenced-based form of intervention for patients with axSpA is questionable, primarily due to the lack of well-designed studies specific to this patient population. Currently, one can extrapolate from the literature pertaining to non-specific low back pain and other forms of arthritis; however, there are inherent problems with this, given the disease-specific nature of axial SpA. Nonetheless, CAM may play an important role in symptom management for patients who have not attained optimal response to conventional treatments or who may wish to augment traditional treatment with various complementary and alternative therapies. For the most part, CAM approaches are considered safe when provided by trained and competent healthcare professionals; however, some therapies are not without risks and need to be approached with caution.

Although a number of limitations regarding study design have been identified in the reviewed literature pertaining to non-pharmacological management for AS, there is opportunity for further research into this important area of AS care. The positive impact of non-pharmacological treatment on pain reduction, spinal mobility, fatigue, function, and quality of life, alongside conventional pharmacological management will ensure optimal outcomes in this unique patient population.

References

1. Sieper J, van der Heijde D. Review: nonradiographic axial spondyloarthritis: new definition of an old disease? Arthritis Rheum 2013;65(3):543–51.
2. Deodhar A, Reveille JD, van den Bosch F, et al. The concept of axial spondyloarthritis: joint statement of the spondyloarthritis research and treatment network and the Assessment of SpondyloArthritis international Society in response to the US Food and Drug Administration's comments and concerns. Arthritis Rheumatol 2014;66(10):2649–56.
3. Boonen A, Sieper J, van der Heijde D, et al. The burden of non-radiographic axial spondyloarthritis. Semin Arthritis Rheum 2015;44(5);556–62.
4. Brionez TF, Assassi S, Reveille JD, et al. Psychological correlates of self-reported functional limitation in patients with ankylosing spondylitis. Arthritis Res Ther 2009;11(6):R182.
5. Kilic G, Kilic E, Ozgocmen S. Relationship between psychiatric status, self-reported outcome measures, and clinical parameters in axial spondyloarthritis. Medicine 2014;93(29):e337.
6. Braun J, van den Berg R, Baraliakos X, et al. 2010 update of the ASAS/EULAR recommendations for the management of ankylosing spondylitis. Ann Rheum Dis 2011;70(6):896–904.
7. Ozgocmen S, Akgul O, Altay Z, et al. Expert opinion and key recommendations for the physical therapy and rehabilitation of patients with ankylosing spondylitis. Int J Rheum Dis 2012;15(3):229–38.
8. van der Heijde D, van der Linden S, Bellamy N, Calin A, Dougados M, Khan MA. Which domains should be included in a core set for endpoints in ankylosing spondylitis? Introduction to the ankylosing spondylitis module of OMERACT IV. J Rheumatol 1999;26(4):945–7.

9. Doward LC, Spoorenberg A, Cook SA, et al. Development of the ASQoL: a quality of life instrument specific to ankylosing spondylitis. Ann Rheum Dis 2003;62(1):20–6.
10. Kiltz U, van der Heijde D, Boonen A, et al. Development of a health index in patients with ankylosing spondylitis (ASAS HI): final result of a global initiative based on the ICF guided by ASAS. Ann Rheum Dis 2013;72:A124–5.
11. Poddubnyy D, Haibel H, Listing J, et al. Baseline radiographic damage, elevated acute-phase reactant levels, and cigarette smoking status predict spinal radiographic progression in early axial spondylarthritis. Arthritis Rheum 2012;64(5):1388–98.
12. Poddubnyy D, Sieper J. Similarities and differences between nonradiographic and radiographic axial spondyloarthritis: a clinical, epidemiological and therapeutic assessment. Curr Opin Rheumatol 2014;26(4):377–83.
13. Elyan M, Khan MA. Does physical therapy still have a place in the treatment of ankylosing spondylitis? Curr Opin Rheumatol 2008;20(3):282–6.
14. O'Dwyer T, O'Shea F, Wilson F. Exercise therapy for spondyloarthritis: a systematic review. Rheumatol Int 2014;34(7):887–902.
15. Dagfinrud H, Kvien TK, Hagen KB. Physiotherapy interventions for ankylosing spondylitis. Cochrane Database Syst Rev 2008(1):CD002822.
16. Passalent LA. Physiotherapy for ankylosing spondylitis: evidence and application. Curr Opin Rheumatol 2011;23(2):142–7.
17. Dagfinrud H, Halvorsen S, Vollestad NK, Niedermann K, Kvien TK, Hagen KB. Exercise programs in trials for patients with ankylosing spondylitis: do they really have the potential for effectiveness? Arthritis Care Res 2011;63(4):597–603.
18. Santos H, Brophy S, Calin A. Exercise in ankylosing spondylitis: how much is optimum? J Rheumatol 1998;25(11):2156–60.
19. Uhrin Z, Kuzis S, Ward MM. Exercise and changes in health status in patients with ankylosing spondylitis. Arch Intern Med 2000;160(19):2969–75.
20. Durmus D, Alayli G, Uzun O, et al. Effects of two exercise interventions on pulmonary functions in the patients with ankylosing spondylitis. Joint Bone Spine 2009;76(2):150–5.
21. Durmus D, Alayli G, Cil E, Canturk F. Effects of a home-based exercise program on quality of life, fatigue, and depression in patients with ankylosing spondylitis. Rheumatol Int 2009;29(6):673–7.
22. Aytekin E, Caglar NS, Ozgonenel L, Tutun S, Demiryontar DY, Demir SE. Home-based exercise therapy in patients with ankylosing spondylitis: effects on pain, mobility, disease activity, quality of life, and respiratory functions. Clin Rheumatol 2012;31(1):91–7.
23. Ortancil O, Sarikaya S, Sapmaz P, Basaran A, Ozdolap S. The effect(s) of a six-week home-based exercise program on the respiratory muscle and functional status in ankylosing spondylitis. J Clin Rheumatol 2009;15(2):68–70.
24. Rodriguez-Lozano C, Juanola X, Cruz-Martinez J, et al. Outcome of an education and home-based exercise programme for patients with ankylosing spondylitis: a nationwide randomized study. Clin Exp Rheumatol 2013;31(5):739–48.
25. Sveaas SH, Berg IJ, Provan SA, et al. Efficacy of high intensity exercise on disease activity and cardiovascular risk in active axial spondyloarthritis: a randomized controlled pilot study. PloS One 2014;9(9):e108688.
26. Niedermann K, Sidelnikov E, Muggli C. Effect of cardiovascular training on fitness and perceived disease activity in people with ankylosing spondylitis. Arthritis Care Res 2013;65(11):1844–52.
27. Silva EM, Andrade SC, Vilar MJ. Evaluation of the effects of global postural reeducation in patients with ankylosing spondylitis. Rheumatol Int 2012;32(7):2155–63.
28. Teodori RM, Negri JR, Cruz MC, Marques AP. Global postural re-education: a literature review. Rev Bras Fisioter 2011;15(3):185–9.
29. Fernandez-de-Las-Penas C, Alonso-Blanco C, Morales-Cabezas M, Miangolarra-Page JC. Two exercise interventions for the management of patients with ankylosing spondylitis: a randomized controlled trial. Am J Phys Med Rehabil 2005;84(6):407–19.
30. Fernandez-de-Las-Penas C, Alonso-Blanco C, Alguacil-Diego IM, Miangolarra-Page JC. One-year follow-up of two exercise interventions for the management of patients with ankylosing spondylitis: a randomized controlled trial. Am J Phys Med Rehabil 2006;85(7):559–67.
31. Altan L, Korkmaz N, Dizdar M, Yurtkuran M. Effect of Pilates training on people with ankylosing spondylitis. Rheumatol Int 2012;32(7):2093–9.
32. Rosu MO, Topa I, Chirieac R, Ancuta C. Effects of Pilates, McKenzie and Heckscher training on disease activity, spinal motility and pulmonary function in patients with ankylosing spondylitis: a randomized controlled trial. Rheumatol Int 2014;34(3):367–72.
33. Lee EN, Kim YH, Chung WT, Lee MS. Tai chi for disease activity and flexibility in patients with ankylosing spondylitis—a controlled clinical trial. Evidence-based complementary and alternative medicine. Evid Based Complement Alternat Med 2008;5(4):457–62.
34. Lubrano E, D'Angelo S, Parsons WJ, et al. Effectiveness of rehabilitation in active ankylosing spondylitis assessed by the ASAS response criteria. Rheumatology 2007;46(11):1672–5.
35. Viitanen JV, Suni J, Kautiainen H, Liimatainen M, Takala H. Effect of physiotherapy on spinal mobility in ankylosing spondylitis. Scand J Rheumatol 1992;21(1):38–41.
36. Band DA, Jones SD, Kennedy LG. Which patients with ankylosing spondylitis derive most benefit from an inpatient management program? J Rheumatol 1997;24(12):2381–4.
37. Helliwell PS, Abbott CA, Chamberlain MA. A randomised trial of three different physiotherapy regimes in ankylosing spondylitis. Physiotherapy 1996;82:85–90.
38. Bulstrode SJ, Barefoot J, Harrison RA, Clarke AK. The role of passive stretching in the treatment of ankylosing spondylitis. Br J Rheumatol 1987;26(1):40–2.
39. Kjeken I, Bo I, Ronningen A, et al. A three-week multidisciplinary in-patient rehabilitation programme had positive long-term effects in patients with ankylosing spondylitis: randomized controlled trial. J Rehab Med 2013;45(3):260–7.
40. Staalesen Strumse YA, Nordvag BY, Stanghelle JK, et al. Efficacy of rehabilitation for patients with ankylosing spondylitis: comparison of a four-week rehabilitation programme in a Mediterranean and a Norwegian setting. J Rehab Med 2011;43(6):534–42.
41. Altan L, Bingol U, Aslan M, Yurtkuran M. The effect of balneotherapy on patients with ankylosing spondylitis. Scand J Rheumatol 2006;35(4):283–9.
42. Colina M, Ciancio G, Garavini R, Conti M, Trotta F, Govoni M. Combination treatment with etanercept and an intensive spa rehabilitation program in active ankylosing spondylitis. Int J Immunopathol Pharmacol 2009;22(4):1125–9.
43. Yurtkuran M, Ay A, Karakoc Y. Improvement of the clinical outcome in ankylosing spondylitis by balneotherapy. Joint Bone Spine 2005;72(4):303–8.
44. Aydemir K, Tok F, Peker F, Safaz I, Taskaynatan MA, Ozgul A. The effects of balneotherapy on disease activity, functional status, pulmonary function and quality of life in patients with ankylosing spondylitis. Acta Reumatol Port 2010;35(5):441–6.
45. Van Tubergen A, Boonen A, Landewe R, et al. Cost effectiveness of combined spa-exercise therapy in ankylosing spondylitis: a randomized controlled trial. Arthritis Rheum 2002;47(5):459–67.
46. van Tubergen A, Landewe R, van der Heijde D, et al. Combined spa-exercise therapy is effective in patients with ankylosing spondylitis: a randomized controlled trial. Arthritis Rheum 2001;45(5):430–8.
47. Ciprian L, Lo Nigro A, Rizzo M, et al. The effects of combined spa therapy and rehabilitation on patients with ankylosing spondylitis being treated with TNF inhibitors. Rheumatol Int 2013;33(1):241–5.
48. Codish S, Dobrovinsky S, Abu Shakra M, Flusser D, Sukenik S. Spa therapy for ankylosing spondylltis at the Dead Sea. Israel Med Assoc J 2005;7(7):443–6.
49. Karapolat H, Eyigor S, Zoghi M, Akkoc Y, Kirazli Y, Keser G. Are swimming or aerobic exercise better than conventional exercise in ankylosing spondylitis patients? A randomized controlled study. Eur J Physical Rehab Med 2009;45(4):449–57.

50. Dundar U, Solak O, Toktas H, et al. Effect of aquatic exercise on ankylosing spondylitis: a randomized controlled trial. Rheumatol Int 2014;34(11):1505–11.
51. Shehata M, Schwarzmeier JD, Hilgarth M, et al. Effect of combined spa-exercise therapy on circulating TGF-beta1 levels in patients with ankylosing spondylitis. Wien Klin Wochenschr 2006;118(9–10):266–72.
52. Lubrano E, D'Angelo S, Parsons WJ, et al. Effects of a combination treatment of an intensive rehabilitation program and etanercept in patients with ankylosing spondylitis: a pilot study. J Rheumatol 2006;33(10):2029–34.
53. Masiero S, Poli P, Bonaldo L, et al. Supervised training and home-based rehabilitation in patients with stabilized ankylosing spondylitis on TNF inhibitor treatment: a controlled clinical trial with a 12-month follow-up. Clin Rehab 2013;28(6):562–72.
54. Lubrano E, Spadaro A, Amato G, et al. Tumour necrosis factor alpha inhibitor therapy and rehabilitation for the treatment of ankylosing spondylitis: a systematic review. Semin Arthritis Rheum 2015;44(5):542–50.
55. Oosterveld FG, Rasker JJ, Floors M, et al. Infrared sauna in patients with rheumatoid arthritis and ankylosing spondylitis. A pilot study showing good tolerance, short-term improvement of pain and stiffness, and a trend towards long-term beneficial effects. Clin Rheumatol 2009;28(1):29–34.
56. Gemignani G, Olivieri I, Ruju G, Pasero G. Transcutaneous electrical nerve stimulation in ankylosing spondylitis: a double-blind study. Arthritis Rheum 1991;34(6):788–9.
57. Turan Y, Bayraktar K, Kahvecioglu F, et al. Is magnetotherapy applied to bilateral hips effective in ankylosing spondylitis patients? A randomized, double-blind, controlled study. Rheumatol Int 2014;34(3):357–65.
58. Tarner IH, Muller-Ladner U, Uhlemann C, Lange U. The effect of mild whole-body hyperthermia on systemic levels of TNF-alpha, IL-1beta, and IL-6 in patients with ankylosing spondylitis. Clin Rheumatol 2009;28(4):397–402.
59. Barlow J. How to use education as an intervention in osteoarthritis. Best Pract Res Clin Rheumatol 2001;15(4):545–58.
60. Barlow J, Wright C, Sheasby J, Turner A, Hainsworth J. Self-management approaches for people with chronic conditions: a review. Patient Educ Couns 2002;48(2):177–87.
61. Nolte S, Osborne RH. A systematic review of outcomes of chronic disease self-management interventions. Qual Life Res 2013;22(7):1805–16.
62. Lorig K, Lubeck D, Kraines RG, Seleznick M, Holman HR. Outcomes of self-help education for patients with arthritis. Arthritis Rheum 1985;28(6):680–5.
63. Riemsma RP, Kirwan JR, Taal E, Rasker JJ. Patient education for adults with rheumatoid arthritis. Cochrane Database Syst Rev 2003(2):CD003688.
64. Kennedy CA, Beaton DE, Warmington K, Shupak R, Jones C, Hogg-Johnson S. Prescription for education: development, evaluation, and implementation of a successful interprofessional education program for adults with inflammatory arthritis. J Rheumatol 2011;38(10):2247–57.
65. Du S, Yuan C, Xiao X, Chu J, Qiu Y, Qian H. Self-management programs for chronic musculoskeletal pain conditions: a systematic review and meta-analysis. Patient Educ Couns 2011;85(3):e299–310.
66. Scholten C, Brodowicz T, Graninger W, et al. Persistent functional and social benefit 5 years after a multidisciplinary arthritis training program. Arch Phys Med Rehab 1999;80(10):1282–7.
67. Taal E, Riemsma RP, Brus HL, Seydel ER, Rasker JJ, Wiegman O. Group education for patients with rheumatoid arthritis. Patient Educ Couns 1993;20(2–3):177–87.
68. Warsi A, LaValley MP, Wang PS, Avorn J, Solomon DH. Arthritis self-management education programs: a meta-analysis of the effect on pain and disability. Arthritis Rheum 2003;48(8):2207–13.
69. Thompson B, Rapley TJ, Broderick W, May CR, Kay LJ. Education for people with ankylosing spondylitis: current practice in the UK. British Society for Rheumatology and British Health Professionals in Rheumatology Annual Meeting, Glasgow, 2009, p. i51.
70. Kraag G, Stokes B, Groh J, Helewa A, Goldsmith C. The effects of comprehensive home physiotherapy and supervision on patients with ankylosing spondylitis—a randomized controlled trial. J Rheumatol 1990;17(2):228–33.
71. Barlow JH, Barefoot J. Group education for people with arthritis. Patient Educ Couns 1996;27(3):257–67.
72. Kjeken I, Dagfinrud H, Mowinckel P, Uhlig T, Kvien TK, Finset A. Rheumatology care: involvement in medical decisions, received information, satisfaction with care, and unmet health care needs in patients with rheumatoid arthritis and ankylosing spondylitis. Arthritis Rheum 2006;55(3):394–401.
73. Kang R, Passalent L, Morton R, et al. Utilization of an informational needs assessment to develop an education program for patients with ankylosing spondylitis and related axial spondyloarthritis. Ann Rheum Dis 2013;72:1037–8.
74. Cooksey R, Brophy S, Husain MJ, Irvine E, Davies H, Siebert S. The information needs of people living with ankylosing spondylitis: a questionnaire survey. BMC Musculoskelet Disord 2012;13:243.
75. Hay MC, Cadigan RJ, Khanna D, et al. Prepared patients: internet information seeking by new rheumatology patients. Arthritis Rheum 2008;59(4):575–82.
76. Diaz JA, Griffith RA, Ng JJ, Reinert SE, Friedmann PD, Moulton AW. Patients' use of the Internet for medical information. J Gen Intern Med 2002;17(3):180–5.
77. Lorig KR, Ritter PL, Laurent DD, Plant K. Internet-based chronic disease self-management: a randomized trial. Medical Care 2006;44(11):964–71.
78. van Echteld I, Cieza A, Boonen A, et al. Identification of the most common problems by patients with ankylosing spondylitis using the international classification of functioning, disability and health. J Rheumatol 2006;33(12):2475–83.
79. National Center for Complementary and Integrative Health. Complementary, alternative, or integrative health: what's in a name? NCCIH, 2015, https://nccih.nih.gov/health/whatiscam.
80. Chatfield SM, Dharmage SC, Boers A, et al. Complementary and alternative medicines in ankylosing spondylitis: a cross-sectional study. Clin Rheumatol 2009;28(2):213–17.
81. Braun J, Brandt J, Listing J, et al. Treatment of active ankylosing spondylitis with infliximab: a randomised controlled multicentre trial. Lancet 2002;359(9313):1187–93.
82. Rudwaleit M, Listing J, Brandt J, Braun J, Sieper J. Prediction of a major clinical response (BASDAI 50) to tumour necrosis factor alpha blockers in ankylosing spondylitis. Ann Rheum Dis 2004;63(6):665–70.
83. Braun BM, Simonson SJ. Introduction to Massage Therapy, 3rd edn. Baltimore, Wolters Kluwer, 2008.
84. Furlan AD, Brosseau L, Imamura M, Irvin E. Massage for low back pain. Cochrane Database Syst Rev 2002(2):CD001929.
85. Chunco R. The effects of massage on pain, stiffness, and fatigue levels associated with ankylosing spondylitis: a case study. Int J Ther Massage Bodywork 2011;4(1):12–17.
86. Han JS. Acupuncture and endorphins. Neurosci Lett 2004;361(1–3):258–61.
87. Lee SC, Yin SJ, Lee ML, Tsai WJ, Sim CB. Effects of acupuncture on serum cortisol level and dopamine beta-hydroxylase activity in normal Chinese. Am J Chinese Med 1982;10(1–4):62–9.
88. Samuels N, Gropp C, Singer SR, Oberbaum M. Acupuncture for psychiatric illness: a literature review. Behav Med 2008;34(2):55–64.
89. Pomeranz B. Scientific research into acupuncture for the relief of pain. J Altern Complement Med 1996;2(1):53–60; discussion 73–5.
90. Furlan AD, van Tulder MW, Cherkin DC, et al. Acupuncture and dry-needling for low back pain. Cochrane Database Syst Rev 2005(1):CD001351.
91. Walker BF, French SD, Grant W, Green S. Combined chiropractic interventions for low-back pain. Cochrane Database Syst Rev 2010(4):CD005427.

92. Rose KA, Kim WS. The effect of chiropractic care for a 30-year-old male with advanced ankylosing spondylitis: a time series case report. J Manipul Physiolog Ther 2003;26(8):E1–9.
93. McDermaid C, Mior S. Ankylosing spondylitis presenting to a chiropractic office: a report of two cases. J Can Chiropr Assoc 2000;44(2):87–97.
94. Chiropractic in Canada. Clinical Guidelines for Chiropractic Practice in Canada. Proceedings of a Consensus Conference commissioned by the Canadian Chiropractic Association, Mississauga, Ontario, 1993, http://www.chiro.org/links/full/canada/contraindications.html.
95. Carter S, Lories RJ. Osteoporosis: a paradox in ankylosing spondylitis. Curr Osteoporos Rep 2011;9(3):112–15.
96. Klingberg E, Lorentzon M, Mellstrom D, et al. Osteoporosis in ankylosing spondylitis—prevalence, risk factors and methods of assessment. Arthritis Res Ther 2012;14(3):R108.
97. Magrey M, Khan MA. Osteoporosis in ankylosing spondylitis. Curr Rheumatol Rep 2010;12(5):332–6.
98. Sambrook PN, Geusens P. The epidemiology of osteoporosis and fractures in ankylosing spondylitis. Ther Adv Musculoskelet Dis 2012;4(4):287–92.
99. Ji W, Li J, Lin Y, et al. Report of 12 cases of ankylosing spondylitis patients treated with *Tripterygium wilfordii*. Clin Rheumatol 2010;29(9):1067–72.
100. Oltean H, Robbins C, van Tulder MW, Berman BM, Bombardier C, Gagnier JJ. Herbal medicine for low-back pain. Cochrane Database Syst Rev 2014;12:CD004504.
101. Cameron M, Gagnier JJ, Chrubasik S. Herbal therapy for treating rheumatoid arthritis. Cochrane Database Syst Rev 2011(2):CD002948.

CHAPTER 20

Treatment: NSAIDs

Jonathan Chan and Nigil Haroon

Introduction to non-steroidal anti-inflammatory drugs

NSAIDs are widely used in a variety of musculoskeletal conditions, including AS, osteoarthritis, and RA, due to their effectiveness as analgesics and anti-inflammatories. Until the advent of biologic therapies, NSAIDs were the only effective pharmacological treatment available for AS and they continue to be widely used as a first-line therapy. Though NSAIDs are largely thought to be little more than analgesics in the armamentarium of RA therapy, they play a more prominent role in the treatment of AS due to their impressive efficacy. Furthermore, there is some evidence of their role in potentially modifying spinal radiographic progression, though this is still an area of evolving research. Many clinicians are nonetheless cautious about using NSAIDs because of their side-effect profile. Nearly all NSAID trials discussed in this chapter were conducted in AS patients fulfilling the mNY criteria and not in other forms of axSpA, including nr-axSpA. However, it can probably be extrapolated from the AS trials that NSAIDs have a similar efficacy for the whole group of axSpA. Indeed, patients in the European Community (EC) with a diagnosis of nr-axSpA are treated in a similar fashion to patients with AS and typically must fail NSAID therapy before a TNF-blocker is considered (for more details see Chapter 22).

Pharmacology

The class of medications we group together as NSAIDs encompasses a variety of structurally different compounds that share the ability to block prostaglandin synthesis. Arachidonic acid becomes transformed into prostaglandins, prostacyclins, and thromboxanes through prostaglandin endoperoxide synthase (PTGS), also known as cyclooxygenase (COX). A number of these compounds are involved in the inflammatory response through increasing local blood flow, hyperalgesia, and vascular permeability. The predominant mechanism of NSAIDs is to inhibit the COX enzyme. The two most well-studied isotypes of COX are termed COX-1 and COX-2. COX-1 is constitutively present in most tissues and functions as a 'housekeeping' enzyme to regulate the normal function of the GI tract, endothelium, platelet aggregation, and kidneys. COX-2 is only constitutively present in brain, kidney, bone, and female reproductive organs, but is otherwise undetectable in most other tissues. It is only during a state of inflammation that COX-2 becomes more widely expressed (1).

Though COX inhibition is thought to be the predominant effect of NSAIDs, a number of non-prostaglandin-mediated effects have also been postulated. These may explain to some extent why some patients report a superior response to one NSAID but not another. NSAIDs are able to insert themselves into cell membranes and are thought to disrupt transmembrane transport and oxidative phosphorylation, thus disturbing cellular function (2, 3). Non-acetylated NSAIDs are able to inhibit neutrophil function by decreasing the expression of L-selectin, thus interfering with their ability to adhere to endothelial cells (4). In vitro, NSAIDs such as aspirin have been demonstrated to reduce expression of inducible nitric oxide synthase through an inhibition of NFκB. This results in a reduction of nitric oxide that otherwise would contribute to inflammation through vasodilation and vascular permeability (5).

NSAIDs are rapidly absorbed after oral ingestion, attaining a peak plasma level at 1–4 hours. In the blood, they are highly protein bound until metabolized by the liver, and eventually renally excreted.

Evidence for NSAID use in ankylosing spondylitis

A number of RCTs support the efficacy of NSAIDs in reducing pain intensity and improving patient function (6–10). Many trials use the BASDAI and BASFI as outcome measures, and NSAIDs have been shown to improve these gauges of disease severity. More recent trials have also confirmed the effectiveness of NSAIDs in attaining composite measures, such as ASAS criteria for partial remission (ASAS-PR) and ASAS improvement criteria (ASAS 20 and 40). A few studies have demonstrated a mild reduction in CRP among patients treated with NSAIDs compared to placebo (11). One cross-sectional study of over 1000 AS patients in Germany and Austria reported that 20% of patients reported complete resolution of pain and 34% had a 50% reduction in pain (12). A systematic review of RCTs evaluating the efficacy of NSAIDs/TNFs compared with placebo demonstrated that both NSAIDs and TNFs have a medium to large effect on pain, physical function, and patient global assessment, although, in this study, NSAIDs had no significant effect on acute-phase reactants (13).

Because most trials of TNFi involve patients who have pain refractory to NSAID use, very few trials have compared the efficacy of NSAIDs head to head with TNFi. In the Infliximab for Treatment of Axial Spondyloarthritis (INFAST) trial, Sieper et al. (14, 15) studied the effect of naproxen and placebo compared with the combination of infliximab and naproxen in patients with early axSpA who had ≤3 years of disease duration. Interestingly, both groups had similar ASAS 20 responses at week 28 (73 vs 81%, $p = 0.30$), though more stringent measures of disease activity, such as ASAS-PR and ASDAS major improvement, favoured combination therapy. Partial remission was achieved by 35% of patients in the naproxen arm, which was much higher than in previous trials where remission rates were roughly 15%. This may have been due to the fact that patients had short disease duration and required BME on MRI as part of the inclusion criteria (14, 15).

Compared with non-specific mechanical back pain, NSAIDs demonstrate drastically different efficacy in ameliorating symptoms. Eighty percent of patients with AS report at least good improvement of their symptoms, and up to 15% of patients with active AS who are treated with NSAIDs are able to achieve ASAS-PR. In contrast, only 15% of patients with mechanical back pain derive good clinical response from NSAID therapy (16). As a result, responsiveness to NSAIDs has been included in the ASAS classification criteria.

Within many RCTs, the majority of improvement from NSAIDs occurred within the first 2–4 weeks of treatment, although therapy for up to 28 weeks may result in a further slight decrease in BASDAI. Many of these trials suggest that a higher response is achieved with patients of younger age, shorter disease duration, and male gender (17).

There is some evidence that NSAIDs have a small effect on reducing BME noted on MRI. An open-label trial of etoricoxib 90 mg showed a reduction in 13/60 BME lesions within the SI joints and spine when comparing baseline MRI to repeat MRI at 6 weeks. Unfortunately there was no control group in this study and it is difficult to know what proportion of BME lesions would have spontaneously resolved (18).

While NSAIDs are first-line therapy for the treatment of axial symptoms, they are also first-line therapy for peripheral symptoms, including peripheral arthritis, enthesitis, and dactylitis. A number of RCTs support the use of NSAIDs in the treatment of peripheral arthritis due to PsA (19, 20). Treatment recommendations from the GRAPPA have also suggested the use of NSAIDs for mild cases of enthesitis and dactylitis, but acknowledge that this is based on expert opinion as there is a paucity of evidence in this area (21, 22).

Daily maximum recommended doses of NSAIDs are shown in Box 20.1. A number of trials have assessed the efficacy of NSAIDs used above these doses. Van der Heijde et al. studied the efficacy of etoricoxib 120 mg, etoricoxib 90 mg, and naproxen 1000 mg in AS patients (8). Etoricoxib 120 mg had an equivalent efficacy to etoricoxib 90 mg with respect to pain, patient's global assessment, BASFI, BASDAI, nocturnal back pain, and morning stiffness at weeks 6 and 52. There was no statistically significant increase in the number of adverse events with this higher dose, although the number of cardiovascular thrombotic events was numerically higher (among 294 patients there were four events in the etoricoxib 120 mg, one in the etoricoxib 90 mg, and 0 in the naproxen 1000 mg groups). Similarly, Dougados et al. studied the efficacy of meloxicam 22.5 mg, meloxiam 15 mg, piroxicam 20 mg, and placebo in patients with AS (6). The higher dose of meloxicam did not show superior efficacy over meloxicam 15 mg or piroxicam with respect to patient overall assessment; however, there was a statistically significant reduction in study drug discontinuation. There was no significant difference in adverse events between the meloxicam groups during the trial. From these studies we can conclude that there may be a minimal benefit with higher doses of NSAIDs, but it is difficult to draw any conclusions with regards to adverse events since these studies did not follow patients beyond 1 year and were not powered to detect outcomes such as cardiac events. Additionally, there is no evidence to support the use of combination therapy with more than one NSAID and such therapy likely increases the risk of adverse events.

Box 20.1 Maximum daily doses of NSAIDs and corresponding half-lives

1) COX-2 inhibitors
   a. Celecoxib 400 mg, 8–12 hours
   b. Etoricoxib 90 mg, 22 hours
2) Acetic acid derivatives:
   a. Indomethacin 150 mg, 2 hours
   b. Diclofenac 150 mg, 2 hours*
   c. Aceclofenac 200 mg, 4 hours
3) Proprionic acid derivatives:
   a. Ketoprofen 200 mg, 1.5–2.5 hours
   b. Ibuprofen 2400 mg, 1.8–3.5 hours
   c. Naproxen 1000 mg, 10–18 hours
4) Enolic acid derivatives:
   a. Meloxicam 15 mg, 20 hours
   b. Piroxicam 20 mg, 30–60 hours
   c. Phenylbutazone 600 mg, 50–100 hours

*Recent Health Canada advisory, based on reports of increased cardiovascular side-effects of diclofenac, recommends a maximum daily dose of 100 mg.

Comparative efficacy of NSAIDs in ankylosing spondylitis

A number of studies have compared the efficacy of NSAIDs of differing pharmacological classes. One study assessed 1331 AS patients from the UK and described the prevalence of different NSAID usage, drug survival, efficacy, and toxicity. The researchers found that indomethacin scored the highest for efficacy, pain relief, stiffness relief, and survival (23). However, other comparisons in retrospective trials of celecoxib, meloxicam, diclofenac, naproxen, ketoprofen, indomethacin, rofecoxib, ibuprofen, and piroxicam have not demonstrated any clear differences (12).

More recently, a number of head-to-head comparisons using RCTs have demonstrated equivalent effect and thus all groups of NSAIDs are generally thought to have comparable efficacy (7, 9, 24–26). A possible exception was the RCT mentioned in the section 'Evidence for NSAID use in ankylosing spondylitis' comparing etoricoxib 90 mg, etoricoxib 120 mg, naproxen 1000 mg, and placebo (8). All NSAID groups were found to be superior to placebo with respect to the study's primary outcomes of improvement of spine pain VAS (–41.5, –41.6, –33.7, and –12.6, respectively), patient's global assessment of disease activity (–27.9, –26.6, –20.9, and –3.4, respectively), and mean BASDAI on VAS (–28.6, –28.5, –23.6, and –6.4, respectively). Both etoricoxib 90 mg and 120 mg groups had a superior response to naproxen that was statistically significant in all primary outcomes, though the absolute clinical difference was small. Additionally, there was no major difference in the frequency of adverse events, although in the extension phase of the trial, five patients from the two etoricoxib groups experienced serious cardiac thrombotic events, while none was seen in the naproxen group. COX-2 selective inhibitors such as celecoxib and rofecoxib have not been shown to have superior efficacy to other non-selective NSAIDs. Though this trial showed superior efficacy for etoricoxib, we hope that future studies can lend further strength to this finding.

NSAIDs and disease modification in ankylosing spondylitis

There is a suggestion that NSAIDs may have a disease-modifying effect in patients with AS. There are several theoretical arguments in favour of this concept. Patients with AS have a significantly higher upregulation of COX-2 within synovial tissues compared with patients with osteoarthritis, RA, and PsA. Zygoapophyseal joints obtained at the time of surgery from AS patients have higher prostaglandin E2 (PGE2) expression compared to autopsy controls (27). AS is associated with *PTGER4* that codes for EP4, the receptor for PGE2 (28). EP4 knockout mice have reduced bone resorption (29), though the effects of PTGER4 polymorphism in AS are not yet well understood. Both COX-2 knockout and COX-2 inhibitor-treated mice demonstrate reduced callous formation, possibly related to suppression of osteoblasts. Evidence from the spinal fusion literature and mouse fracture healing models also support a possible effect of NSAIDs in reducing bone formation (30, 31).

This hypothesis was tested by Wanders et al. in an RCT that assessed whether continuous NSAID use was associated with a decreased progression of syndesmophyte formation (32). Patients had completed a 6-week RCT comparing celecoxib 100 mg twice a day (BID), ketoprofen 100 mg BID, and placebo and underwent a 2- to 14-day washout period. They were then randomized to receive continuous celebrex 100 mg BID treatment for 2 years or on-demand NSAID treatment. Patients could increase celebrex to 200 mg BID or switch to another type of NSAID if necessary. Of 215 patients who were randomized, 96 completed the study in the continuous treatment arm and 86 in the on-demand treatment arm, and complete sets of radiographs were available in 76 and 74 patients, respectively. After 2 years, there was a significant difference in the proportion of patients without radiographic progression, measured using the mSASSS, as well as fewer patients with ≥ 3 units of progression in favour of the continuous treatment group. Despite the fact that baseline characteristics in both groups were not statistically different, the baseline characteristics for many variables of disease severity, including baseline mSASSS, time-averaged pain at night, and physician's global assessment, were slightly higher in the on-demand group. Additionally, the mean difference in the mean daily dosage between the two groups was small (243 vs 201 mg) though statistically significant. A further post-hoc subgroup analysis of this study demonstrated that this effect was only found in patients with elevated acute-phase reactants (CRP and/or ESR) (33).

To study this question within a cohort design, a novel NSAID index for assessing NSAID use was developed (34). This ASAS-approved NSAID index can be calculated for any NSAID based on the maximum recommended dose mentioned in Box 20.1 and the actual patient exposure. If patients have taken 50% of the recommended dose (e.g. 500 mg per day of naproxen instead of 1000 mg per day) for the entire period of observation, the NSAID index for the patient would be 50, as opposed to 100 if the full dose was taken for the entire period. Similarly, if the full dose of 1000 mg of naproxen was taken for only 50% of the observation period, the NSAID index would again be 50. Thus the index quantitates the total NSAID exposure and not the regularity of NSAID intake.

Poddubnyy et al. assessed the impact of NSAIDs on radiographic progression among both AS and nr-axSpA patients from the GESPIC using this NSAID index (35). Patients with high (index ≥ 50) and low (index < 50) NSAID index were compared. There was a numerically lower rate of progression in AS patients within the high NSAID index group (mean mSASSS change 0.02 ± 1.39) compared with the low index group (mean mSASSS change 0.96 ± 2.78) which did not reach significance (p = 0.142) after 2 years. After adjusting for known predictors of radiographic progression, including baseline mSASSS, CRP, and smoking, there was a significant reduction in the number of patients with ≥2 mSASSS units of progression (with OR = 0.15, p = 0.045). This difference was most evident among patients with both baseline syndesmophytes and elevated CRP, whilst NSAIDs had no significant impact on mSASSS worsening among patients without baseline risk factors for radiographic progression. Within the nr-axSpA group, there was no difference in mSASSS progression or on rate of progression to AS.

Sieper et al. recently reported the results of an RCT assessing mSASSS progression after 2 years with continuous versus on-demand diclofenac treatment in the Effects of Non-Steroidal Anti-Inflammatory Drugs on Radiographic Damage in Ankylosing Spondylitis (ENRADAS) study (36). The mean NSAID index (0–100) of diclofenac in the continuous arm was 75 and 44 in the on-demand arm. This study found that there was a numerical worsening of mSASSS progression in the continuous arm but no significant difference between the two groups. Additionally, the on-demand treatment arm had a numerically higher baseline mSASSS and CRP, but these were not statistically different. It is not known if these results refute the findings of previous trials or if this disease-modifying effect is only seen with certain classes of NSAIDs. The results of various studies assessing whether NSAIDs have a DMARD effect are summarized in Table 20.1.

From these studies, it seems the decision to recommend continuous NSAID use is predominantly driven by adequate control of patients' symptoms. In patients with risk factors for radiographic progression, such as smoking, baseline syndesmophytes, and elevated acute-phase reactants, there may be a rationale for continuous use of NSAIDs, though further studies are required to determine whether this benefit is seen in a larger sample size of patients, whether there is a coxib class effect, and whether the potential risks of adverse events outweigh the benefits of therapy.

Safety/adverse effects

A number of RCTs support the safety of NSAIDs when used in patients with AS; however, there is a lack of data assessing the long-term (more than 1 year) safety of these medications. Potential adverse effects include an increased risk of cardiovascular events, GI toxicity, renal failure, heart failure, hypertension, elevated liver enzymes, bleeding, and skin-related reactions. Other rare adverse events include bronchospasm, aplastic anaemia, aseptic meningitis, and cognitive dysfunction.

Table 20.1 NSAIDs and disease-modifying effects in AS

Study	NSAID	Dose tested	Number of AS patients	DMARD effect	Comments
Wanders et al. 2005 (32)	Cel	RCT	150	Yes	
Kroon et al. 2012 (33)	Cel		150	Yes	Post-hoc analysis of patients from Wanders et al. study with elevated time-averaged acute-phase reactants, ASDAS, and BASDAI
Haroon et al. 2013 (88)	NS	H vs L	334	No	Analysis correcting for TNFi effect and baseline acute-phase reactants and mSASSS
Poddubnyy et al. 2012 (35)	NS	H vs L	88	No	
Poddubnyy et al. 2012 (35) sub-analysis	NS	H vs L	18	Yes	Subgroup analysis of patients with baseline syndesmophytes and elevated ESR
Sieper et al. 2015 (36)	Dcl	RCT	122	No	

NS, Non-selective; Cel, celecoxib; Dcl, diclofenac; H, high NSAID index; L, low NSAID index; RCT, randomized controlled trial; ESR, erythrocyte sedimentation rate; CRP, C-reactive protein; mSASSS, modified Stoke Ankylosing Spondylitis Spinal Score.

Cardiac risk

The potential for NSAIDs to increase the risk of serious cardiovascular events was first brought to mainstream media attention when the selective COX-2 inhibitor rofecoxib was removed from the market. A long-term placebo controlled trial (37) of both celecoxib 400 mg and 800 mg per day for the prevention of colonic adenomas demonstrated an increased risk of cardiac events, whereas two other long-term trials of celecoxib (38, 39) at these doses did not show an increased risk. Furthermore, celecoxib 800 mg per day did not demonstrate higher cardiac risk when compared to diclofenac 150 mg or ibuprofen 2400 mg per day in the Celecoxib Long-term Arthritis Safety Study (CLASS) trial (40). A large meta-analysis involving RCTs of NSAIDs versus placebo and NSAIDs versus other NSAIDs (41) demonstrated an increase in major vascular events with the use of coxibs (relative risk (RR) 1.37) and diclofenac (RR 1.41). Ibuprofen demonstrated a numerically higher rate of major vascular events that did not meet significance (RR 1.44, $p = 0.14$), and naproxen did not increase either major vascular events or mortality. Among 1000 patients with low cardiac risk who are treated with a coxib or diclofenac for 1 year, it is estimated that NSAID use results in three additional major vascular events and one additional death. If these 1000 patients have a high baseline risk for cardiac events of roughly 2% per year, it is estimated that there will be an excess of eight vascular events per year, with two deaths. Another systematic review comparing the cardiac risk of various NSAIDs supported the relative safety of naproxen and suggested that all other NSAIDs increase cardiac risk to some degree (42). Thus if an NSAID must be given in a patient with an increased risk of cardiac disease, naproxen would be the preferred agent. Additionally, NSAIDs should be avoided in patients with congestive heart failure, as they are estimated to double the risk of hospitalization in these patients.

All of these trials demonstrated low rates of cardiac events in young patients and those without cardiac risk factors, such as hyperlipidaemia and hypertension. Given the fact that AS patients tend to be younger and with fewer comorbidities, these patients are thought to be at low risk for GI and cardiovascular side-effects (43). However, as patients accumulate additional comorbidities with time, the decision to continue long-term NSAID treatment must be made on a case-by-case basis. Additionally, it is not known whether the risk of treatment with NSAIDs is preferable to the risk of a TNFi.

As most studies assessing the cardiac risk of NSAIDs have not been done in patients with AS, it is uncertain if these results are entirely generalizable to SpA patients. For example, Watson et al. published a study demonstrating that naproxen was found to decrease the risk of thromboembolic cardiovascular events in patients with RA (44). Specifically, there was a 39% reduction in risk of myocardial infarction, sudden death, and stroke compared with non-naproxen use. This was not seen in other non-naproxen NSAIDs such as ibuprofen and diclofenac. Similarly, Lindhardsen et al. assessed the cardiovascular risk of NSAIDs in RA patients using a Danish nationwide cohort study (45). Though NSAIDs as a whole increased the risk with an HR of 1.22, this was lower in comparison to controls that had an HR of 1.51. This risk was predominantly elevated with the use of rofecoxib (HR 1.57) and diclofenac (HR 1.35), while other NSAIDs such as ibuprofen, naproxen, nabumatone, piroxicam, ketoprofen, etodolac, and celecoxib did not show an increased risk in RA patients. Conversely, piroxicam, etodolac, rofecoxib, and diclofenac all demonstrated increased risk in control patients. Unfortunately for both of these trials, no adjustment was made for the types of therapy patients were on for the treatment of their RA.

A number of studies have documented an increased rate of cardiac events in patients with AS, but it is not known whether this increased risk is due to comorbidities such as smoking, AS-associated inflammation, or therapies such as NSAIDs.

A recent Canadian population-based study of AS patients demonstrated a reduction in vascular mortality among those treated with traditional NSAIDs but not with coxibs (46). It was hypothesized that in AS patients, the anti-inflammatory effect of NSAIDs outweighed any increased cardiac risk—though it was also recognized that this might be due to a selection bias, as patients who are prescribed NSAIDs might have a lower cardiovascular risk. Furthermore, patients not on NSAIDs may in fact have more severe disease and instead be treated with a TNFi. Similarly, increased systemic inflammation as measured by CRP has been found to be a strong independent predictor of major cardiovascular events (47–54). NSAIDs have been demonstrated to reduce CRP levels and it is possible the anti-inflammatory effect of these medications may help to neutralize the potential cardiac risk.

Another population-based study assessed the risk of ischaemic heart disease (IHD) and acute myocardial infarction (AMI) in AS patients compared with population controls. They found that only female patients with AS had an increased risk of IHD that lost significance after adjustment for NSAID use (55). This effect was most striking among patients using COX-2 inhibitors, whereas patients using naproxen had a numerically lower frequency of IHD and AMI that did not reach significance. There was no increased risk of AMI in AS patients, regardless of NSAID use. In contrast, a nationwide case control study from Taiwan compared the risk of stroke and major adverse cardiac events (MACE) endpoints between AS patients who either did not use NSAIDs, or had a medical possession rate (MPR) of NSAIDs of <80%, or had an MPR ≥ 80% (56). Patients treated with COX-2 inhibitors had a significant reduction in the frequency of cardiac disease, with an OR of 0.08 (0.01–0.92) at 24 months; however, this effect lost significance at 36 months.

Finally, a recently published meta-analysis of RCTs compared traditional NSAIDs and COX-2 inhibitors with placebo among patients with axSpA (10). While the analysis supported the clinical efficacy of NSAIDs, it did not find a significant difference in the frequency of withdrawals due to adverse events between NSAID and placebo groups at 12 weeks (n = 1836 from eight trials). Additionally, this study did not demonstrate a difference in harm between naproxen and other types of NSAIDs (n = 646), nor was there a dose response effect on benefit or harm.

Gastrointestinal risk

As part of their mechanism of action, NSAIDs block both COX-1 and 2. COX-1 is involved in the formation of gastric mucosal protective prostaglandins such as PGE2. As a result, patients treated with NSAIDs are at increased risk of GI toxicity. Mild side-effects include nausea, abdominal pain, and diarrhoea. More severe side-effects include symptomatic ulcers, GI bleeding, and GI perforation. These more serious side-effects occur in roughly 1% of patients treated with NSAIDs (57). Among non-NSAID users, the incidence of hospitalization due to complicated peptic ulcer disease is 1 case per 1000 people per year (58). The use of NSAIDs is estimated to increase this number by an additional 3 cases per 1000 people per year. Hospitalization due to a major GI bleed is associated with a mortality rate of 5% (59). This risk returns to baseline within 1 month of stopping the medication.

Guidelines from the American College of Gastroenterology suggest classifying patients as being high, medium, or low risk (60). Risk factors include age more than 65 years, high-dose NSAID use, a history of uncomplicated ulcer, and concurrent use of aspirin, glucocorticoids, or anticoagulants. High-risk patients are those with a history of complicated peptic ulcer disease or more than two risk factors. Medium-risk patients have one to two risk factors and low-risk patients have no risk factors. Table 20.2 summarizes these recommendations. The risk of GI toxicity associated with NSAID use can be greatly reduced by selecting a COX-2 inhibitor selective NSAID or concomitant therapy with either a proton pump inhibitor (PPI), or a prostaglandin E1 analogue misoprostol, or a high-dose histamine 2 receptor antagonist (H_2RA).

COX-2 inhibitor

A number of RCTs have demonstrated the reduced GI toxicity associated with COX-2 inhibitors compared with traditional NSAIDs (61–65). Furthermore, celebrex 200 mg BID had a lower frequency of GI events compared with the combination of diclofenac 75 mg BID and omeprazole 20 mg daily (66). If patients are treated with a COX-2 inhibitor, the addition of a protective agent can add further benefit (67). In patients taking celebrex 200 mg BID for 6 months, it is estimated that 16.5% will develop gastric ulcers on endoscopy, though this risk was reduced to less than 5% with the addition of a PPI.

Table 20.2 American College of Gastroenterology guidelines (60) with regard to prevention of NSAID-related ulcers

	GI risk		
	Low	**Moderate**	**High**
Low cardiovascular risk	NSAID alone (least ulcerogenic NSAID at the lowest effective dose)	NSAID + PPI/ misoprostol	Alternative therapy if possible or COX-2 inhibitor + PPI/ misoprostol
High cardiovascular risk	Naproxen + PPI/ misoprostol	Naproxen + PPI/ misoprostol	Avoid NSAIDs and COX-2 inhibitors. Use alternative therapy

PPI, Proton pump inhibitor.

Source: Lanza FL, Chan FK, Quigley EM. Guidelines for prevention of NSAID-related ulcer complications. Am J Gastroenterol. 2009 Mar;104(3):728–38.

Enteric coated NSAIDs and H_2RA

While many patients report improved tolerability with enteric coated or buffered NSAIDs, there is no evidence to suggest they can prevent NSAID-related gastric or duodenal ulceration (68–70). The concomitant use of standard-dose H_2RA has been shown to prevent duodenal ulcers but was not effective in reducing gastric ulcer complications (71); however, double-dose H_2RA (famotidine 40 mg BID) has been shown to decrease the risk of both gastric and duodenal ulcers (72). Though the use of H_2RAs has the least efficacy of current prevention strategies, this may be the most cost-effective method.

Misoprostol

A number of RCTs and meta-analysis have highlighted the superior efficacy of misoprostol over both placebo and H_2RAs. A Cochrane review in 2002 (70) demonstrated that both high- and low-dose misoprostol (800 and 400 μg per day, respectively) resulted in a 53% reduction in duodenal ulcers and a 74% reduction in gastric ulcers compared with placebo. Misoprostol was also able to reduce clinically evident ulcer complications such as severe GI bleeding but was associated with diarrhoea in a dose-related fashion. It is important to note that the majority of studies assessing the GI toxicity of NSAIDs demonstrate that 30–50% of patients develop GI ulcers evident on endoscopy; however, only 10% of patients treated with NSAIDs have symptomatic ulcers and far fewer have complications such as GI bleeding. When comparing the efficacy of misoprostol with 30 mg of lansoprazole, misoprostol resulted in a numerically lower rate of gastric ulcers that was not statistically significant (73). Lower doses of misoprostol (200 and 100 μg four times a day (QID)) are also associated with a reduction in duodenal ulcers, though this was not seen with 50 μg QID (74). Misoprostol is very effective at reducing the risk of NSAID-related GI bleeding; unfortunately, many patients do not tolerate the drug's side-effects of diarrhoea and abdominal pain when used at a full dose.

Proton pump inhibitors (PPIs)

PPIs are a popular concomitant medication to reduce the risk of GI toxicity. Omeprazole 20 mg was found to have superior efficacy compared with ranitidine 150 mg BID, placebo, and misoprostol 400 μg per day (75, 76). Additionally, patients treated with COX-2 inhibitors demonstrated further benefit with regards to ulcer prevention when treated with esomeprazole 20 mg and 40 mg, with both doses of PPI having similar reduction rates of ulcer complications (67). Almost all studies evaluating the efficacy of PPIs in preventing GI toxicity have relied on endoscopic diagnosis of ulcers. Only one trial among *Helicobacter pylori*-positive patients treated with NSAIDs utilized GI bleeding as a clinical endpoint (77). Nonetheless, observational studies and secondary analysis of RCTs support the efficacy of PPIs in reducing the risk of GI bleeds. PPIs are generally well tolerated when compared to misoprostol and thus have become the more popular form of gastric protection. There are, however, some concerns regarding the long-term use of these medications. A number of meta-analyses of cohort studies have suggested an increased risk of infections such as *Clostridium difficile* (78–80), as well as the malabsorption of nutrients such as calcium and magnesium (81–83).

Helicobacter pylori infection

Patients requiring long-term NSAID use may be at further risk of GI bleeding if there is concomitant *H. pylori* infection. A meta-analysis of the risk of GI bleeding related to *H. pylori* infection, NSAID use, and both *H. pylori* and NSAID use indicated a RR of 1.79, 4.85, and 6.13, respectively (84). Chan et al. demonstrated that treatment of *H. pylori* had an equivalent effect on preventing recurrent GI bleeds compared with omeprazole 20 mg in patients taking low-dose aspirin (77). Among patients taking other NSAIDs, omeprazole was found to be superior to *H. pylori* eradication. The American College of Gastroenterology guidelines recommend that all patients requiring long-term NSAID treatment should be screened for *H. pylori* infection and treated if found positive.

Hepatotoxicity

Though NSAIDs are known to increase transaminases, the incidence of severe liver failure is exceedingly rare and many gastroenterology guidelines do not suggest regular monitoring for liver disease in patients using NSAIDs. In patients with a history of liver cirrhosis, clinicians must be more cautious. The risk of liver injury is highest during the first prescription of an NSAID compared to subsequent prescriptions. Roughly 5 cases of liver injury per 100 000 population can be attributable to the use of NSAIDs (58).

Renal risk

In healthy individuals, inhibition of prostaglandin synthesis does not have a significant effect on renal function or blood pressure. However, patients with concomitant kidney disease have an upregulation of their renin–aldosterone–angiotensin system and are dependent on prostaglandin synthesis for the maintenance of renal blood flow. In these situations, renal prostaglandins act as renal vasodilators. When NSAIDs inhibit the function of COX enzymes, the kidneys may experience a variety of adverse effects, including acute kidney injury, nephrotic syndrome, electrolyte and acid/base imbalance, papillary necrosis, chronic interstitial nephritis, hypertension, and oedema. The most common adverse event related to NSAID use is mild pedal oedema, which can occur in up to 5% of patients. With the exception of papillary necrosis, most of the adverse events will resolve within 1 week of discontinuation of the NSAID. Cumulatively, all renal-related adverse events occur in roughly 1% of patients treated with NSAIDs (85, 86). Papillary necrosis is the only permanent renal complication associated with NSAID use and is very rare. The risk of hospitalization due to renal failure that is attributable to NSAID use is roughly 4–8 cases per 100 000 patients per year (58). This risk may be increased with advancing age, chronic kidney disease (≥ stage 3), volume-depleted states, heart failure, severe hypercalcaemia, and medications such as angiotensin-converting enzyme inhibitors (ACEi) and angiotensin II receptor antagonists (ARBs) (87). Though there is no renal protective agent that can be concomitantly prescribed, severe long-term renal damage is rare if caution is used in patients at high risk of renal impairment.

Drug interactions

NSAIDs may interact with other medications by a variety of mechanisms such as decreased renal perfusion, increased bleeding risk and inhibition of CYP-2C9. Medications that may be affected include anticoagulants (increased plasma levels of warfarin), antiplatelet agents (ibuprofen and naproxen may interfere with the cardioprotective effect of aspirin), antihypertensives (such as ACEi), calcineurin inhibitors, digoxin, diuretics, glucocorticoids, lithium, selective serotonin reuptake inhibitors, and MTX (when used for chemotherapy at high doses). It should be noted that there is no significant interaction between NSAIDs and MTX in low doses that is typically used to treat rheumatic conditions.

Conclusion

NSAIDs continue to be a cornerstone therapy for the treatment of AS. Not only are they effective for axial and peripheral symptoms, but also there is some evidence to suggest that they may have some disease-modifying effect particularly in patients with elevated acute-phase reactants. Though they are generally thought to be safe, especially in young patients with no comorbidities, there continues to be uncertainty regarding the safety of taking these medications for many decades. Additionally, it is not known whether other treatment strategies such as a biologic medication would have a preferential risk profile.

References

1. Dubois RN, Abramson SB, Crofford L, et al. Cyclooxygenase in biology and disease. FASEB J 1998;12(12):1063–73.
2. Abramson SB, Weissmann G. The mechanisms of action of nonsteroidal antiinflammatory drugs. Arthritis Rheum 1989;32(1):1–9.
3. Brooks PM, Day RO. Nonsteroidal antiinflammatory drugs—differences and similarities. N Engl J Med 1991;324(24):1716–25.
4. Diaz-Gonzalez F, Gonzalez-Alvaro I, Campanero MR, et al. Prevention of in vitro neutrophil-endothelial attachment through shedding of L-selectin by nonsteroidal antiinflammatory drugs. J Clin Invest 1995;95(4):1756–65.
5. Amin AR, Vyas P, Attur M, et al. The mode of action of aspirin-like drugs: effect on inducible nitric oxide synthase. Proc Natl Acad Sci USA 1995;92(17):7926–30.

6. Dougados M, Gueguen A, Nakache JP, et al. Ankylosing spondylitis: what is the optimum duration of a clinical study? A one year versus a 6 weeks non-steroidal anti-inflammatory drug trial. Rheumatology (Oxford) 1999;38(3):235–44.
7. Dougados M, Behier JM, Jolchine I, et al. Efficacy of celecoxib, a cyclooxygenase 2-specific inhibitor, in the treatment of ankylosing spondylitis: a six-week controlled study with comparison against placebo and against a conventional nonsteroidal antiinflammatory drug. Arthritis Rheum 2001;44(1):180–5.
8. van der Heijde D, Baraf HS, Ramos-Remus C, et al. Evaluation of the efficacy of etoricoxib in ankylosing spondylitis: results of a fifty-two-week, randomized, controlled study. Arthritis Rheum 2005;52(4):1205–15.
9. Barkhuizen A, Steinfeld S, Robbins J, West C, Coombs J, Zwillich S. Celecoxib is efficacious and well tolerated in treating signs and symptoms of ankylosing spondylitis. J Rheumatol 2006;33(9):1805–12.
10. Kroon FP, van der Burg LR, Ramiro S, et al. Non-steroidal anti-inflammatory drugs (NSAIDs) for axial spondyloarthritis (ankylosing spondylitis and non-radiographic axial spondyloarthritis). Cochrane Database Syst Rev 2015;7:CD010952.
11. Benhamou M, Gossec L, Dougados M. Clinical relevance of C-reactive protein in ankylosing spondylitis and evaluation of the NSAIDs/coxibs' treatment effect on C-reactive protein. Rheumatology (Oxford) 2010;49(3):536–41.
12. Zochling J, Bohl-Buhler MH, Baraliakos X, Feldtkeller E, Braun J. Nonsteroidal anti-inflammatory drug use in ankylosing spondylitis—a population-based survey. Clin Rheumatol 2006;25(6):794–800.
13. Escalas C, Trijau S, Dougados M. Evaluation of the treatment effect of NSAIDs/TNF blockers according to different domains in ankylosing spondylitis: results of a meta-analysis. Rheumatology (Oxford) 2010;49(7):1317–25.
14. Sieper J, Lenaerts J, Wollenhaupt J, et al. Efficacy and safety of infliximab plus naproxen versus naproxen alone in patients with early, active axial spondyloarthritis: results from the double-blind, placebo-controlled INFAST study, part 1. Ann Rheum Dis 2014;73(1):101–7.
15. Sieper J, Lenaerts J, Wollenhaupt J, et al. Maintenance of biologic-free remission with naproxen or no treatment in patients with early, active axial spondyloarthritis: results from a 6-month, randomised, open-label follow-up study, INFAST part 2. Ann Rheum Dis 2014;73(1):108–13.
16. Amor B, Dougados M, Listrat V, et al. Are classification criteria for spondylarthropathy useful as diagnostic criteria? Rev Rhum Eng Ed 1995;62(1):10–15.
17. Cinar M, Dinc A, Simsek I, et al. Evaluation of the short term efficacy of NSAIDs on patients with active ankylosing spondylitis in daily practice: a 3-month, longitudinal, observational study. Rheumatol Int 2010;30(3):331–40.
18. Jarrett SJ, Sivera F, Cawkwell LS, et al. MRI and clinical findings in patients with ankylosing spondylitis eligible for anti-tumour necrosis factor therapy after a short course of etoricoxib. Ann Rheum Dis 2009;68(9):1466–9.
19. Soriano ER, McHugh NJ. Therapies for peripheral joint disease in psoriatic arthritis. A systematic review. J Rheumatol 2006;33(7):1422–30.
20. Zochling J, van der Heijde D, Burgos-Vargas R, et al. ASAS/EULAR recommendations for the management of ankylosing spondylitis. Ann Rheum Dis 2006;65(4):442–52.
21. Helliwell PS. Therapies for dactylitis in psoriatic arthritis. A systematic review. J Rheumatol 2006;33(7):1439–41.
22. Ritchlin CT, Kavanaugh A, Gladman DD, et al. Treatment recommendations for psoriatic arthritis. Ann Rheum Dis 2009;68(9):1387–94.
23. Calin A, Elswood J. A prospective nationwide cross-sectional study of NSAID usage in 1331 patients with ankylosing spondylitis. J Rheumatol 1990;17(6):801–3.
24. Batlle-Gualda E, Figueroa M, Ivorra J, Raber A. The efficacy and tolerability of aceclofenac in the treatment of patients with ankylosing spondylitis: a multicenter controlled clinical trial. Aceclofenac Indomethacin Study Group. J Rheumatol 1996;23(7):1200–6.
25. Villa Alcazar LF, de Buergo M, Rico Lenza H, Montull Fruitos E. Aceclofenac is as safe and effective as tenoxicam in the treatment of ankylosing spondylitis: a 3 month multicenter comparative trial. Spanish Study Group on Aceclofenac in Ankylosing Spondylitis. J Rheumatol 1996;23(7):1194–9.
26. Sieper J, Klopsch T, Richter M, et al. Comparison of two different dosages of celecoxib with diclofenac for the treatment of active ankylosing spondylitis: results of a 12-week randomised, double-blind, controlled study. Ann Rheum Dis 2008;67(3):323–9.
27. Syrbe U, Bleil J, Maier R, Appel H, Sieper J (eds). Analysis of Inflammatory Markers Within Facet Joints of Patients Within Ankylosing Spondylitis. San Diego, American College of Rheumatology, 2013.
28. Evans DM, Spencer CC, Pointon JJ, et al. Interaction between ERAP1 and HLA-B27 in ankylosing spondylitis implicates peptide handling in the mechanism for HLA-B27 in disease susceptibility. Nat Genet 2011;43(8):761–7.
29. Miyaura C, Inada M, Suzawa T, et al. Impaired bone resorption to prostaglandin E2 in prostaglandin E receptor EP4-knockout mice. J Biol Chem 2000;275(26):19819–23.
30. Reuben SS, Ablett D, Kaye R. High dose nonsteroidal anti-inflammatory drugs compromise spinal fusion. Can J Anaesth 2005;52(5):506–12.
31. Spiro AS, Beil FT, Baranowsky A, et al. BMP-7-induced ectopic bone formation and fracture healing is impaired by systemic NSAID application in C57BL/6-mice. J Orthop Res 2010;28(6):785–91.
32. Wanders A, Heijde D, Landewe R, et al. Nonsteroidal antiinflammatory drugs reduce radiographic progression in patients with ankylosing spondylitis: a randomized clinical trial. Arthritis Rheum 2005;52(6):1756–65.
33. Kroon F, Landewe R, Dougados M, van der Heijde D. Continuous NSAID use reverts the effects of inflammation on radiographic progression in patients with ankylosing spondylitis. Ann Rheum Dis 2012;71(10):1623–9.
34. Dougados M, Simon P, Braun J, et al. ASAS recommendations for collecting, analysing and reporting NSAID intake in clinical trials/epidemiological studies in axial spondyloarthritis. Ann Rheum Dis 2011;70:249–51.
35. Poddubnyy D, Rudwaleit M, Haibel H, et al. Effect of non-steroidal anti-inflammatory drugs on radiographic spinal progression in patients with axial spondyloarthritis: results from the German Spondyloarthritis Inception Cohort. Ann Rheum Dis 2012;71(10):1616–22.
36. Sieper J, Listing J, Poddubunyy D, et al. Continuous versus on demand treatment of ankylosing spondylitis with diclofenac over 2 years does not prevent radiographic progression of the spine—results from a randomized prospective multi-center trial (ENRADAS). EULAR Congress, Rome, 2005.
37. Solomon SD, McMurray JJ, Pfeffer MA, et al. Cardiovascular risk associated with celecoxib in a clinical trial for colorectal adenoma prevention. N Engl J Med 2005 17;352(11):1071–80.
38. ADAPT Research Group. Cardiovascular and cerebrovascular events in the randomized, controlled Alzheimer's Disease Anti-Inflammatory Prevention Trial (ADAPT). PLoS Clin Trials 2006;1(7):e33.
39. Arber N, Eagle CJ, Spicak J, et al. Celecoxib for the prevention of colorectal adenomatous polyps. N Engl J Med 2006;355(9):885–95.
40. White WB, Faich G, Whelton A, et al. Comparison of thromboembolic events in patients treated with celecoxib, a cyclooxygenase-2 specific inhibitor, versus ibuprofen or diclofenac. Am J Cardiol 2002;89(4):425–30.
41. Bhala N, Emberson J, Merhi A, et al. Vascular and upper gastrointestinal effects of non-steroidal anti-inflammatory drugs: meta-analyses of individual participant data from randomised trials. Lancet 2013;382(9894):769–79.
42. McGettigan P, Henry D. Cardiovascular risk with non-steroidal anti-inflammatory drugs: systematic review of population-based controlled observational studies. PLoS Med 2011;8(9):e1001098.

43. Song IH, Poddubnyy DA, Rudwaleit M, Sieper J. Benefits and risks of ankylosing spondylitis treatment with nonsteroidal antiinflammatory drugs. Arthritis Rheum 2008;58(4):929–38.
44. Watson DJ, Rhodes T, Cai B, Guess HA. Lower risk of thromboembolic cardiovascular events with naproxen among patients with rheumatoid arthritis. Arch Intern Med 2002;162(10):1105–10.
45. Lindhardsen J, Gislason GH, Jacobsen S, et al. Non-steroidal anti-inflammatory drugs and risk of cardiovascular disease in patients with rheumatoid arthritis: a nationwide cohort study. Ann Rheum Dis 2013 Jun 8.
46. Haroon NN, Paterson JM, Li P, Inman RD, Haroon N. Patients with ankylosing spondylitis have increased cardiovascular and cerebrovascular mortality: a population-based study. Ann Intern Med 2015;163(6):409–16.
47. Libby P, Ridker PM, Maseri A. Inflammation and atherosclerosis. Circulation 2002;105(9):1135–43.
48. Ridker PM, Cushman M, Stampfer MJ, Tracy RP, Hennekens CH. Inflammation, aspirin, and the risk of cardiovascular disease in apparently healthy men. N Engl J Med 1997;336(14):973–9.
49. Ridker PM, Hennekens CH, Buring JE, Rifai N. C-reactive protein and other markers of inflammation in the prediction of cardiovascular disease in women. N Engl J Med 2000;342(12):836–43.
50. Ridker PM, Rifai N, Clearfield M, et al. Measurement of C-reactive protein for the targeting of statin therapy in the primary prevention of acute coronary events. N Engl J Med 2001;344(26):1959–65.
51. Danesh J, Wheeler JG, Hirschfield GM, et al. C-reactive protein and other circulating markers of inflammation in the prediction of coronary heart disease. N Engl J Med 2004;350(14):1387–97.
52. Hansson GK, Libby P. The immune response in atherosclerosis: a double-edged sword. Nat Rev Immunol 2006;6(7):508–19.
53. Ridker PM, Danielson E, Fonseca FA, et al. Rosuvastatin to prevent vascular events in men and women with elevated C-reactive protein. N Engl J Med 2008;359(21):2195–207.
54. Ridker PM, Rifai N, Rose L, Buring JE, Cook NR. Comparison of C-reactive protein and low-density lipoprotein cholesterol levels in the prediction of first cardiovascular events. N Engl J Med 2002;347(20):1557–65.
55. Essers I, Stolwijk C, Boonen A, et al. Ankylosing spondylitis and risk of ischaemic heart disease: a population-based cohort study. Ann Rheum Dis 2016;75(1):203–9.
56. Tsai WC, Ou TT, Yen JH, Wu CC, Tung YC. Long-term frequent use of non-steroidal anti-inflammatory drugs might protect patients with ankylosing spondylitis from cardiovascular diseases: a nationwide case-control study. PLoS One 2015;10(5):e0126347.
57. Lanas A, Benito P, Alonso J, et al. Safe prescription recommendations for non steroidal anti-inflammatory drugs: consensus document ellaborated by nominated experts of three scientific associations (SER-SEC-AEG). Reumatol Clin 2014;10(2):68–84.
58. Hernandez-Diaz S, Garcia-Rodriguez LA. Epidemiologic assessment of the safety of conventional nonsteroidal anti-inflammatory drugs. Am J Med 2001;110(Suppl 3A):20S–7S.
59. Lanas A, Perez-Aisa MA, Feu F, et al. A nationwide study of mortality associated with hospital admission due to severe gastrointestinal events and those associated with nonsteroidal antiinflammatory drug use. Am J Gastroenterol 2005;100(8):1685–93.
60. Lanza FL, Chan FK, Quigley EM. Guidelines for prevention of NSAID-related ulcer complications. Am J Gastroenterol 2009;104(3):728–38.
61. Bensen WG, Fiechtner JJ, McMillen JI, et al. Treatment of osteoarthritis with celecoxib, a cyclooxygenase-2 inhibitor: a randomized controlled trial. Mayo Clin Proc 1999;74(11):1095–105.
62. Emery P, Zeidler H, Kvien TK, et al. Celecoxib versus diclofenac in long-term management of rheumatoid arthritis: randomised double-blind comparison. Lancet 1999;354(9196):2106–11.
63. Laine L, Harper S, Simon T, et al. A randomized trial comparing the effect of rofecoxib, a cyclooxygenase 2-specific inhibitor, with that of ibuprofen on the gastroduodenal mucosa of patients with osteoarthritis. Rofecoxib Osteoarthritis Endoscopy Study Group. Gastroenterology 1999;117(4):776–83.
64. Simon LS, Weaver AL, Graham DY, et al. Anti-inflammatory and upper gastrointestinal effects of celecoxib in rheumatoid arthritis: a randomized controlled trial. JAMA 1999;282(20):1921–8.
65. Goldstein JL, Correa P, Zhao WW, et al. Reduced incidence of gastroduodenal ulcers with celecoxib, a novel cyclooxygenase-2 inhibitor, compared to naproxen in patients with arthritis. Am J Gastroenterol 2001;96(4):1019–27.
66. Chan FK, Lanas A, Scheiman J, Berger MF, Nguyen H, Goldstein JL. Celecoxib versus omeprazole and diclofenac in patients with osteoarthritis and rheumatoid arthritis (CONDOR): a randomised trial. Lancet 2010;376(9736):173–9.
67. Scheiman JM, Yeomans ND, Talley NJ, et al. Prevention of ulcers by esomeprazole in at-risk patients using non-selective NSAIDs and COX-2 inhibitors. Am J Gastroenterol 2006;101(4):701–10.
68. Lanza FL, Royer GL Jr, Nelson RS. Endoscopic evaluation of the effects of aspirin, buffered aspirin, and enteric-coated aspirin on gastric and duodenal mucosa. N Engl J Med 1980;303(3):136–8.
69. McCarthy DM. Sucralfate. N Engl J Med 1991;325(14):1017–25.
70. Rostom A, Dube C, Wells G, et al. Prevention of NSAID-induced gastroduodenal ulcers. Cochrane Database Syst Rev 2002(4):CD002296.
71. Koch M, Dezi A, Ferrario F, Capurso I. Prevention of nonsteroidal anti-inflammatory drug-induced gastrointestinal mucosal injury. A meta-analysis of randomized controlled clinical trials. Arch Intern Med 1996;156(20):2321–32.
72. Laine L, Kivitz AJ, Bello AE, Grahn AY, Schiff MH, Taha AS. Double-blind randomized trials of single-tablet ibuprofen/high-dose famotidine vs. ibuprofen alone for reduction of gastric and duodenal ulcers. Am J Gastroenterol 2012;107(3):379–86.
73. Graham DY, Agrawal NM, Campbell DR, et al. Ulcer prevention in long-term users of nonsteroidal anti-inflammatory drugs: results of a double-blind, randomized, multicenter, active- and placebo-controlled study of misoprostol vs lansoprazole. Arch Intern Med 2002;162(2):169–75.
74. Lanza FL, Fakouhi D, Rubin A, et al. A double-blind placebo-controlled comparison of the efficacy and safety of 50, 100, and 200 micrograms of misoprostol QID in the prevention of ibuprofen-induced gastric and duodenal mucosal lesions and symptoms. Am J Gastroenterol 1989;84(6):633–6.
75. Hawkey CJ, Karrasch JA, Szczepanski L, et al. Omeprazole compared with misoprostol for ulcers associated with nonsteroidal antiinflammatory drugs. Omeprazole versus Misoprostol for NSAID-induced Ulcer Management (OMNIUM) Study Group. N Engl J Med 1998;338(11):727–34.
76. Yeomans ND, Tulassay Z, Juhasz L, et al. A comparison of omeprazole with ranitidine for ulcers associated with nonsteroidal antiinflammatory drugs. Acid Suppression Trial: Ranitidine versus Omeprazole for NSAID-associated Ulcer Treatment (ASTRONAUT) Study Group. N Engl J Med 1998;338(11):719–26.
77. Chan FK, Chung SC, Suen BY, et al. Preventing recurrent upper gastrointestinal bleeding in patients with *Helicobacter pylori* infection who are taking low-dose aspirin or naproxen. N Engl J Med 2001;344(13):967–73.
78. Leonard J, Marshall JK, Moayyedi P. Systematic review of the risk of enteric infection in patients taking acid suppression. Am J Gastroenterol 2007;102(9):2047–56; quiz 57.
79. Kwok CS, Arthur AK, Anibueze CI, Singh S, Cavallazzi R, Loke YK. Risk of *Clostridium difficile* infection with acid suppressing drugs and antibiotics: meta-analysis. Am J Gastroenterol 2012;107(7):1011–19.
80. Janarthanan S, Ditah I, Adler DG, Ehrinpreis MN. *Clostridium difficile*-associated diarrhea and proton pump inhibitor therapy: a meta-analysis. Am J Gastroenterol 2012;107(7):1001–10.
81. Yu EW, Bauer SR, Bain PA, Bauer DC. Proton pump inhibitors and risk of fractures: a meta-analysis of 11 international studies. Am J Med 2011;124(6):519–26.

82. Khalili H, Huang ES, Jacobson BC, Camargo CA Jr, Feskanich D, Chan AT. Use of proton pump inhibitors and risk of hip fracture in relation to dietary and lifestyle factors: a prospective cohort study. BMJ 2012;344:e372.
83. Hess MW, Hoenderop JG, Bindels RJ, Drenth JP. Systematic review: hypomagnesaemia induced by proton pump inhibition. Aliment Pharmacol Ther 2012;36(5):405–13.
84. Huang JQ, Sridhar S, Hunt RH. Role of *Helicobacter pylori* infection and non-steroidal anti-inflammatory drugs in peptic-ulcer disease: a meta-analysis. Lancet 2002;359(9300):14–22.
85. Whelton A, Hamilton CW. Nonsteroidal anti-inflammatory drugs: effects on kidney function. J Clin Pharmacol 1991;31(7):588–98.
86. Whelton A. Nephrotoxicity of nonsteroidal anti-inflammatory drugs: physiologic foundations and clinical implications. Am J Med 1999;106(5B):13S–24S.
87. Gooch K, Culleton BF, Manns BJ, et al. NSAID use and progression of chronic kidney disease. Am J Med 2007;120(3):280.e1–7.
88. Haroon N, Inman RD, Learch TJ, et al. The impact of tumor necrosis factor alpha inhibitors on radiographic progression in ankylosing spondylitis. Arthritis Rheum 2013;65(10):2645-54.

CHAPTER 21

Treatment: DMARDs

Denis Poddubnyy and Hildrun Haibel

Introduction to DMARDs

The term 'disease-modifying antirheumatic drug' (DMARD) comprises a heterogeneous group of drugs which act more than symptomatically in the treatment of inflammatory joint diseases, particularly RA (1). Disease-modifying property in RA usually means an ability to halt or to retard joint destruction. Using this definition, two groups of DMARDs can be defined: (1) synthetic ('classical' DMARDs such as SSZ, MTX, and leflunomide) and (2) biological—a heterogeneous group of novel drugs (also called *biologics*), usually monoclonal antibodies or soluble receptors targeting certain molecules related to inflammation, such as TNFα and IL-6. This chapter discusses currently available data on the efficacy of synthetic DMARDs in AS/ axSpA. The role of biologics in axSpA is discussed in Chapter 22.

It is evident that the previous use of the term 'disease modification' in RA cannot be directly applied to axSpA, since the morphological substrate of structural damage in axSpA is not joint destruction but rather new bone formation in the axial skeleton. Nonetheless, we use the historical and widely accepted term 'DMARDs' in the context of axSpA, despite the lack of evidence for disease modification with this drug class. Moreover, even a symptomatic efficacy of DMARDs in axSpA is questionable. According to the current ASAS/EULAR recommendations for the management of AS (2), which could be generalized to the entire group of axSpA, classical DMARDs are generally not recommended for the treatment of axial manifestations due to lack of proven efficacy, but might be considered as an option in the case of peripheral arthritis. However, due to weak evidence, even in the case of peripheral involvement in axSpA, a DMARD trial is not mandatory prior to TNFi therapy (3). Nonetheless, up to one-third of patients with axSpA do DMARDs (mostly SSZ and MTX) (4–6), indicating that this drug class is still considered by rheumatologists as an option for the treatment of active axSpA.

Sulfasalazine

SSZ has a long history as a therapeutic agent for the treatment of AS. Especially prior to the introduction of TNFi, SSZ was often considered as a drug of choice if NSAIDs had failed. Not surprisingly, therefore, the vast majority of studies investigating efficacy of SSZ in AS were conducted in the 1980s and early 1990s. In 2005, a Cochrane review summarizing data from 11 placebo-controlled studies with SSZ in AS was published (7). In 2014, an update of this review was performed (8); however, no new trials could be included. The pooled analysis showed that the difference between the intervention groups was significant only for ESR and morning stiffness, favouring SSZ over placebo, but not for the other variables (7, 8). Importantly, none of the included trials used composite outcome variables such as ASAS 20, ASAS 40, or ASAS-PR, which are currently standard outcome assessments in clinical trials. BASDAI, BASFI, BASMI, and radiographic progression were also not assessed in these trials, making interpretation of the results in relation to symptom- or disease-modifying properties of SSZ in AS difficult or even not possible. However, a few trials showed some effect of SSZ compared to placebo on peripheral arthritis in AS, as reflected by a significant reduction of the swollen joint count (9, 10). A trend toward better 3-month response to SSZ in patients with axSpA and peripheral joint swelling, and a significantly better 3-year drug survival than in patients without swollen joints at baseline were observed in a Norwegian multicentre longitudinal observational study (the Norwegian Disease-Modifying Antirheumatic Drug Register—NOR-DMARD) (11). There is no evidence to date indicating that SSZ might have an effect on other peripheral manifestations such as enthesitis (12, 13) or dactylitis. In one RCT, a reduction of occurrence of recurrent AAU in patients with AS associated with SSZ treatment was reported (14).

The Cochrane review included only studies performed in AS. So far, no studies with SSZ (nor for the other DMARDs) in nr-axSpA have been performed. There is, however, a placebo-controlled study with SSZ that included a broader population of patients with axSpA (15). In the entire population of 230 patients with axSpA and symptom duration of less than 5 years, after 24 weeks of treatment there were no differences between SSZ and placebo in any outcome parameter (BASDAI, spinal pain, BASFI, spinal mobility, swollen joint count, enthesitis, acute-phase reactants). Interestingly, SSZ was associated with significant reduction of BASDAI, spinal pain, and morning stiffness only in a subgroup of patients without peripheral arthritis (15).

Most recently, two studies in axSpA with SSZ as a comparator for a TNFi (ETN) have been conducted (16, 17). In the Ankylosing Spondylitis Study Comparing Enbrel and Sulfasalazine Dosed Weekly (ASCEND), patients with AS were randomly assigned either to ETN 50 mg once weekly or to SSZ up to 3 g per day. Although ETN was clearly superior to SSZ (75.9% of ETN-treated patients achieved the ASAS 20 response at week 16—the primary endpoint), a substantial proportion (52.9%, $p < 0.001$) of SSZ-treated patients achieved the same response. Similarly, ASAS 40 response at week 16 was achieved by 59.8% versus 32.6% of patients treated with ETN versus SSZ, respectively ($p < 0.001$), and ASAS-PR by 33.3% versus 15.5% of patients, respectively ($p < 0.001$) (16). Unfortunately, there was no clear placebo arm in this study in order to assess the clinical effect attributable to SSZ itself.

In the second trial—Effects of Etanercept versus Sulfasalazine in Early Axial Spondyloarthritis (ESTHER)—patients with axSpA (including both nr-axSpA and AS with symptom duration up to 5 years and active inflammation in the axial skeleton as detected by MRI) were treated with ETN 25 mg twice weekly or with SSZ up to 3 g per day for 48 weeks. At week 48, more patients in the ETN group compared to the SSZ group demonstrated a good clinical response, as defined by ASAS 40 (70% vs 31%, $p = 0.001$) or ASAS-PR (50% vs 19%, $p = 0.006$). Also, reduction of inflammation on MRI was more prominent in the ETN group (17). Again, in this study there was no placebo group, and therefore it is not clear whether the clinical response observed in the SSZ group was due to the anti-inflammatory properties of SSZ or represented the level of response that would be seen with a placebo.

There are two open-label studies indicating a possible clinical efficacy of mesalazine (also known as 5-aminosalicylic acid—5-ASA—an active metabolite and probably also an active moiety of SSZ) in AS/SpA (18, 19), but this was not confirmed in a later study (20).

Taking all these data together, we cannot exclude that SSZ might be beneficial in a certain proportion of axSpA patients in the treatment of both peripheral and axial manifestations. However, this proportion seems to be quite small (which might explain borderline results of placebo-controlled trials) and no factors predicting efficacy of SSZ in axSpA are known. Furthermore, SSZ is clearly less effective than TNFi in axSpA. For patients in whom there is a contraindication or unavailability of TNFi, a trial of SSZ might be undertaken, with the recognition of the small treatment effects, as discussed.

Methotrexate

It might be surprising, but there is virtually no evidence in support of MTX use in axSpA. A Cochrane review initially performed in 2004 and updated in 2013 identified only three RCTs with MTX in AS (21, 22). In these trials, MTX was tested in relatively low dosages between 7.5 and 10 mg per week given for a time period between 12 and 24 weeks. There was no beneficial effect of MTX in two of these trials (23, 24), while in one study with a high percentage of patients with concurrent peripheral arthritis, a better response in some of the outcome variables was found (25).

In the trial by Altan et al. (23), a significant difference between the placebo and MTX groups was found only in physician global assessment, while patient-reported parameters related to disease activity and function demonstrated no difference. In the study by Roychowdhury et al. (24), no significant differences were found between the MTX and the placebo group and there was no change from baseline of BASDAI, BASMI, and CRP levels. In the study by Gonzalez-Lopez et al. (25), the primary outcome measure was a composite index of improvement in five of the following scales: severity of morning stiffness, physical well-being, BASDAI, BASFI, HAQ-S, and physician and patient global assessment of disease activity. At week 24, 53% of patients in the MTX group ($n = 17$) had a treatment response, compared with 17% in the placebo group ($n = 18$, $p = 0.03$) (25). However, for secondary outcomes, including those outcome parameters used for response judgement and mentioned above, no statistically significant differences were found between the treatment groups (25). In another open-label study with MTX given intramuscularly at a dose of 12.5 mg per week for 1 year to 34 patients with AS, 53% (most of them with peripheral arthritis) were considered as responders at the end of the treatment period (26).

Again, as in the studies with SSZ, none of the studies mentioned above used standard ASAS outcome parameters. Further, the dosages of MTX (7.5–12.5 mg per week) tested in these studies were low compared to those currently used for the treatment of RA (15–25 mg per week). To determine whether the lack of evidence of MTX for the treatment of AS might be due to inadequate dosing regimens, a more recent 16-week open-label trial of MTX given in a dose of 20 mg per week subcutaneously was conducted. This trial did not show any effect on axial and only some statistically non-significant improvement in peripheral symptoms (27). No studies with MTX have been conducted to date in nr-axSpA nor in the entire axSpA spectrum, and no studies in AS included structural damage as an outcome parameter. There are also no studies investigating efficacy of combined therapy (e.g. SSZ with MTX) on signs and symptoms of axSpA.

One open-label trial compared SSZ, MTX 10 mg per week, and the combination given for 6 months for their impact on active sacroiliitis on MRI in 55 patients with early axSpA. No significant influence on active sacroiliitis was found in any treatment group (28).

Beyond clinical efficacy of MTX itself, there is also a relevant question of whether addition of MTX to a TNFi in axSpA might increase efficacy of the latter or increase the drug survival over time. Several studies have demonstrated that addition of MTX to a TNFi does not significantly affect the clinical response, the course of inflammation on MRI, and TNFi dosing intervals (29–31). Also no influence of MTX on pharmacokinetics and pharmacodynamics in AS has been found (32). There is only one small open-label study in AS, which could show some increase in treatment response to infliximab associated with MTX (33).

In two large observational studies (the Danish Registry for Biologic Therapies in Rheumatology (DANBIO) and NOR-DMARD), use of MTX was not associated with better retention rates (drug survival) of TNFi in AS and no additional clinical effect of MTX could be shown (5, 34). Notably, TNFi survival was generally better in AS than in RA (34). This might be related to a generally lower prevalence of anti-drug antibodies, including neutralizing antibodies in AS; whether or not MTX is able to influence anti-drug antibody formation in AS still has to be determined.

In the most recent study, however, performed in the Swedish Biologics Register (Antirheumatic Therapies in Sweden—ARTIS), use of synthetic DMARDs (mainly MTX) was associated with better retention of TNFi therapy both in AS and uSpA. The effect was slightly more pronounced for AS (HR 0.71 vs 0.82 in uSpA) and present both for MTX and other DMARDs in AS, while in the uSpA the authors could find an effect only for MTX (35).

The available data would indicate that there is no evidence that MTX might be effective in axial disease and only marginal evidence exists in support of MTX use in the case of peripheral involvement. Efficacy of a combination therapy (e.g. MTX plus SSZ) remains uncertain. Benefits of MTX addition to TNFi in axSpA remain uncertain.

Other DMARDs

Leflunomide was investigated in AS (but not in nr-axSpA) in two trials, with negative results (36, 37). However, some positive effect was seen in a subgroup of patients with the presence of peripheral arthritis (36).

There was no clinical effect of gold salts (auranofin) (38) and antimalarial drugs (39) in respective clinical trials in AS. Penicillamine was effective in reduction of axial and peripheral symptoms of AS in one open-label trial (40), but there was no effect in a subsequent controlled trial (41). There was some improvement of peripheral arthritis and ESR associated with intravenous cyclophosphamide in one small open-label trail in AS (42). There are to date no published results of clinical trials investigating azathioprine and cyclosporine efficacy in axSpA.

It is relevant to include commentary on thalidomide and pamidronate, although these drugs cannot be regarded as classical DMARDs. Thalidomide has been tested for the treatment of AS patients in several open-label trials with some success, but is regarded as too toxic for widespread use (43–45). Clinical trials with pamidronate, a bisphosphonate, provided contradictory results in AS. Clinical effect of pamidronate in active AS was demonstrated for the first time in a small open-label study (46). In a subsequent 6-month RCT from the same group, pamidronate given in a dose of 60 mg intravenously once a month was superior to 10 mg pamidronate monthly, with a significant improvement of function and pain (47). However, following open-label studies, using the same dosing regimen of pamidronate provided rather negative or inconclusive results (48–51) which precludes any strong conclusion regarding efficacy of this kind of therapy in axSpA.

Conclusion

In axSpA there is little evidence to support the use of DMARDs in active disease, with the majority of studies performed in advanced AS. SSZ is the best investigated DMARD in axSpA. The positive clinical effect of SSZ, if any, seems to be more prominent in the presence of peripheral arthritis, although there may a certain proportion of patients with axial disease who might benefit from SSZ therapy. SSZ and to a further extent other DMARDs are less effective than TNFi. No disease-modifying properties, for example retardation of structural damage progression in the spine, have been demonstrated for DMARDs in axSpA to date.

References

1. Haibel H, Specker C. Disease-modifying anti-rheumatic drugs in rheumatoid arthritis and ankylosing spondylitis. Clin Exp Rheumatol 2009;27:S159–63.
2. Braun J, van den Berg R, Baraliakos X, et al. 2010 update of the ASAS/EULAR recommendations for the management of ankylosing spondylitis. Ann Rheum Dis 2011;70:896–904.
3. van der Heijde D, Sieper J, Maksymowych WP, et al. 2010 Update of the international ASAS recommendations for the use of anti-TNF agents in patients with axial spondyloarthritis. Ann Rheum Dis 2011;70:905–8.
4. Rudwaleit M, Haibel H, Baraliakos X, et al. The early disease stage in axial spondylarthritis: results from the German Spondyloarthritis Inception Cohort. Arthritis Rheum 2009;60:717–27.
5. Glintborg B, Ostergaard M, Krogh NS, et al. Predictors of treatment response and drug continuation in 842 patients with ankylosing spondylitis treated with anti-tumour necrosis factor: results from 8 years' surveillance in the Danish nationwide DANBIO registry. Ann Rheum Dis 2010;69:2002–8.
6. Relas H, Kautiainen H, Puolakka K, et al. Survival of disease-modifying antirheumatic drugs used as the first antirheumatic medication in the treatment of ankylosing spondylitis in Finland. A nationwide population-based register study. Clin Rheumatol 2014;33:1135–8.
7. Chen J, Liu C. Sulfasalazine for ankylosing spondylitis. Cochrane Database Syst Rev 2005;2:CD004800.
8. Chen J, Lin S, Liu C. Sulfasalazine for ankylosing spondylitis. Cochrane Database Syst Rev 2014;11:CD004800.
9. Clegg DO, Reda DJ, Abdellatif M. Comparison of sulfasalazine and placebo for the treatment of axial and peripheral articular manifestations of the seronegative spondylarthropathies: a Department of Veterans Affairs cooperative study. Arthritis Rheum 1999;42:2325–9.
10. Dougados M, vam der Linden S, Leirisalo-Repo M, et al. Sulfasalazine in the treatment of spondylarthropathy. A randomized, multicenter, double-blind, placebo-controlled study. Arthritis Rheum 1995;38:618–27.
11. Fagerli KM, van der Heijde D, Heiberg MS, et al. Is there a role for sulphasalazine in axial spondyloarthritis in the era of TNF inhibition? Data from the NOR-DMARD longitudinal observational study. Rheumatology (Oxford) 2014;53:1087–94.
12. Lehtinen A, Leirisalo-Repo M, Taavitsainen M. Persistence of enthesopathic changes in patients with spondylarthropathy during a 6-month follow-up. Clin Exp Rheumatol 1995;13:733–6.
13. Genc H, Duyur Cakit B, Nacir B, et al. The effects of sulfasalazine treatment on enthesal abnormalities of inflammatory rheumatic diseases. Clin Rheumatol 2007;26:1104–10.
14. Benitez-Del-Castillo JM, Garcia Sanchez J, Iradier T, et al. Sulfasalazine in the prevention of anterior uveitis associated with ankylosing spondylitis. Eye (Lond) 2000;14(Pt 3A):340–3.
15. Braun J, Zochling J, Baraliakos X, et al. Efficacy of sulfasalazine in patients with inflammatory back pain due to undifferentiated spondyloarthritis and early ankylosing spondylitis: a multicentre randomised controlled trial. Ann Rheum Dis 2006;65:1147–53.
16. Braun J, van der Horst-Bruinsma IE, Huang F, et al. Clinical efficacy and safety of etanercept versus sulfasalazine in patients with ankylosing spondylitis: a randomized, double-blind trial. Arthritis Rheum 2011;63:1543–51.
17. Song IH, Hermann K, Haibel H, et al. Effects of etanercept versus sulfasalazine in early axial spondyloarthritis on active inflammatory lesions as detected by whole-body MRI (ESTHER): a 48-week randomised controlled trial. Ann Rheum Dis 2011;70:590–6.
18. Dekker-Saeys BJ, Dijkmans BA, Tytgat GN. Treatment of spondyloarthropathy with 5-aminosalicylic acid (mesalazine): an open trial. J Rheumatol 2000;27:723–6.
19. Thomson GT, Thomson BR, Thomson KS, et al. Clinical efficacy of mesalamine in the treatment of the spondyloarthropathies. J Rheumatol 2000;27:714–8.
20. van Denderen JC, van der Horst-Bruinsma I, Bezemer PD, et al. Efficacy and safety of mesalazine (Salofalk) in an open study of 20 patients with ankylosing spondylitis. J Rheumatol 2003;30:1558–60.
21. Chen J, Veras MM, Liu C, et al. Methotrexate for ankylosing spondylitis. Cochrane Database Syst Rev 2013;2:CD004524.
22. Chen J, Liu C. Methotrexate for ankylosing spondylitis. Cochrane Database Syst Rev 2004;3:CD004524.
23. Altan L, Bingol U, Karakoc Y, et al. Clinical investigation of methotrexate in the treatment of ankylosing spondylitis. Scand J Rheumatol 2001;30:255–9.
24. Roychowdhury B, Bintley-Bagot S, Bulgen DY, et al. Is methotrexate effective in ankylosing spondylitis? Rheumatology (Oxford) 2002;41:1330–2.
25. Gonzalez-Lopez L, Garcia-Gonzalez A, Vazquez-Del-Mercado M, et al. Efficacy of methotrexate in ankylosing spondylitis: a randomized, double blind, placebo controlled trial. J Rheumatol 2004;31:1568–74.
26. Sampaio-Barros PD, Costallat LT, Bertolo MB, et al. Methotrexate in the treatment of ankylosing spondylitis. Scand J Rheumatol 2000;29:160–2.
27. Haibel H, Brandt HC, Song IH, et al. No efficacy of subcutaneous methotrexate in active ankylosing spondylitis: a 16-week open-label trial. Ann Rheum Dis 2007;66:419–21.
28. Kabasakal Y, Kitapcioglu G, Yargucu F, et al. Efficacy of SLZ and MTX (alone or combination) on the treatment of active sacroiliitis in early AS. Rheumatol Int 2009;29:1523–7.
29. Breban M, Ravaud P, Claudepierre P, et al. Maintenance of infliximab treatment in ankylosing spondylitis: results of a one-year randomized

controlled trial comparing systematic versus on-demand treatment. Arthritis Rheum 2008;58:88–97.
30. Li EK, Griffith JF, Lee VW, et al. Short-term efficacy of combination methotrexate and infliximab in patients with ankylosing spondylitis: a clinical and magnetic resonance imaging correlation. Rheumatology (Oxford) 2008;47:1358–63.
31. Marzo-Ortega H, McGonagle D, Jarrett S, et al. Infliximab in combination with methotrexate in active ankylosing spondylitis: a clinical and imaging study. Ann Rheum Dis 2005;64:1568–75.
32. Ternant D, Mulleman D, Lauferon F, et al. Influence of methotrexate on infliximab pharmacokinetics and pharmacodynamics in ankylosing spondylitis. Br J Clin Pharmacol 2012;73:55–65.
33. Perez-Guijo VC, Cravo AR, Castro Mdel C, et al. Increased efficacy of infliximab associated with methotrexate in ankylosing spondylitis. Joint Bone Spine 2007;74:254–8.
34. Heiberg MS, Koldingsnes W, Mikkelsen K, et al. The comparative one-year performance of anti-tumor necrosis factor alpha drugs in patients with rheumatoid arthritis, psoriatic arthritis, and ankylosing spondylitis: results from a longitudinal, observational, multicenter study. Arthritis Rheum 2008;59:234–40.
35. Lie E, Kristensen LE, Forsblad-d'Elia H, et al. The effect of comedication with conventional synthetic disease modifying antirheumatic drugs on TNF inhibitor drug survival in patients with ankylosing spondylitis and undifferentiated spondyloarthritis: results from a nationwide prospective study. Ann Rheum Dis 2015;74:970–8.
36. Haibel H, Rudwaleit M, Braun J, et al. Six months open label trial of leflunomide in active ankylosing spondylitis. Ann Rheum Dis 2005;64:124–6.
37. van Denderen JC, van der Paardt M, Nurmohamed MT, et al. Double blind, randomised, placebo controlled study of leflunomide in the treatment of active ankylosing spondylitis. Ann Rheum Dis 2005;64:1761–4.
38. Grasedyck K, Schattenkirchner M, Bandilla K. [The treatment of ankylosing spondylitis with auranofin (Ridaura).] Z Rheumatol 1990;49:98–9.
39. Williamson L, Illingworth H, Smith D, et al. Oral quinine in ankylosing spondylitis: a randomized placebo controlled double blind crossover trial. J Rheumatol 2000;27:2054–5.
40. Bernacka K, Tytman K, Sierakowski S. Clinical application of D-penicillamine in ankylosing spondylitis: a 9-month study. Med Interne 1989;27:295–301.
41. Steven MM, Morrison M, Sturrock RD. Penicillamine in ankylosing spondylitis: a double blind placebo controlled trial. J Rheumatol 1985;12:735–7.
42. Sadowska-Wroblewska M, Garwolinska H, Maczynska-Rusiniak B. A trial of cyclophosphamide in ankylosing spondylitis with involvement of peripheral joints and high disease activity. Scand J Rheumatol 1986;15:259–64.
43. Breban M, Gombert B, Amor B, et al. Efficacy of thalidomide in the treatment of refractory ankylosing spondylitis. Arthritis Rheum 1999;42:580–1.
44. Huang F, Gu J, Zhao W, et al. One-year open-label trial of thalidomide in ankylosing spondylitis. Arthritis Rheum 2002;47:249–54.
45. Wei JC, Chan TW, Lin HS, et al. Thalidomide for severe refractory ankylosing spondylitis: a 6-month open-label trial. J Rheumatol 2003;30:2627–31.
46. Maksymowych WP, Jhangri GS, Leclercq S, et al. An open study of pamidronate in the treatment of refractory ankylosing spondylitis. J Rheumatol 1998;25:714–17.
47. Maksymowych WP, Jhangri GS, Fitzgerald AA, et al. A six-month randomized, controlled, double-blind, dose-response comparison of intravenous pamidronate (60 mg versus 10 mg) in the treatment of nonsteroidal antiinflammatory drug-refractory ankylosing spondylitis. Arthritis Rheum 2002;46:766–73.
48. Haibel H, Brandt J, Rudwaleit M, et al. Treatment of active ankylosing spondylitis with pamidronate. Rheumatology (Oxford) 2003;42:1018–20.
49. Grover R, Shankar S, Aneja R, et al. Treatment of ankylosing spondylitis with pamidronate: an open label study. Ann Rheum Dis 2006;65:688–9.
50. Toussirot E, Le Huede G, Lohse A, et al. Transient efficacy of pulse pamidronate treatment in active spondylarthropathies: an open study of 35 cases. Clin Exp Rheumatol 2006;24:348.
51. Cairns AP, Wright SA, Taggart AJ, et al. An open study of pulse pamidronate treatment in severe ankylosing spondylitis, and its effect on biochemical markers of bone turnover. Ann Rheum Dis 2005;64:338–9.

CHAPTER 22

Treatment: biologics

Juergen Braun and Irene E. van der Horst-Bruinsma

Introduction to biologics

According to classification criteria which have been developed in the last years (1–4) and earlier (5), the spectrum of SpA covers axSpA, which includes nr-axSpA and AS, and peripheral SpA, which overlaps with PsA. Management recommendations for many forms of SpA have been recently published (6–9). Treatment of patients with axSpA with active disease starts with a sufficient dose of NSAIDs for a period of at least 4 weeks and preferably longer, in combination with exercise. In the case of peripheral SpA, several DMARDs (see Chapter 21) can be given, but these drugs are not efficacious in axial disease. In case of insufficient response to NSAIDs for axSpA, biologic treatment can be added (6). The biologics most commonly used are TNF blocking agents, but some other biologic agents seem to be beneficial in axial diseases as well, such as secukinumab (SEC) (an IL-17 blocker) (Table 22.1). However, these new drugs have not yet been approved for axSpA at the time of writing this chapter.

Table 22.1 Biologics used for the treatment of SpA

TNF-blocking agents	AS	nr-axSpA*	PsA	Undifferentiated peripheral SpA
Infliximab 5 mg per kg iv every 6 weeks*	+++	++	+++	(+)
Etanercept 50 mg per week sc	+++	+++	+++	(+)
Adalimumab 40 mg every 2 weeks sc	+++	+++	+++	+
Golimumab 50 mg every 4 weeks sc	+++	+++	+++	–
Certolizumab 200 mg every 2 weeks sc*	+++	+++	+++	?
Ustekinumab (anti-IL-12) 90 mg every 3 months sc*	(+)	?	+++	?
Secukinumab (anti-IL-17) 150 mg every 4 weeks sc*	++	?	++	?
Brodalumab (anti-IL-17R) 280 mg every 2 weeks*	?	?	+	?
Ixekizumab (anti-IL-17) 75 mg every 4 weeks*	?	?	?	?
Clazikizumab (anti-IL-23) 100 mg every 4 weeks	?	?	+	?

? No data; – not efficacious; (+) limited data, probably efficacious; + some efficacy in at least one controlled trial; ++ efficacious but not yet approved; +++ efficacious and approved; * approval only in the EC, not the USA; iv, intravenous; sc, subcutaneous. Non-efficacious in axSpA: rituximab, apremilast, abatacept, tocilizumab, sarilumab, anakinra.

Treatment of axial spondyloarthritis with biologics

The early phase of TNF-blockers in spondyloarthritis

A first rationale to inhibit TNFα in SpA developed when strong expression of TNFα mRNA and protein was described in inflamed SI joints of patients with AS—the biopsy material had been obtained by CT-guided biopsies which were taken in conjunction with local corticosteroid injections (10, 11). At that time, it had just become clear that the chimeric monoclonal antibody *infliximab* had the capacity to substantially improve synovitis in patients with RA (12). In the following years it became also clear that inhibition of TNFα worked for severe manifestations of CD (13) and for psoriasis (14). In a small case series it was reported that also the CD-associated arthritis improved on anti-TNF therapy (15). The clinical results of the first pilot studies with infliximab (16–18) strongly suggested that a major clinical improvement was also possible in patients with active AS, and that was formally proven by the RCT that followed shortly thereafter (19). The results of a trial with the soluble 75-kDa TNF receptor *ETN* first suggested that this was likely to be a class effect (20).

Even though RA and AS are obviously rather different rheumatic diseases in many aspects (21–23), TNFα blockade seemed to work in both, for example for synovitis, enthesitis, and osteitis. However, there is the clinical impression (and some data would support that) that TNF blockers work better in SpA than in RA, and this may not relate to differences in dosage (25). This difference might also be due to the fact that DMARDs work well in RA but not in SpA, so there is more improvement to gain due to TNF blockers alone in SpA, whereas in RA these drugs are normally combined. The observation that the retention rates are higher in SpA would also be supportive of that notion (26). A major difference between RA and AS clearly is that RA is rather osteodestructive, while AS is more osteoproliferative. Accordingly, the different effect of TNF blockade on erosions, on the one hand, and new bone formation, on the other hand, could have been predicted. However, in PsA, anti-TNF therapy was clearly shown to inhibit radiographic progression (27).

TNF blockers for the treatment of axial spondyloarthritis

Five tumour-necrosis-factor antagonists (aTNF) are now approved for patients with active AS (and also for active PsA) in most countries worldwide, including the EC and the USA: *adalimumab, certolizumab, ETN, golimumab*, and *infliximab*, More recently, adalimumab (28), certolizumab (29), ETN (30), and golimumab (31) have also been approved for the treatment of nr-axSpA (according to the ASAS classification criteria) in the EC and many other countries worldwide, but not yet in the USA. In addition to a certain level of patient symptoms (currently scored by the BASDAI, which should be ≥4) for the indication of nr-axSpA, the presence of objective signs of inflammation, such as elevated CRP and active inflammation in the SI joint and/or spine on MRI, is mandatory in the EC approval, while for the treatment of AS, only an elevated BASDAI is asked for, although the presence of positive CRP and MRI have also been shown to be predictive for a good response to TNF-blocker therapy in AS patients.

There is good evidence that all these agents reduce the clinical signs and symptoms of most patients with axSpA, including r-axSpA and nr-axSpA (28–33), and they also reduce very effectively CRP serum levels and axial inflammation, as detected by MRI (34). Indeed, given a similar level of inflammation at baseline, the response to TNF blockers is similar in patients with AS and nr-axSpA (29). It has been shown that TNF blockers are also effective in patients with peripheral arthritis (35) and enthesitis and EAMs in the eye, skin, and gut (36). Most TNF blockers work well for most EAMs of axSpA, except for ETN which has no efficacy for IBD.

In AS, but also in RA and PsA, the development of antibodies against TNF blockers, especially infliximab and adalimumab, is found to be related to loss of efficacy. These antibodies can develop within 6 months of treatment but can also occur later, and are associated with lower serum through levels of the drug (37–41). Currently there is no clear evidence that combining a TNF-blocker with a conventional DMARD, such as MTX, can reduce such an effect of antidrug antibodies on efficacy and side-effects, while this seems to be different in RA and possibly also in PsA (for more details see Chapter 21). The drug survival of TNF blockers was shown to be superior in AS patients treated with DMARDs in a registry (42). This may be especially the case in patients with peripheral arthritis.

Recently, the first anti-TNF biosimilar for infliximab has been approved not only for AS (43) and RA but also for psoriasis, PsA, and chronic IBDs (extrapolation). Similar efficacy and safety have been documented, and interchangeability (switching) seems possible, but many rheumatologists and societies ask for more data. Immunogenicity does not seem to be different for this agent.

Anti-TNF therapy works especially well in the early stages of axSpA patients with short disease duration and/or young age (44). It is possible to predict the success of TNF blockers in patients with axSpA based on age, CRP level, HLA-B27 status, and other parameters (45). There is potential to discontinue or reduce dosages especially in patients treated early (46). However, more studies are ongoing regarding how to best identify patients in whom the TNF-blocker dosage can be reduced or the injection interval be prolonged. Long-term therapy over several years was shown to be successful in many patients (47, 48). However, it is unclear whether an early anti-TNF-based intervention will reduce or inhibit bone formation. Some evidence in favour of this (49–51) has still to be confirmed in larger prospective trials.

The very same anti-TNF agents have also been shown to work in PsA on both a short-term (15, 52–54) and a longer term basis over 2 years (55) and at 5 years, as recently reported for golimumab (56). Furthermore, structural damage is inhibited in PsA (57, 58)—and

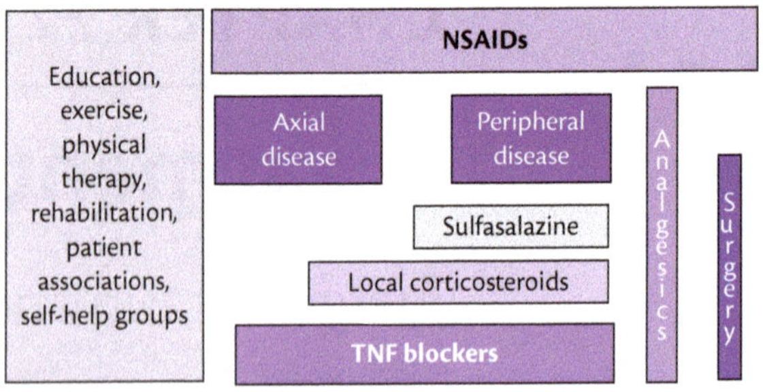

Fig. 22.1 (See colour plate section). ASAS/EULAR recommendations for the management of AS.

Reproduced from Ann Rhuem Dis, Zochling, J et al., 65, 442–52, 2006 with permission from BMJ Publishing Group Ltd. Reproduced from Ann Rhuem Dis, Braun et al., 70, 896–904, 2011 with permission from BMJ Publishing Group Ltd.

this is more relevant for osteodestructive rather than osteoproliferative changes. The safety profile of TNF blockers has been good with longer term follow-up studies (59–61), and there are no major differences between agents, with the exception of tuberculosis which occurs less often with ETN, but appropriate screening strategies have largely overcome this relative disadvantage (62).

Because of the well-documented efficacy of TNF blockers in the major rheumatic diseases, the clinical endpoints of remission and low disease activity have been placed much in the foreground of patient care, especially in RA in recent years. In contrast, that was not so much discussed for PsA and AS. However, for the recently reported Tight Control of Psoriatic Arthritis (TICOPA) trial, a strategy was developed that used minimal disease activity as the central action point (63). Based mostly on expert opinion, treatment to target aims have been formulated both for axSpA and PsA, with clinical remission and normalization of an elevated CRP as the primary targets (64). Since there is some evidence that CRP and ASDAS values have a significant influence on radiographic progression in AS (65), these are currently the best candidates for treatment decisions, even though the clinical cutoff of BASDAI ≥ 4 is still the basis to start anti-TNF therapy in axSpA (7, 66).

ASAS/EULAR recommendations for the management of axSpA have been specified with regard to treatment with TNF blockers (7) (Fig. 22.1). Patients can be classified either by the mNY criteria for AS or by the ASAS criteria for axSpA, including patients with nr-axSpA. If the axial manifestations are leading, TNF-blocker therapy can be started if the patient fails two NSAIDs, the BASDAI is ≥4, and indication for TNF blocker is confirmed by an expert, mostly based on the presence of objective signs of inflammation (Fig. 22.2).

Taken together, anti-TNF agents are rather efficient in patients with SpA, including PsA. Since not all patients are responsive to anti-TNF treatment, there is a need to better understand the cellular and molecular mechanisms that govern the disease to potentially find new pathways that will allow benefit to more patients (Fig. 22.3). Since ustekinumab (UST), targeting IL-23 and IL-12, and secukinumab, targeting IL-17, have been primarily developed in psoriasis and PsA, this is a natural starting point.

The IL-17/IL-23 axis

Genetic studies were the first to link the IL-17/IL-23 axis to SpA (67), and there is evidence that immune-mediated diseases such as AS and psoriasis have common genetic traits, including the IL-23R (68). PsA associations with single nucleotide polymorphisms

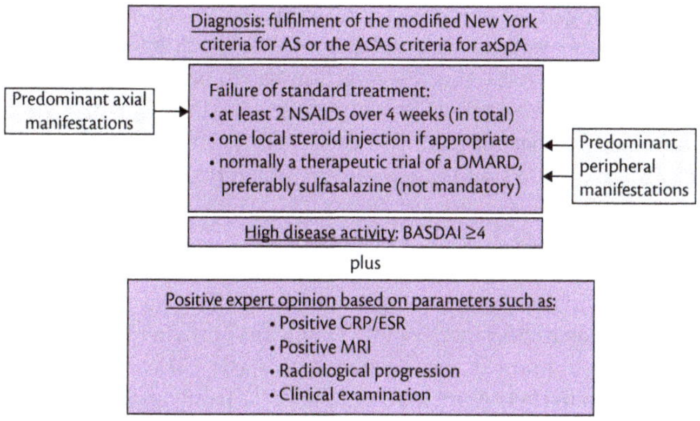

Fig. 22.2 ASAS recommendations for the use of anti-TNF agents in patients with axSpA.

Reproduced from Ann Rheum Dis, van der Heijde D et al., 70, 905–8, 2011 with permission from BMJ Publishing Group Ltd.

in IL-23R as well as TRAF3IP2 (Act1), a molecule downstream of the IL-17R, have linked the IL-23/IL-17 axis to disease pathology in psoriasis (69).

As pointed out in an earlier review some years ago, type 17 helper T cells (Th17)—at this point in time still a novel third class of T cells—and their major cytokine, IL-17, are essential for the defence against certain fungi, extracellular bacteria, and *Mycobacterium tuberculosis*, while defective control of Th17 cells and production of IL-17 are prominent in chronic inflammation and several immune-mediated inflammatory disorders (70). Furthermore, IL-23 was shown to be critical in an animal model of enthesitis by acting on specific IL-23R resident T cells which allow entheses to respond to IL-23 in the absence of further cellular recruitment and to elaborate inflammatory mediators (71).

The differentiation of naïve T cells into the Th17 phenotype is facilitated by the presence of a cytokine milieu containing a combination of TGFβ and IL-6 (72). Subsequently, as a hallmark of Th17 development, the transcription factor RORγt is expressed and activated. Thus the differentiation of Th17 cells places the Th17 lineage in close relationship with CD4+CD25+Foxp3+ Treg cells. Later stages of Th17 cell differentiation, such as clonal expansion, and phenotype stabilization with IL-17 production also rely on expression of IL-23, a potent inducer of IL-17 (72). However, under certain circumstances, IL-17 can also be produced in the absence of IL-23 and, vice versa, IL-23 can have biologic activities independently of IL-17. Thus IL-23 activates Th17, which produces IL-17, activating DCs to produce IL-12, hence stimulating Th1 cells to fight pathogens and cause inflammation (72).

Blood samples of AS patients have reported increased IL-17 and/or IL-23 activity (73)—including enrichment of circulating IL-17-secreting IL-23R-positive γ/δ T cells (74); this was in part connected to established hypotheses on HLA-B27 homodimers (75) and the unfolded protein response (76). The cytokines IL-17 and IL-23 have also been detected in spinal (77, 78) and synovial biopsies (79); however, in these human tissue samples, IL-17 was mostly not produced by T cells but rather by cells of the innate immune system.

Taken together, there is strong evidence that the IL-17/IL-23 axis plays a role in the pathogenesis of SpA, and this is substantiated by the effect of biologic agents blocking these cytokines.

Clinical responses to blockade of IL-23

In addition to IL-23 and the Th17 pathway, IL-12 has been identified as an important component of the Th1 inflammatory pathway, suggesting that this cytokine may also be a key mediator of psoriasis. *UST* is a fully human immunoglobulin G1κ (IgG1κ) monoclonal antibody against common subunit p40 of IL-12 and IL-23 (80). UST has been approved for psoriasis and PsA by the European Medicines Agency (EMA) and the FDA.

In an RCT with patients suffering from plaque psoriasis, the primary endpoint, PASI 75 at 12 weeks, was achieved in 67% of those who received 45-mg and 81% of those who received 90-mg doses

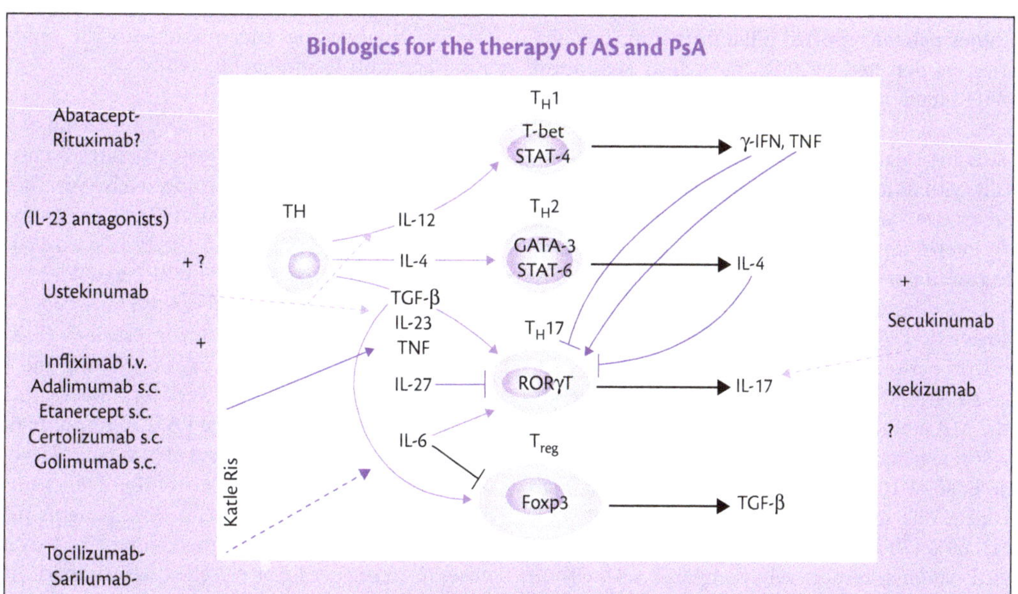

Fig. 22.3 (See colour plate section). Biologics for the therapy of AS and PsA. + Efficacy proven; – no efficacy in clinical trials; ?, not tested or results not unequivocal.

Adapted from Steinman L, Nat Med 13:144 (2007), IV ANOV I, (2006), Tato CM Nature 44 1:166 (2006).

of UST every 4 weeks, compared to 2% on placebo (81). In another RCT on moderate-to-severe psoriasis, patients received UST 45 mg or 90 mg at weeks 0 and 4, and then every 12 weeks, or placebo (Phoenix 1). Again, 67.1% and 66.4% versus 3.1% of patients on placebo achieved PASI 75 at week 12. Thereafter, dosing every 12 weeks maintained efficacy for 1 year or more in most patients (69). Dosing intensification (Phoenix 2) improved clinical response rates in patients who partially responded to initial treatment (82). In another phase III trial (Accept) on patients with psoriasis, UST was superior to ETN at the primary endpoint of 12 weeks: the percentage of patients achieving PASI 75 was 68% and 74% on UST, while 57% improved on ETN (83).

The data in PsA are overall less impressive, but there is evidence that UST works also in PsA (84–87). In an early study in active PsA, 42% of patients treated with UST reached ACR 20 at week 12 compared to only 10% on placebo (84). In the following RCT in active PsA (PSUMMIT 1), ACR 20 responses at week 24 were more often seen in patients treated with UST than with placebo: 42% and 50% versus 23%, respectively (85). In the other trial (PSUMMIT 2), patients with active PsA despite treatment with conventional and/or biologic agents were randomized and also stratified by site, weight (≤ 100 kg or > 100 kg), and MTX use to receive UST 45 mg or 90 mg at weeks 0 and 4, and then q12 weeks or placebo (86). Significantly more UST-treated (44% combined) than placebo-treated (20%) patients achieved ACR 20 at week 24. There is also evidence that UST inhibits radiographic progression in PsA (87).

There is limited evidence from one open proof-of-concept study that UST also works in AS (88). In a prospective open-label trial with no placebo group, UST administered in a dose of 90 mg subcutaneously at baseline, at week 4 and week 16, substantially improved 20 patients with active AS, as defined by a BASDAI score of ≥ 4, despite previous treatment with NSAIDs. The primary endpoint, an ASAS 40 response at week 24, was reached by as many as 65% of patients, and ASAS-PR by 30%. A total of 50% and 20% of the patients achieved the ASDAS clinically important improvement and major improvement, respectively, while 35% of patients had an ASDAS 'inactive disease' (ASDAS < 1.3), all at week 24. Significant improvement of other patient-reported outcome parameters and active inflammation as detected by MRI, as well as significant reduction of NSAID intake, were reported. The clinical response correlated with reduction of inflammation and of the serum CRP level. That pilot study is clearly positive, but controlled trials are needed—potentially with different dosage regimens, since the time to reach a good response was longer than with anti-TNF agents (88). It is especially interesting in that regard that UST also works in CD—importantly also in patients who had not responded to TNF blockade (89, 90). UST does not seem to work well in RA, indicating that the pathogenetic link between axSpA, psoriasis, and CD might be stronger than between axSpA and RA.

Guselkumab is an anti-IL-23-specific monoclonal antibody directed against the p19 subunit. Early data are available in patients with moderate-to-severe plaque psoriasis (91). Patients randomized to receive a single dose of 10, 30, 100, or 300 mg of guselkumab or placebo achieved a 75% improvement in PASI scores at week 12 in 50% (10 mg), 60% (30 and 100 mg), and 100% (300 mg) of guselkumab-treated patients, respectively, compared with 0% on placebo, and improvements were maintained through week 24 (91). Currently there are no data on the efficacy of this drug in SpA.

Taken together, blocking IL-23 works very well for psoriasis and relatively well for PsA and also for AS. Blocking IL-12 seems to be less important, but this question has to be further clarified. More studies and analyses will hopefully reveal which patients are most likely to benefit from this treatment. Furthermore, the optimal dosage of UST and other anti-IL-23 compounds clearly needs more study.

Blocking IL-17

Genetic and immunohistologic studies in diseased tissues have pointed to an important role of IL-17 and Th17 cells in the pathogenesis of autoimmune disorders such as psoriasis, IBD, and SpA (92). In addition to IL-17A, members of the IL-17 family include IL-17B, IL-17C, IL-17D, IL-17E (IL-25), and IL-17F. To elicit its functions, IL-17 binds to a type I cell surface receptor called IL-17R, of which there are at least three variants–IL17RA, IL17RB, and IL17RC. Th17 cells are producers of the proinflammatory cytokine IL-17A as well as other effector cytokines, including IL-22. Recent research has shown that IL-17A is also expressed by multiple lineages of the innate immune system, including mast cells, neutrophils, DCs, γδ-T cells, macrophages, and NK cells. IL-17A acts on keratinocytes to increase expression of chemokines involved in recruiting myeloid DCs, Th17 cells, and neutrophils to the lesion site. The inhibition of IL-17A as a therapeutic target can be expected to exert different physiological effects than the suppression of Th17 cell activity (93). At present, no anti-IL-17 biologic agent has been approved.

First clinical data are available on *SEC*, a recombinant, highly selective, fully human monoclonal anti-IL-17A antibody of the IgG1κ isotype. In an early study on patients suffering from active CD, SEC was not effective and higher rates of adverse events were noted compared with placebo (94). In three clinical studies on (1) patients with Behçet's uveitis (SHIELD), (2) patients with active, non-infectious, non-Behçet's uveitis (INSURE), and(3) patients with quiescent, non-infectious, non-Behçet's uveitis (ENDURE), patients were treated with different dosages of SEC. After completion or early termination of the trial, there were no statistically significant differences in uveitis recurrence between the SEC and placebo. However, patients treated with SEC tended to use immunosuppressants less frequently (95).

Patients with moderate to severe plaque psoriasis who had received subcutaneous doses of SEC 3 × 75 mg or 3 × 150 mg every 4 weeks had higher PASI 75 response rates versus placebo at week 12: 82% and 97% versus 9%, respectively (96); these response rates were maintained over 36 weeks (97). Recently, two controlled trials (Efficacy of Response and Safety of Two Fixed Secukinumab Regimens in Psoriasis (ERASURE) and Full Year Investigative Examination of Secukinumab versus Etanercept Using Two Dosing Regimens to Determine Efficacy in Psoriasis (FIXTURE)) on SEC in plaque psoriasis, using dosages of 300 mg and 150 mg subcutaneously administered once a week for 5 weeks, then every 4 weeks, versus placebo or ETN showed PASI 75 response rates of the higher dose of SEC at week 12 of about 80% versus placebo (5%) and ETN (44%), suggesting a strong effect of IL-17 blockade (98).

In the pilot study with active PsA, patients fulfilling CASPAR criteria were randomly assigned to receive two intravenous SEC doses of 10 mg per kg or placebo 3 weeks apart. ACR 20 responses at weeks 6, 12, and 24 were higher in the SEC group but not significantly superior to placebo: about 40% versus about 20% (99).

A phase 3 trial in active PsA showed improved physical function and fatigue and increased work productivity (100).

A small pilot study in patients with active AS showed an ASAS 20 response at week 6 in 59% of patients treated with SEC in a dose of 2 × 10 mg per kg given intravenously 3 weeks apart versus 24% on placebo (101). An RCT in this indication showed that a weekly dose of 150 mg subcutaneously was effective at rapidly reducing signs and symptoms without unexpected safety findings (102). In addition, patients who received a loading dose of intravenous treatment with SEC of 10 mg per kg, followed by a subcutaneous dose every 4 weeks, showed rapid and sustained improvement in signs and symptoms of AS (103) up to 52 weeks and in patient-reported outcomes such as fatigue and work disability. Spinal and SI inflammation as assessed by MRI also improved significantly. SEC was also effective in AS patients who were TNF-experienced in both phase 3 trials (102, 103).

Other agents targeting IL-17, *brodalumab* and *ixekizumab* (104–106), have been shown to work in psoriasis (104,106) and PsA (105), respectively. In PsA, brodalumab, an anti-IL-17R antibody, shows a significant clinical response with continued improvement from weeks 12 to 52 (107). No data for these agents are available yet for axSpA.

Taken together, blocking IL-17 works very well for psoriasis and relatively well for PsA and AS. More subgroup analyses will hopefully reveal which patients are most likely to benefit from this treatment. More dosing data are also clearly needed.

Other biologics

There is some evidence that there is an association between the IL-1 family gene cluster and SpA (108). The first non-TNF biologic tested in AS was the IL-1R antagonist *anakinra*, with conflicting results (109–111). Altogether, the effects were clearly not strong, but it seems possible that individual patients may have some benefit. However, controlled data are not available.

Anakinra was also tested in an open study in PsA, and 4/20 patients achieved an ACR 50 response, but only six completed week 24 (112). No controlled data of anakinra in PsA are available.

Rituximab, a chimeric monoclonal antibody against the protein CD20 which is primarily found on the surface of B cells, was studied in a dosage of 1000 mg administered intravenously at baseline and at week 2 in 20 patients with active AS, ten of which had never received TNF blockers, and in ten this treatment had failed (113). The primary endpoint, an ASAS 20% improvement, was reached by 50% of the anti-TNF-naive patients, while the anti-TNF failure group showed no response, exceeding that to be expected from placebo (30% ASAS 20). Among the nine patients who responded, five flared after week 24 and were successfully retreated (114). Data from a French registry-based study were largely similar to the German experience (115).

In a small open Austrian trial there seemed to be some efficacy of rituximab also in PsA (116). In the absence of controlled data, these results suggest that there may be some efficacy of therapies directed against B cells in AS and PsA. More studies are needed, but getting funding for such studies is difficult because the patent of rituximab runs out soon.

Abatacept, a fusion protein composed of the Fc region of the immunoglobulin IgG1 fused to the extracellular domain of CTLA-4, was tested in patients with active AS in a prospective open-label pilot phase 2 study (117). It was administered in a dosage of 10 mg per kg intravenously on days 1, 15, and 29 and every 28 days thereafter up to week 24 in anti-TNF-naive patients with an inadequate response to TNFα inhibitors. The primary endpoint, an ASAS 40 response, was reached by 13% and 0% of patients, respectively. No further studies have been performed.

In PsA one controlled trial with abatacept was performed (118). In the group receiving the usual dose of abatacept of 10 mg per kg on days 1, 15, and 29 and then once every 28 days thereafter, patients had the highest ACR 20 response rate of 48% versus placebo 19%. However, no further studies were performed.

In the original immunohistological study where the presence of abundant TNF in the SI joints was reported (10), the expression of also some IL-6 had been described. After some conflicting case reports (119), the two large trials in AS performed with *tocilizumab* (120) and *sarilumab* (121), targeting IL-6 and the IL-6R, respectively, were both negative in terms of efficacy, highlighting again the fact that there are important differences between the inflammatory process in AS and RA, which, however, remain poorly defined at present. The data of IL-6 inhibition in PsA are very limited; one positive case report has been published (122).

A small study with *apremilast*, an oral phosphodiesterase inhibitor, in 38 AS patients failed to meet the target outcome measure (123), but it did show clinically meaningful improvement in PsA (124), with improvement of physical function (125).

In conclusion, several biologics, such as anakinra, rituximab, abatacept, apremilast, and tocilizumab that clearly work in RA, do not work in SpA, with some possible differences between AS and PsA. In contrast, TNFi are clearly efficacious in both axSpA and PsA, and this has made rather dramatic changes in the management of these diseases. Furthermore, there are several new compounds that hold promise, such as 'pure' IL-23 inhibitors (e.g. guselkumab) and JAK inhibitors (e.g. tofacitinib), which are in different development states. Several companies are testing antibodies with two target qualities such as anti-TNFα and anti IL-17 on the cell surface.

References

1. Rudwaleit M, Landewé R, van der Heijde D, et al. The development of Assessment of SpondyloArthritis international Society (ASAS) classification criteria for axial spondyloarthritis (part I): classification of paper patients by expert opinion including uncertainty appraisal. Ann Rheum Dis 2009;68(6):770–6.
2. Rudwaleit M, van der Heijde D, Landewe R, et al. The development of Assessment of SpondyloArthritis international Society classification criteria for axial spondyloarthritis (part II): validation and final selection. Ann Rheum Dis 2009;68(6):777–83.
3. van der Linden S, Valkenburg HA, Cats A. Evaluation of diagnostic criteria for ankylosing spondylitis. A proposal for modification of the New York criteria. Arthritis Rheum 1984;27(4):361–8.
4. Rudwaleit M, van der Heijde D, Landewé R, et al. The Assessment of SpondyloArthritis international Society classification criteria for peripheral spondyloarthritis and for spondyloarthritis in general. Ann Rheum Dis 2011;70(1):25–31.
5. Taylor W, Gladman D, Helliwell P, et al. Classification criteria for psoriatic arthritis: development of new criteria from a large international study. Arthritis Rheum 2006;54(8):2665–73.
6. Braun J, et al. 2010 Update of the ASAS/EULAR recommendations for the management of ankylosing spondylitis. Ann Rheum Dis 2011;70(6):896–904.
7. van der Heijde D, et al. 2010 Update of the international ASAS recommendations for the use of anti-TNF agents in patients with axial spondyloarthritis. Ann Rheum Dis 2011;70(6):905–8.

8. Gossec L, Smolen JS, Gaujoux-Viala C, et al. European League Against Rheumatism recommendations for the management of psoriatic arthritis with pharmacological therapies. Ann Rheum Dis 2012;71(1):4–12.
9. Smolen JS, Braun J, Dougados M, et al. Treating spondyloarthritis, including ankylosing spondylitis and psoriatic arthritis, to target: recommendations of an international task force. Ann Rheum Dis 2014;73(1):6–16.
10. Braun J, Bollow M, Neure L, et al. Use of immunohistologic and in situ hybridization techniques in the examination of sacroiliac joint biopsy specimens from patients with ankylosing spondylitis. Arthritis Rheum 1995;38(4):499–505.
11. Braun J, Bollow M, Seyrekbasan F, et al. Computed tomography guided corticosteroid injection of the sacroiliac joint in patients with spondyloarthropathy with sacroiliitis: clinical outcome and followup by dynamic magnetic resonance imaging. J Rheumatol 1996;23(4):659–64.
12. Elliott MJ, Maini RN, Feldmann M, et al. Randomised double-blind comparison of chimeric monoclonal antibody to tumour necrosis factor alpha (cA2) versus placebo in rheumatoid arthritis. Lancet 1994;344(8930):1105–10.
13. van Dullemen HM, van Deventer SJ, Hommes DW, et al. Treatment of Crohn's disease with anti-tumor necrosis factor chimeric monoclonal antibody (cA2). Gastroenterology 1995;109(1):129–35.
14. van Dullemen HM, van Deventer SJ, Hommes DW, et al. Treatment of Crohn's disease with anti-tumor necrosis factor chimeric monoclonal antibody (cA2). Gastroenterology 1995;109(1):129–35.
15. Mease PJ, Goffe BS, Metz J, VanderStoep A, Finck B, Burge DJ. Etanercept in the treatment of psoriatic arthritis and psoriasis: a randomised trial. Lancet 2000;356(9227):385–90.
16. Brandt J, Haibel H, Cornely D, et al. Successful treatment of active ankylosing spondylitis with the anti-tumor necrosis factor alpha monoclonal antibody infliximab. Arthritis Rheum 2000; 43(6):1346–52.
17. Van den Bosch F, Kruithof E, De Vos M, De Keyser F, Mielants H. Crohn's disease associated with spondyloarthropathy: effect of TNF-alpha blockade with infliximab on articular symptoms. Lancet 2000;356(9244):1821–2.
18. Stone M, Salonen D, Lax M, Payne U, Lapp V, Inman RD. Clinical and imaging correlates of response to treatment with infliximab in patients with ankylosing spondylitis. J Rheumatol 2001;28(7):1605–14.
19. Braun J, Brandt J, Listing J, et al. Treatment of active ankylosing spondylitis with infliximab: a randomised controlled multicentre trial. Lancet 2002;359(9313):1187–93.
20. Gorman JD, Sack KE, Davis JC Jr. Treatment of ankylosing spondylitis by inhibition of tumor necrosis factor alpha. N Engl J Med 2002;346(18):1349–56.
21. Braun J, Sieper J, Pincus T. A systematic comparison between rheumatoid arthritis and ankylosing spondylitis: an introduction. Clin Exp Rheumatol 2009 ;27(4 Suppl 55):S1–2.
22. Cross MJ, Smith EU, Zochling J, March IM. Differences and similarities between ankylosing spondylitis and rheumatoid arthritis: epidemiology. Clin Exp Rheumatol 2009 ;27(4 Suppl 55):S36–42.
23. Inman RD, El-Gabalawy HS. The immunology of ankylosing spondylitis and rheumatoid arthritis: a tale of similarities and dissimilarities. Clin Exp Rheumatol 2009;27(4 Suppl 55):S26–32.
24. Maksymowych WP, Brown MA. Genetics of ankylosing spondylitis and rheumatoid arthritis: where are we at currently, and how do they compare? Clin Exp Rheumatol 2009;27(4 Suppl 55):S20–5.
25. Heiberg MS, Koldingsnes W, Mikkelsen K, et al. The comparative one-year performance of anti-tumor necrosis factor alpha drugs in patients with rheumatoid arthritis, psoriatic arthritis, and ankylosing spondylitis: results from a longitudinal, observational, multicenter study. Arthritis Rheum 2008;59(2):234–40.
26. Biggioggero M, Favalli EG. Ten-year drug survival of anti-TNF agents in the treatment of inflammatory arthritides. Drug Dev Res 2014;75(Suppl 1):S38–41.
27. Kavanaugh A, McInnes IB, Mease P, et al. Clinical efficacy, radiographic and safety findings through 5 years of subcutaneous golimumab treatment in patients with active psoriatic arthritis: results from a long-term extension of a randomised, placebo-controlled trial (the GO-REVEAL study). Ann Rheum Dis 2014;73(9):1689–94.
28. Sieper J, et al. Efficacy and safety of adalimumab in patients with non-radiographic axial spondyloarthritis: results of a randomised placebo-controlled trial (ABILITY-1). Ann Rheum Dis 2013;72(6):815–22.
29. Landewe R, et al. Efficacy of certolizumab pegol on signs and symptoms of axial spondyloarthritis including ankylosing spondylitis: 24-week results of a double-blind randomised placebo-controlled phase 3 study. Ann Rheum Dis 2014;73(1):39–47.
30. Dougados M, van der Heijde D, Sieper J, et al. Symptomatic efficacy of etanercept and its effects on objective signs of inflammation in early nonradiographicaxial spondyloarthritis: a multicenter, randomized, double-blind, placebo-controlled trial. Arthritis Rheumatol 2014;66(8):2091–102.
31. Sieper J, van der Heijde D, Dougados M, et al. A randomized, double-blind, placebo-controlled, sixteen-week study of subcutaneous golimumab in patients with active nonradiographic axial spondyloarthritis. Arthritis Rheumatol 2015;67(10):2702–12.
32. Braun J, et al. Clinical efficacy and safety of etanercept versus sulfasalazine in patients with ankylosing spondylitis: a randomized, double-blind trial. Arthritis Rheum 2011;63(6):1543–51.
33. Braun J, Deodhar A, Inman RD, et al. Golimumab administered subcutaneously every 4 weeks in ankylosing spondylitis: 104-week results of the GO-RAISE study. Ann Rheum Dis 2011;71(5):661–7.
34. Braun J, Baraliakos X, Hermann KG, et al. Golimumab reduces spinal inflammation in ankylosing spondylitis: MRI results of the randomised, placebo- controlled GO-RAISE study. Ann Rheum Dis 2012;71(6):878–84.
35. Braun J, et al. Clinical efficacy of etanercept versus sulfasalazine in ankylosing spondylitis subjects with peripheral joint involvement. J Rheumatol 2012;39(4):836–40.
36. van der Horst-Bruinsma IE, Nurmohamed MT. Management and evaluation of extra-articular manifestations in spondyloarthritis. Ther Adv Musculoskelet Dis 2012;4(6):413–22.
37. de Vries MK, Brouwer E, van der Horst-Bruinsma IE, et al. Decreased clinical response to adalimumab in ankylosing spondylitis is associated with antibody formation. Ann Rheum Dis 2009;68(11):1787–8.
38. de Vries MK, Wolbink GJ, Stapel SO, et al. Decreased clinical response to infliximab in ankylosing spondylitis is correlated with anti-infliximab formation. Ann Rheum Dis 2007;66(9):1252–4.
39. Kneepkens EL, Wei JC, Nurmohamed MT, et al. Immunogenicity, adalimumab levels and clinical response in ankylosing spondylitis patients during 24 weeks of follow-up. Ann Rheum Dis 2013;74(2):396–401.
40. Bartelds GM, Krieckaert CL, Nurmohamed MT, et al. Development of antidrug antibodies against adalimumab and association with disease activity and treatment failure during long-term follow-up. JAMA 201113;305(14):1460–8.
41. Vogelzang EH, Kneepkens EL, Nurmohamed MT, et al. Anti-adalimumab antibodies and adalimumab concentrations in psoriatic arthritis; an association with disease activity at 28 and 52 weeks of follow-up. Ann Rheum Dis 2014;73(12):2178–82.
42. Lie E, Kristensen LE, Forsblad-d'Elia H, et al. The effect of comedication with conventional synthetic disease modifying antirheumatic drugs on TNF inhibitor drug survival in patients with ankylosing spondylitis and undifferentiated spondyloarthritis: results from a nationwide prospective study. Ann Rheum Dis 2015;74(6):970–8.
43. Park W, et al. A randomised, double-blind, multicentre, parallel-group, prospective study comparing the pharmacokinetics, safety, and efficacy of CT-P13 and innovator infliximab in patients with ankylosing spondylitis: the PLANETAS study. Ann Rheum Dis 2013;72(10):1605–12.
44. Barkham N, Keen HI, Coates LC, et al. Clinical and imaging efficacy of infliximab in HLA-B27-positive patients with magnetic resonance imaging-determined early sacroiliitis. Arthritis Rheum 2009; 60(4):946–54.
45. Vastesaeger N, van der Heijde D, Inman RDet al. Predicting the outcome of ankylosing spondylitis therapy. Ann Rheum Dis 2011;70(6):973–81.
46. Braun J, Sieper J. Remission and possible discontinuation of biological therapy in axial spondyloarthritis. Clin Exp Rheumatol 2013 ;31(4 Suppl 78):S33–6.

47. Baraliakos X, et al. Persistent clinical efficacy and safety of infliximab in ankylosing spondylitis after 8 years—early clinical response predicts long-term outcome. Rheumatology (Oxford) 2011;50(9):1690–9.
48. Baraliakos X, et al. Long-term outcome of patients with active ankylosing spondylitis with etanercept-sustained efficacy and safety after seven years. Arthritis Res Ther 2013;15(3):R67.
49. Braun J, et al. The effect of two golimumab doses on radiographic progression in ankylosing spondylitis: results through 4 years of the GO-RAISE trial. Ann Rheum Dis 2014;73(6):1107–13.
50. Baraliakos X, Haibel H, Listing J, Sieper J, Braun J. Continuous long-term anti-TNF therapy does not lead to an increase in the rate of new bone formation over 8 years in patients with ankylosing spondylitis. Ann Rheum Dis 2014;73(4):710–15.
51. Haroon N, Inman RD, Weisman MH, et al. The impact of TNF-inhibitors on radiographic progression in ankylosing spondylitis. Arthritis Rheum 2013;65:2645–54.
52. Antoni C, Krueger GG, de Vlam K, et al. Infliximab improves signs and symptoms of psoriatic arthritis: results of the IMPACT 2 trial. Ann Rheum Dis 2005;64(8):1150–7.
53. Mease PJ, Gladman DD, Ritchlin CT, et al. Adalimumab for the treatment of patients with moderately to severely active psoriatic arthritis: results of a double-blind, randomized, placebo-controlled trial. Arthritis Rheum 2005;52(10):3279–89.
54. Mease PJ, Fleischmann R, Deodhar AA, et al. Effect of certolizumab pegol on signs and symptoms in patients with psoriatic arthritis: 24-week results of a phase 3 double-blind randomised placebo-controlled study (RAPID-PsA). Ann Rheum Dis 2014;73(1):48–55.
55. Kavanaugh A, McInnes IB, Mease PJ, et al. Clinical efficacy, radiographic and safety findings through 2 years of golimumab treatment in patients with active psoriatic arthritis: results from a long-term extension of the randomised, placebo-controlled GO-REVEAL study. Ann Rheum Dis 2013;72(11):1777–85.
56. Kavanaugh A, McInnes IB, Mease P, et al. Clinical efficacy, radiographic and safety findings through 5 years of subcutaneous golimumab treatment in patients with active psoriatic arthritis: results from a long-term extension of a randomised, placebo-controlled trial, the GO-REVEAL study. Ann Rheum Dis 2014;73(9):1689–94.
57. Haroon M, Gallagher P, Fitzgerald O, et al. Diagnostic delay of more than 6 months contributes to poor radiographic and functional outcome in psoriatic arthritis. Ann Rheum Dis 2015;74(6):1045–50.
58. van der Heijde D, Fleischmann R, Wollenhaupt J, et al. Effect of different imputation approaches on the evaluation of radiographic progression in patients with psoriatic arthritis: results of the RAPID-PsA 24-week phase III double-blind randomised placebo-controlled study of certolizumab pegol. Ann Rheum Dis 2014;73(1):233–7.
59. Furst DE, Keystone EC, Braun J, et al. Updated consensus statement on biological agents for the treatment of rheumatic diseases, 2011. Ann Rheum Dis 2012; 71(Suppl 2):i2–45.
60. Kay J, Fleischmann R, Keystone E, et al. Golimumab 3-year safety update: an analysis of pooled data from the long-term extensions of randomised, double-blind, placebo-controlled trials conducted in patients with rheumatoid arthritis, psoriatic arthritis or ankylosing spondylitis. Ann Rheum Dis 2015;74(3):538–46.
61. Kay J, et al. Golimumab 5-year safety: an analysis of pooled data from the long term extensions of rnadomized, double blind, placebo-controlled studies in rheumatoid arthritis, psoriatic arthritis and ankylosing spondylitis. Arthritis Rheum 2014;(Suppl): S198.
62. Tubach F, Salmon D, Ravaud P, et al. Research Axed on Tolerance of Biotherapies Group. Risk of tuberculosis is higher with anti-tumor necrosis factor monoclonal antibody therapy than with soluble tumor necrosis factor receptor therapy: the three-year prospective French Research Axed on Tolerance of Biotherapies registry. Arthritis Rheum 2009;60:1884–94.
63. Coates L, Moverley A, McParland L, et al. Effect of tight control of inflammation in early psoriatic arthritis (TICOPA): a multicentre, open-label, randomised controlled trial. Lancet 2014;383:S36.
64. Smolen JS, Braun J, Dougados M, et al. Treating spondyloarthritis, including ankylosing spondylitis and psoriatic arthritis, to target: recommendations of an international task force. Ann Rheum Dis 2014;73(1):6–16.
65. Ramiro S, van der Heijde D, van Tubergen A, et al. Higher disease activity leads to more structural damage in the spine in ankylosing spondylitis: 12-year longitudinal data from the OASIS cohort. Ann Rheum Dis 2014;73(8):1455–61.
66. Kiltz U, et al. Treatment of ankylosing spondylitis in patients refractory to TNF-inhibition: are there alternatives? Curr Opin Rheumatol 2012;24(3): 252–60.
67. Robinson PC, Brown MA. Genetics of ankylosing spondylitis. Mol Immunol 2014;57(1):2–11.
68. Parkes M, Cortes A, van Heel DA, Brown MA. Genetic insights into common pathways and complex relationships among immune-mediated diseases. Nat Rev Genet 2013;14(9):661–73.
69. Suzuki E, Mellins ED, Gershwin ME, Nestle FO, Adamopoulos IE. The IL-23/IL-17 axis in psoriatic arthritis. Autoimmun Rev 2014;13(4–5):496–502.
70. Miossec P, Korn T, Kuchroo VK. Interleukin-17 and type 17 helper T cells. N Engl J Med 2009;361:888–98.
71. Sherlock JP, Joyce-Shaikh B, Turner SP, et al. IL-23 induces spondyloarthropathy by acting on ROR-γt+ CD3+CD4–CD8– entheseal resident T cells. Nat Med 2012;18:1069–76.
72. Korn T, Bettelli E, Oukka M, Kuchroo VK. IL-17 and Th17 cells. Annu Rev Immunol 2009;27:485–517.
73. Shen H, Goodall JC, Hill Gaston JS. Frequency and phenotype of peripheral blood Th17 cells in ankylosing spondylitis and rheumatoid arthritis. Arthritis Rheum 2009;60:1647–56.
74. Kenna TJ, Davidson SI, Duan R, et al. Enrichment of circulating interleukin-17-secreting interleukin-23 receptor-positive γ/δ T cells in patients with active ankylosing spondylitis. Arthritis Rheum 2012;64:1420–9.
75. Bowness P, Ridley A, Shaw J, et al. Th17 cells expressing KIR3DL2+ and responsive to HLA-B27 homodimers are increased in ankylosing spondylitis. J Immunol 2011;186:2672–80.
76. Zeng L, Lindstrom MJ, Smith JA. Ankylosing spondylitis macrophage production of higher levels of interleukin-23 in response to lipopolysaccharide without induction of a significant unfolded protein response. Arthritis Rheum 2011;63:3807–17.
77. Appel H, Maier R, Wu P, et al. Analysis of IL-17(+) cells in facet joints of patients with spondyloarthritis suggests that the innate immune pathway might be of greater relevance than the Th17-mediated adaptive immune response. Arthritis Res Ther 2011;13:R95.
78. Appel H, Maier R, Bleil J, et al. In situ analysis of interleukin-23- and interleukin-12-positive cells in the spine of patients with ankylosing spondylitis. Arthritis Rheum 2013;65(6):1522–9.
79. Noordenbos T, Yeremenko N, Gofita I, et al. Interleukin-17-positive mast cells contribute to synovial inflammation in spondylarthritis. Arthritis Rheum 2012;64:99–109.
80. Krueger GG, Langley RG, Leonardi C, et al. A human interleukin-12/23 monoclonal antibody for the treatment of psoriasis. N Engl J Med 2007;356(6):580–92.
81. Leonardi CL, Kimball AB, Papp KA, et al. Efficacy and safety of ustekinumab, a human interleukin-12/23 monoclonal antibody, in patients with psoriasis: 76-week results from a randomised, double-blind, placebo-controlled trial (PHOENIX 1). Lancet 2008;371(9625):1665–74.
82. Papp KA, Langley RG, Lebwohl M, et al. Efficacy and safety of ustekinumab, a human interleukin-12/23 monoclonal antibody, in patients with psoriasis: 52-week results from a randomised, double-blind, placebo-controlled trial (PHOENIX 2). Lancet 2008;371(9625):1675–84.
83. Griffiths CE, Strober BE, van de Kerkhof P, et al. Comparison of ustekinumab and etanercept for moderate-to-severe psoriasis. N Engl J Med 2010;362(2):118–28.

84. Gottlieb A, Menter A, Mendelsohn A, et al. Ustekinumab, a human interleukin 12/23 monoclonal antibody, for psoriatic arthritis: randomised, double-blind, placebo-controlled, crossover trial. Lancet 2009;373(9664):633–40.
85. McInnes IB, Kavanaugh A, Gottlieb AB, et al. Efficacy and safety of ustekinumab in patients with active psoriatic arthritis: 1 year results of the phase 3, multicentre, double-blind, placebo-controlled PSUMMIT 1 trial. Lancet 2013;382(9894):780–9.
86. Ritchlin C, Rahman P, Kavanaugh A, et al. Efficacy and safety of the anti-IL-12/23 p40 monoclonal antibody, ustekinumab, in patients with active psoriatic arthritis despite conventional non-biological and biological anti-tumour necrosis factor therapy: 6-month and 1-year results of the phase 3, multicentre, double-blind, placebo-controlled, randomised PSUMMIT 2 trial. Ann Rheum Dis 2014;73(6):990–9.
87. Kavanaugh A, Ritchlin C, Rahman P, et al. Ustekinumab, an anti-IL-12/23 p40 monoclonal antibody, inhibits radiographic progression in patients with active psoriatic arthritis: results of an integrated analysis of radiographic data from the phase 3, multicentre, randomised, double-blind, placebo-controlled PSUMMIT-1 and PSUMMIT-2 trials. Ann Rheum Dis 2014;73(6):1000–6.
88. Poddubnyy D, Hermann KG, Callhoff J, Listing J, Sieper J. Ustekinumab for the treatment of patients with active ankylosing spondylitis: results of a 28-week, prospective, open-label, proof-of-concept study (TOPAS). Ann Rheum Dis 2014;73(5):817–23.
89. Sandborn WJ, Gasink C, Gao LL, et al. Ustekinumab induction and maintenance therapy in refractory Crohn's disease. N Engl J Med 2012;367(16):1519–28.
90. Sandborn WJ, Feagan BG, Fedorak RN, et al. A randomized trial of ustekinumab, a human interleukin-12/23 monoclonal antibody, in patients with moderate-to-severe Crohn's disease. Gastroenterology 2008;135(4):1130–41.
91. Sofen H, Smith S, Matheson RT, et al. Guselkumab (an IL-23-specific mAb) demonstrates clinical and molecular response in patients with moderate-to-severe psoriasis. J Allergy Clin Immunol 2014;133(4):1032–40.
92. Fitzgerald O, Winchester R. Editorial: emerging evidence for critical involvement of the interleukin-17 pathway in both psoriasis and psoriatic arthritis. Arthritis Rheumatol 2014;66(5):1077–80.
93. Patel DD, Lee DM, Kolbinger F, Antoni C. Effect of IL-17A blockade with secukinumab in autoimmune diseases. Ann Rheum Dis 2013;72(Suppl 2):ii116–23.
94. Hueber W, Sands BE, Lewitzky S, et al. Secukinumab, a human anti-IL-17A monoclonal antibody, for moderate to severe Crohn's disease: unexpected results of a randomised, double-blind placebo-controlled trial. Gut 2012;61(12):1693–700.
95. Dick AD, Tugal-Tutkun I, Foster S, et al. Secukinumab in the treatment of noninfectious uveitis: results of three randomized, controlled clinical trials. Ophthalmology 2013;120(4):777–87.
96. Rich P, Sigurgeirsson B, Thaci D, et al. Secukinumab induction and maintenance therapy in moderate-to-severe plaque psoriasis: a randomized, double-blind, placebo-controlled, phase II regimen-finding study. Br J Dermatol 2013;168:402–11.
97. Papp KA, Langley RG, Sigurgeirsson B, et al. Efficacy and safety of secukinumab in the treatment of moderate-to-severe plaque psoriasis: a randomized, double-blind, placebo-controlled phase II dose-ranging study. Br J Dermatol 2013;168(2):412–21.
98. Langley RG, Elewski BE, Lebwohl M, et al. Secukinumab in plaque psoriasis—results of two phase 3 trials. N Engl J Med 2014;371(4):326–38.
99. McInnes IB, Sieper J, Braun J, et al. Efficacy and safety of secukinumab, a fully human anti-interleukin-17A monoclonal antibody, in patients with moderate-to-severe psoriatic arthritis: a 24-week, randomised, double-blind, placebo-controlled, phase II proof-of-concept trial. Ann Rheum Dis 2014;73(2):349–56.
100. Strand V, Mease PJ, McInne IB, et al. Secukinumab, an interleukin-17A monoclonal antibody, improves physical function, quality of life and work productivity in patients with active psoriatic arthritis: results from a phase 3, randomized, controlled. Arthritis Rheum 2014;(Suppl):S240–1.
101. Baeten D, Baraliakos X, Braun J, et al. Anti-interleukin-17A monoclonal antibody secukinumab in treatment of ankylosing spondylitis: a randomised, double-blind, placebo-controlled trial. Lancet 2013;382(9906):1705–13.
102. Baeten DL, et al. Secukinumab, a monoclonal antibody to interleukin-17A, significantly improves signs and symptoms of active ankylosing spondylitis: results of a 52 week phase 3, randomized, placebo-controlled trial with intravenous loading and subcutaneous maintenance dosing. Arthritis Rheum 2014;(Suppl): S360.
103. Sieper J, et al. Secukinumab, a monoclonal antibody to interleukin-17A, significantly improves signs and symptoms of active ankylosing spondylitis: results of a phase 3, randomized, placebo-controlled trial with subcutaneous loading and maintenance dosing. Arthritis Rheum 2014;(Suppl):S232.
104. Papp KA, Leonardi C, Menter A, et al. Brodalumab, an anti-interleukin-17-receptor antibody for psoriasis. N Engl J Med 2012;366(13):1181–9.
105. Mease PJ, Genovese MC, Greenwald MW, et al. Brodalumab, an anti-IL17RA monoclonal antibody, in psoriatic arthritis. N Engl J Med 2014;370(24):2295–306.
106. Leonardi C, Matheson R, Zachariae C, et al. Anti-interleukin-17 monoclonal antibody ixekizumab in chronic plaque psoriasis. N Engl J Med 2012;366(13):1190–9.
107. Genovese MC, et al. Clinical response in subjects with psoriatic arthritis following one year treatment with brodalumab, an anti-interleukin-17 receptor antobody. Arthritis Rheum 2014;(Suppl):S687.
108. van der Paardt M, van der Horst-Bruinsma IE, Crusius JBA, et al. Interleukin-1 beta and interleukin-1 receptor antagonist gene polymorphisms in the susceptibility to ankylosing spondylitis. Rheumatology 2002;41:1419–23.
109. Tan AL, Marzo-Ortega H, O'Connor P, Fraser A, Emery P, McGonagle D. Efficacy of anakinra in active ankylosing spondylitis: a clinical and magnetic resonance imaging study. Ann Rheum Dis 2004;63(9):1041–5.
110. Bennett AN, Tan AL, Coates LC, Emery P, Marzo-Ortega H, McGonagle D. Sustained response to anakinra in ankylosing spondylitis. Rheumatology (Oxford) 2008;47(2):223–4.
111. Haibel H, Rudwaleit M, Listing J, Sieper J. Open label trial of anakinra in active ankylosing spondylitis over 24 weeks. Ann Rheum Dis 2005;64(2):296–8.
112. Jung N, Hellmann M, Hoheisel R, et al. An open-label pilot study of the efficacy and safety of anakinra in patients with psoriatic arthritis refractory to or intolerant of methotrexate (MTX). Clin Rheumatol 2010;29(10):1169–73.
113. Song IH, Heldmann F, Rudwaleit M, et al. Different response to rituximab in tumor necrosis factor blocker-naive patients with active ankylosing spondylitis and in patients in whom tumor necrosis factor blockers have failed: a twenty-four-week clinical trial. Arthritis Rheum 2010;62(5):1290–7.
114. Song IH, Heldmann F, Rudwaleit M, et al. One-year follow-up of ankylosing spondylitis patients responding to rituximab treatment and re-treated in case of a flare. Ann Rheum Dis 2013;72(2):305–6.
115. Wendling D, Dougados M, Berenbaum F, et al. Rituximab treatment for spondyloarthritis. A nationwide series: data from the AIR registry of the French Society of Rheumatology. J Rheumatol 2012;39(12):2327–31.
116. Jimenez-Boj E, Stamm TA, Sadlonova M, et al. Rituximab in psoriatic arthritis: an exploratory evaluation. Ann Rheum Dis 2012;71(11):1868–71.
117. Song IH, Heldmann F, Rudwaleit M, et al. Treatment of active ankylosing spondylitis with abatacept: an open-label, 24-week pilot study. Ann Rheum Dis 2011;70:1108–10.
118. Mease P, Genovese MC, Gladstein G, et al. Abatacept in the treatment of patients with psoriatic arthritis: results of a six-month, multicenter, randomized, double-blind, placebo-controlled, phase II trial. Arthritis Rheum 2011;63(4):939–48.

119. Henes JC, Horger M, Guenaydin I, Kanz L, Koetter I. Mixed response to tocilizumab for ankylosing spondylitis. Ann Rheum Dis 2010;69(12):2217–18.
120. Sieper J, Porter-Brown B, Thompson L, Harari O, Dougados M. Assessment of short-term symptomatic efficacy of tocilizumab in ankylosing spondylitis: results of randomised, placebo-controlled trials. Ann Rheum Dis 2014;73:95–100.
121. Sieper J, Braun J, Kay J, et al. Sarilumab for the treatment of ankylosing spondylitis: results of a phase II, randomised, double-blind, placebo-controlled study (ALIGN). Ann Rheum Dis 2015;74(6):1051–7 .
122. Hughes M, Chinoy H. Successful use of tocilizumab in a patient with psoriatic arthritis. Rheumatology (Oxford) 2013;52(9):1728–9.
123. Pathan E, Abraham S, Van Rossen E, et al. Efficacy and safety of apremilast, an oral phosphodiesterase 4 inhibitor, in ankylosing spondylitis. Ann Rheum Dis 2013;72(9):1475–80.
124. Wells A, et al. A phase 3 randomized, controlled trial of apremilast, an oral phosphodiestrease 4 inhibitor, for treatment of psoriatic arthritis: long-term (52 week) improvements in physical function. Arthritis Rheum 2014;(Suppl): S264.
125. Kavanaugh A, et al. Apremilast, an oral phosphodiestrease 4 inhibitor, is associated with long-term (52 week)improvement in measures of disease activity in patients with psoriatic arthritis: results from 3 phase 3 randomized, controlled trials. Arthritis Rheum 2014;(Suppl):S239.

CHAPTER 23

Treatment: spinal surgery

Heinrich Boehm and Y. Raja Rampersaud

Introduction

Despite remarkable progress in understanding the pathological processes and in alleviating symptoms by TNFα blocking medication, the mechanism that converts flexible tissue into bone still cannot be completely prevented or reversed. In axSpA, components of motion segments, such as zygoapophyseal joints, intervertebral discs, and spinal ligaments, can ossify in varying sequence, extent, and location between the ilium and the occiput, resulting in AS. Throughout this process, the spinal column is vulnerable to kyphotic deformity due to the inescapable influence of gravity, body weight, and muscle action and a preponderance of life's flexion-based activities. Areas with low fusion tendency, such as the atlanto-axial joints and post-traumatically weakened spots of a formerly ankylosed vertebral block (Andersson's lesion), can endanger the patient's spinal cord, by instability, dislocation, and compression. Whereas acute trauma rarely escapes adequate attention, progressive kyphosis after minor trauma or simple repetitive stresses often are diagnosed late. Conservative treatment options are lacking and surgical consideration in these advanced disease states is required.

Regardless of indication, surgery in the AS patient is a difficult decision for the patient, rheumatologist and surgeon, that requires multidisciplinary consideration: effective long-term medication with TNFα blockers needs to be discontinued preoperatively (1), LFN washed out, and long-term anticoagulant therapy for cardiovascular comorbidities may require bridging.

For an individual with AS whose oxygen exchange is hindered by lack of intercostal breathing and whose immunological system might be hampered by steroids or biologics, conventional open surgery for the posterior spine, and possibly additional open thoracotomy from the front, are associated with high risk of morbidity and the possibility of mortality. However, now less invasive access techniques are evolving that do allow and extend surgical options, even for the severely endangered and elderly AS patients.

Surgical treatment is electively indicated for spinal deformity when a horizontal axis of vision can only be achieved by compensatory flexion of the knees while the hip joints are maximally extended. A patient with global kyphotic deformity in AS is endangered twice: due to the impaired range of vision, he/she is more prone to accidents, and, in case of an impact, his/her spine is much more susceptible to fracture. Trauma and its sequelae affect a stiff bamboo spine much more than a normal spine with shock-absorbing articulations and thus represents an important and often urgent indication for surgery. Another indication is intractable mechanical pain and danger of neurological deficit arising from incompletely fused, secondarily unstable motion segments.

Despite artificial discs and 'non-fusion techniques', until now there has been no surgical option to restore mobility within the spinal column of AS patients. In some cases, consideration is being given to whether localized minimally invasive surgical intervention/correction combined with anti-TNFα agents is effective in at least delaying disease and/or deformity progression in adjacent segments. Although not proven, the rationale here would be to reduce mechanical pain and overload on compensatory regions and the rest of the mobile spine (Fig. 23.1).

In the typical patient, however, all surgical efforts aim at restoring the decompensated posture, eradicating the painful instability of a formerly fused spine, and decompressing the spinal cord and roots for associated neurological dysfunction.

Analysis of the deformity

In addition to true thoracic hyperkyphosis, loss of lumbar lordosis as well as short-curved angulations at the cervico-thoracic and thoraco-lumbar junctions are other reasons for decompensation of posture in an AS patient (Fig. 23.2). As long as hip joints can be overextended, global kyphosis can be compensated to some extent by rotation of the pelvis (Fig. 23.2C). Whenever a long-standing painless mild deformity decompensates, special attention should be paid to the hip joints.

Should arthritis and flexion contracture of one or both hips be found, this should be treated first by joint replacement (Fig. 23.3). Often this suffices to restore sagittal balance; if not, spinal surgery should be considered.

In principle, surgery aims at correcting at the site of deformity by cutting the bony bridges of malaligned vertebrae, restoring anatomy, and securing it by metallic implants until new bone formation yields a biological long-term solution. Realignment can be accomplished focally (i.e. at a single level) in post-traumatic kyphosis and Andersson's lesions; however, in long-curved kyphosis with slight deformity at each individual level, correction of each malfused segment is impractical. Thus the main goal of the analysis of the deformity is surgical planning in order to identify which type of compensatory localized overcorrection, and at which particular spinal area(s), will result in the optimal realignment. The question therefore should not be whether one osteotomy type is better than another, but rather the optimal balance between safety, immediate restoration of posture, and long-term result. Sometimes different osteotomy types need to be combined (Figs 23.4 and 23.5). In addition, attention must be paid to lack of residual motion, particularly at the occipito-cervical junction, to ensure that realignment does not result in a non-functional, fixed upward gaze.

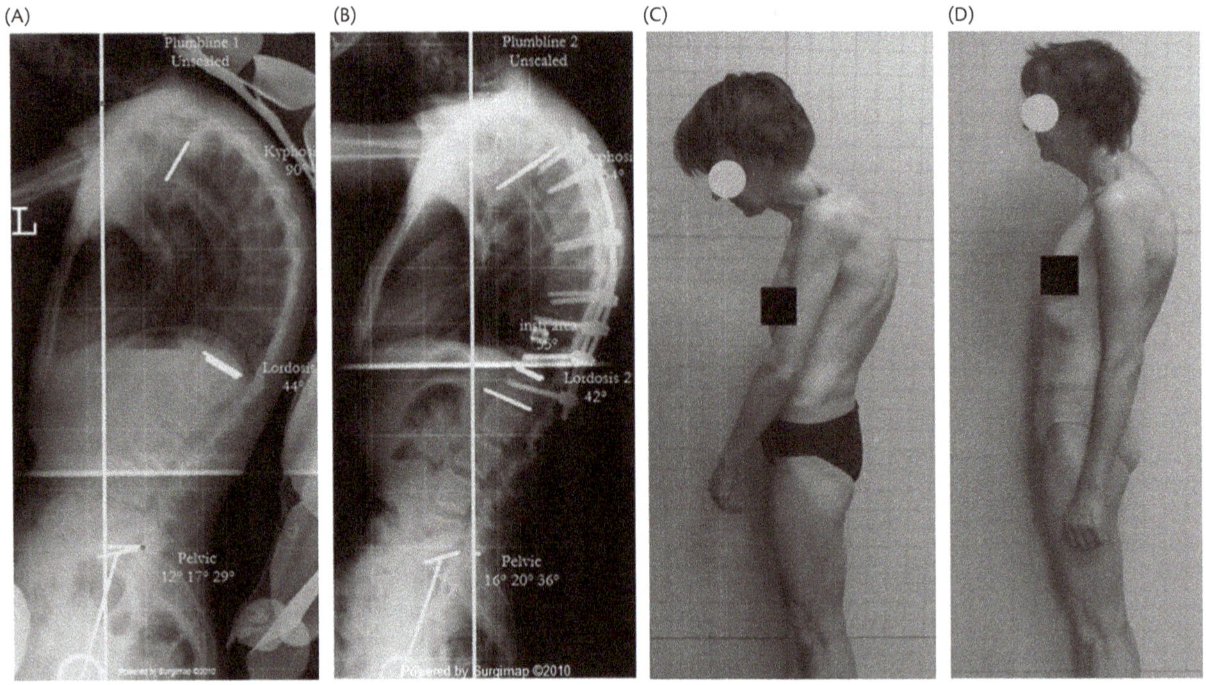

Fig. 23.1 Preserving motion in AS. Improving load distribution in the still-mobile cervical and lumbar spine by minimally invasive correction of the hyperkyphotic thoracic spine. Before surgery, the still-mobile cervical and lumbar spine is compensating for the thoracic hyperkyphosis of 90 degrees by extension (A, C) to the maximum. At 4 years postoperatively (B, D), the correction to 54 degrees in the thoracic kyphosis could be maintained. The patient reports markedly reduced pain in the neck and lumbar spine, while the range of motion is increased.

Important clinical parameters

For preoperative evaluation as well as long-term postoperative follow-up, a few simple measurements should be routinely performed. The position of the head relative to the body is documented as the distance from occiput to the wall in a patient standing maximally erect at a wall (Fig. 23.3A, e). In case of residual mobility the measurements should be performed with the head midway between the flexion–extension range. The axis of vision is reflected by the chin–brow angle (Fig. 23.3A, fgh). We feel it easier to use the 'AS spectacles' (Fig. 23.3A, a): the arms of the frame are extended, telescoping beyond the ears, and angulated 90 degrees. The angle bcd in Fig. 23.3B to the plumb-line represents the amount of deviation from horizontal vision and thus the amount to be corrected. When used during the routine lateral standing X-ray, the film of the truncal spine stores the information of the axis of vison without exposing the head.

Whenever an additional hip component in addition to spinal deformity is suspected, video documentation from the lateral side

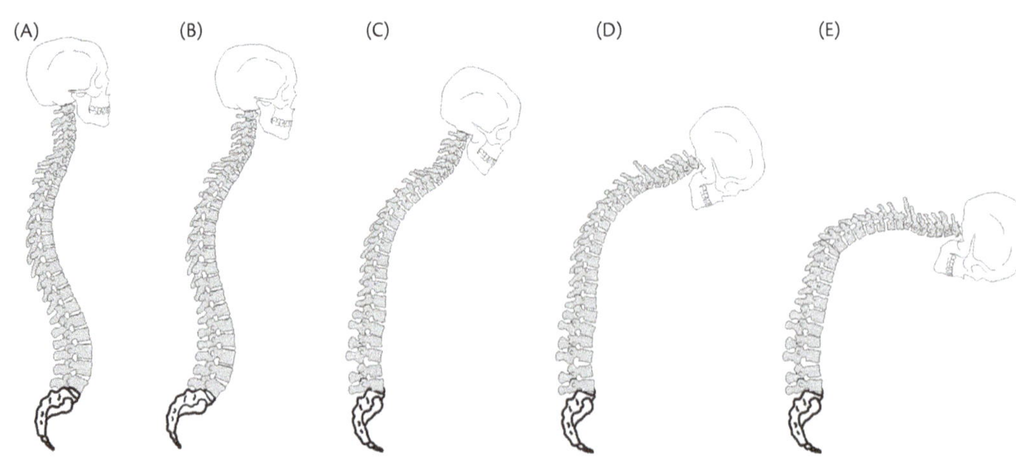

Fig. 23.2 Types of deformity in axSpA. (A) Ankylosis in normal-anatomic posture. (B) Normal anatomic ankylosis of the spinal column, but the trunk is rotated forward due to hip problems (flexion contracture inducing pelvic tilt of 20 degrees). The fused spinal column cannot compensate and thus is rotated together with the pelvis. (C) Hip joints without disease allowing hyperextension and retroversion of the pelvis. In spite of 20-degree pelvic retroversion, loss of lumbar lordosis enforces imbalance of the trunk. (D) Additional kyphosis of the cervical spine adds to the severity of deformity. (E) Severe global kyphosis due to addition of 'true' hyperkyphosis of the thoracic spine.

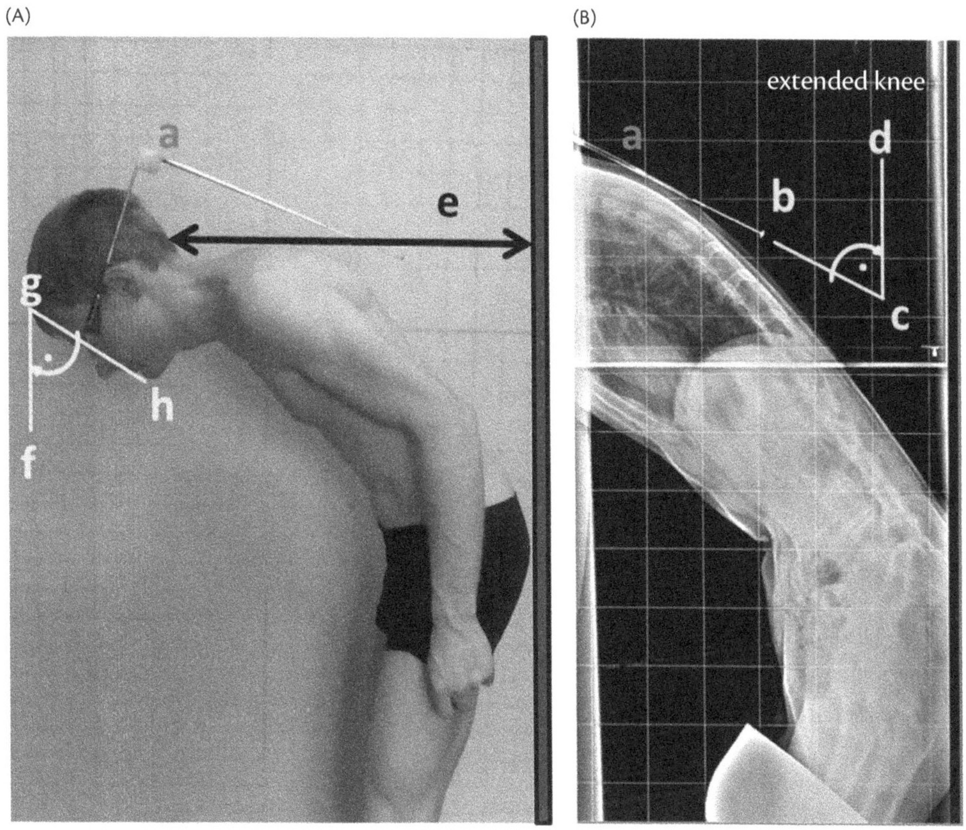

Fig. 23.3 (See colour plate section). Documentation of deranged posture clinically on standing photograph (A) and lateral X-ray (B). 'AS-spectacles', angulated and telescoping extensions on a spectacles frame, (a) allow documentation and measurement of visual axis without X-ray exposure of the head. On standing X-ray, the angle bcd between extension of the frame and the plumb-line indicates how many degrees are lost from horizontal vision. If performed standing with knees and hips extended maximally, one lateral X-ray of the trunk stores all information on global sagittal imbalance. In the case discussed, there is no thoracic hyperkyphosis and deformity derives exclusively from loss of lumbar lordosis and hip joints fused in flexion. Occiput–wall distance (e) is a measure of sagittal trunk imbalance. Chin–brow-angle fgh similar to the AS-spectacles indicates position of head and visual axis, respectively.

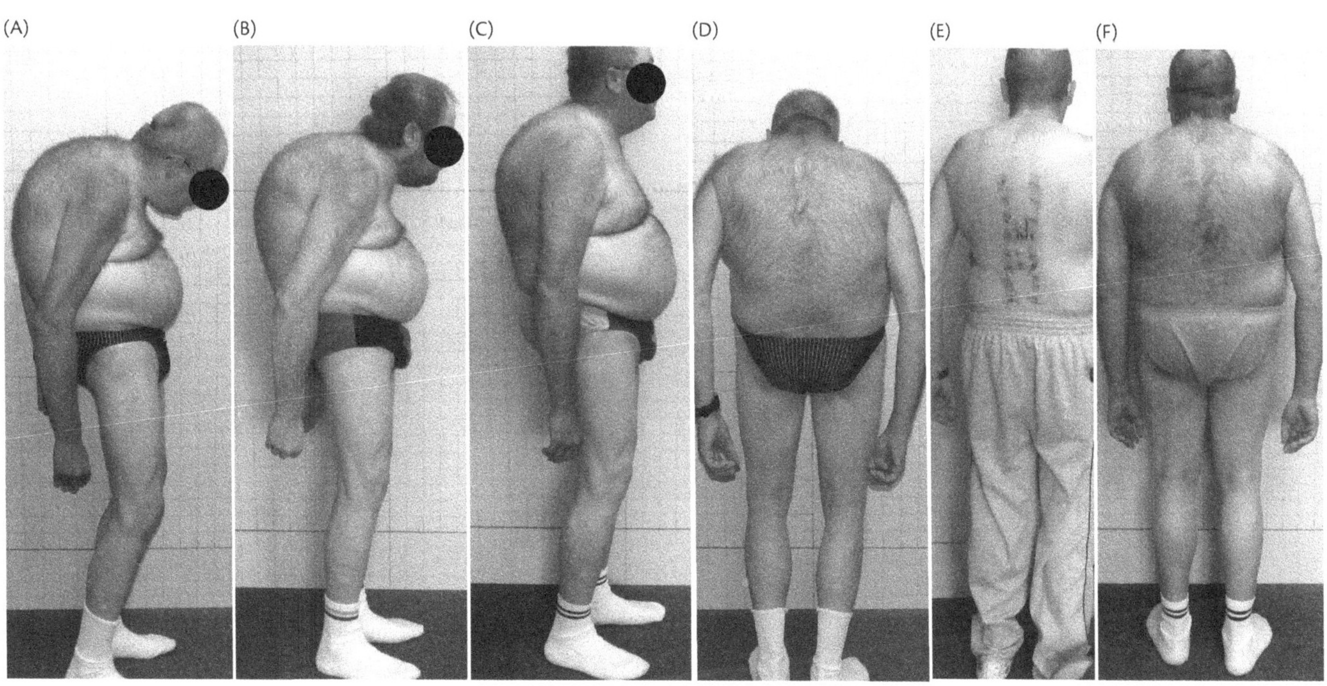

Fig. 23.4 (A) A male, aged 37 years old, with complete ankylosis of all spine segments in global kyphosis, hips overextendable. Chin on chest deformity does not allow positioning of the patient for thoraco-lumbar surgery. (B) Cervico-thoracic extension osteotomy first. (C) Three years after thoraco-lumbar double osteotomy Th11/12 and L1–L2. (D) Same patient preoperatively viewed from posterior. (E) Patient immediately after thoraco-lumbar miDVO-R. Bilateral horizontal stab incisions depict entrance points of fixation screws and rods. Two 3-cm-long midline incisions represent the approach for the two posterior microscope-assisted osteotomies; a 4-cm incision at the left side stems from the thoracoscopic anterior osteotomies and cage-assisted fusions. (F) No loss of correction at 3 years postoperatively. Erector muscles are maintained fully through minimally invasive access technique.

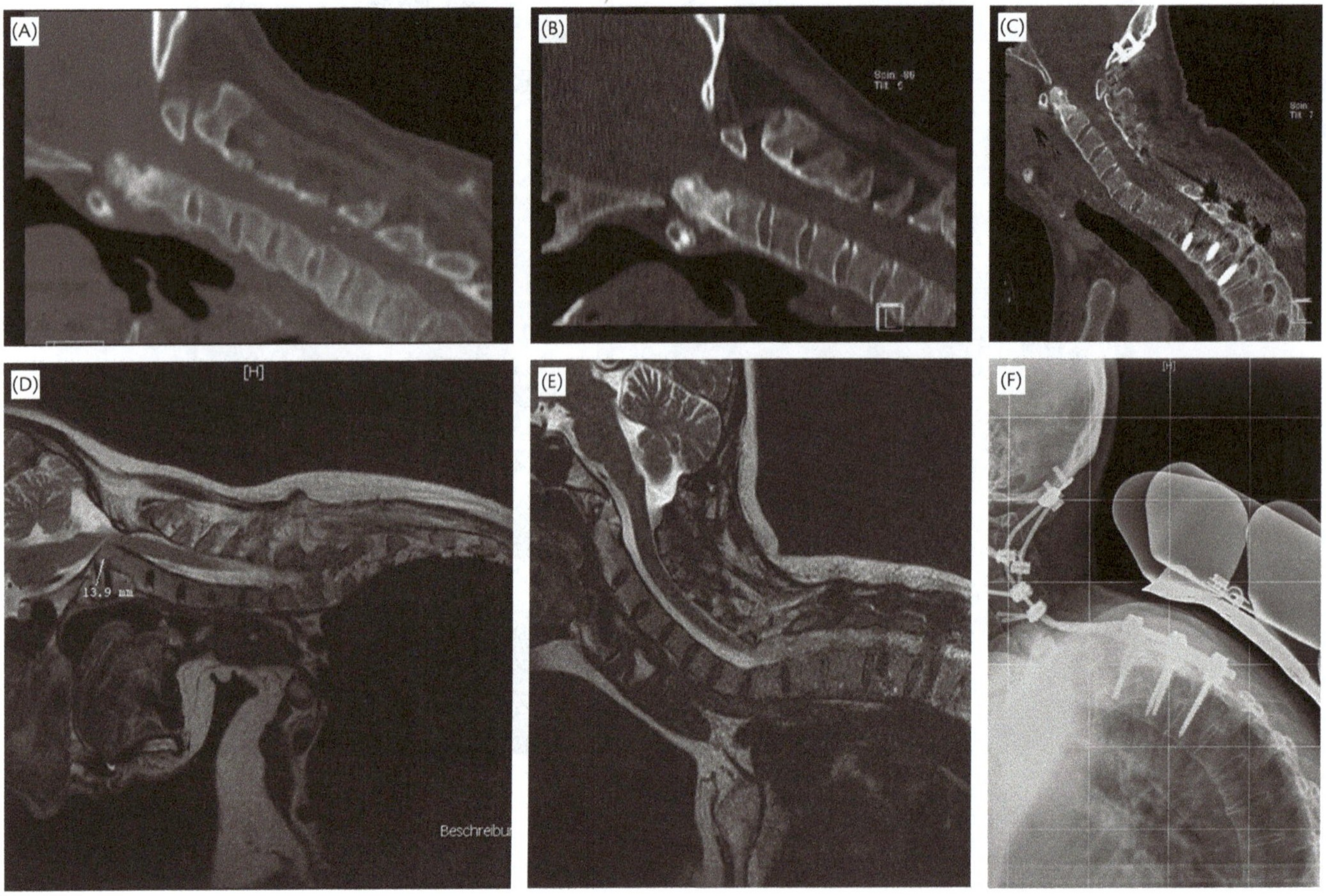

Fig. 23.5 Upper row: atlanto-axial instability in AS. Within 1 year during rapid increase of kyphosis in cervico-thoracic region, the only remaining mobile segment C1–C2 progressed from translational instability (A) to cranial settling (B). The tip of the odontoid passes posteriorly in relation to the clivus. Concomitantly, the arc of C1 moves caudally in relation to the axis. (C) After operative reduction and stabilization, relative position of odontoid, anterior arc of C1, and clivus is normalized. In the same sitting, cervico-thoracic kyphosis was corrected. Lower row: another patient, showing influence of deformity and correction on cervical viscera. (D) Chin on chest deformity with head in horizontal position and atlanto-axial dislocation plus compression of medulla. (E) T2W MRI after surgery: medulla and brain stem are indirectly decompressed by reduction, CSF space is restored, and after extension osteotomy at C7 the chin–sternum relation is normalized. (F) Lateral X-ray, with posterior occipito-thoracic instrumentation outlining the restored skeletal contour.

during walking reveals the 'functional amount of kyphosis', which can exceed to some extend the values of standing with extended knees and hips. Should angular deformity be present, sequelae of spinal stenosis such as myelopathy and claudication have to be ruled out.

Diagnostic imaging

Conventional X-ray (CR)

A conventional standing X-ray of the thoracic and lumbar spine ('whole spine') taken in a standardized manner with both arms supported is the most important imaging modality for preoperative evaluation and follow-up. To avoid unnecessary X-ray exposure and to allow judgement of global posture, both proximal femurs and the cervico-thoracic junction should be visible on a single image.

Magnetic resonance imaging

CRs lack sufficient visualization of transitional zones to the occiput, chest cage, and sacrum. A preoperative MRI fills that gap and allows depiction of anomalies in bone and soft tissue, namely post-traumatic alterations, stenosis, myelopathy, syringomyelia, and the 'empty dura' of the AS-associated cauda equina syndrome (Fig. 23.6).

Peridiscal destruction typical in Andersson's lesions can pose problems in differential diagnosis to pyogenic spondylitis and tumours (see section 'Management of fractures'). In those cases, additional T1 sequences without and with contrast are valuable (2). Whenever a significant change does occur in the type or level of long-standing 'inflammatory pain', or when kyphosis starts to progress again rapidly, osteoporotic fractures should be ruled out by adding a turbo inversion recovery magnitude (TIRM) sequence to the MR evaluations (3). Long before CR or CT allows diagnosis, the oedema in the MRI can be diagnostic and prevent the patient and the physician from delayed or wrong treatment.

Preceding surgery to the upper cervical spine, MR angiography allows sufficient visualization of the vertebral arteries and their topographic relations to atlas, axis, or dura.

MRI is indispensable in cases of postoperative neurological deterioration due to its ability to depict haematoma, dural lesions, alterations of the spinal cord, and infections (4).

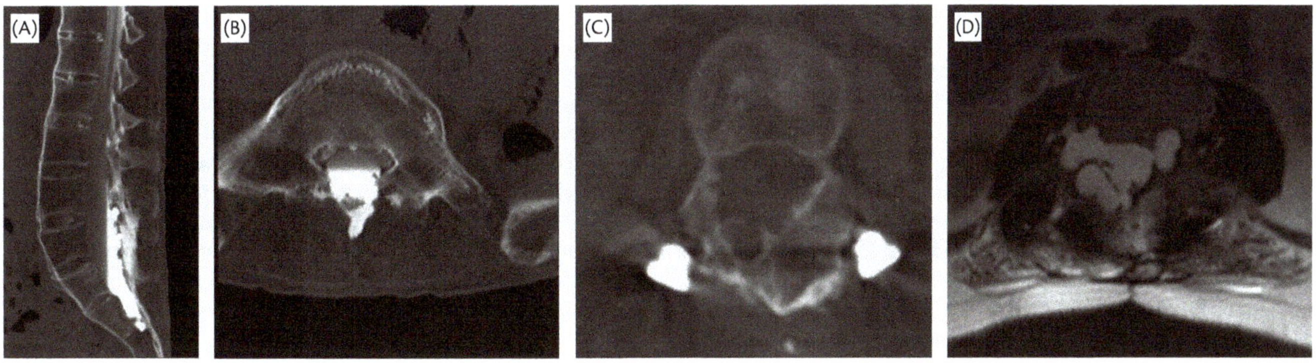

Fig. 23.6 (A) Cauda equina syndrome after long-standing SpA in a 69-year-old male whose spine is ankylosed without deformity, with no previous surgery and progressive loss of sphincter control and walking ability. (B) This post-myelogram CT scan of the same patient, in supine position, shows fluid level and contrast dye extruding into laminae, with impression of 'empty dura', since all fascicles adhere to the inner aspect of dura. (C) Axial CT scan of a male aged 60 years who experienced loss of muscle power of the right leg, with difficulty in walking, commencing 10 years after uneventful thoraco-lumbar extension osteotomy. (D) MRI of a 44-year-old female, 13 years after lumbar osteotomy, experiencing difficulty in walking and bladder control for the last 2 years.

Computed tomography

A computer tomogram yields a much higher spatial resolution of bone than MRI. It is valuable to answer specific questions regarding stenosis and post-traumatic changes of the spinal column, and indispensable in patients who cannot have MRI (e.g. those on cardiac defibrillators). For routine preoperative assessment, CT imaging is not necessary, unless there is uncertainty regarding occipito-cervical ankylosis.

Methods: options and planning of correction

General aspects

The spinal cord is very susceptible to distraction and compression. All manoeuvres on the supporting bone therefore should minimize changes in length and translation of the canal. This is best achieved when the axis of rotation of the osteotomized column is situated near the centre of the spinal canal. Correction of a kyphosis under these specifications always requires surgical creation of a gap posterior to the cord by resection of bony elements such as lamina, ossified joints, spinal process, and sometimes pedicles. The length of this gap determines the amount of achievable correction when closed (5).

If the disc space at the level of the gap can open, such as in cases with exclusively posterior ossification, the anterior column allows for an indirect correction (Fig. 23.7C, D). In a bamboo spine, however, forceful opening of the syndesmophytic bridges could result in uncontrolled anterior distraction and/or translation effects. When required, direct operative division of the anterior column, be it from an approach from the back or the front, is the better and safer option.

The location of the deformity determines the best site for correction. In those cases where more than one region requires osteotomy and where it is not possible to perform all in one anaesthesia, it is advisable to work from the bottom to the top. This strategy presents the additional option of lumbar overcorrection in order to compensate a more cranial hyperkyphosis, avoiding the specific risks of following the opposite route (6). Whenever contractures of a hip are diagnosed, those should be treated first.

The more near the pelvis a site of correction is situated, the bigger is the lever arm of the cranial spine and the effect of backward rotation of the trunk. However, in the case of a true thoracic hyperkyphosis, the cosmetic effect remains unsatisfactory, since a rotated hump still appears as a hump (Fig. 23.4C). Due to anatomical barriers and/or higher risk, deformities in the mid-cervical region, the high thoracic region (Fig. 23.4A–C), and in the lumbar spine

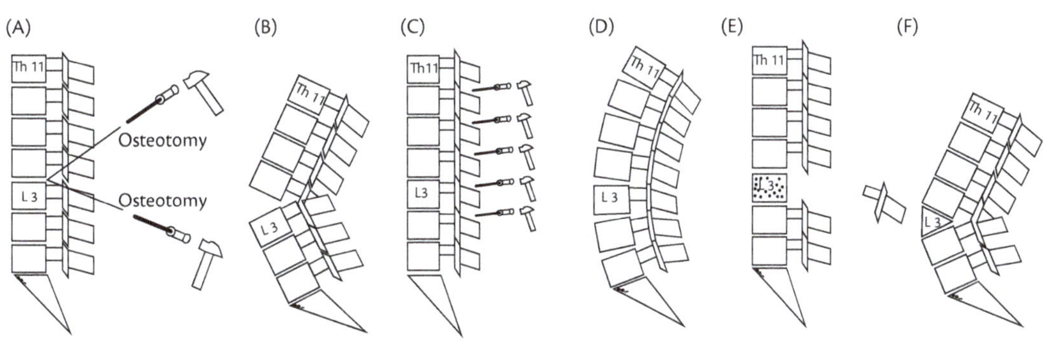

Fig. 23.7 Standard types of spinal osteotomies. (A) Bone resection in SPO. (B) The resulting situation after osteoclasis of anterior bony bridgings is an open wedge osteotomy. (E) Principle of pedicle subtraction osteotomy (PSO). After removal of lamina and pedicles as well as parts of the posterior wall, the correction is possible without direct division of anterior structures. (F) Anterior-based wedge vertebra as a result of successful correction: closing wedge osteotomy. (C) Between these techniques is the Zielke method, where up to five V-shaped narrow SPOs are performed, hoping that those close either by gaping of not yet fused discs, as in (D), or by compression of the osteopenic posterior vertebral body.

the AS-specific adhesions of cauda equina (see section 'The cauda equine syndrome in spondyloarthritis') can necessitate a deviation from the rule regarding the optimal location of the osteotomy.

In the cranio-cervical area, the C1–C2 segment has the lowest potential for ossification of all motion segments of an AS spine. Unfortunately, the biomechanical overload to the last remaining mobile segment adds to the increased stresses of a sagittally imbalanced head (Fig. 23.5A, B). Anterior dislocation of the atlas versus the axis with concomitant compression of the medulla oblongata can occur and endanger the patient vitally (Fig. 23.5D). The respiratory and vasomotor centres that are located in that area are in danger even more than, for example, in an RA patient with the same mechanical problem, since the latter usually has shock-absorbing mobile segments left.

In early stages and pure instability, a posterior-only reduction and fusion from occiput to the mid-cervical spine is sufficient. In neglected cases, when bony anterior bridges are blocking correction and clinical examination or MRI confirms medullar compression and signal change, an anterior (i.e. trans-oral) release/decompression is necessary.

In the thoracic and lumbar spine, due to the long lever arm of a rigid spine and inactivity-ridden erector muscles, the corrected spinal column requires a very stable fixation until bony healing has taken place. Since the mechanical quality of bone in AS is reduced, the stabilizing forces need to be distributed on at least six anchoring points at either side of the osteotomy. In conventional open surgery this requires an incision from the mid-thoracic region to the sacrum and deflection of the paraspinal muscles at the whole length, 3 cm from the midline to both sides. The resulting wound adds to the invasivity of the lamina resection necessary for osteotomy. Consequently, minimal access surgery techniques, if they are as safe as conventional methods and if as effective in respect of the correcting potential, would be of substantial advantage.

Types of osteotomy

Regardless of the type of approach, the main goal of surgery is, first, to safely resect bony structures around the spinal cord; second, to change the position of the adjacent vertebral column partners; third, to fix the readapted vertebrae mechanically stable by means of implants, and—finally and most importantly—to enable new rapid bone formation to biologically stabilize and maintain the corrected position long term. Basically, there are four concepts (7): the Smith-Petersen osteotomy (SPO) (8), pedicle subtraction osteotomy (PSO) (9), dorsal lordosating spondylodesis (DLS), and the concept of posterior plus anterior direct osteotomies and reconstruction of the bony defect by minimally invasive approach techniques (see section 'Minimally invasive dorso-ventral osteotomy and reconstruction (miDVO-R)').

Smith-Petersen osteotomy

The SPO, described in 1945 (8), aims at creating an anterior opening wedge (Fig. 23.7). The spinous process and lamina are resected in an angular manner (Fig. 23.7B). By extension manoeuvres of the spine, closure of the gap in the posterior column is enforced. The correction, pivoting on the area of the posterior wall, then occurs by rupture of structures of the anterior column—either by opening of the persisting or former disc space or by creating an extension fracture of the vertebral body. Besides uncontrolled osteoclasis effects, mechanical instability and dislocation, a main risk of this osteotomy is impingement of the exiting nerve roots between the pedicles. This is why not more than 30–35 degrees of correction can be reached by one SPO.

In the true bamboo spine, a safe and controlled correction via SPO could only be achieved by an additional surgery in which the ossified discs at the correcting level are divided through an anterior approach to the spine. Anterior osteotomies performed in conventional technique, however, necessitate a major surgery in lateral positioning of the patient preceding the posterior correction. For this reason, most spinal surgeons these days resort to the posterior-only technique of PSO.

Pedicle subtraction osteotomy

During PSO, an extended defect of at least the complete lamina is created (see Fig. 23.7E, F). Then both pedicles and a part of the posterior vertebral body are removed or decancellated ('egg-shell procedure') (10). Ideally afterwards the column hinges at the anterior wall, and by shortening of the posterior side and closure of the defect an angular correction of up to 45 degrees can be achieved. One drawback of the PSO is the extended bony wound and the corresponding blood loss. The second is the anterior location of the axis of rotation. This results in a substantial shortening of the spinal canal, with the risk of buckling of the dura and the danger of neurological deficit in up to 12% of cases (11). In areas cranial to the conus therefore the cord might get compressed when the posterior gap is closed. Another and perhaps the most important drawback is the weakening of the anterior column, which may result in fracture during closure of the osteotomy and persisting mechanical instability. Pain, often severe on movements, would result until bony healing has taken place. In up to 23% of patients, healing of the PSO did not fuse (12, 13), which means painful pseudoarthrosis, loss of correction, and even danger of neurological deficit. SPO and PSO result in a local overcorrection to compensate a long multilevel deformity (14). In severe kyphosis, two PSOs may be necessary, doubling the blood loss, often by 4 L (15), which may result in a complete exchange of circulating blood. Since the second PSO needs to be localized some segments cranial to the first and thus approaching the thoracic cord, the neurological risk is increased as well.

Dorsal lordosating spondylodesis (DLS)

In between SPO and PSO is the technique of DLS, described by Puschel and Zielke in 1982 (16). It differs from the technique of Ponte, who described resection of unfused joints (17). It aims at posterior closure with or without anterior opening after V-shaped osteotomies in the region of the former joints. Up to six osteotomies, each around 7 mm wide, sum up to the total correction (see Fig. 23.7C, D). On average, 9 degrees of correction can be gained in each level of a Zielke osteotomy/DLS (18, 19).

An advantage of DLS and of SPO (see Fig. 23.7D–F) is the fact that the axis of rotation lies in the anterior part of the spinal canal. This renders the vertebral body mechanically stable, the neural foramen high, and the posterior canal only mildly shortened.

The disadvantages of the SPO and the DLS are that both are not reaching the anterior column and thus rely on indirect effects for correction: either an opening/rupture of the annulus or via osteoclasis by intentionally fracturing the fused anterior column by an extension manoeuvre on the spine during surgery (20). Due to the uncertainties and dangers of both techniques, they should be restricted to the spondyloarthritic type (the posterior elements, but not discs are ossified). In cases where in osteopenic bone the anterior column does not open but the vertebral body gives in posteriorly, the nerve root foramen is narrowed. The danger of nerve root impingement rises significantly in those cases of DLS, and this restricts the amount of correction and the method. Whenever a bamboo spine needs to be corrected and a PSO is not performed, an additional osteotomy from the anterior side is unavoidable to remain on the safe side.

Minimally invasive dorso-ventral osteotomy and reconstruction (miDVO-R)

In order to rule out shortcomings and hazards of the different conventional methods while combining their advantages, one of the authors (HB) developed a less invasive technique for osteotomy and reconstruction (5, 21). This was made possible due to rapid progress in recent years regarding minimally invasive solutions for approach to the posterior and anterior spine, as well as safe video-assisted control of surgical steps, and percutaneous techniques for spinal fixation. Instead of achieving everything from one extended posterior opening, as in PSO, the new concept approaches the important—but usually small-sized—anterior areas for osteotomy via small incisions through optimal routes. The simultaneous access to the spine in prone position allows a titrated resection of as little bone as necessary, an excellent visual control during correction, and, by means of percutaneously placed implants, an optimal fixation (Fig. 23.8).

The miDVO-R consists of six intraoperative steps:

a) Percutaneous placement of anchoring screws posteriorly (Fig. 23.8C)
b) Minor access, microscope-assisted posterior osteotomy
c) Thoracoscopically and/or retroperitoneoscopically assisted anterior osteotomy (Fig. 23.8D)
d) Correction by repositioning of the patient (Fig. 23.8D)
e) Posterior fixation by percutaneous implantation of fixation rods
f) Anterior reconstruction of the defect by cage and bone graft.

Regarding (b): through a midline incision of 3–4 cm length, the spinous process and lamina of the vertebra cranial to the osteotomized level is partially removed under vision of the operating microscope. In the manner of a Zielke osteotomy, the resection laterally is extended in a V-shaped manner to both foraminae.

Regarding (c): the division of an ankylosed disc requires an exposure area of only 1 square inch at the antero-lateral aspect

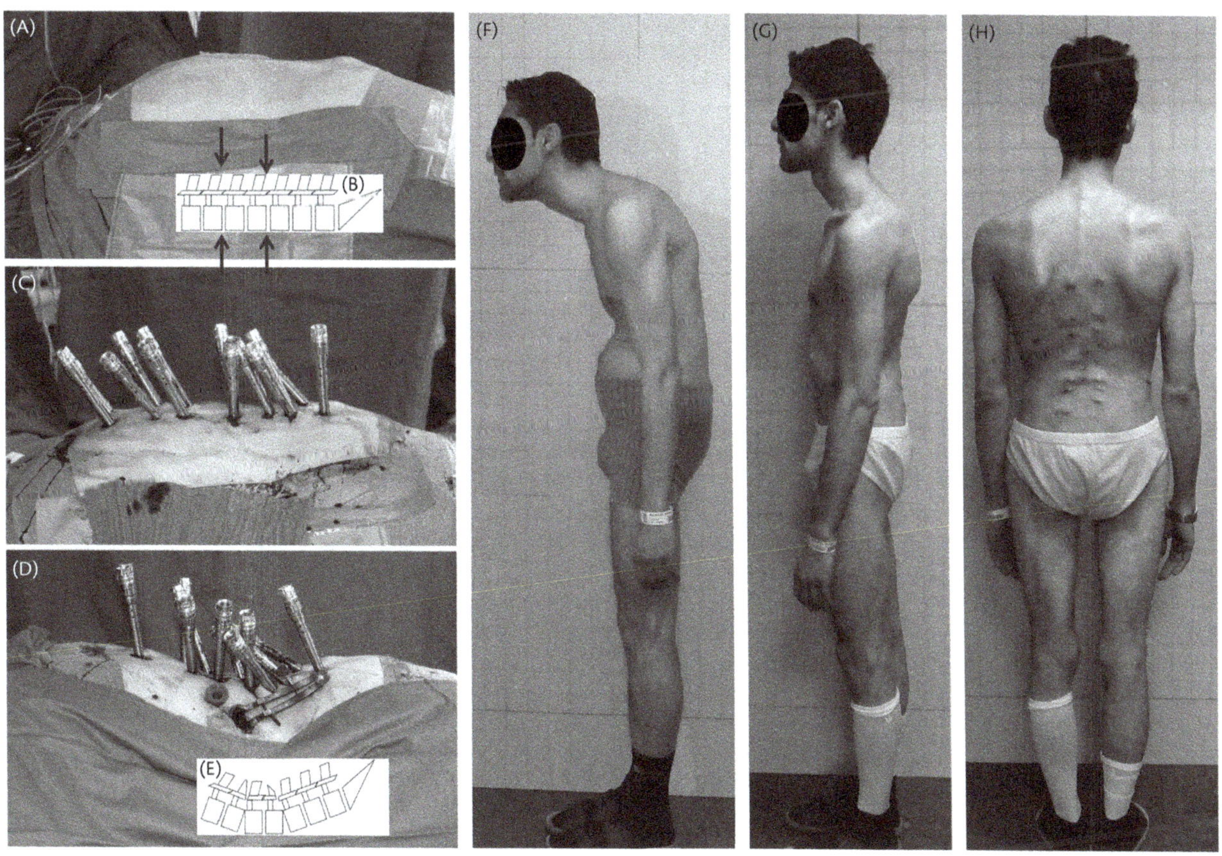

Fig. 23.8 (See colour plate section). MiDVO-R. (A) Patient positioned prone on the operative table after sterile draping. (B) Schematic of the posterior and anterior sites of osteotomies (arrows). (C) After percutaneous implantation of fixation screws and before osteotomies. (D) Change from C-shape to S-shape of the spine: microscope-assisted posterior and thoracoscopic/retroperitoneal anterior osteotomies performed, allowing correction. (E) Schematic of correction to Th12/L1 and L2/L3. (F) The same patient preoperatively in maximum extension. (G) Postoperative situation viewed from the side. (H) Directly postoperative, viewed from the back: stab incisions from screw implantation, two small incisions from posterior osteotomies, and laterally at the left side the thoracoscopic entry and at the right side the retroperitoneoscopic entry can be seen.

of the spine. The thoracoscopically assisted approach through an intercostal space and the chest cage after deflating the lung allows securing all intrathoracic and prevertebral structures and afterwards the reopening of the former disc space. In the same manner, under endoscopical control, the peritoneal sac can be mobilized anteriorly and the disc of L2–L3 or L3–L4 exposed and divided.

Regarding (d): under the influence of gravity and change of the position of the operating table, the posterior osteotomy closes while the corresponding disc anteriorly opens. The main advantage of the anterior osteotomy is that the axis of correction remains at the level of the canal. This ensures the smallest geometrical changes in length for the dura and cord as well as the height of the intervertebral foramen.

Regarding (e): in case of one single osteotomy, titanium rods of adequate length are introduced into the screws from cranial to caudal and fixed by locking screws. Should a second osteotomy be necessary, short rods are introduced temporarily to stabilize the corrected level and points (b), (c) (retroperitoneally), (d), and (e) are repeated.

Regarding (f): after definitive implantation of the fixating rods posteriorly, the anterior corrective sites are controlled again and the defects filled with a metal cage and bone harvested during (b). For further details see reference (21).

Specifics of the corrective osteotomy of the cervico-thoracic region

Due to the forward angulation of the head and neck inherent to that indication, an approach to the anterior cervical spine usually is barred (Fig. 23.5D). For this reason, the correction needs to be performed from posterior. The technique basically is a mélange of SPO, in regard to posterior resection and indirect anterior opening, and PSO, regarding the removal of the pedicles of C7 (22–24). In our experience, this is the osteotomy with the highest rate of—usually transient—postoperative neurological deficit: particularly after long-standing deformity, traction on the nerve roots C7 and C8 unavoidably occurs during correction and can cause muscular weakness and sensory loss for months.

Corrective and stabilizing procedures for the cranio-cervical junction

The ankylosing process in AS usually proceeds in a cephalad direction, including the second cervical vertebra. The C1–C2 joints might be spared completely or affected by varying amounts of restriction. Due to the fact that the atlanto-occipital joints tend to fuse early, all mechanical load is concentrating on one remaining mobile segment. In spite of the disease-related tendency for fusion, the biomechanical overload often leads to elongation and wear of stabilizing ligaments and joint capsules (Fig. 23.5A, B, D). The disordered sagittal balance of an AS patient whose position of the head must be held against gravity (Fig. 23.4A) is adding to this overload. In consequence, there is a tendency for anterior translation of the head/C1 against C2 and the remaining spine which can lead to substantial narrowing of the canal and damage to the medulla/spinal cord (Fig. 23.5D). Attempts of nature to reduce instability via new bone formation can hinder or prevent reduction and necessitate additional operative measures.

In early and mobile stages, surgery is sufficient from posterior only, where the occiput and the lower cervical spine provide good anchoring points for rod-screw systems (Fig. 23.5C, F). If after mechanical stabilization the surface of the bone is decorticated, rapid bony fusion ensures a cure long term.

With late interventions, surgery needs to be much more extended: via approach through the mouth, the obstacles in the atlanto-axial region or in the joint area need to be removed. Probably not as a rheumatoid process but as a sequel of mechanical irritation, retrodental cysts can develop and reach relevant space-occupying size. Detected too late, they get filled with fibrin and turn solid. Whereas in early stages, mechanical stabilization alone solves the problem, a solidified cyst needs removal in the neurologically compromised patient. This requires extension of the transoral procedure via resection of the odontoid and direct decompression of the anterior medulla. It underlines the importance of including the head/neck area in the routine check-up of the rheumatologist.

Results

From 1994 to 2014, a total of 437 surgical corrective interventions in 334 AS patients have been performed in Bad Berka Spine Centre, Thuringia, Germany. Including additional osteotomies at other spine regions, revisions for pseudoarthrosis, implant failure, loss of correction, and infections, the overall number of surgeries in this patient group amounted to 487, or 1.4 surgeries per patient in a time period of up to 20 years. Counting only corrective measures in different spinal regions and disregarding surgeries for complications, every AS patient had on average 1.3 corrective procedures over a time period of maximum 20 years. Probably reflecting the difference in severity of the disease, there were 37 females and 297 males. The mean age at time of surgery of all patients was 53.3 years (85 the oldest and 26 years the youngest patient). The patients older than 76 mainly were acute trauma cases ($n = 53$) with neurological deficit in 40% and cervical location of the fracture in 55%.

Listing the spine locations from occiput to pelvis, 6.2% (27 patients) of all indications were atlanto-axial instabilities and dislocations, of which 12 patients required transoral decompression of the medulla in addition to occipito-cervical fusion from posterior, according to the procedures described in the section 'Corrective and stabilizing procedures for the cranio-cervical junction'. Spinal stenosis and instability/dislocation in a not yet fused segment in the subaxial cervical spine required surgical intervention in 6.4% of the cases.

Corrective osteotomies for angular deformities at the neck–chest junction (see section 'Specifics of the corrective osteotomy of the cervico-thoracic region') were necessary in 26.3% (115 patients) (Fig. 23.5C–F), occasionally in combination with treatment of an additional atlanto-axial problem.

Regional thoracic problems in AS requiring localized surgery were rare—4.5% and constituting mainly Andersson's lesions and stenoses around zygoapophyseal joints that did not fuse completely.

Global kyphosis of the thoracic and lumbar spine with or without Andersson's lesions represent the major indication for extension osteotomies (50.8%, 222 patients), but since severe AS deformities tend to affect the whole spine, 28 of those (12.6%) needed an additional cervico-thoracic osteotomy.

Isolated corrective or stabilizing surgery to the lumbar spine was necessary or sufficing in only 3.4% of patients. Indications mainly were stenosis or progressive kyphosis of other origin like haematogenous pyogenic spondylitis.

The lumbo-sacral junction and the sacrum in only 2.5% (11 patients) of the 437 surgeries needed treatment. Post-traumatic deformity and mechanical pain due to neglected insufficiency fractures of the cranial sacrum in those cases were the pathological substrate.

In 204 patients requiring osteotomy during the whole period of 21 years, only one region was corrected, in 54 patients two regions, and in eight patients three regions (atlanto-axial, cervico-thoracic, and thoraco-lumbar). It is interesting that there seem to be slightly different populations: the group of cervico-thoracic osteotomy patients were on average 6 years older at the time of surgery, with females contributing only 7.6%, whereas thoraco-lumbar-only patients on average were 48 years old, with 12% of female gender.

The crucial criterion for deformity surgery of the spine is the long-term outcome: again, excluding all acute trauma cases, we therefore examined a subgroup with more than 10 years' follow-up.

Long-term results of deformity surgery

The mechanically stable healing of an osteotomy by bony fusion under optimal conditions needs 8–12 months. As soon as this is achieved the risk of complications, such as loss of correction and implant failure within the instrumented area, nears zero. The behaviour of spine regions outside the surgical site is difficult to predict. Whether their kyphosing tendency just reflects natural history or is modified by the surgical change of posture cannot yet be answered. Removal of implants is only necessary in case of late infection, which in our series so far occurred at a rate of 0.69%. In order to recognize AS-related problems of other relevant areas of the spine and hips, regular orthopaedic assessment in 5- to 7-year intervals is advisable. Besides looking for possible changes in other spinal areas, such as hyperkyphosis and cranio-cervical instability, hip and knee function as well as muscle status should be checked and specific rehabilitation programmes initiated if necessary.

Unfortunately, a detailed analysis of our operative AS patients is still missing. However, a small subgroup of 20 thoraco-lumbar osteotomy patients has been prospectively collected for an MD thesis (25) and continuously followed for 10–13 years. In this group, one to three V-shaped opening wedge osteotomies from a conventional open posterior approach were combined with thoracoscopically assisted anterior osteotomy and reconstruction of the defect. The data are as follows: two patients died after 4 and 5 years due to unrelated causes: myocardial infarction and carcinoma of the lung. Two patients after 2 and 5 unproblematic postoperative years with bony healing did not return for further follow-up. In the 16 remaining patients (14 male, 2 female, average age 46 years) 2.5 posterior and 1.1 anterior osteotomies on average were performed, yielding a height gain of ø 7.6 cm, an improvement of thoracic kyphosis of ø 15.1 degrees, and an increase of lumbar lordosis of ø25 degrees. The sagittal balance improved from 104.9 ± 55.7 mm to 20.2 ± 13. 2 mm after 10 years.

The estimated blood loss in those patients who were operated on before the era of minimal invasive osteotomy on average amounted to 1505 ml. With two dural tears and one fractured pedicle there were three intraoperative complications. One patient postoperatively deteriorated neurologically to Frankel C, but recovered completely.

Not surgery related but nevertheless a severe AS complication occurred 8 years postoperatively in one patient of this prospective series: starting with numbness in one leg, an AS-specific cauda equine syndrome developed, which after 13 years deteriorated to muscle weakness, impeding walking (Fig. 23.6C). In spite of this severe impairment, this patient was very satisfied with the results of surgery and the gain in quality of life. At minimum 10 years, all 16 patients available for follow-up claimed they would choose surgical correction of their deformity again.

Complications

Since spinal surgery in non-traumatic cases of axSpA is elective in almost all cases, the rate and severity of complications is crucial.

Pulmonary embolism represents the most eminent lethal threat, due to lengthy surgical procedures and lack of mobility of the chest cage with fused rib–vertebral joints. In our whole series of 437 mostly complex corrective procedures in 334 patients with global kyphosis, three patients at the end of surgery during transfer from the operative table developed circulatory arrest. While after resuscitation two recovered completely and without sequelae, the third patient, in spite of immediate thrombolytic therapy, did not recover and died within 36 hours postoperatively.

A second patient of 77 years, after uneventful transoral decompression and posterior cranio-cervical fusion for severe compression of the medulla oblongata due to C1–C2 instability and stenosis, was found dead without warning signs within 30 days postoperatively.

Complete paralysis of the spinal cord occurred in two patients: one intraoperatively and the other gradually during the first 24 hours postoperatively. New and persisting postoperative radicular and myelopathic disturbances had to be registered in five patients. Temporary radicular impairment, mostly after cervico-thoracic correction and affecting the C7 or C8 nerve root, occurred in 8% of extension osteotomies in that area. All recovered to normal function, but some required up to 7 months for complete restitution. Directly after osteotomies at the level of L2–L4, radicular symptoms in the lower extremities occurred at a rate of 12%, affecting mainly the stability of the knee. All but four of those completely recovered within the first 2 postoperative weeks.

In spite of utmost care regarding positioning of the patient on the operative table, adverse effects of weight-related pressure on skin and nerve plexus cannot be completely avoided. If occurring in spite of special padding, it is usually not severe and recovery rapid and complete. The intraoperative loss of blood, in particular during conventional open procedures such as PSO of the thoraco-lumbar spine, can amount to several litres (7, 15). This can be markedly reduced by the minimally invasive technique of miDVO-R, with an average blood loss of 813 ml.

Long-lasting postoperative pain on movement or exertion usually is elicited by insufficient mechanical stability. Osteopenia in AS, too few anchoring points of the instrumentation, and/or insufficient stability of the anterior spinal column can be the cause.

In all cases where during the first weeks after surgery the patient does not feel pain-free and if implant loosening starts, an early additional anterior operative stabilization is advisable. One should not wait until a pseudoarthrosis develops and the posterior fixation needs to be changed as well, since the success of the corrective surgery is then at risk (12, 13).

Patients with AS are more in danger of postoperative wound infections, in particular after conventional open approaches. Reasons might be nutritional after long-lasting administration of non-steroidal antirheumatics (NSARs), or impaired immune response after treatment with DMARDs or TNFα inhibitors. Surgical revision and debridement can salvage the instrumentation and thus the success of the whole procedure, and should be performed without hesitation.

Management of fractures in ankylosing spondylitis

Background

Several studies have demonstrated that AS patients have a significantly higher risk of spinal fractures during their lifetime compared with those without an ankylosed spine (26, 27). A recent Danish case-controlled study demonstrated a five-fold higher risk of clinical spine fracture and a 35% increased risk of non-vertebral fracture, with excess risk peaking early, in the first 2.5 years of AS disease (28). In a review of the literature, Fatemi et al. noted that the prevalence of vertebral fracture in AS patients ranges from 0.4 to 32.4% (29). Interestingly, despite successful antirheumatic treatment of AS with disease-modifying drugs, a Swedish national registry study by Robinson et al. found that the incidence of cervical spinal fractures related to AS is steadily rising (30).

The reasons for this increased risk are multifactorial, with the pathophysiological and secondary consequences that occur in AS leading to increased risk of falls and vulnerability of the spine to fracture (29). The spinal changes of AS often lead to spinal kyphosis, which can impact horizontal gaze that requires lower extremity compensation, thereby resulting in abnormal gait and biomechanics. Furthermore, Fatemi and colleagues noted that imbalance and incoordination due to vestibular impairments (including side-effects from AS medications) may be increased in AS patients (29). Consequently, negotiating simple transfer such as in and out of a bath-tub could pose a significant challenge to someone with the impairments present in AS subjects. Most notable, however, is that the consequence of ossification of both supportive and elastic spinal soft tissues: (1) does not allow the normal absorption of forces imparted on the spine with any type of trauma: (2) typically leads to kyphotic deformity that shifts the head and/or centre of gravity forward and increases the loading moment applied to the head and spine, which is further compounded by long rigid spinal segments, and (3)the associated osteoporosis that weakens the spine both result in the fact that even the most trivial trauma or repetitive stresses can lead to a spinal fracture in AS patients (29, 31).

Due to this unique scenario, AS fractures characteristically occur due to a hyperextension mechanism, propagate transversely, and involve the anterior and posterior columns of the spine (Figs 23.9 and 23.10), with varying degrees of distraction and translation. They tend to occur through or just below the ankylosed intervertebral disc space. AS fractures are often unstable as a result of the two long rigid spinal segments above and below the fracture (akin to a long bone (e.g. femur) fracture), and as such there is typically displacement with a high associated degree of neurological sequelae.

General considerations

A systematic review of AS fractures by Westerveld et al. combined data on 345 AS fracture patients from 76 articles (published between 1980 and 2007) (31). The mean patient age was 59 years (32–82) and the majority of AS fractures occur in males (90%), in the cervical spine (81%), and resulted from low-energy trauma (66%), such as a fall from standing or less. In the Westerveld report, neurological deficits were present in 67.2% of patients. Approximately half of the deficits were complete spinal cord injuries, a rate that is significantly higher than that of complete spinal cord injuries reported in the non-AS spinal trauma population (32). Of concern, 14% of patients suffered a secondary deterioration, reportedly due to the grossly unstable nature of the fracture, and subsequent inadequate immobilization, with fracture mobility/displacement, inconsiderate transfers, and application of a hard collar on the cervical spine with pre-existing kyphotic deformity (i.e. inadvertently conforming the spine to normal alignment), or in some cases following surgical or non-surgical intervention. In addition, AS patients are prone to delayed neurological deterioration due to epidural haematoma formation from ruptured epidural veins, and the cancellous, osteoporotic bone of the vertebral fracture may cause compressive epidural haematoma (32). This frequency of neurological deterioration is unheard of in the non-ankylosed spine trauma population and points to the particular complexities and significant precautions required when managing the fractured AS spine.

The average mortality rate associated with AS fractures is approximately 20%, which is extremely high considering that the reported mortality in individuals treated surgically for traumatic spinal fractures is less than 1% (31). In particular for cervical spine injuries, the mortality rates for patients with AS and spinal cord injuries range from 35% to 50%, compared with rates of 4–16% for the general population of spinal cord injury patients (11). In a study by Robinson et al., it was reported that a patient in Sweden with a surgically treated subaxial cervical fracture without AS has a mean survival of 218 months, compared to a mean survival of 52 months in their series of 41 prospectively followed AS cervical fracture patients (33). The authors found that survival was significantly affected (negatively) by older age, smoking, and the presence of a complete spinal cord injury. Mortality is most commonly associated with respiratory complications (31). However, other catastrophic complications specific to the kyphotic AS patient such as aortic injury and tracheal disruption are typically fatal (31). Based on current data, for minimally ambulatory patients the general medical complication and mortality rate seemed to be higher in conservatively treated patients compared to surgically treated patients (31, 32). This is likely due to the ability of aggressive and early mobilization and rehabilitation (including respiratory care) afforded by surgical stabilization (33).

Given the high-risk nature of AS fractures, the persistence of a high rate of delayed or missed diagnosis remains a significant concern. In the review by Westerveld et al., a delay in diagnosis occurred in 20% of patient, half of which were due to the injury not being initially recognized by the physician ('doctor's delay') and the other half due to patient delay in their decision to seek medical attention ('patient's delay'). This is an ongoing issue, which is clearly multifactorial in its origin, and warrants further discussion. First, AS vertebral fractures often occur with trivial trauma, and thus the physician's index of suspicion may not be appropriately raised. Second, patients with AS commonly have neck and/or back pain, and thus pain from a fracture could be attributed (by both patient and physician) to their AS. Third, given the highly abnormal structure of the vertebral column in patients with AS and fractures which are often at the base of the neck (i.e. cervico-thoracic junction), fracture identification can be difficult on the basis of plain radiographs. In addition, commonly used c-spine imaging rules for assessing patients in the emergency room do not explicitly identify the AS patient as high risk (34). For example, the most sensitive algorithm, the Canadian C-spine Rule (CCR), states an age of 65 or older as high risk, warranting imaging; however, the mean age of AS fractures is 59 (31, 34). The CCR algorithm also notes that

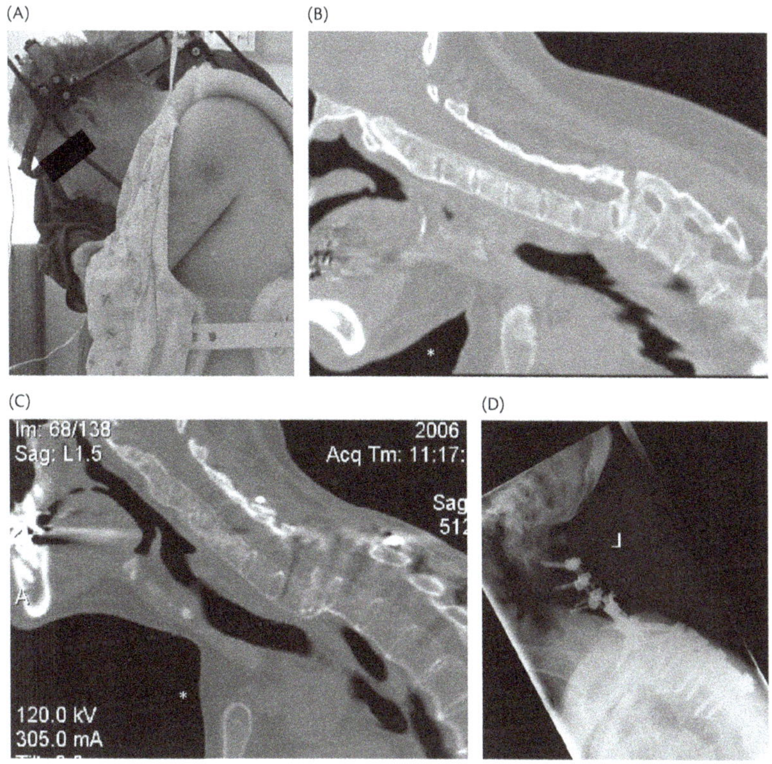

Fig. 23.9 (A) Clinical picture of a 65-year-old male who tripped and fell 2 months prior and suffered from progressive neck pain, neck flexion, and loss of horizontal gaze. He eventually saw his rheumatologist and was noted to have a new chin-on-chest deformity, ataxic gait, and right hand weakness. He was admitted to hospital and had radiographs, a CT, and subsequent surgical consultation on the same day. Neurological examination confirmed evidence of spinal cord dysfunction (i.e., cervical myelopathy). (B) CT demonstrating typical bony features of AS, including occipito-cervical ankylosis and a transverse fracture below the C7 to T1 disc space, through the T1 pedicle, with posterior distraction. He also had a small posterior haematoma with cord compression. Asterisk denotes minimal space between his chin and sternum. He was placed in a halo-vest and then underwent urgent posterior decompression, bilateral pedicle subtraction, realignment, and multilevel cervico-thoracic screw-rod stabilization. During surgery, as a result of no anterior integrity of the spinal column, he translated during correction of his deformity. Fortunately, he remained neurologically stable, as the translation occurred after wide multilevel decompression of the cord above and below the fracture, thus mitigating compression from the translation that would have otherwise rendered him paralyzed. At long-term follow-up he had persistent hand weakness, but good neurological improvement in his lower extremities. (C) Mid-sagittal CT demonstrating lateral radiographs, 4 years post-surgical treatment, demonstrating the translation of C7 on T1 and solid fusion across the fracture site. As denoted by the asterisk, and compared to pre-surgery CT, there was significant improvement of his chin-on-chest deformity. (D) Lateral radiographs demonstrating the C2 to T4 instrumentation.

the rules do not apply to individuals with known vertebral disease; however, AS is not explicitly listed and would be dependent on the emergency room physician to routinely enquire about a history of AS, which may be unknown to undiagnosed patient; recognize kyphotic alignment or enquire about a change in alignment; and recognize the radiographic features of AS on a plain X-ray. *Due to often-irreversible neurologic consequences and possible associated mortality, it is universally recommended by the spine surgical/trauma community that any new complaint of spinal pain in a patient with or suspected of having spinal ankylosis, particularly following the scenario of any trauma (regardless of how trivial, or even a near fall) or increase in physical activity, is to be considered secondary to a fracture until proven otherwise.* In such cases, advanced imaging with CT and MRI is strongly recommended before discharging the patient (29).

Management

Acute fractures

In most series, and for the reasons noted (instability, neurological deficits, inability to mobilize), surgical management is typically more commonly recommended than non-surgical treatment. In addition, due to the aforementioned associated morbidity and mortality, initial management in an intensive care or monitored setting is recommended for all AS fracture patients. A trial of non-surgical treatment is typically indicated for patients who are neurologically normal, able to ambulate, with no evidence of fracture translation and/or distraction and no evidence of a compressive epidural haematoma on CT and MR imaging. In addition, some patients may absolutely refuse to consider surgical intervention and thus are treated non-surgically against medical advice. Non-surgical treatment typically involves halo-vest treatment for cervical and upper thoracic (T3 and above) fractures, and, for thoraco-lumbar injuries, a custom molded cervical or thoracic-lumbar-sacral orthosis (CTLSO/TLSO) and supportive measures for 6 months or more, with frequent follow-up. Non-surgical treatment is relatively contraindicated in those with more significant deformity that precludes functional fitting of the orthosis, or who are at significant risk for increased pulmonary complications. Patients are typically followed up for a minimum of 1–2 years to ensure solid healing of the facture and no progressive deformity. It is deliberate that the word 'conservative' treatment is not used in this scenario; as noted, there are significant risks associated with what has been outlined

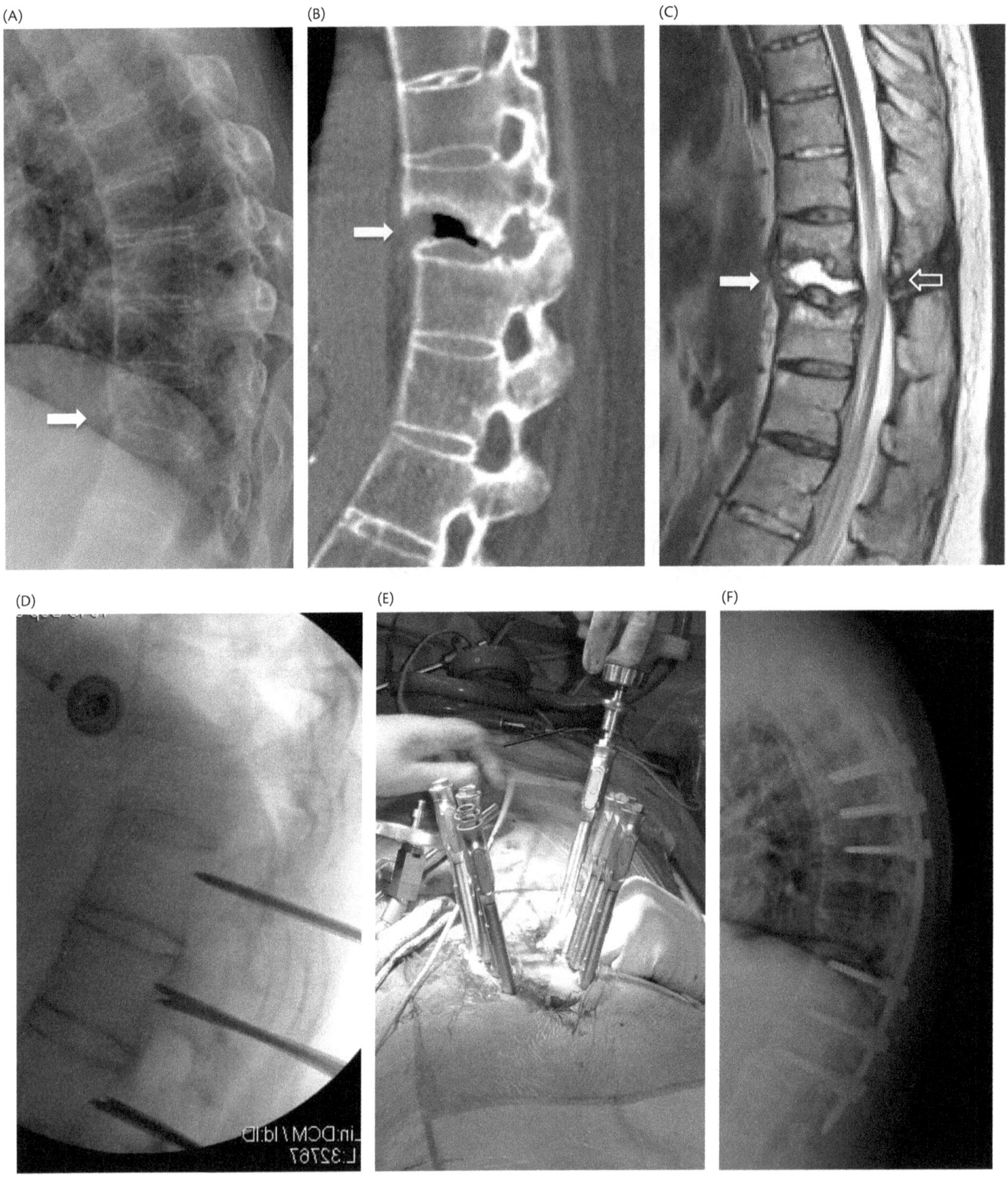

Fig. 23.10 (A) Standing lateral thoracic radiographs from a 60-year-old male with acute pain after a fall while walking 1 week ago. Progressive mechanical pain brought him to the emergency room. He was neurologically intact. As indicated by the arrow, there is a break and slight translation in the line of the ossified anterior longitudinal ligament at T8–9 with no distraction. (B) Supine mid-sagittal CT demonstrating gross anterior distraction (arrow) and slight increase in translation indication instability. This is a good example of the instability and possible dangers that can occur in AS fractures with postural change. In this case, the extension moment that occurs with the supine position results in anterior distraction. (C) Supine mid-sagittal T2W MRI demonstrates fluid in the fracture site and a small, minimally compressive, posterior haematoma. Surgical management by percutaneous fixation was recommended. (D) Lateral intraoperative fluoroscopic image demonstrating reduction of the fracture and position of percutaneous trocars into the pedicles three levels below the fracture. (E) Intraoperative picture demonstrating percutaneous pedicle screw extenders that enable percutaneous passage of the stabilization rods into the pedicle screws. This patient mobilized immediately after surgery and was discharged from hospital 3 days post-surgery with no complications. (F) Post-operative lateral thoracic radiograph 2 years following surgery, with evidence of fusion. For this type of case, the patient is placed on a kyphosing spinal frame to prevent the effect noted in B and C. In addition, appropriate contouring of the rod is required to prevent an extension moment and fracture displacement during rod reduction.

as non-surgical (i.e. conservative) treatment, which may in fact be greater than those associated with surgical treatment, other than the specific indications noted. In a comparative study comparing 25 patients with thoraco-lumbar fractures with a minimum 2-year follow-up, Lu et al. noted eight patients with a delay in diagnosis (i.e. non-treatment) that resulted in pseudoarthrosis in all cases, and progressive neurological deficits in four cases. Of the 11 patients who received conservative treatment with bracing, successful fracture union was achieved in only three cases, compared to all six cases treated with early surgery (35). In a series reported by Whang et al., the authors noted that the four deaths that occurred were all directly related to the use of halo-vest orthosis (36). These results, albeit from limited case series, certainly support the findings of Westerveld that suggest AS patients with unstable spinal fractures should receive early surgical management to prevent further catastrophic sequelae.

For all the biomechanical and medical reasons noted, surgical management of AS fracture patients is always a complex endeavour. Although a variety of surgical interventions and approaches are available, the specific technical details of surgery are beyond the scope of this chapter. In general, the surgery is recommended to be performed from a posterior surgical approach with multiple levels of fixation above and below the fracture (typically a minimum of three levels on either side) to compensate for the long rigid lever arms and osteoporotic bone (Figs 23.9 and 23.10). Due to the gross instability and a posterior approach, the anaesthetic process and transfer of the patient to a prone position can be the most dangerous aspect of the case. These patients require great anaesthesia precautions, with awake fibreoptic intubation, and for cervical spine injuries, especially with a spinal cord injury, patients often require prolonged endotracheal intubation, with some requiring tracheostomy to enable pulmonary toileting and successful weaning from a ventilator. Appropriately contoured tables that accommodate pre-existing spinal deformity and allow a supine-to prone position without losing support of a neurologically stable position (confirmed while the patient is awake in the supine position) enable the greatest degree of safety during prone positioning. Otherwise, an unsupported segment of spine can lead to inadvertent fracture translation and permanent neurological injury during prone positioning. Conventional open posterior approaches to the spine as well as decompression of a haemorrhagic epidural space are typically associated with a high degree of blood loss, associated haemodynamic instability, and for those with spinal cord injuries, adequate blood pressure support for spinal cord perfusion during and after surgery (31–33). In addition, as a result of the lost segmental spinal motion and gross instability, the avoidance of secondary spinal cord injuries from spinal translation during any surgical reduction manoeuvres (of the spine or the spinal rods to the pedicle screw fixation) or attempted correction of any pre-existing deformity through the fracture can present significant technical challenges (Fig. 23.9).

In addition to the medical complications, the kyphotic aspect of the AS spine carries with it a higher rate of wound problems (higher tension and dehiscence) and risk for surgical-site infection (31, 33). As a means of partially reducing the perioperative risk of surgical management, a subset of thoraco-lumbar AS fractures are increasingly being managed by percutaneous methods of spinal fixation. Percutaneous fixation can be done either primarily in the scenario of a neurologically intact patient (Fig. 23.10) with a reduced or reducible fracture, or with hybrid procedures, with a limited open procedure for decompression/reduction of the spinal canal as required and percutaneous fixation above and below.

Chronic fractures

In a subset of patients, fractures may be missed for prolonged periods of time. In this situation, radiographs typically show destructive lesions that occur in the vertebral bodies and intervertebral discs—a finding first described by Andersson in 1937 (37). Since then they have been termed Andersson's lesions, spondylodiscitis, destructive vertebral lesions, and spinal pseudoarthrosis.

The prevalence of peridiscal lesion in AS ranges from 1–28 per 100 cases, and such lesions must be differentiated between inflammatory (non-traumatic) and post-fracture (traumatic or insufficiency) lesions (38). In a review by Park et al., the criteria for an inflammatory lesion were noted to be narrowing of the disc space, erosion of the end-plate, and abnormal radiodensity of the adjacent vertebral body but without severe vertebral destruction; those for a fracture lesion appear more like a fracture pseudoarthroses and demonstrate sclerosis and hypertrophy of the bone adjacent to the disc, with accompanying intervertebral disc destruction and osteolysis of the vertebral body (Fig. 23.11) (38).

Furthermore, in their series, Park et al. noted that inflammatory lesions were more common and originated in the vertebral column in the presence of incomplete bony ankylosis, and were not accompanied by instability at the apex of the lesion, or by fracture of the posterior column (38). In addition, patients with inflammatory lesions did not report trauma and had more inflammatory-type pain (i.e. that improved with activity). Conversely, traumatic lesions occurred when bony ankylosis was relatively well developed compared to the inflammatory lesions and patients had typical mechanical pain (i.e. that is worse with activity or motion of the spine).

Inflammatory lesions typically respond to the general anti-inflammatory management of AS, whereas traumatic lesions require non-surgical or surgical management, as described. Typically, these latter patients have been active without negative neurological sequelae for some time; thus, if their symptoms are manageable (activity modification and analgesics), a trial of bracing (6–12 months) treatment is recommended (Fig. 23.11) (38). Surgical management is recommend, regardless of the duration of symptoms (38–42), for patients who experience failed non-surgical management, who have progressive deformity (i.e. focal increase in kyphosis) that is functionally significant or unacceptable to the patient, or who have evidence of instability (translation > 3–4 mm on standing versus supine imaging) with risk of neurological injury, or established related neurological symptoms or signs (static or dynamic deficit). The surgical techniques required range from simple posterior stabilization and fusion to complex osteotomies, such as those described in this chapter (Figs 23.9 and 23.11).

Prevention

In the face of significant risk of morbidity and mortality, it is paramount that AS patients, their care-providers, and their healthcare providers be actively engaged in primary prevention strategies to avoid the possible devastating complication of fracture in association with their disease process. Patients with AS should be encouraged to install activity aids (e.g. bath rails, shower seats) and other fall-prevention strategies, such as night lights and removal of loose

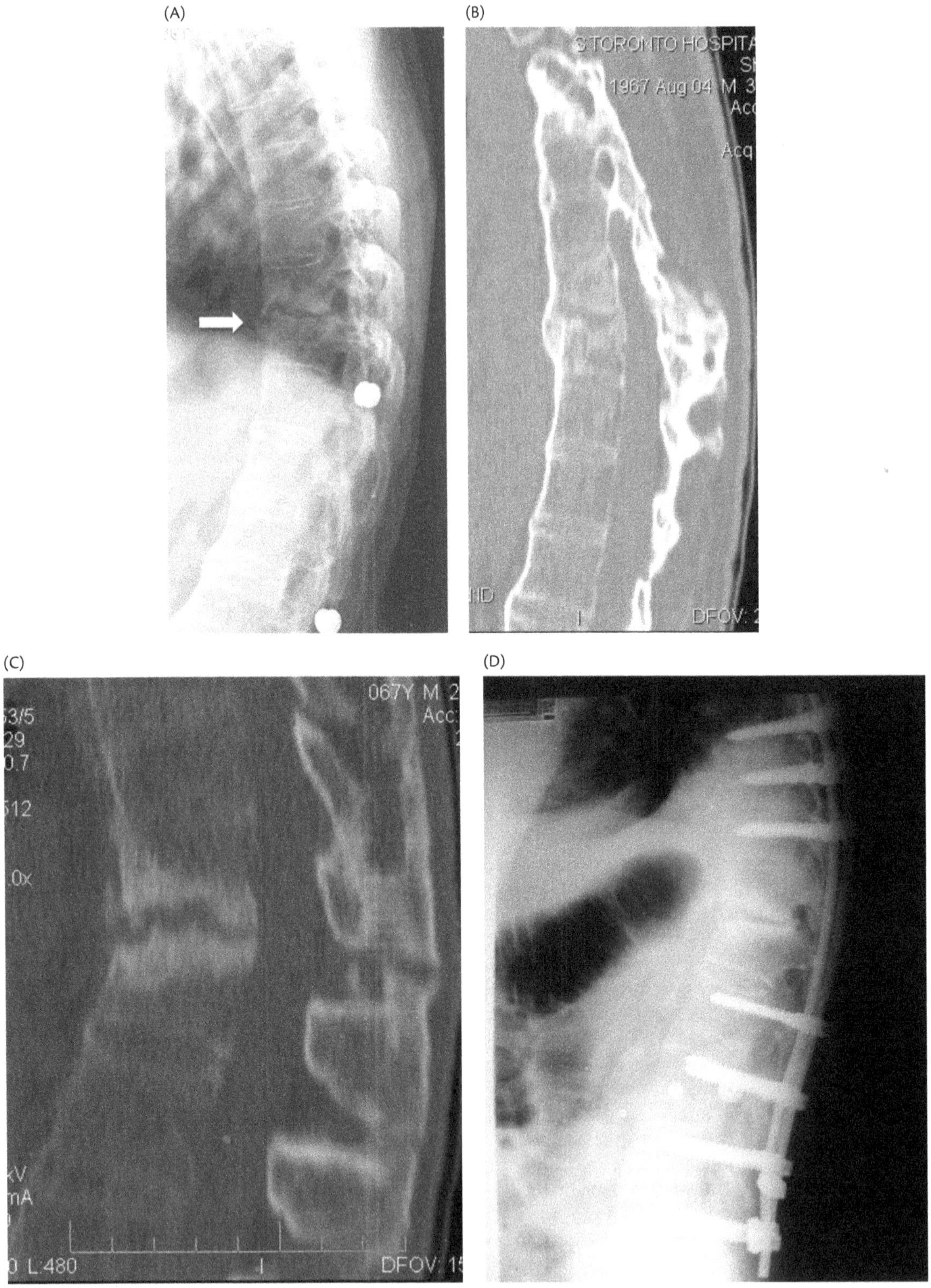

Fig. 23.11 (A) Lateral thoracic radiograph in a 38-year-old male demonstrating minimal kyphotic deformity and a mid-thoracic traumatic/insufficiency Andersson's lesion. He reported a 3-month history of acute onset mechanical mid-thoracic pain, but could not recall any traumatic or near-traumatic event. His symptoms were manageable and he was treated in a TLSO for 6 months, at which time he was pain free. (B) Mid-sagittal CT at 12 months demonstrates that bridging ossification occurred anteriorly and in the posterior spinal elements. (C) In this case, a more chronic and destructive Andersson's lesion is noted in a 68-year-old male with over a 1-year history of progressive rest and mechanical (dominant) pain. He recalled having a minor fall several weeks before his pain began, but thought nothing of it at the time. He did not have any global kyphotic deformity and underwent surgery with a small Smith–Peterson osteotomy at the posterior fracture site and multilevel stabilization (D).

rugs. Excessive use of alcohol should be avoided, as should contact sports and high-impact activity (32). Furthermore, secondary prevention efforts include regional education directed at emergency medical services staff (frontline and hospital based) regarding the need for a high degree of suspicion of fracture in these patient; recommendation of the use of a medical alert bracelet; and when identified or possible, early surgical referral may prevent delayed sequelae of acute and chronic AS fractures.

The cauda equina syndrome in spondyloarthritis

Not every neurological deficit is caused by compression of the cord. Though published more than 50 years ago (43), the AS-associated cauda equina syndrome is not well known (Fig. 23.6), usually has an insidious onset with distal sensory loss, and can deteriorate to all features of the cauda equina syndrome, including incontinence and loss of walking ability (44). Pathoanatomically, the fibres of the cauda equina become adherent to the dura and move to the periphery. In MRI and post- myelogram CT scans, an 'empty dura' occurs (Fig. 23.6B).

Besides avoiding frustrating investigations in other directions, the diagnosis is important whenever corrective surgery to the lumbar spine of an AS patient is considered: in long-standing AS, the periosteum of the vertebral arch can be fused completely with the dura. Particularly when methods are applied that require substantial shortening of the canal, as PSO, the risk of injury to cauda fibres is high. Preoperative planning in such cases should embark on safer techniques and locations at or above the conus for osteotomy. In late stages (after conservative or operative treatment), extended dural ectasias can develop (Fig. 23.6).

Deformity summary

Unlike the situation during inflammatory disease states when an AS patient usually is under close observation by a rheumatologist, later on in 'burned out' ankylosis the patient tends to rarely consult a doctor because of spine problems. This might be a main reason why data about late deformity and operative options, plus their outcomes, are scarce. In this chapter we present data from a prospectively collected series of all AS patients treated operatively in one institution.

Due to the variations in disease activity and ossifying process around peripheral joints and spine segments under the influence of gravity, substantially different orthopaedic problems can arise. A thorough analysis of every deranged posture of an AS patient therefore seems advisable, with particular attention on instability and stenosis in the cranio-cervical junction. Surgery should be advised in cases of myelopathy due to stenosis or instability. The latter—in long-standing cases presenting as Andersson's lesion—often is accompanied by severe mechanical pain. Another indication is loss of ability to see straight ahead without compensatory flexion of the knees. Whereas in less severe deformities, corrective surgery yields very good results and short rehabilitation periods, severe deformities and neglected instabilities demand complex procedures, with combinations of different osteotomies and higher complication and reoperation rates.

Options for osteotomies for posteriorly fused spines with persisting disc spaces anteriorly are the Smith-Petersen 'opening wedge osteotomy' and the Zielke 'dorsal lordosating spondylodeses'. They rely on indirect opening of the anterior column and therefore their outcomes are difficult to predict. For an anteriorly fused bamboo spine PSO at present is the gold standard. However, PSO relies on acute overcorrection in one or maximally two sites for a multisegmental kyphosis, requires invasive posterior approaches, and is associated with significant blood loss and pseudoarthrosis rates. Minimally invasive techniques for approach, implantation of fixation devices, and video-controlled posterior and anterior osteotomy seem to have less blood loss, lower pseudoarthrosis rates, and allow choosing corrective sites well above the conus and a combination of osteotomies. However, there has only been experience with this technique since 2006, and it is technically demanding.

Long-term data of 16 patients followed prospectively for 10 years show these patients retained a height gain of ø 7.6 cm, an improvement of thoracic kyphosis of ø 15.1 degrees, an increase of lumbar lordosis of 25 degrees, and a sagittal balance of 20.2 ± 13.2 mm after over 100 mm preoperatively. All retrieved patients after 10 years were highly satisfied with the surgical correction and would choose this treatment again.

Surgical correction for global kyphosis in AS is a valuable, but demanding treatment option that can improve substantially the quality of life of those patients and should be chosen before disabling severe deformity has developed.

Trauma summary

Patients with AS are at significantly higher risk of sustaining a spinal fracture; for those with a fracture, the risk of morbidity, such as spinal cord injury, and mortality is also dramatically higher than the general population. The reasons for this are multifactorial, with the pathophysiological and secondary consequences that occur in AS leading to increased risk of falls and vulnerability of the spine to fracture, often due to trivial trauma. In addition, AS fractures are often missed and have a high risk of delayed neurological sequelae and/or spinal deformity. New or sudden increase in spinal pain or deformity in the AS patient should be considered a fracture, until proven otherwise by advanced imaging. In general, surgical management is recommended for the majority of AS patients with fracture.

References

1. Kruger K, Albrecht K, Rehart S, Scholz R. [Recommendations of the German Society for Rheumatology on the perioperative approach under therapy with DMARDs and biologicals in inflammatory rheumatic diseases.] Z Rheumatol 2014;73:77–84.
2. Bollow M. [Magnetic resonance imaging in ankylosing spondylitis (Marie-Struempell-Bechterew disease).] RoFo 2002;174:1489–99.
3. Kiltz U, Rudwaleit M, Sieper J, et al. [German Society for Rheumatology S3 guidelines on axial spondyloarthritis including Bechterew's disease and early forms: 3 Clinical symptoms.] Z Rheumatol 2014;73(Suppl 2):28–39.
4. Rasker JJ, Prevo RL, Lanting PJ. Spondylodiscitis in ankylosing spondylitis, inflammation or trauma? A description of six cases. Scand J Rheumatol 1996;25:52–7.
5. Böhm H, Shousha M. Spondyloarthritis. In: Rehart S, Sell, S (eds) Operative Orthopädische Rheumatologie. Stuttgart, Thieme, 2015, pp 225–40.
6. Van Royen BJ. A new technique for correction of an iatrogenic extension deformity in ankylosing spondylitis. Spine 2002;27:332–3.
7. Ravinsky RA, Ouellet JA, Brodt ED, Dettori JR. Vertebral osteotomies in ankylosing spondylitis-comparison of outcomes following closing

wedge osteotomy versus opening wedge osteotomy: a systematic review. Evid Based Spine Care J 2013;4:18–29.
8. Smith-Petersen MN, Larson CB, Aufranc OE. Osteotomy of the spine for correction of flexion deformity in rheumatoid arthritis. J Bone Joint Surg 1945;27:1–11.
9. Bridwell KH, Lewis SJ, Rinella A, Lenke LG, Baldus C, Blanke K. Pedicle subtraction osteotomy for the treatment of fixed sagittal imbalance. Surgical technique. J Bone Joint Surg 2004;86(A Suppl 1):44–50.
10. Thomasen E. Vertebral osteotomy for correction of kyphosis in ankylosing spondylitis. Clin Orthop Rel Res 1985;194:142–52.
11. Buchowski JM, Bridwell KH, Lenke LG, et al. Neurologic complications of lumbar pedicle subtraction osteotomy: a 10-year assessment. Spine 2007;32:2245–52.
12. Kim YJ, Bridwell KH, Lenke LG, Cheh G, Baldus C. Results of lumbar pedicle subtraction osteotomies for fixed sagittal imbalance: a minimum 5-year follow-up study. Spine 2007;32:2189–97.
13. O'Neill KR, Lenke LG, Bridwell KH, et al. Clinical and radiographic outcomes after 3-column osteotomies with 5-year follow-up. Spine 2014;39:424–32.
14. Cho KJ, Bridwell KH, Lenke LG, Berra A, Baldus C. Comparison of Smith-Petersen versus pedicle subtraction osteotomy for the correction of fixed sagittal imbalance. Spine 2005;30:2030–7.
15. Zhang HQ, Huang J, Guo CF, Liu SH, Tang MX. Two-level pedicle subtraction osteotomy for severe thoracolumbar kyphotic deformity in ankylosing spondylitis. Eur Spine J 2013;23(1):234–41.
16. Puschel J, Zielke K. [Corrective surgery for kyphosis in Bekhterev's disease—indication, technique, results (author's transl).] Z Orthop Ihre Grenzgeb 1982;120:338–42.
17. Geck MJ, Macagno A, Ponte A, Shufflebarger HL. The Ponte procedure: posterior only treatment of Scheuermann's kyphosis using segmental posterior shortening and pedicle screw instrumentation. J Spinal Disord Tech 2007;20:586–93.
18. Bohm H, Hehne HJ, Zielke K. [Correction of Bechterew kyphosis.] Der Orthopade 1989;18:142–54.
19. Hehne HJ, Zielke K, Bohm H. Polysegmental lumbar osteotomies and transpedicled fixation for correction of long-curved kyphotic deformities in ankylosing spondylitis. Report on 177 cases. Clin Orthop Rel Res1990;258:49–55.
20. Liu H, Yang C, Zheng Z, et al. Comparison of Smith-Petersen osteotomy and pedicle subtraction osteotomy for the correction of thoracolumbar kyphotic deformity in ankylosing spondylitis: a systematic review and meta-analysis. Spine 2015;40:570–9.
21. Böhm H. Thorakolumbale Aufrichtungsspondylodese bei Morbus Bechterew. In: Sell S, Rehart S (eds) Operationsatlas Orthopädische Rheumatologie. Stuttgart, Georg Thieme, 2013, pp 159–64.
22. Mason C, Cozen L, Adelstein L. Surgical correction of flexion deformity of the cervical spine. Calif Med 1953;79:244–6.
23. McMaster MJ. A technique for lumbar spinal osteotomy in ankylosing spondylitis. J Bone Joint Sur Br 1985;67:204–10.
24. Urist MR. Osteotomy of the cervical spine; report of a case of ankylosing rheumatoid spondylitis. J Bone Joint Surg Am 1958; 40-A:833–43.
25. El Meshtawy M. Value of endoscopic spinal surgery in management of thoracic and thoracolumbar kyphosis. MD thesis. Assiut, Assiut University, Department of Orthopedic Surgery, 2003.
26. Finkelstein JA, Chapman JR, Mirza S. Occult vertebral fractures in ankylosing spondylitis. Spinal Cord 1999;37:444–7.
27. Feldtkeller E, Vosse D, Geusens P, et al. Prevalence and annual incidence of vertebral fractures in patients with ankylosing spondylitis. Rheumatol Int 2006;26:234–9.
28. Prieto-Alhambra D, Muñoz-Ortego J, De Vries F, et al. Ankylosing spondylitis confers substantially increased risk of clinical spine fractures: a nationwide case-control study. Osteoporos Int 2015;26(1):85–91.
29. Fatemi G, Gensler LS, Learch TJ, Weisman MH. Spine fractures in ankylosing spondylitis: a case report and review of imaging as well as predisposing factors to falls and fractures. Semin Arthritis Rheum 2014;44(1):20–4.
30. Robinson Y, Sanden B, Olerud C. Increased occurrence of spinal fractures related to ankylosing spondylitis: a prospective 22-year cohort study in 17,764 patients from a national registry in Sweden. Patient Saf Surg 2013;7:2.
31. Westerveld LA, Verlaan JJ, Oner FC. Spinal fractures in patients with ankylosing spinal disorders: a systematic review of the literature on treatment, neurological status and complications. Eur Spine J 2009;18(2):145–56.
32. Jacobs WB, Fehlings MG. Ankylosing spondylitis and spinal cord injury: origin, incidence, management, and avoidance. Neurosurg Focus 2008;24:E12.
33. Robinson Y, Robinson AL, Olerud C. Complications and survival after long posterior instrumentation of cervical and cervicothoracic fractures related to ankylosing spondylitis or diffuse idiopathic skeletal hyperostosis. Spine (Phila Pa 1976) 2015;40(4):E227–33.
34. Michaleff ZA, Maher CG, Verhagen AP, Rebbeck T, Lin CW. Accuracy of the Canadian C-spine rule and NEXUS to screen for clinically important cervical spine injury in patients following blunt trauma: a systematic review. CMAJ 2012;184(16):E867–76.
35. Lu ML, Tsai TT, Lai PL, et al. A retrospective study of treating thoracolumbar spine fractures in ankylosing spondylitis. Eur J Orthop Surg Traumatol 2014;24(Suppl 1):S117–23.
36. Whang PG, Goldberg G, Lawrence JP, et al. The management of spinal injuries in patients with ankylosing spondylitis or diffuse idiopathic skeletal hyperostosis: a comparison of treatment methods and clinical outcomes. J Spinal Disord Tech 2009;22(2):77–85.
37. Andersson O. Rontgenbilden vid spondylarthritis ankylopoetica. Nord Med 1937;14:2000–2.
38. Park YS, Kim JH, Ryu JA, Kim TH. The Andersson lesion in ankylosing spondylitis: distinguishing between the inflammatory and traumatic subtypes. J Bone Joint Surg Br 2011;93(7):961–6.
39. Wang G, Sun J, Jiang Z, Cui X. The surgical treatment of Andersson lesions associated with ankylosing spondylitis. Orthopedics 2011;34(7):e302–6.
40. Qian BP, Qiu Y, Wang B, et al. Pedicle subtraction osteotomy through pseudarthrosis to correct thoracolumbar kyphotic deformity in advanced ankylosing spondylitis. Eur Spine J 2012;21(4):711–18.
41. Kim KT, Lee SH, Suk KS, Lee JH, Im YJ. Spinal pseudarthrosis in advanced ankylosing spondylitis with sagittal plane deformity: clinical characteristics and outcome analysis. Spine (Phila Pa 1976) 2007;32(15):1641–7.
42. Chang KW, Tu MY, Huang HH, Chen HC, Chen YY, Lin CC. Posterior correction and fixation without anterior fusion for pseudoarthrosis with kyphotic deformity in ankylosing spondylitis. Spine (Phila Pa 1976) 2006;31(13):E408–13.
43. Bowie EA, Glasgow GL. Cauda equina lesions associated with ankylosing spondylitis. Br Med J 1961;2:24–7.
44. Jordan AS, Spencer DG, Howe GB, Manolios N. Cauda equina syndrome in ankylosing spondylitis. J Clin Rheumatol 2013;19:163.

CHAPTER 24

Patient registries

Elisabeth Lie, Tore Kristian Kvien, and Mikkel Østergaard

Definition and rationale

A patient registry has been defined as 'an organized system that uses observational study methods to collect uniform data (clinical and other) to evaluate specified outcomes for a population defined by a particular disease, condition, or exposure, and that serves one or more predetermined scientific, clinical, or policy purposes' (1). There is no clear-cut distinction between longitudinal observational (cohort) studies, clinical databases, and patient registries, and some entities can certainly fit into more than one of these terms. Patient registries typically apply longitudinal observational methodology, and the legislative borders between registries, clinical databases, and longitudinal observational studies vary between countries. This chapter deals with systems that have most typically been described and organized as registries. Three longitudinal cohort studies within the axSpA field do, however, warrant particular mention, namely the Dutch–Belgian–French Outcome in Ankylosing Spondylitis International Study (OASIS) started in 1996 (2), the German Spondyloarthritis Inception Cohort (GESPIC) set up in 2000 (3), and the French DESIR cohort recruiting from 2007 to 2010, the acronym originating from 'outcome of recent undifferentiated spondyloarthritis' (in French, Devenir des Spondyloarthropathies Indifférenciées Récentes) (4). All three cohorts have been the basis for important studies of the epidemiology, diagnosis, and disease course of axSpA in general and AS in particular (2, 3, 5–8).

Patient registries can be either disease-based, that is encompassing all patients with a particular (group of) disease(s) within a defined geographical area, or exposure-/medication-based, such as the Spanish biologics registry BIOBADASER, including patients with rheumatic diseases treated with biologic DMARDs (9, 10). The purpose of a patient registry could be one or several things, including to describe the natural history of disease, to determine clinical effectiveness or cost-effectiveness of healthcare products and services, to measure or monitor safety and harm, and to measure quality of care (1). Data sources for registries include patient-reported data, clinician-reported data, extraction of data from medical charts and electronic health records (EHRs), as well as linkage to institutional, organizational, or administrative databases and other patient registries (1). The existing registries within the field of axSpA have to varying degrees applied these different approaches to obtain the relevant outcome and background/covariate data.

Registries versus randomized controlled trials

Since the 1940s, RCTs have constituted the gold standard for assessment of efficacy of therapeutic interventions in medicine. The ideal methodology is a randomized placebo-controlled trial with prespecified primary and secondary study endpoints and with participants, study personnel, and outcome assessors fully blinded for treatment allocation. With randomization it is expected that the probability of the outcome in the treated group is the same as in the untreated group had the untreated group been assigned to treatment—the groups are said to be interchangeable (11). The randomization process thus eliminates confounding by balancing observed and unobserved covariates across groups.

However, RCTs are costly to execute, and also have certain notable limitations. The inclusion criteria are often rather restrictive, including requirements of disease activity above a certain level, and they are often a means to specifically recruit patients that are expected to show response to treatment. In addition, most RCTs have several exclusion criteria, for example regarding age and comorbidities. In sum, this means that the results from RCTs may not be generalizable to the majority of patients treated in clinical practice (12, 13). Also, the study protocols of RCTs often include inflexible dosing schedules and restrictions regarding concomitant drug therapies. Furthermore, it has been suggested that the efficacy results of clinical trials may be biased by a phenomenon referred to as the Hawthorne effect (14). In this setting, the Hawthorne effect may be defined as an additional clinical improvement as a result of the increased medical attention associated with participation in a clinical trial (14). Another important limitation of RCTs is the short observation period of most trials, while the rheumatic diseases are chronic in nature. With short duration as well as limited sample sizes, most often based on power to detect differences in efficacy, RCTs are generally ill-suited to address rare adverse events and detect insidious side-effects.

Even though clinical trials remain the optimal method to assess new drug therapies, patient registries and longitudinal observational studies may in several ways provide information that is complementary to the knowledge obtained from RCTs. First, the potential for large cohorts and long follow-up time brings the opportunity to detect rare adverse events that unveil over time. Importantly, the safety of drugs can be assessed in patients exposed to the drugs in clinical practice, including patients with comorbidities.

Second, registries and observational studies constitute the preferred method for studying effectiveness, that is how well a drug performs in a real-life clinical setting, and are also important for pharmacoeconomic analyses (15, 16). In general, registries are associated with far lower costs than RCTs, and the purpose of a registry is often broad, allowing a multitude of research questions to be addressed, depending on the size of the registry and the diversity of (outcome) data available. However, the lack of a placebo group and random allocation to treatment is a challenge when using observational study and registry data to assess effectiveness and safety of drugs. In the absence of a placebo arm, one may not be certain that an observed improvement is caused by the intervention and is not due to 'regression towards the mean' or a placebo-like effect. With non-random assignment to treatment, any comparator group is likely to have different background covariates. Channelling occurs when drug therapies with similar indications are preferentially prescribed to groups of patients with different baseline prognoses, and is a source of bias when making comparisons. Further, if a covariate is associated with the outcome of question, the situation is often referred to as confounding by indication. The differences in background covariates can be adjusted for, and bias consequently reduced, by use of various techniques such as matching, stratification, multivariate adjustment, inverse probability of treatment weighting (IPTW), and methods based on the propensity score (matching, stratification, weighting, adjustment) (11, 17, 18).

Registries across the world

Following the availability of biologic DMARDs for the treatment of RA in 1999, so-called biologics registries were established in many European countries and in other parts of the world (19, 20). Most developed countries, and many developing countries, have disease-and/or medication-based registries encompassing patients with axSpA. The following sections describe just a few of these registries.

Examples of disease-based registries

Spondyloarthritis Research Consortium of Canada (SPARCC) was established to address important gaps of knowledge in SpA, regarding both genetics and pathogenesis, as well as clinical and imaging outcomes and outcome measures (21, 22). To address these issues, SPARCC developed a registry or database of patients with AS and nr-axSpA, as well as other forms of SpA. The registry includes registration of a wide range of SpA features, comorbidities, clinical examination, patient questionnaires, and laboratory measures (21).

In a joint effort, the Spondylitis Association of America (SAA), Spondyloarthritis Research and Treatment Network (SPARTAN), and SPARCC have sought to combine three existing SpA longitudinal cohorts/registries in North America (20, 23). The three entities are the Prospective Study of Outcomes in Ankylosing Spondylitis (PSOAS), the Toronto University Health Network Spondylitis Program (which is also part of the SPARCC registry), and the Program to Understand the Longterm Outcomes in Spondyloarthritis (PULSAR). PSOAS was started in 2002, with the main aim to study genetic markers of AS severity, and more than 1000 patients have been enrolled (20, 23, 24). PSOAS includes genetic, serological, and radiographic data, as well as a wide range of clinical variables and outcomes. Patients are followed longitudinally with regular study visits, which include extensive standardized clinical, psychological, and sociodemographic instruments (20, 23). Since 2001, a large number of patients with axSpA, including AS, have been followed longitudinally in the Toronto University Health Network Spondylitis Program, with much of the same data collected as described for PSOAS (20, 23). More than 100 new patients with AS have been added to the cohort each year, and follow-up visits are scheduled every 6 months (23). PULSAR, which was started in 2007, is a prospective registry of patients with SpA within the US Department of Veterans Affairs healthcare system (20, 23). Upon entry to the registry, the patients are carefully clinically phenotyped, and blood samples are collected and stored for future analysis. The Veterans Affairs healthcare system yields the possibility to capture a wide range of health data, and follow-up also includes standardized SpA-specific metrology data and patient-reported outcome measures (23).

The Spanish National Spondyloarthropathies Registry (Registro Español de Espondiloartritis de la Sociedad Española de Reumatologia, REGISPONSER) was launched in 2004 by the Spondyloarthropathies Study Group of the Spanish Society of Rheumatology and includes a selected group of rheumatology centres committed to recruiting at least 100 consecutive SpA patients, each over a period of 12 months (25–27). The registry is internet-based, and the collected cross-sectional data include sociodemographic information, details on diagnosis, clinical examination, patient-reported outcomes, radiography, laboratory tests, and treatment information. Since 2005, the REGISPONSER protocol has been exported to several other countries, with formation of the Ibero-American Registry of Spondyloarthritis (Registro Ibero-Americano de Espondiloartrites, RESPONDIA) (20). After the Spanish REGISPONSER, the largest registry participating in RESPONDIA is the Brazilian Registry of Spondyloarthritis (20, 28).

The Scotland Registry for Ankylosing Spondylitis (SIRAS) includes approximately 2000 patients who are followed longitudinally for 2 years, with an extensive data collection (29). There is also a Korean spondyloarthritis registry—the Observation Study of Spondyloarthropathy Registry (OSKAR)—with longitudinal follow-up of patients with AS and other SpA (30). Data collected in the registry include demographics and disease characteristics, HLA-B27 genotyping, EAMs and comorbidities, patient-reported outcomes including BASDAI and BASFI, and radiographic data (20, 30).

Examples of medication-based registries

Sweden has a long tradition of maintaining population-based registries, and several national and regional rheumatology registries have been established since the mid-1990s. The Swedish biologics registry, ARTIS, was established in late 1999 and is a branch of the Swedish Rheumatology Quality Register (31–33). The ARTIS registry is a nationwide registry that includes patients with rheumatic diseases starting treatment with biologic DMARDs (i.e. incident users of biologic DMARDs). The registry coverage for patients with SpA treated with ETN or adalimumab has recently been estimated at 86% (34). The Swedish Rheumatology Association holds ownership to and overall responsibility for the registry. Direct electronic, web-based registrations have been gradually implemented since 2003. Two relatively large regional registries report to the ARTIS registry, namely the STURE (Stockholm TNFα Follow-up Registry) in the Stockholm region in eastern Sweden, and the SSATG (South Swedish Arthritis Treatment Group) registry in southern Sweden (31, 32). The data collection includes both safety and effectiveness outcomes, and patients are followed up at 3, 6, 12, 18, 24 months, and so on. All Swedish residents have a unique personal identification number that is recorded in all medical files, all rheumatology registries (including ARTIS), and all national health and census registries. Hence, linkage of ARTIS to valuable data sources such as the National Patient Registry (data on in-patient and out-patient care), the Cause of Death Registry, and the National Cancer Registry has been used to retrieve reliable data regarding safety outcomes (32). There is no unexposed comparator group within ARTIS, but relevant control groups can be extracted from the National Patient Registry. This methodology has been used to study a range of safety issues in patients with RA (32).

The Danish biologics registry, DANBIO, was established in 2000 and includes patients with RA, PsA, and AS (35). From 2005, patients on synthetic DMARDs have been registered as well, and these patients make up an internal comparator population. DANBIO has included patients with PsA and AS since 2000, and in 2003 the BASDAI, BASFI, and BASMI were included as outcome measures for patients with axial disease (35). In 2005, an online version of the registry was launched as well, based on an open-source software that has later been adopted by the Swiss Clinical Quality Management (SCQM) registry and the Icelandic ICEBIO registry (35). As for the Swedish registry, the online registration not only makes the maintenance of the registry more efficient, it also constitutes a useful clinical follow-up tool, and patients can enter data on patient-reported outcomes directly into the system by use of touch screens in the waiting rooms (35). From 2006, the registration of patients on biologic DMARDs in DANBIO has been mandatory, and the completeness for this part of the registry has been estimated to around 92% (35). More than 1500 AS patients receiving biologic DMARDs and more than 1000 AS patients receiving synthetic DMARDs are registered in DANBIO. Study visits are generally not prescheduled but take place approximately every 6 months. Linkage to other data sources such as the national cancer registry and the hospitalization registry is possible in a similar manner as for the Swedish biologics registry (35).

The British Society for Rheumatology Biologics Registry (BSRBR) has been running since 2001 and is one of the world's largest biologics registries (36, 37). The primary aim of the registry has been to investigate the long-term outcomes in patients with RA treated with biologic agents, with a focus on safety issues (37, 38). Sample size calculations were made based on the ability to detect a two-fold increased risk of lymphoma, and samples needed equated to recruitment of 4000 patients with RA for each biologic agent, with 5 years of follow-up per patient (38). Data from the Office for National Statistics are additionally used to ascertain deaths and cases of cancer (38). Between 2002 and 2006, the BSRBR recruited a small cohort of patients with AS starting treatment with their first TNFi (39). In 2012, the BSRBR-AS was relaunched, with plans to recruit patients with axSpA treated with TNFi, as well as a comparator cohort of patients not treated with these drugs, through 2016 (29). As of April 2015, more than 1250 patients had been included in this second phase of the BSRBR-AS. In both phases, a wide range of clinical data, including, BASDAI and BASFI, have been collected at regular intervals.

The Spanish Biologics Registry BIOBADASER (Base de Datos de Productos Biológicos de la Sociedad Española de Reumatología) was established in 2000 by the Spanish Society for Rheumatology to investigate the long-term safety of biologic DMARDs in rheumatic diseases (9, 40). In phase 1 of the registry the number of participating centres was unrestricted. About 100 centres participated, and the coverage was estimated at around 50%. In order to achieve higher data quality, the number of participating centres was reduced to 14 in July 2006, and this marked the beginning of the second phase of the registry, titled BIOBADASER 2.0 (9). The 14 centres were selected based on successful participation in phase I of the registry and are all large public hospitals (9, 41). The data collection, which is online and based on a specifically designed software solution, includes registration of 'relevant adverse events' as defined by the study protocol, the severity and outcome of such events, and any concomitant medication used at the time of occurrence. Further, the data collection includes relevant confounding factors and data related to discontinuation and duration of treatment (9). There are no set time points for patient evaluation, but there are specific guidelines for how to registry data. Since 2008, the procedure has also included yearly direct contact with registered patients for additional validation (41).

Examples of registry-based research in axial spondyloarthritis

Epidemiology of AS and AS severity

In a cross-sectional study of 1316 patients with AS from the REGISPONSER, published in 2011, Almodóvar et al. compared disease characteristics of patients who had first-degree relatives with SpA ('familial AS') versus those who did not ('sporadic AS'). They found that the former group of patients were more often female, younger at symptom onset, and more often HLA-B27 positive, and a larger proportion had a history of uveitis (27). A study of 402 AS patients from the North American PSOAS compared demographics and disease characteristics, including radiographic scores, between patients with juvenile onset of symptoms, defined as ≤16 years of age (n = 79) and patients with adult/older onset (n = 323) (42). Except from a somewhat higher proportion of women in the juvenile onset group (32.9% vs 22.9%), the groups were similar. However, by multivariable analyses, adjusting for multiple covariates, radiographic hip score was higher and need for total hip arthroplasty more frequent in the juvenile group, while the radiographic spine score was lower (42). In another study, also from PSOAS, Lee et al. looked at gender differences in clinical and radiographic characteristics among patients with AS (43). As in the Spanish REGISPONSER, a family history of AS in a first-degree relative was more common among female AS patients, and age at AS onset was also somewhat lower. Furthermore, radiographic severity (Bath Ankylosing Spondylitis Radiographic Index (BASRI) spine score) was worse among men. Function, measured by BASFI, was similar in males and females, but when adjusting for BASRI spine score, BASFI scores were worse in females (43).

Radiographic severity has also been the focus of other studies from PSOAS. Ward et al. studied the association between occupational activities and radiographic damage measured by BASRI spine score in a cohort of 397 patients with AS, and found that exposure to jobs with whole-body vibration, and jobs requiring more dynamic flexibility and extent flexibility, were associated with worse radiographic scores (24). The same group also studied clinical and immunogenetic predictors of radiographic severity, and found independent associations with male sex, current smoking, older age at onset, and several HLA genotypes (*HLA-B*4100, DRB1*0804, DQA1*0401, DQB1*0603*, and *DPB1*0202*) (44). Conversely, the genotype *DRB1*0801* was a strong negative predictor of BASRI spine score. Kim et al. used cross-sectional and longitudinal data from the Korean OSKAR registry to study the association between radiographic damage of the cervical and lumbar spine and heterozygosity versus homozygosity for HLA-B27 among HLA-B27-positive patients with AS. There was no statistically significant difference either for radiographic damage score cross-sectionally or for radiographic progression over 5 years (30).

Genetic association studies

Several genetics papers have come out of the SPARCC registry. In 2006, Maksymowych et al. published the finding of an association of AS with several single nucleotide polymorphisms (SNPs) in the *IL1* gene region in a study of 394 patients with AS and 446 controls (45). Later, in a larger study, association with SNPs in the *IL23R* locus was demonstrated, and found to be independent of concurrent psoriasis and IBD in AS patients (46). In 2009, the group published association between AS and a specific *ERAP1* (a non-major histocompatibility complex encoding an endoplasmatic reticulum aminopepdidase) haplotype (47).

Effectiveness of TNF inhibitors

Several European biologics registers have reported effectiveness results for TNFi treatment in AS (Fig. 24.1). One large study, including 842 patients with AS treated with their first TNFi, came out of the DANBIO registry (48). The estimated 1- and 2-year drug survival rates were 74% and 63%, respectively. Clinical response was defined as either 50% or 20 mm (2 units) improvement in BASDAI, and 63% achieved such a response at least once over the first 6 months (48). In a later DANBIO publication, which included 1436 patients with AS, it was reported that BASDAI response was achieved by 54% of patients within the first 6 months (49).

Lord et al. reported effectiveness results in 261 patients with AS who were included in the BSRBR between 2002 and 2006 and who had at least 6 months follow-up data. BASDAI50 response at 6 months was achieved by 52% of patients, and the mean improvement in BASDAI score was 3.6 units (39). The Register of Biologic Treatment in Finland (ROB-FIN) group published TNFi effectiveness results in 229 patients with AS in 2007 and found an ASAS 20 response rate of 79% (50). A study of 310 patients with AS from the Czech national biologics registry ATTRA found 1- and 3-year retention rates of 84% and 72%, respectively, and 65.9% reaching a BASDAI score < 4 at 6 months from a mean baseline BASDAI of 6.4 (51).

In a publication from the SCQM registry, Ciurea et al. compared disease burden and response to TNFi treatment in patients with r- and nr-axSpA. At 1 year, 48.9% of 239 patients with r-axSpA versus 34.6% of 54 patients with nr-axSpA achieved a BASDAI 50 response, while 48.1% versus 29.6% reached an ASAS 40 response (52). In a publication from the regional SSATG registry of 112 patients with axSpA other than AS, 49% of patients achieved BASDAI 50 response at 6 months (53). Fagerli et al. reported 3-month response rates among patients with axSpA included in the NOR-DMARD. BASDAI 50 and ASAS 40 responses were achieved by 48.0% and 43.1%, respectively, of the 339 patients who were DMARD naïve, with similar response rates observed in a smaller group of patients who had previously been treated with SSZ (54).

Predictors of TNF inhibitor response and retention

The study from DANBIO, referred to in the section Effectiveness of TNF inhibitors, also investigated both predictors of TNFi retention and BASDAI response. Male sex, lower level of fatigue, and elevated CRP at baseline were independently associated with better drug survival, while elevated CRP, lower BASFI at baseline, and younger age were independent predictors of BASDAI response

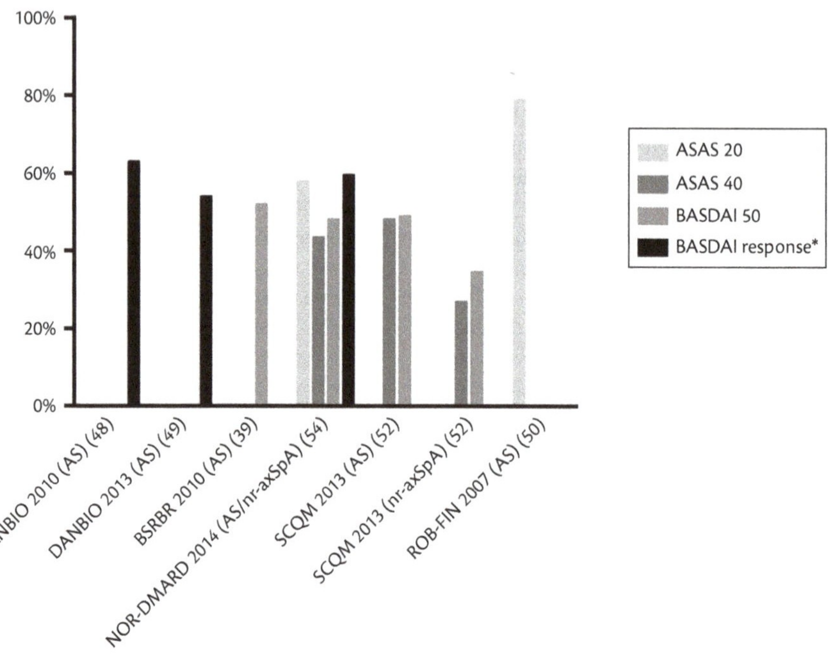

Fig. 24.1 TNFi response rates reported for axSpA in European biologics registers. Reference number is given in parentheses. Asterisk denotes response defined as 50% and/or 2 units (20 mm) of improvement in BASDAI.

(48). In the BSRBR study, Lord et al. analysed baseline predictors of BASDAI 50 response at 6 months and found that male sex, higher BASDAI, lower BASFI, elevated inflammatory markers, and comedication with MTX or any DMARD were independently associated with achieving BASDAI 50 response, while current smoking was a negative predictor (39). A study from the SCQM registry sought to specifically study the effect of current smoking on TNFi response. Current smoking was found to be a negative predictor of response versus never smoking, adjusted for a range of other factors previously shown to be predictors of TNFi response (55). A study of 243 patients with AS in the SSATG registry showed that male sex and peripheral arthritis were associated with better drug survival (56).

TNF inhibitor switching

The effectiveness of treatment with a second and third TNFi has been studied in DANBIO, from which results for 432 patients treated with a second and 137 patients treated with a third TNFi were reported (Fig. 24.2). Retention to therapy was reduced for the second and third TNFi compared to the first (47% and 49% vs 58%, respectively, at 2 years), and the proportions achieving BASDAI response (50% or 20 mm improvement) were 37% and 30%, respectively, versus 54% for the first TNFi (49). An earlier, smaller study for NOR-DMARD, including 77 patients treated with a second TNFi, found 3-month BASDAI 50 and ASAS 40 response rates of 28% and 31%, respectively, and, similarly to results from the DANBIO study, poorer retention to therapy of the second TNFi compared to the first (57). With regard to effectiveness of the second TNFi, no clear relation with reason for discontinuation of the first TNFi was found in either study (49, 57).

Safety of TNF inhibitors

Important information regarding the safety of TNFi has come out of some of the major biologics registers, but these studies have with few exceptions been performed solely in patients with RA (58–61). One exception is a publication from DANBIO by Dreyer et al. that investigated the risk of cancer in arthritis patients exposed to TNFi, and the study included 861 AS patients treated and 136 AS patients never treated with these drugs (62). For patients with AS, the standardized incidence ratio (SIR) (95% CI) versus the general population was 0.82 (0.41–1.64), and also there was no signal of increased risk for patients with RA and PsA. Site-specific SIRs and HRs versus patients not exposed to TNFi were only reported for patients with RA, due to small numbers for the other diseases (62).

Several publications from the Spanish biologics registry BIOBADASER have also included patients with AS/SpA when addressing various safety issues related to TNFi treatment (63–66). Carmona et al. analysed cancer rates in patients with rheumatic diseases exposed to TNFi, and patients with AS (761 patients, 2288 patient-years) constituted the second largest patient group (63). The study did not find higher cancer rates compared to the background Spanish population. SIRs for all-site malignancy and specific cancer types for RA, AS, and PsA were included in the publication (63). Another BIOBADASER study found significantly increased risk of hospitalization due to varicella zoster virus infections (shingles and chickenpox) in rheumatic patients exposed to

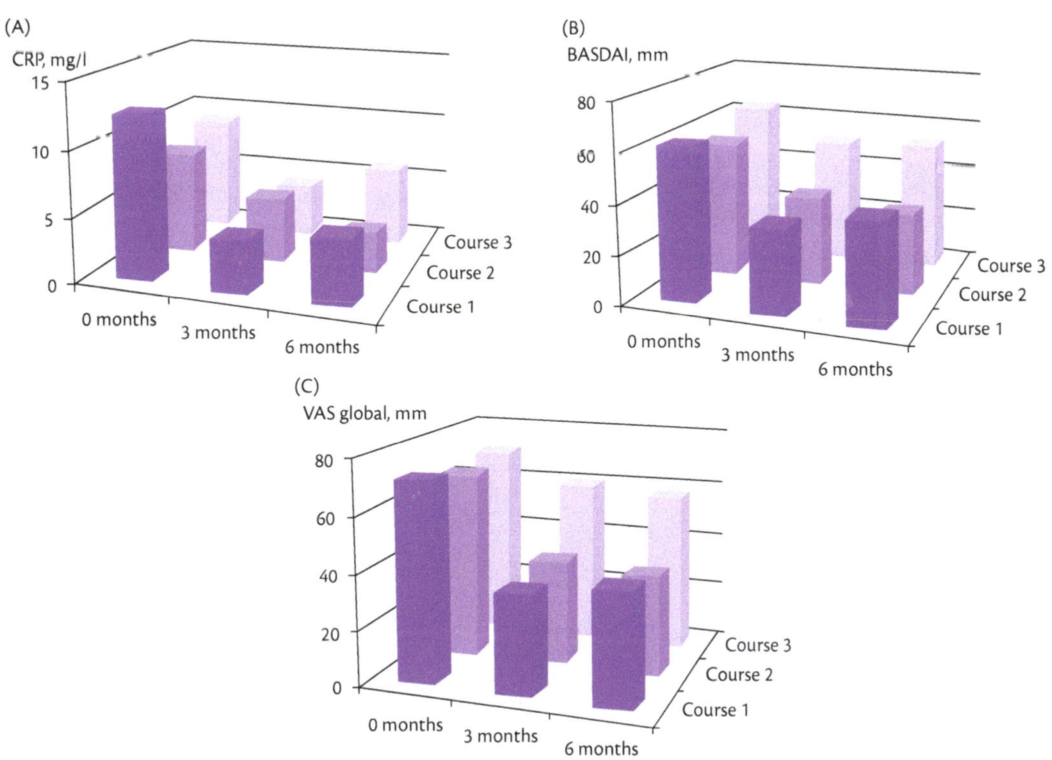

Fig. 24.2 Disease activity for switchers at baseline, 3 months, and 6 months during biologic treatment course 1 (dark purple), course 2 (purple), and course 3 (light purple) (n = 432). Columns show medians. Study from the Danish Biologics Registry DANBIO.

From: Glintborg B et al, Ann Rheum Dis 2013;72(7):1149–55. Copyright BMJ Publishing Group Ltd, reproduced with permission.

TNFi compared to the general population, with an SIR (95% CI) of 9 (3–20) for shingles and 19 (5–47) for chickenpox (64). Peña-Sagredo et al. addressed the association between TNFi treatment and non-*typhi Salmonella* infection, and found no increased risk of such infection, but increased risk of severe complications, suggesting increased risk of disseminated *Salmonella* infection (65). Finally, in a case series on demyelinating disease from 21 425 patient-years of follow-up from patients in BIOBADASER (including 2870 patient-years in patients with AS), a total of 14 cases were found, of which two occurred in patients with AS (66).

Working status and work disability

Verstappen et al. studied the working status of patients with RA, AS, and PsA treated with TNFi and included in BSRBR, and 229 patients with AS were included, of whom 41% were work-disabled at baseline. During follow-up, 4.0% (5 of 125) of working AS patients became work disabled, and 8.5% (8 of 94) work-disabled AS patients started to work again (67). A study of 139 patients with AS from the SSATG registry examined proportions on sick leave and disability pension before and after treatment with TNFi, with data retrieved from the Swedish Social Insurance Agency; they found a decline in proportion of patients on sick leave during the first 12 months of treatment, while the proportion on disability pension remained unchanged (68).

TNF inhibitors in ankylosing spondylitis versus other diagnoses

A large number of registry-based studies have compared outcomes with TNFi treatment in AS and other rheumatic diseases, in particular RA. In the publication from the Czech ATTRA registry (see section 'Effectiveness of TNF inhibitors'), Pavelka et al. reported significantly longer drug survival for patients with AS compared to patients with RA, with a larger difference observed among men than women (51). Similarly, a study from the Brazilian biologics registry BIOBADABRASIL compared 372 patients with AS and 901 patients with RA treated with their first TNFi, and found that drug survival was better in AS, with an HR (95% CI) of 1.62 (1.14–2.31) (adjusted for sex and corticosteroid use) (69). A study from BIOBADASER published in 2006 compared drug survival rates of 4006 patients with RA and 1524 patients with various types of SpA (of whom 657 were diagnosed with AS), and the rates were consistently higher for patients with AS and other SpA at 1, 2, and 3 years (70). Using data from NOR-DMARD, Heiberg et al. compared retention to therapy and HRQoL outcomes in TNFi-treated patients with AS, RA, and PsA, and found superior retention to therapy in AS and PsA versus RA, and somewhat greater improvements in HRQoL in AS compared to RA (71, 72).

Other studies on treatment of axial spondyloarthritis

A non-randomized single-centre Czech study within the ATTRA registry compared the effectiveness, safety, and cost of reduced versus standard dose TNFi treatment in 244 AS patients who had achieved low disease activity on treatment (73). Over 6 months there was no significant difference in disease activity measures or rates of relapse and adverse events, but there was a substantial difference in costs (mean (95% CI) net monetary benefit €–3354 (€–4989 to –1666)) (Fig. 24.3).

The effect of comedication with conventional synthetic DMARDs on TNFi drug survival was addressed in a study from the Swedish biologics registry ARTIS. The study included 1365 patients with AS and 1155 patients with uSpA, of whom 40.8% and 50.3%, respectively, used comedication at baseline. Comedication was

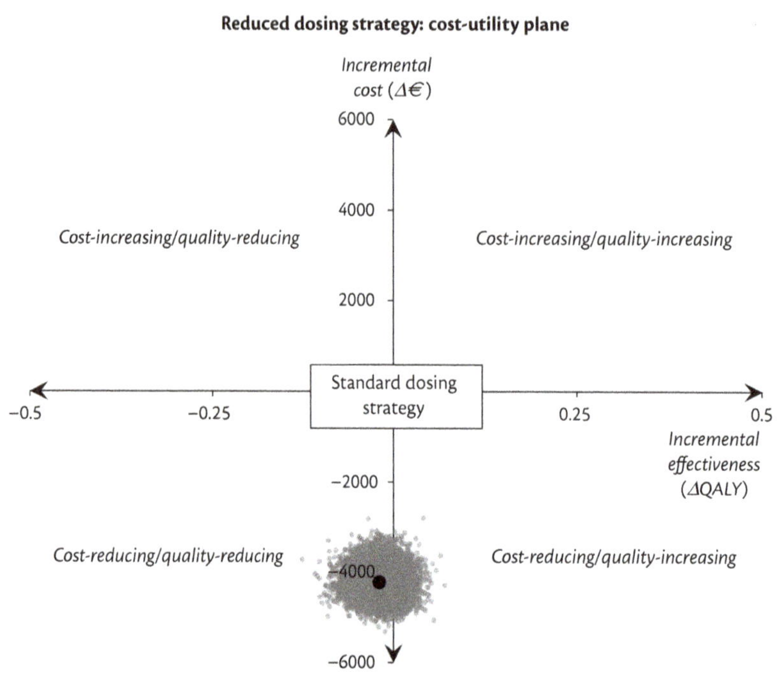

Fig. 24.3 Cost-utility plane: reduced versus standard dosing strategy. QALY, Quality-adjusted life year. Study from the Czech Biologics Registry ATTRA.
From: Zavada J et al, Ann Rheum Dis 2014. Published online first: 27 Aug 2014. doi: 10.1136/annrheumdis-2014-20520. Copyright BMJ Publishing Group Ltd., reproduced with permission.

Table 24.1 Baseline characteristics of patients with AS starting TNFi, across registries

	ARAD (75)	DANBIO (48)	ATTRA (51)	BSRBR (39)	SCQM (52)	ARTIS (74)	BIOBADABRASIL (69)
n	354	842	310	261	363	1365	372
Age (years)	45.1	41*	36.8	43*	–	43.8	43.7
Percentage males	71.8	72	76.8	81.6	74.7	72.9	80.1
Disease duration (years)	18.5	5*	8.1	13*	12.2*	14.0*	10.5
Percentage HLA-B27+	–	–	–	–	83.9	–	71.7
Percentage on MTX	14.1	40.7	–	34.5	–	31.4	32.5
Percentage on any DMARD	20.3	–	–	44.4	–	40.8	43.0
BASDAI	7.6	5.9*	6.4	7.6*	5.8*	–	5.6
BASFI	–	5.0*	5.4	7.9*	4.0*	–	–
CRP (mg/L)	31.8	14*	31.0	23*	11*	13*	–
Patient global (0–100)	–	67	–	–	70*	57.5	–

Reference number is given in parentheses. Values are means unless otherwise indicated. *Median value.

TNF, Tumour necrosis factor; MTX, methotrexate; DMARD, disease modifying anti-rheumatic drug; BASDAI, Bath Ankylosing Spondylitis Disease Activity Index; BASFI, Bath Ankylosing Spondylitis Functional Index; CRP, C-reactive protein; ARAD, Australian Rheumatology Association Database; DANBIO, Danish Biologics Register; ATTRA, Czech biologics register; BSRBR, British Society for Rheumatology Biologics Register; SCQM, Swiss Clinical Quality Management; ARTIS, Anti-Rheumatic Treatment in Sweden; BIOBADABRASIL, Brazilian Registry of Biological Therapies in Rheumatic Diseases.

most frequently MTX, followed by SSZ. By multivariable analysis, comedication was associated with superior drug survival both in AS (HR (95% CI) 0.71 (0.59–0.85)) and uSpA (HR (95% CI) 0.82 (0.69–0.97)) (74). Sensitivity analysis in a subgroup of patients, with available information on whether the conventional synthetic DMARD was used before start of the TNFi or initiated simultaneously as comedication, revealed that the difference versus comedication non-users was somewhat more pronounced in those treated with DMARD before TNFi and who continued it as comedication, and was also present in patients who stopped conventional synthetic DMARD treatment when starting TNFi treatment.

Oldroyd et al. reported on the baseline characteristics (Table 24.1) of 354 patients with AS included in the Australian Rheumatology Association Database (ARAD) and exposed to biologic therapy. Compared to participants in RCTs on biologic DMARDs, the patients in the registry were older and had longer disease duration and higher baseline disease activity, measured by BASDAI. The ARAD patients also had a high frequency of comorbidities, with 66% reporting at least one comorbid condition and 46% reporting more than one, and 24 of 198 patients (6.8%) with available data had a previous malignancy (non-melanoma skin cancer in 15 of 24 patients) (75).

A study from NOR-DMARD assessed the effectiveness of SSZ in 181 patients with axSpA. Drug survival over 3 years was poor, and the clinical responses were generally modest, but somewhat better response was observed in patients with swollen joints at baseline. By Cox regression analysis, absence of joint swelling, higher CRP, and higher BASDAI back pain score at baseline were independently associated with discontinuation of SSZ (54).

The importance of patient registries in axial spondyloarthritis

As described in this chapter, the number and range of patient registries covering axSpA is large and has been steadily growing over the past couple of decades. The registries have been and will continue to be essential to provide knowledge on the epidemiology and disease course, and are also a potential basis for studies of the genetics of axSpA, which may again fuel research on the pathogenesis of the disease. The ASAS classification criteria for axSpA, published in 2009, have strengthened the concept of axSpA as one disease with a spectrum from non-radiographic to radiographic disease (i.e. AS) (76, 77). The main body of the knowledge regarding epidemiology and disease course as well as genetics is currently from studies only including patients with AS, and much less is known about patients with nr-axSpA, a group that may or may not later in the disease course develop radiographic changes to meet the definition of AS.

The main objective of all the major treatment registries for inflammatory arthritis established since the introduction of biologic DMARDs has been to assess the safety of these new drugs, and it is within this area that the biologics registries have contributed the most. However, as the brief summary in this chapter shows, the main body of this research has been conducted on patients with RA. Thus there is a need for studies addressing the same safety issues in patients with other diseases, including axSpA, as well as a need for confirmation of previously published results in independent cohorts and registries. Also, with new therapies being introduced, some with SpA (and/or other conditions such as psoriasis and PsA) rather than RA as the main therapeutic area, having large and robust patient registries capable of effective pharmacosurveillance in SpA will continue to be important.

Registry data are also important to confirm, or sometimes to modify and even refute, efficacy results from clinical trials. The magnitude of benefit from treatment shown in clinical trials may not always be reproducible in clinical practice. Furthermore, some research questions are less likely to become subject to specific trials or observational studies, and data from treatment registries may then be of high value. The large numbers of patients included in most registries can also be beneficial in some cases. Effectiveness results from treatment registries may also generate hypotheses that can be further addressed in RCTs or specifically designed longitudinal observational studies. However, the less standardized data collection, limited availability of appropriate comparator groups, and frequent lack of prespecified effectiveness objectives are factors that must be considered when planning analyses and interpreting results. Adjustment techniques to account for channelling bias and methods for imputation of missing data can only to a certain degree make up for the inherent limitations of treatment registries. RCTs are essential to establish superiority of a certain treatment or treatment strategy over another, and cannot be replaced by any type of observational study design. Registries can and should be data sources for studies of treatment effectiveness, but should not replace investigator-initiated interventional research and more specific longitudinal observational studies.

References

1. Gliklich R, Dreyer N, Leavy M (eds). Registries for Evaluating Patient Outcomes: A User's Guide, 3rd edn. Rockville, Agency for Healthcare Research and Quality, 2014, AHRQ Publication no. 13(14)-EHC111. http://www.effectivehealthcare.ahrq.gov/registries-guide-3.cfm.
2. Ramiro S, Stolwijk C, van Tubergen A, et al. Evolution of radiographic damage in ankylosing spondylitis: a 12 year prospective follow-up of the OASIS study. Ann Rheum Dis 2015;74(1):52–9.
3. Rudwaleit M, Haibel H, Baraliakos X, et al. The early disease stage in axial spondylarthritis: results from the German Spondyloarthritis Inception Cohort. Arthritis Rheum 2009;60(3):717–27.
4. Dougados M, d'Agostino MA, Benessiano J, et al. The DESIR cohort: a 10-year follow-up of early inflammatory back pain in France: study design and baseline characteristics of the 708 recruited patients. Joint Bone Spine 2011;78(6):598–603.
5. Essers I, Ramiro S, Stolwijk C, et al. Characteristics associated with the presence and development of extra-articular manifestations in ankylosing spondylitis: 12-year results from OASIS. Rheumatology (Oxford) 2015;54(4):633–40.
6. Poddubnyy D, Haibel H, Listing J, et al. Cigarette smoking has a dose-dependent impact on progression of structural damage in the spine in patients with axial spondyloarthritis: results from the German Spondyloarthritis Inception Cohort (GESPIC). Ann Rheum Dis 2013;72(8):1430–2.
7. Molto A, Paternotte S, van der Heijde D, Claudepierre P, Rudwaleit M, Dougados M. Evaluation of the validity of the different arms of the ASAS set of criteria for axial spondyloarthritis and description of the different imaging abnormalities suggestive of spondyloarthritis: data from the DESIR cohort. Ann Rheum Dis 2015;74(4):746–51.
8. Blachier M, Canoui-Poitrine F, Dougados M, et al. Factors associated with radiographic lesions in early axial spondyloarthritis. Results from the DESIR cohort. Rheumatology (Oxford) 2013;52(9):1686–93.
9. Spanish Registry of Adverse Events of Biological Therapies in Rheumatic Diseases (BIOBADASER). https://biobadaser.ser.es/biobadaser/eng/index.html.
10. Carmona L, de la Vega M, Ranza R, et al. BIOBADASER, BIOBADAMERICA, and BIOBADADERM: safety registers sharing commonalities across diseases and countries. Clin Exp Rheumatol 2014;32(5 Suppl 85):S163–7.
11. Choi HK, Seeger JD. Observational research in rheumatic disorders. Rheum Dis Clin North Am 2004;30(4):685–99.
12. Zink A, Strangfeld A, Schneider M, et al. Effectiveness of tumor necrosis factor inhibitors in rheumatoid arthritis in an observational cohort study: comparison of patients according to their eligibility for major randomized clinical trials. Arthritis Rheum 2006;54(11):3399–407.
13. Greenberg JD, Kishimoto M, Strand V, et al. Tumor necrosis factor antagonist responsiveness in a United States rheumatoid arthritis cohort. Am J Med 2008;121(6):532–8.
14. Wolfe F, Michaud K. The Hawthorne effect, sponsored trials, and the overestimation of treatment effectiveness. J Rheumatol 2010;37(11):2216–20.
15. Bombardier C, Maetzel A. Pharmacoeconomic evaluation of new treatments: efficacy versus effectiveness studies? Ann Rheum Dis 1999;58(Suppl 1):I82–5.
16. van Vollenhoven RF, Severens JL. Observational studies: a valuable source for data on the true value of RA therapies. Clin Rheumatol 2011;30(Suppl 1):S19–24.
17. Kurth T, Walker AM, Glynn RJ, et al. Results of multivariable logistic regression, propensity matching, propensity adjustment, and propensity-based weighting under conditions of nonuniform effect. Am J Epidemiol 2006;163(3):262–70.
18. Lunt M, Solomon D, Rothman K, et al. Different methods of balancing covariates leading to different effect estimates in the presence of effect modification. Am J Epidemiol 2009;169(7):909–17.
19. Zink A, Askling J, Dixon WG, Klareskog L, Silman AJ, Symmons DP. European biologicals registers: methodology, selected results and perspectives. Ann Rheum Dis 2009;68(8):1240–6.
20. Reveille JD. A registry of ankylosing spondylitis registries and prospects for global interfacing. Curr Opin Rheumatol 2013;25(4):468–76.
21. Gladman DD, Rahman P, Cook RJ, et al. The Spondyloarthritis Research Consortium of Canada registry for spondyloarthritis. J Rheumatol 2011;38(7):1343–8.
22. Spondyloarthritis Research Consortium of Canada (SPARCC). http://www.sparcc.ca.
23. Caplan L, Clegg DO, Inman RD. Ankylosing spondylitis clinical registries: principles, practices and possibilities. Am J Med Sci 2013;345(6):437–9.
24. Ward MM, Reveille JD, Learch TJ, Davis JC Jr, Weisman MH. Occupational physical activities and long-term functional and radiographic outcomes in patients with ankylosing spondylitis. Arthritis Rheum 2008;59(6):822–32.
25. Collantes E, Zarco P, Munoz E, et al. Disease pattern of spondyloarthropathies in Spain: description of the first national registry (REGISPONSER) extended report. Rheumatology (Oxford) 2007;46(8):1309–15.
26. Almodóvar R, Zarco P, Collantes E, et al. Relationship between spinal mobility and disease activity, function, quality of life and radiology. A cross-sectional Spanish registry of spondyloarthropathies (REGISPONSER). Clin Exp Rheumatol 2009;27(3):439–45.
27. Almodóvar R, Font P, Zarco-Montejo P, et al. Phenotypic differences between familial versus sporadic ankylosing spondylitis: a cross-sectional Spanish registry of spondyloarthropathies (REGISPONSER). Clin Exp Rheumatol 2011;29(5):822–7.
28. Skare TL, Leite N, Bortoluzzo AB, et al. Effect of age at disease onset in the clinical profile of spondyloarthritis: a study of 1424 Brazilian patients. Clin Exp Rheumatol 2012;30(3):351–7.
29. University of Aberdeen, Epidemiology Research, Spondyloarthritis. http://www.abdn.ac.uk/iahs/research/epidemiology/spondyloarthritis.php.
30. Kim TJ, Sung IH, Lee S, et al. HLA-B27 homozygosity has no influence on radiographic damage in ankylosing spondylitis: Observation Study of Korean spondyloArthropathy Registry (OSKAR) data. Joint Bone Spine 2013;80(5):488–91.
31. van Vollenhoven RF, Askling J. Rheumatoid arthritis registries in Sweden. Clin Exp Rheumatol 2005;23(5 Suppl 39):S195–200.
32. Askling J, Fored CM, Geborek P, et al. Swedish registers to examine drug safety and clinical issues in RA. Ann Rheum Dis 2006;65(6):707–12.
33. Eriksson JK, Askling J, Arkema EV. The Swedish Rheumatology Quality Register: optimisation of rheumatic disease assessments using register-enriched data. Clin Exp Rheumatol 2014;32(5 Suppl 85):S147–9.
34. Wadstrom H, Eriksson JK, Neovius M, Askling J. How good is the coverage and how accurate are exposure data in the Swedish Biologics Register (ARTIS)? Scand J Rheumatol 2015;44(1):22–8.

35. Hetland ML. DANBIO—powerful research database and electronic patient record. Rheumatology (Oxford) 2011;50(1):69–77.
36. British Society for Rheumatology Biologics Register (BSRBR). http://www.rheumatology.org.uk/resources/bsr_biologics_registers/default.aspx.
37. Silman A, Symmons D, Scott DG, Griffiths I. British Society for Rheumatology Biologics Register. Ann Rheum Dis 2003;62(Suppl 2):ii28–9.
38. Hyrich KL, Watson KD, Isenberg DA, Symmons DP. The British Society for Rheumatology Biologics Register: 6 years on. Rheumatology (Oxford) 2008;47(10):1441–3.
39. Lord PA, Farragher TM, Lunt M, Watson KD, Symmons DP, Hyrich KL. Predictors of response to anti-TNF therapy in ankylosing spondylitis: results from the British Society for Rheumatology Biologics Register. Rheumatology (Oxford) 2010;49(3):563–70.
40. Gomez-Reino JJ, Carmona L, Valverde VR, Mola EM, Montero MD. Treatment of rheumatoid arthritis with tumor necrosis factor inhibitors may predispose to significant increase in tuberculosis risk: a multicenter active-surveillance report. Arthritis Rheum 2003;48(8):2122–7.
41. Carmona L, Descalzo MA, Ruiz-Montesinos D, Manero-Ruiz FJ, Perez-Pampin E, Gomez-Reino JJ. Safety and retention rate of off-label uses of TNF antagonists in rheumatic conditions: data from the Spanish registry BIOBADASER 2.0. Rheumatology (Oxford) 2011;50(1):85–92.
42. Gensler LS, Ward MM, Reveille JD, Learch TJ, Weisman MH, Davis JC Jr. Clinical, radiographic and functional differences between juvenile-onset and adult-onset ankylosing spondylitis: results from the PSOAS cohort. Ann Rheum Dis 2008;67(2):233–7.
43. Lee W, Reveille JD, Davis JC Jr, Learch TJ, Ward MM, Weisman MH. Are there gender differences in severity of ankylosing spondylitis? Results from the PSOAS cohort. Ann Rheum Dis 2007;66(5):633–8.
44. Ward MM, Hendrey MR, Malley JD, et al. Clinical and immunogenetic prognostic factors for radiographic severity in ankylosing spondylitis. Arthritis Rheum 2009;61(7):859–66.
45. Maksymowych WP, Rahman P, Reeve JP, Gladman DD, Peddle L, Inman RD. Association of the IL1 gene cluster with susceptibility to ankylosing spondylitis: an analysis of three Canadian populations. Arthritis Rheum 2006;54(3):974–85.
46. Rahman P, Inman RD, Gladman DD, Reeve JP, Peddle L, Maksymowych WP. Association of interleukin-23 receptor variants with ankylosing spondylitis. Arthritis Rheum 2008;58(4):1020–5.
47. Maksymowych WP, Inman RD, Gladman DD, Reeve JP, Pope A, Rahman P. Association of a specific ERAP1/ARTS1 haplotype with disease susceptibility in ankylosing spondylitis. Arthritis Rheum 2009;60(5):1317–23.
48. Glintborg B, Ostergaard M, Krogh NS, Dreyer L, Kristensen HL, Hetland ML. Predictors of treatment response and drug continuation in 842 patients with ankylosing spondylitis treated with anti-tumour necrosis factor: results from 8 years' surveillance in the Danish nationwide DANBIO registry. Ann Rheum Dis 2010;69(11):2002–8.
49. Glintborg B, Ostergaard M, Krogh NS, et al. Clinical response, drug survival and predictors thereof in 432 ankylosing spondylitis patients after switching tumour necrosis factor alpha inhibitor therapy: results from the Danish nationwide DANBIO registry. Ann Rheum Dis 2013;72(7):1149–55.
50. Konttinen L, Tuompo R, Uusitalo T, et al. Anti-TNF therapy in the treatment of ankylosing spondylitis: the Finnish experience. Clin Rheumatol 2007;26(10):1693–700.
51. Pavelka K, Forejtova S, Stolfa J, et al. Anti-TNF therapy of ankylosing spondylitis in clinical practice. Results from the Czech national registry ATTRA. Clin Exp Rheumatol 2009;27(6):958–63.
52. Ciurea A, Scherer A, Exer P, et al. Tumor necrosis factor alpha inhibition in radiographic and nonradiographic axial spondyloarthritis: results from a large observational cohort. Arthritis Rheum 2013;65(12):3096–106.
53. Gulfe A, Kapetanovic MC, Kristensen LE. Efficacy and drug survival of anti-tumour necrosis factor-alpha therapies in patients with non-radiographic axial spondyloarthritis: an observational cohort study from Southern Sweden. Scand J Rheumatol 2014;43(6):493–7.
54. Fagerli KM, van der Heijde D, Heiberg MS, et al. Is there a role for sulphasalazine in axial spondyloarthritis in the era of TNF inhibition? Data from the NOR-DMARD longitudinal observational study. Rheumatology (Oxford) 2014;53(6):1087–94.
55. Ciurea A, Scherer A, Weber U, et al. Impaired response to treatment with tumour necrosis factor alpha inhibitors in smokers with axial spondyloarthritis. Ann Rheum Dis 2016;75(3):532–9.
56. Kristensen LE, Karlsson JA, Englund M, Petersson IF, Saxne T, Geborek P. Presence of peripheral arthritis and male sex predicting continuation of anti-tumor necrosis factor therapy in ankylosing spondylitis: an observational prospective cohort study from the South Swedish Arthritis Treatment Group Register. Arthritis Care Res (Hoboken) 2010;62(10):1362–9.
57. Lie E, van der Heijde D, Uhlig T, et al. Effectiveness of switching between TNF inhibitors in ankylosing spondylitis: data from the NOR-DMARD register. Ann Rheum Dis 2011;70(1):157–63.
58. Askling J, van Vollenhoven RF, Granath F, et al. Cancer risk in patients with rheumatoid arthritis treated with anti-tumor necrosis factor alpha therapies: does the risk change with the time since start of treatment? Arthritis Rheum 2009;60(11):3180–9.
59. Galloway JB, Hyrich KL, Mercer LK, et al. Anti-TNF therapy is associated with an increased risk of serious infections in patients with rheumatoid arthritis especially in the first 6 months of treatment: updated results from the British Society for Rheumatology Biologics Register with special emphasis on risks in the elderly. Rheumatology (Oxford) 2011;50(1):124–31.
60. Strangfeld A, Hierse F, Rau R, et al. Risk of incident or recurrent malignancies among patients with rheumatoid arthritis exposed to biologic therapy in the German biologics register RABBIT. Arthritis Res Ther 2010;12(1):R5.
61. Greenberg JD, Kremer JM, Curtis JR, et al. Tumour necrosis factor antagonist use and associated risk reduction of cardiovascular events among patients with rheumatoid arthritis. Ann Rheum Dis 2011;70(4):576–82.
62. Dreyer L, Mellemkjaer L, Andersen AR, et al. Incidences of overall and site specific cancers in TNFα inhibitor treated patients with rheumatoid arthritis and other arthritides—a follow-up study from the DANBIO Registry. Ann Rheum Dis 2013;72(1):79–82.
63. Carmona L, Abasolo L, Descalzo MA, et al. Cancer in patients with rheumatic diseases exposed to TNF antagonists. Semin Arthritis Rheum 2011;41(1):71–80.
64. Garcia-Doval I, Perez-Zafrilla B, Descalzo MA, et al. Incidence and risk of hospitalisation due to shingles and chickenpox in patients with rheumatic diseases treated with TNF antagonists. Ann Rheum Dis 2010;69(10):1751–5.
65. Peña-Sagredo JL, Farinas MC, Perez-Zafrilla B, et al. Non-*typhi Salmonella* infection in patients with rheumatic diseases on TNF-alpha antagonist therapy. Clin Exp Rheumatol 2009;27(6):920–5.
66. Fernandez-Espartero MC, Perez-Zafrilla B, Naranjo A, et al. Demyelinating disease in patients treated with TNF antagonists in rheumatology: data from BIOBADASER, a pharmacovigilance database, and a systematic review. Semin Arthritis Rheum 2011;40(4):330–7.
67. Verstappen SM, Watson KD, Lunt M, McGrother K, Symmons DP, Hyrich KL. Working status in patients with rheumatoid arthritis, ankylosing spondylitis and psoriatic arthritis: results from the British Society for Rheumatology Biologics Register. Rheumatology (Oxford) 2010;49(8):1570–7.
68. Kristensen LE, Petersson IF, Geborek P, et al. Sick leave in patients with ankylosing spondylitis before and after anti-TNF therapy: a population-based cohort study. Rheumatology (Oxford) 2012;51(2):243–9.

69. Fafa BP, Louzada-Junior P, Titton DC, et al. Drug survival and causes of discontinuation of the first anti-TNF in ankylosing spondylitis compared with rheumatoid arthritis: analysis from BIOBADABRASIL. Clin Rheumatol 2015;34(5):921–7.
70. Carmona L, Gomez-Reino JJ. Survival of TNF antagonists in spondylarthritis is better than in rheumatoid arthritis. Data from the Spanish registry BIOBADASER. Arthritis Res Ther 2006;8(3):R72.
71. Heiberg MS, Koldingsnes W, Mikkelsen K, et al. The comparative one-year performance of anti-tumor necrosis factor alpha drugs in patients with rheumatoid arthritis, psoriatic arthritis, and ankylosing spondylitis: results from a longitudinal, observational, multicenter study. Arthritis Rheum 2008;59(2):234–40.
72. Heiberg MS, Nordvag BY, Mikkelsen K, et al. The comparative effectiveness of tumor necrosis factor-blocking agents in patients with rheumatoid arthritis and patients with ankylosing spondylitis: a six-month, longitudinal, observational, multicenter study. Arthritis Rheum 2005;52(8):2506–12.
73. Zavada J, Uher M, Sisol K, et al. A tailored approach to reduce dose of anti-TNF drugs may be equally effective, but substantially less costly than standard dosing in patients with ankylosing spondylitis over 1 year: a propensity score-matched cohort study. Ann Rheum Dis 2016;75(1):96-102.
74. Lie E, Kristensen LE, Forsblad-d'Elia H, Zverkova-Sandstrom T, Askling J, Jacobsson LT. The effect of comedication with conventional synthetic disease modifying antirheumatic drugs on TNF inhibitor drug survival in patients with ankylosing spondylitis and undifferentiated spondyloarthritis: results from a nationwide prospective study. Ann Rheum Dis 2015;74(6):970–8.
75. Oldroyd J, Schachna L, Buchbinder R, et al. Ankylosing spondylitis patients commencing biologic therapy have high baseline levels of comorbidity: a report from the Australian rheumatology association database. Int J Rheumatol 2009;2009:268569.
76. Rudwaleit M, van der Heijde D, Landewe R, et al. The development of Assessment of SpondyloArthritis international Society classification criteria for axial spondyloarthritis (part II): validation and final selection. Ann Rheum Dis 2009;68(6):777–83.
77. Deodhar A, Reveille JD, van den Bosch F, et al. The concept of axial spondyloarthritis: joint statement of the spondyloarthritis research and treatment network and the Assessment of SpondyloArthritis international Society in response to the US Food and Drug Administration's comments and concerns. Arthritis Rheumatol 2014;66(10):2649–56.

CHAPTER 25

Cost-of-illness and economic evaluations in axial spondyloarthritis

Annelies Boonen

Introduction to health economics

In the second half of the twentieth century the paradigm of outcome assessment in medicine shifted from outcomes that were relevant according to physicians towards outcomes that are relevant from the perspective of patients, and outcomes that provide information on costs and the budget impact for society.

In rheumatological inflammatory diseases, traditionally physicians focused on biopathological aspects of the disease, such as the markers of inflammation in blood and assessment of radiographic damage. One of the first instruments in rheumatology to assess patients' life impact was the patient-reported HAQ, whose development was presented in a publication in 1982 (1, 2). Since then, the field of patient-reported outcomes has grown substantially, to such an extent that initiatives were undertaken to improve the validity of patient-reported outcomes, and to achieve consensus on preferred reporting to enhance comparability across studies. Currently, accounting for patients' preferences in healthcare has become almost as important as evidence-based practices.

Parallel with the attention on the life impact of ill health, the first cost-of-illness (COI) study in rheumatology was published in 1965 (3), and the first cost-effectiveness study was a randomized trial in 1988 which showed that oral gold salts were cost-effective compared to no treatment in patients with RA (4). Over the years, the number of publications addressing costs in arthritis and spondylitis have steadily increased, and did so even when adjusted for the number of total publications in this field. Over time, a number of guidelines have become available to improve quality and to harmonize the methodology and the reporting of studies. Health economics has taken an indisputable position in medical research and healthcare.

As such, it is not surprising that society has paid increasing attention to the costs of healthcare. Commonly, the expenditures in healthcare are increasing at a rate that is faster than the growth of a country's gross domestic product (GDP) (5). In most societies, healthcare is a public service, paid largely by society, whose budget is not infinite. Moreover, in developed countries, not all healthcare innovations result predictably in true improvements in health. For all these reasons, approaches are needed to provide insight into the financial consequences of healthcare and to assess costs in relation to the effectiveness of new technologies. As such, the area of health economics encompasses two main directions. In the *economy of healthcare*, research concentrates on how society can organize the provision of healthcare, given a limited budget and a specific ideology. Some typical examples concern the amount of budget to be allocated to healthcare, the level of patient out-of-pocket contributions that are considered acceptable, and the role of the GP as a gatekeeper to secondary care. *Economic evaluations*, on the other hand, explore (usually on the individual patient level) to what extent the additional costs associated with new drugs and other innovations in healthcare result in additional health benefits. As such, they are just one of the 'tools' to inform decision makers whether health benefits are worth the costs (Fig. 25.1).

In many countries, economic evaluations have become formally part of the decision whether or not new technology will be reimbursed and made available to clinicians and patients (6). Clinicians cannot ignore such facts anymore and should be aware that inefficient use of healthcare resources will limit access to those that are in need of healthcare. This requires knowledge not only on efficacy, effectiveness, and safety of technologies, but also on their cost-effectiveness. Also the Institute of Medicine recognizes that high-quality healthcare should be efficient and equitable (7). In this chapter, evidence of economic evaluations, but not of the economy of healthcare is addressed. First, evidence of COI and health impact in terms of utilities associated with axSpA are reviewed, and next the available evidence of cost-effectiveness. Each part is preceded by a brief methodological introduction (8, 9).

Perspective of economic analyses

When appraising a health economic evaluation, it is essential to understand the influence of the perspective or point of view of the

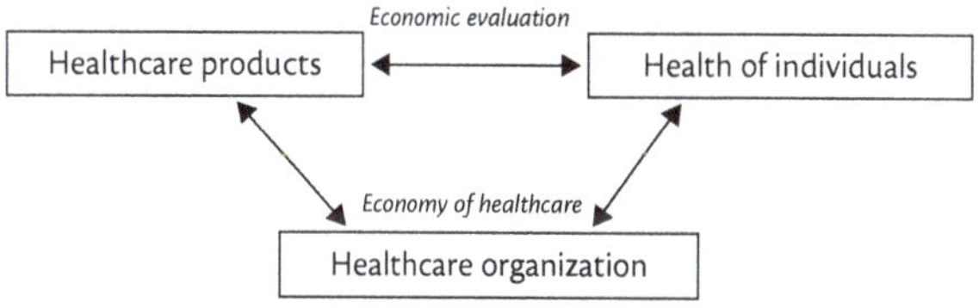

Fig. 25.1 Economic evaluation investigate how healthcare technologies rprovide returns in either economic benefits or health benefits (micro level). The economy of healthcare is the science that investigates how society can optimally organize healthcare given a political ideology and (usually) limited budgets (macro level).

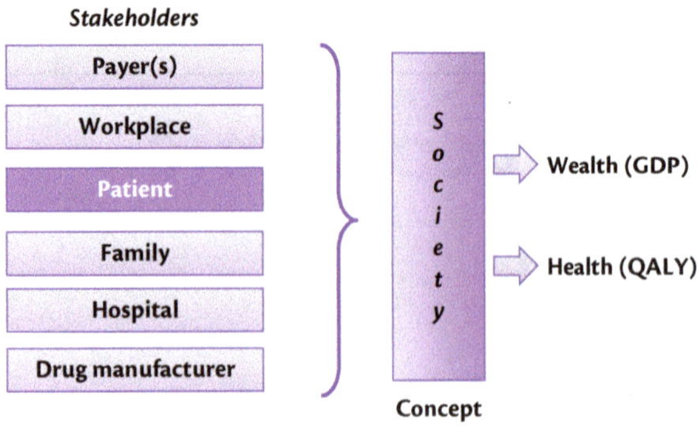

Fig. 25.2 An economic evaluation can be performed from different perspectives. In each perspective, different costs (type of categories and cost per unit) and health benefits can be of interest. The societal perspective is the umbrella and most relevant for healthcare providers.

analysis. The costs and benefits of interest are usually not those that are relevant from the patients' point of view, but usually relevant from the point of view of the hospital, the healthcare payer, or society. For each of these perspectives, different categories of costs and resources can be important, and even if similar resources are relevant, the price of the unit of the resource might be different. For example, a reduction of the hospitalization days may be an outcome of interest for the hospital, the payer, and society, but the cost relevant for each of these perspectives will be different, as for the hospital it will be the profit after deducting the expenditures, for the payer it will be the negotiated tariff, and for society it will be the true cost of all activities during one hospital day (Fig. 25.2).

For healthcare providers, the societal perspective should be the most relevant, as it addresses costs and benefits of the disease or its treatment, independent of the actual payer. Therefore, from a true societal perspective, not only the medical services delivered to or used by the patient, but also the need for help from caregivers and loss of worker productivity for society should be valued, and the costs should not be 'negotiated tariffs' but the true calculation of the costs of the service or product provided to the patients and the true value of the lost worker productivity due to the disease. The health benefit from the societal perspective is the societal utility (or societal value attached to health states) and the societal QALY, which is the integration of utility over time.

Cost-of-illness

General methodological aspects of cost-of-illness studies

COI studies aim to estimate the cost consequences of a disease. A distinction can be made between prevalence and lifetime studies, in which the costs for the latter studies consider the entire course of illness, including diagnosis and death. In prevalence COI studies, the period over which the costs are collected needs to be provided. When reporting results, costs are often extrapolated to a 1-year time frame. Such extrapolations are of course liable to systematic errors. Results can be presented as the costs per patient or as the costs per total number of patients in a country or specified setting. To interpret the latter, data on the epidemiology of the disease have to be available. Data can be retrieved either from questionnaires on resource utilization or costs, completed by the patient, or drawn from existing databases. Typical large data sources to provide costs are insurance claims and hospital databases. Ideally, first resources are collected, and then total costs can be calculated by summing the product of the number of each resource used by its unit costs, thus:

$$\textit{Cost-of-illness} = \sum_{i-j}^{n} (\textit{nb resources}_i \times \textit{unit cost of resource}_i)$$

As indicated, the type of resource as well as the specific monetary value of each resource depends on the 'perspective' taken. Furthermore, when collecting the resources and/or costs, it can be decided to focus on the costs of the index disease or to collect the costs associated with overall health. Given the extra-articular manifestations (EAMs) and possible other comorbidities associated with AS, and the difficulty in attributing healthcare use and expenditures to a particular disease, it is advisable to assess overall and not the disease-specific resource utilization and costs. Moreover, this will facilitate comparison with reference population data and with other diseases.

Although several classifications have been proposed to categorize the different types of resources and costs, the classic categories that can be distinguished are shown in Box 25.1.

A challenge in costing data is the timing of the study and international transferability. COI studies can differ among countries because patterns of healthcare provision and magnitude of interference with worker productivity might differ, but mainly because the 'cost' of the resource and of lost productivity between countries differs. For the costing issue, consumer price indices can help to adjust for differential timing, and purchasing power parities for differences in purchasing power across countries.

Box 25.1 Categories of health resources and costs that are classically assessed in COI studies from a societal perspective

Direct resources or costs are related to the diagnosis, treatment, and care of the person affected by the disease.

Direct healthcare resources or costs include resources or costs prescribed in the healthcare setting, and comprise consultations to professionals, medications, technical procedures, hospitalization, and formal care.

Direct non-healthcare resources or costs are not formally prescribed in the healthcare system. They are sometimes also referred to as patient and family costs. Examples are transportation costs, informal care, and CAM (unless reimbursed).

Indirect or productivity costs reflect productivity loss in paid or unpaid work.

The measurement of *loss of paid work* raises theoretical issues (10):

- The 'friction cost' method accounts for illness-related absence from work until the worker is substituted by a colleague or a person looking for work (friction period).
- The 'human capital' approach accounts for the illness-related absence from work until the age of retirement (or death, whichever comes first).
- As there is as yet no valid approach to measure actual loss of productivity when attending work while being ill (presenteeism), it is currently recommended not to include at-work productivity loss based on simple patient-reported presenteeism.

Loss of unpaid work can be measured as the hours associated with tasks in and around the house which either cannot be performed or are taken over by caregivers or household help (while avoiding double counting).

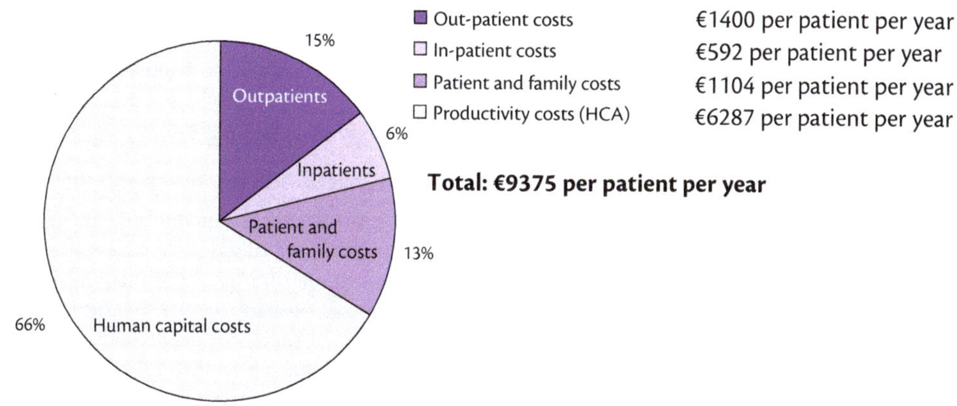

Fig. 25.3 Total societal cost-of-illness and contribution of the different cost-categories for AS in the pre-biologic era.

COI studies are first of all useful to understand the economic burden of a disease. However, their interpretation as stand-alone data is not straightforward as a universal benchmark is not available. Therefore comparison with COI of other diseases or of the general population, but also evolution of costs over time, is often more interesting. In such comparisons, the cost-categories that contribute to (evolution of or difference in) overall costs can be identified. The second, and perhaps more important reason to collect data on resource utilization and costs is that these data are essential in cost-effectiveness analyses whose objective is to compare costs and health benefits of competing treatments.

Cost-of illness studies in axial spondyloarthritis

Overall, 14 COI studies have been published in axSpA. Seven COI studies were performed in the prebiologic era. All studies are prevalent costs, and lifetime cost studies are not available. All studies addressed AS (i.e. radiographic axSpA (r-axSpA)). Studies differed substantially in patients included, study design, type of resource utilized, price/value of unit costs, and whether or not the resource utilization or cost was attributable to AS or overall health. The seven prebiologic studies were all published in 2000 or later (11). The average age of patients in these studies was 47 years and 69% were male. The time horizons (i.e. the time over which costs incurred by patients was measured) varied between 3 months and 3 years. Two studies were from North America and all others from western European countries. Mean total costs (the sum of the total healthcare, patient and family, and productivity (or indirect) costs assessed by the human capital approach (HCA)) were €9375 per patient per year for AS (2006 cost). The human capital productivity costs (which represent productivity loss due to sick leave and work disability) accounted for 66% of the total costs of AS. This large share of productivity costs in the total costs reflected the high burden of the disease on work participation.

The out-patient healthcare expenditures constituted 15% of the overall costs and were due to medication costs, visits to physicians, and non-physician service utilizations. Prescriptions of NSAIDs and DMARDs were almost exclusively placed in the total medication costs, and overall were a small part of costs. In-patient costs were 6% of the overall costs. The direct costs not prescribed by the healthcare system (including patient and family costs) were 13% of the overall costs and were recorded for home-care services, alternative therapies, and devices and aids. While patient time also represented high costs, this was measured by one study only. Patient time can be a surrogate for the unpaid productivity loss, but if reflecting only the 'patient burden', then the cost-category should not be added to direct or indirect costs of disease. When exploring separately the five studies that addressed indirect (or productivity) costs, the average costs of sick leave were €924 (range €388–1079), but average human capital costs were €6278 (range €5111–7725) when using the human capital approach (10) (Fig. 25.3).

Cost drivers in the prebiologic era, as reported by a limited number of studies, were disease activity (BASDAI) and function (BASFI or HAQ), and to a varying extent also age, disease duration, comorbidities, and EAMs. In addition, female gender was associated with higher costs for formal and informal care, and lower education and manual jobs increased the probability and level of productivity costs.

None of these studies provided comparisons with the general population. In an indirect comparison for studies published in the same period, COI of AS was slightly lower for all cost-categories (except for physiotherapy) than in RA. When summarizing studies published in the same period, total COI for RA was estimated to be €14 961 per patient per year (vs €9375 per year for AS), of which €8452 (56% of total) per patient per year were indirect costs (vs €6278 (66% of total) per patient per year for AS). In view of the younger age onset, the lifetime costs of AS will likely be higher compared to RA, but these data are not available. When comparing societal COI of patients with fibromyalgia, chronic low back pain, and AS, costs were €7824 (median: €5145), €8533 (median: €5068), and €3205 (median: €1793) per patient per year, respectively, indicating a much lower economic burden for AS. Although this pattern was seen for all cost-categories, it was slightly more pronounced for the indirect costs (sick leave) which were 33–34% for fibromyalgia and chronic low back pain and 15% of total costs for r-axSpA (12).

Patient out-of-pocket cost or loss of income due to work disability can be substantial and in some countries can lead to relevant impoverishment of patients. One study in three western European countries reported that annual out-of-pocket expenditures for direct (healthcare and non-healthcare) resource use were €431 per patient, and average annual income loss €1371 per patient. Contributions to healthcare costs were highest for Belgian patients and lowest for French patients, while income loss was the highest for Dutch patients (mainly due to the higher proportion of Dutch patients being work disabled). Total patients' costs were associated with higher age and worse physical function (13).

It is currently believed that about 50% of patients with AS in rheumatology care are treated with a biologic at some point in the course of disease. In the literature, proportions of between 25% and 70% have been reported, depending on the country and whether the clinic is a referral centre (14). In the NOR-DMARD registry, the differences in the 2 years' societal costs between patients starting a synthetic DMARD compared to a biologic DMARD were €61 855 (€37 653) as opposed to €115 427 (€109 068), respectively. The higher costs in those starting a biologic were mainly attributable to drug-related (including day care) costs, but also somewhat higher costs of rehabilitation and work disability (15). It should be noted that likely biologics were started in those patients with worse disease and therefore already higher costs at baseline. Two prevalence COI studies in the UK, one being in a GP setting and the other in a rheumatology clinic, reported that medication costs, which were almost negligible in the prebiologic era, accounted for 25% and 70% of the direct healthcare costs, respectively, in settings where biologics were prescribed (16, 17). Notwithstanding, the total costs of the disease remain mainly attributable (88% and 83%) to indirect costs (human capital). Three studies in countries with lower economic welfare (Turkey and Greece) observed a similar pattern, with 88–93% of direct healthcare costs attributable to the costs of biologics (24–35% of prevalent patients being treated with biologics), but indirect costs in one of these studies contributing still 66% of the total costs (18–20). It is worrisome that price of (biologic) drugs are only marginally adjusted to the spending power of the individual country where they are made available, thus hampering access. It is of note that physical functioning and disease activity but also presence of EAMs and comorbidities remained the clinical variables most strongly associated with direct or total costs. Very few studies report on the change in healthcare resource utilization and direct costs related to biologics. One RCT, evaluating the effect of ETN in several western European countries, showed that at entry into the open-label extension study (all patients were at least 16 weeks on ETN), a significant decrease in direct healthcare costs had occurred, mainly due to reduction in the number of visits to the physiotherapist and out-patient physicians before treatment with biologics. It should be noted that biologics were not included in the costs (21). It cannot be excluded that part of the change in direct costs reflects regression to the mean in a group of symptomatic patients that are in high need of healthcare upon entry into the trial. In the Czech Republic the healthcare costs of AS between 2005 and 2008 increased from €1812 to €2588 due to more frequent prescribing of biologics, while there was only a marginal decrease of 6.7% in the indirect costs (22).

Recognizing the relevance of reducing indirect (productivity) costs when trying to receive monetary returns on the additional costs of biologics, a systematic review that included nine studies assessed the influence of biologics on work outcome (23). For presenteeism and absence from work, most comparisons showed improvement in favour of biologic agents, but not all comparisons were statistically significant and they usually concerned before–after (instead of between intervention and non-intervention group) analyses. For work status ($n = 4$), changes were less often favourable, but studies dealt with patients with long-standing AS, lacked power, and had a relatively short follow-up. Observational studies and registries should make more effort to collect high-quality data on work outcomes. Along these lines, in Sweden there is the possibility of linking clinical data to national social security databases and matching patients to controls, which is laudable. These data make clear that despite optimal treatment with biologics, patients with AS still have more sick leave compared to population controls (24).

Utility as the basis for QALY

General methodological aspects of utilities and QALY

A QALY is the product of 'quality' and 'quantity' of health over time and is the preferred outcome to assess health benefits in an economic evaluation. The 'quality' subcomponent should be assessed by a preference-based or utility measure. In the societal perspective, the value or utility for health should reflect society's (and not the patient's) value for health. By consensus, the utility is scaled between zero, a value for health state equal to death, and 1, a value representing perfect health (Fig. 25.4).

Doing so, the societal utilities or QALY are generic measures that allow decision makers to compare health benefits across diseases. The EQ-5D and SF-6D are the most frequently used utility measures and typically represent the societal value for health. They belong to the 'indirect' societal utility measures, in which the value for health is not assigned directly by society for each individual subject's health state, but indirectly through the profiles of health that can be generated by a patient's scores on the EQ and SF. In other words, the patient's score on the EQ or SF can be converted into a utility, using an existing formula that was derived following a large population valuation study. As there is evidence that different cultures can attach different values to health states, some (but not all) indirect utility instruments have national tariffs available. Although the different approaches to assess utilities should provide the same results, in the reality of clinical research, sometimes large difference between instruments are observed (25, 26).

There are several reasons explaining the differences in results between instruments. First, due to different approaches to anchor the health states between zero and 1, instruments differ with regard to the score range, especially for the lowest possible values. For the UK tariff of the EQ-5D, for example, the utility score can go as low as −0.50 (health state worse than death), while the lowest score for the SF-6D would be +0.30. Partly this can explain the larger standard deviation (SD) and contributes to the differences in smallest detectable difference (SDD). Second, the distribution of the instruments is very different, with EQ-5D more skewed with a long left

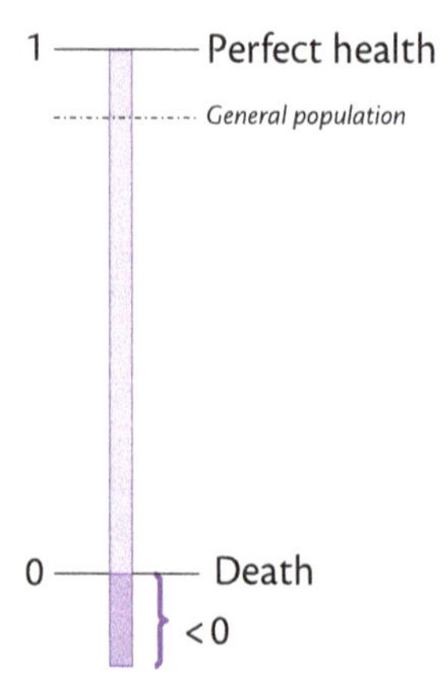

Fig. 25.4 Graphical representation of a utility, which values health on a scale on which zero equals death and 1 equals perfect health.

tail with the lower values. Likely this explains the higher responsiveness of the EQ-5D in the lower values of the scale. Finally, instruments differ in the content, with more items related to functioning in the SF-6D, for example, and in the levels of the item score (3 for EQ and 5 for SF) also contributing to difference in clinimetric properties. Currently, an EQ-D with 5 answer levels (EQ-5D-5L) is being developed (27).

As, increasingly, disease-specific utilities can be relevant for decisions on resources within a disease, and as the patient perspective of health gains more impact, also in economic evaluations, there is currently an initiative to convert the ASAS HI into a societal and patient utility (28).

Utilities in ankylosing spondylitis

Four studies reported on utilities in the prebiologic era (29, 30). All used the EQ-5D, and one additionally the SF-6D. The average value of the utility varied between 0.62 and 0.69. The mean decrease in utility when compared to the general population norm (between 0.75 and 0.89, depending on the instrument) was between −0.1 and −0.3 units below the population norm. BASFI and BASDAI are the most important clinical determinants of utility in AS. When reviewing studies (n = 4) that included patients with active disease and selected for a biologic intervention, average values could be as low as 0.45, substantially lower than in unselected patients. Interventions with biologics reported substantial and sustained improvements in utilities between 0.08 and 0.19, with one study reporting QALY gain after 78 weeks of 0.10 and 0.24 for EQ-5D and SF-6D, respectively, largely depending on the instrument used (31–34). Of note, utility in treated patients remained below the population norm (34).

Further exploration of differences in clinimetrics between SF-6D and EQ-5D showed that both instruments correlated equally with disease-specific activity, functioning, and quality of life, but absolute agreement between EQ-5D and SF-6D (using intra-class correlation (ICC)) is only moderate (35). The SDD in persons with stable disease was 0.36 and 0.17 for EQ-5D and SF-6D, respectively. The ability to detect treatment effect showed standardized effect sizes (ES) that were moderate for EQ-5D and SF-6D (ES: 0.63 and 0.64) in persons with a moderate disease severity (baseline utility was 0.66 (SD 0.21) for EQ-5D and 0.64 (SD 0.11) for SF-6D). It is clear that the potential absolute gain in EQ-5D utilities is much larger when improving disease activity, than for SF-6D utilities. The minimal important difference (MID) was not assessed specifically in AS, but one study reported the MID to be, on average, 0.074 for EQ-5D and 0.041 for SF-6D across 11 chronic conditions, and likely this would also be applicable in AS.

Economic evaluations

General methodological aspects of economic evaluations

Innovations in the field of diagnosis, prognosis, and pharmacological as well as non-pharmacological interventions are usually associated with extra costs. On the other hand, when implementing such innovations in clinical care, benefits are expected in terms of gains in health, but often also as return in costs when improved health reduces health resource utilization or improved paid and unpaid work of the patient. In a full economic evaluation, the difference in costs (expenditures and returns) of the novel strategy is balanced against the changes in health of the new as opposed to the old technology. The result is the so-called incremental cost for the additional effects or benefits. Depending on the way of measuring the effects or benefits in the denominator, and the way of expressing effects (denominator), classically four types of full economic evaluations can be distinguished (Box 25.2, Fig. 25.5).

Box 25.2 Types of economic evaluations: the case of health benefits

In *cost-effectiveness analysis*, health benefits in the denominator are expressed in specific clinical outcomes, such as number of patients in remission and number of patients permanently returned to work.

A *cost-utility analysis* is actually a special form of cost-effectiveness analysis, in which the benefits represent an overall improvement in health, expressed in QALY. Cost-utility analysis has the advantage of comparability between diseases.

In *cost-minimization analysis* the denominator is omitted. This type of evaluation assumes that the new intervention is not associated with a (positive or negative) difference in health, but has only different costs when compared to the alternative technology. The value represents the final money gained (or lost) by the new technology. It is clear that such analyses are only relevant when an innovation is expected to have a different cost. Very few cost-minimization studies are done, as often new technologies will also have some differences in health.

In *cost-benefit analysis*, the change in health (denominator) is expressed in monetary terms. The incremental ratio therefore provides the overall monetary gain or loss to the patient of the new compared to the old technology. Such analyses are more relevant when comparing cost-effectiveness across different sectors, such as investments in health compared to education or climate.

Most healthcare innovations in AS aim to influence the long-term effects (and costs) of the disease. As clinical trials are typically short term, include selected patients, are strongly controlled, and often choose the least effective (instead of the best available) comparator, *trial-based economic evaluations* are less suitable to inform decision makers on long-term consequences for costs and in real life.

Therefore *long-term models* are preferred. The starting point of an economic model is the development and parametrization of a valid mathematical model that represents the course of health of

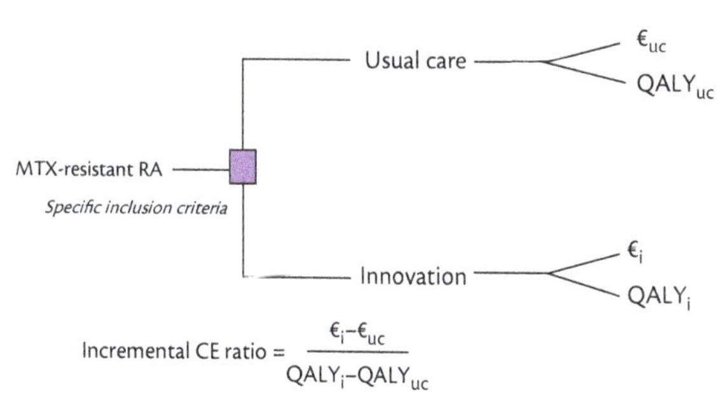

Fig. 25.5 Simplified graphical presentation of the principle of economic evaluation: incremental cost-effectiveness analysis provides the ratio of differences in costs (expenditures and monetary returns) and health benefits (QALY) between innovative and usual care strategies.

patients, accounting for current recommendations of diagnosis and management. Ideally, relevant subgroups of patients (with different courses of health) should be distinguished. Once such model is available and validated, the influence of new diagnostic criteria, markers of prognosis, and pharmacological or non-pharmacological treatments on the course of health can be evaluated. In a last step, the modeled health outcome is linked to costs and utilities (often while considering relevant other characteristics, such as age, disease duration, and prognostic factors), allowing a weighing of the incremental costs and incremental utilities over time in the different arms that are compared in the model. It will be clear that the data on the course of the disease under usual care, the influence of the course of health by the innovative technique or treatment strategy, and finally the relationship between the health and costs and utilities usually require different data sources. To enhance the comparability across data, methods allowing indirect comparison will be needed. To allow for uncertainty with either the structure of the model or the available data to parametrize the model, respective scenario and sensitivity analyses can be performed.

Two types of models allow inclusion of the time factor, one being a Markov model and the other a discrete event simulation (DES). Both approaches have been used in AS. In a Markov model, health states are defined and can change only after a specific and fixed period of time. The number of health states is therefore limited. In a DES, health is modelled over time until specific events (start of treatment, loss of response, adverse event) occur. In addition, DES can explicitly take a patient's history into account, facilitating simulating treatment selection and linking costs and utilities to past and current patients' characteristics.

As the choice of decisions for the structure of the model and the source of data to parameterize the model will likely have important influence on the final cost-effectiveness or cost-utility, recommendations are available that identify the relevant points of choice and provide a specific recommendation. About ten Recommendations for Economic Evaluations have been published so far, and some countries have (in addition) national recommendations. They aim to ensure quality of research and/or transparency in reporting by providing an overview of the key issues that are at stake and by offering for each issue a background and at the same time a generic recommendation on how to approach it. Recently, a task force aimed at achieving consensus on such recommendations and proposed the Consolidated Health Economic Evaluation Reporting Standards (CHEERS) (36). For AS, a working group came together in 2006 within the OMERACT initiative, to reach consensuses on a limited number but key disease-specific issues that should be fulfilled in order to provide reliable cost-effectiveness evaluations in AS (37). Currently, new measures to assess health outcome are available and insight into the 'natural' course of AS has evolved. As a consequence, the previously published recommendations would need an update. Table 25.1 addresses the same key issues identified earlier, but adjusts the specific recommendation according to new insights.

Table 25.1 Key issues identified previously as essential when modelling healthcare innovations in AS (37), with updated proposals and research agenda

Key issue	Tentative proposal	Areas for further research
1. Time horizon/duration of follow-up		
	◆ Taking into account comparability with the RA reference case, results should be reported with a short-term (≤ 2 years) (DMARD and SMARD), medium-term (5 years), and lifetime (DMARDs only) time horizon ◆ Short-/medium-term time horizons should have a realistic link with (observed) evidence of new technology and primary source(s) of effectiveness.	◆ Evidence is needed on long-term effectiveness of treatments, in particular on radiographic outcome, work outcome, rare events (toxicity or rare disease complications), and mortality ◆ Rates at which IBP progresses to axSpA and nr-axSpA evolves to AS are needed
2. Duration of treatment		
	◆ An option for initial non-response resulting in discontinuation of therapy at a specified time point should be included ◆ Sequencing of treatment should be accounted for, as this will be relevant in real life use of the drug	◆ Registries should examine reasons and rates of withdrawal and mortality ◆ Registries should collect data on sequence of treatments given to patients ◆ Criteria for stopping drugs and flares (leading to restarting drug treatment) should be developed and observational data collected
3. Extrapolation of effects beyond treatment and/or trial duration		
	◆ Unless there is overwhelming evidence of long-term benefits of treatment, the main analysis should always be presented assuming that there is no long-term effect	◆ Registries (and open-label studies) should continue to collect data on long-term clinical effects of drugs (and management)
4. Choice of comparator and synthesis of comparisons and treatment strategies where clinical trials do not exist		
	◆ New economic models should always include 'usual care' as recommended in guidelines as the comparator ◆ Absence of head-to-head studies should not restrict comparisons, though appropriate methods and sensitivity analysis should be used when making indirect comparisons	◆ Comparative effectiveness trials should be stimulated ◆ Devise methods for making indirect comparisons, particularly when there is heterogeneity in patient characteristics

(continued)

Table 25.1 Continued

Key issue	Tentative proposal	Areas for further research
5. Measures to model the course of disease		
	◆ In evaluations of treatments, BASDAI and BASFI should be used to model disease progression	◆ As ASDAS showed to be a more accurate measure, this should be included in sensitivity analyses and over time will be used in the base case ◆ It should be considered whether evolution of nr- to r-axSpA should be considered. This would require availability of data on this issue
6. Valuation of health in terms of quality of life or health utilities		
	◆ A generic societal health utility (health state preference) measure should be included in clinical trials and registries	◆ Relationship between changes in clinical measures (BASDAI, BASFI, but also radiographic damage, prognostic factors, occurrence of EAM, and comorbidities) and changes in health utilities in AS should be further explored ◆ Registries and observational datasets should incorporate utilities ◆ Disease-specific utilities from a patient perspective could be developed and used in sensitivity analyses (as this allows for better decisions on treatments within one disease) ◆ Data on process of care and satisfaction/preferences of care might in future become more relevant in assessment of overall 'value of health'
7. Resource utilization and costing		
	◆ Estimates of changes in productivity costs associated with an intervention should be made, but are preferably presented as a separate base-case analysis	◆ Registries and observational datasets should incorporate economic endpoints (work disability—sick leave—resource use) ◆ As friction and human capital methods provide different information, both approaches can be considered. Care should be taken about risk of bias in primary data sources, as many studies that provide data on work outcome suffer from bias (such as insufficient sample size) ◆ Improve methods and consensus on when and how to include at-work productivity loss (or costs) in economic evaluations
8. Population risk stratification—subgroups		
	◆ Clinically relevant subgroups of patients should be analysed and limitations in evidence should be clearly disseminated ◆ Along these lines, it is still advisable to provide separate analyses for nr-axSpA and AS	◆ Relevant subgroups (and their relation) of patients for new interventions/risk assessment with biomarkers in axSpA should be defined
9. Uncertainty analysis		
	◆ Extensive one-way sensitivity analysis should always be performed ◆ Probabilistic sensitivity analysis should be used where description of parameter uncertainty is possible, and methods feasible	◆ Assess how methods such as expected value of information and expected value of individualized care can be used to direct further research in AS most efficiently
10. Model development and reporting		
	◆ Structure of the model should also be presented graphically ◆ Structure of the model should either (1) be agreed upon by experts in axSpA or (2) reflect national or international recommendations for the usual care comparator ◆ All parameters associated with the model should be reported, so that analyses are transparent and reproducible ◆ All assumptions should be reported explicitly. All potential conflicts of interests should be reported, and specific roles of each author disseminated	◆ Strive for a universal model that is managed and updated by an international organization and has open access for use by others

Interpretation of the cost per QALY and budget impact

While interpretation of clinical outcome measures is facilitated by defining the MIDs and thresholds that distinguish between meaningful levels of the outcome, the interpretation of QALY is related to what society is able or prepared to pay for a gain in (time-integrated) health (ƛ). Many approaches have been discussed to provide either a theoretically grounded or evidence-based foundation. In practice, commonly used thresholds (ƛ) are £30 000 per QALY in the UK and the range is between $50 000 and 100 000 in the USA. To account for the unavoidable uncertainty around the point estimate of the incremental cost-effectiveness ratio (iCER), often results are presented as the chance (proportion of repeated analyses) for which the iCER falls within the threshold. In most countries, the iCER provides guidance on the adoption (i.e. reimbursement) of the technology without being used in relation to an absolute threshold. Additional considerations are taken into account during the final appraisal, including ethical reflections, the severity of the disease, whether the technology aims to prevent or treat a health condition, and, last but not least, budget considerations. Notwithstanding, more research into defining MID and acceptable health state for QALY, although challenging, would be valuable.

It should be noted that a cost per QALY presents patient-level information (the average costs to gain one QALY per patient in the specified time interval). It is the result of a cohort-based analysis in which all patients start the treatment at the same point in time. Therefore the iCER cannot inform about the budget impact, as this requires information about the absolute number of patients that receive the medication at a specific point in calendar time. Such a calculation is sometimes done as a separate model, but nowadays also is integrated in conventional modelling, as shown in an example in AS (38).

Overview of current cost-effectiveness studies

In AS (or r-axSpA), 15 cost-effectiveness analyses have been published from 1994 onwards (39). Two addressed non-pharmacotherapy and all others addressed pharmacotherapy with either TNFi or different NSAIDs before continuing a TNFi (n = 1)

A 9-month trial-based cost-effectiveness analysis from the payer's perspective in 144 Dutch patients with AS attending a rheumatology department compared the costs and effects of group physical therapy with unsupervised exercise at home. The study found that for an extra cost of US$409 per patient per year, there was a 5% additional increase in fitness, 7% additional improvement in mobility, and 28% difference in gain in overall global health. Although extra benefits were small and no utility was provided, the extra costs for additional benefits seem acceptable (40). Another 9-month trial-based cost-effectiveness analysis conducted from a societal perspective in 111 Dutch patients with AS, who suffered from limitations in physical functioning despite home or group exercise and received spa exercise in Austria or in the Netherlands, showed an iCER of €7463/QALY (95% CI: 3294–14 686) for SpA in Austria and €18 575 (95% CI: 3267–114 257) for SpA in the Netherlands compared to usual care. Interestingly, when using the SF-6D as an alternative utility to assess QALY in sensitivity analyses, the gain in health was smaller, making the iCER less favourable but still acceptable for the Dutch healthcare system (30).

A Markov model with a 30-year time horizon evaluated the cost-effectiveness from the UK's payer's perspective of etoricoxib relative to celecoxib and non-selective naproxen and diclofenac (all at recommended full doses), in the initial treatment of AS. Patients who failed two NSAIDs were started on a TNFi. The efficacy of the different NSAIDs on AS symptoms and gastrointestinal as well as cardiovascular safety and mortality was modelled. Effect of drugs on BASDAI and BASFI was synthesized with a mixed-treatment comparison meta-analysis of clinical trials and linked to QALY and disease-specific costs. Starting etoricoxib resulted in a small extra health benefit of QALYs over 30 years compared to the other interventions. The probability was more than 99% that etoricoxib had the lowest cost. Etoricoxib was expected to save £13 620 relative to celecoxib, £9957 relative to diclofenac, and £9863 relative to naproxen. By having an improved safety profile and by postponing the start if TNFi, etoricoxib has a higher chance to be cost-effective for the UK payer. The model was repeated from the Norwegian perspective and provided similar results. The manufacturer of etoricoxib was involved in the model and preparation of the manuscript.

Twelve studies on cost-effectiveness of TNFi reported 16 incremental ratios. In 14 of these, the comparator was usual care and the active drug was infliximab (n = 7), ETN (n = 3), adalimumab (n = 1), golimumab (n = 1 plus a revision), various TNFi (n = 1), and a sequence of three TNFi (n = 1) (39, 41, 42, 43, 44). In the remaining studies, different dosing schedules were compared (46). In two studies, iCERs of two or more TNFi were analysed in the same model, but always compared to usual care (39).

In all studies, patients with active AS, defined by BASDAI ≥ 4 were considered, except for one study that addressed dose reduction in patients in remission (44). Three studies were so-called trial-based evaluations (one was a formal RCT, while others matched intervention and control patients in a registry). All other studies were models, of which one was a DES and all others a Markov model. In all models, BADAI and/or BASFI were used to model the course of health over time, except in one study where the HAQ was used. In the modelling studies, data on efficacy and safety of the new intervention were most frequently retrieved from one registration trial, once from real-life register data, and only once was all available literature synthesized. In case a cost-utility was provided, QALY was invariably based on EQ-5D, with one study performing a sensitivity analyses with SF-6D. The time horizon was in eight studies 20 years or longer. The perspective of the base case analyses was exclusively the payer in five studies, while all other studies considered the societal perspective in either the base case or scenario analyses. One economic evaluation used US costs to value resources, one study used Canadian costs, and all other evaluations incorporated costs from western European countries (UK = 5). In five studies, there was no manufacturer involvement.

When summarizing results of the two *short-term* cost-effectiveness models, the base case iCERs were between £32 800 and €189 564 per QALY, respectively. The latter study was one of the earliest cost-effectiveness models in AS and distinguished only a limited number of health states, therefore likely underestimating the beneficial effects of TNF inhibition. In this study, ETN provided a more favourable iCER. Moreover, sensitivity analyses with the best-case scenario resulted in an iCER of €42 914 per QALY. The *long-term models* were even more favourable, with iCERs ranging from €15 157 to €54 815 per QALY. Sensitivity analyses revealed that the reduction of the drug price, the inclusion of direct costs, and the choice of utility measures were the most potent variables changing iCER. Furthermore, estimates were sensitive to the assumptions on long-term health in the treatment and control groups over time, with more favourable iCERs when worsening of BASFI continued at a faster rate in control than in the intervention group. Of interest was the fact that in the analyses comparing golimumab, ETN, and adalimumab to usual care, the manufacturer's publication found the iCER of golimumab was most favourable (£26 597 per QALY), while the independent review group found that ETN had the most favourable iCER (£26 505 per QALY), suggesting bias in the choice of parameters when the manufacturer is involved.

One study compared in an observational cohort the cost and effects of biologics (different compounds) in RA (n = 206), PsA (n = 57), and AS (n = 34) using a before–after analysis. Only drug costs were accounted for availability. The annual costs to achieve an MID were $41 636, $42 077, and $42 147, respectively. The number needed to treat to achieve an MID was 1.94 (RA), 1.88 (PsA), and 2.30 (AS) (43). Before–after studies should be interpreted with care as they lack a true comparator.

Overall, when comparing cost-effectiveness of biologics in AS with those in RA (45), results are much more favourable in AS, especially when considering the studies in RA where a true real-life comparator is used.

Although dosing could be an effective way to reduce costs, only two studies have addressed this issue. A French trial-based cost-effectiveness study with a time horizon of 1 year comprising direct as well as indirect (sick leave) costs compared administration of infliximab every 6 weeks to an 'on-demand' administration, and showed an iCER of €15 842 per additional ASAS responder, of €23 296 for an additional patient in remission, and an incremental cost-utility ratio (iCUR) of €50 706 per QALY for the fixed administration schedule. While conceptualized to prove evidence of the superiority of a fixed dosing, given the reduced dosing and drug costs in the 'on-demand' schedule, one could reverse the question when interpreting the data, and wonder whether patients or rheumatologists would be willing to save healthcare costs for QALYs forgone in the 'on-demand' schedule.

In the Czech Republic, physicians reached consensus to consider careful dose reduction in patients with inactive disease for more than 6 months. In a budget-restricted healthcare system, savings could be used to treat more new active patients. To understand the cost-effectiveness of such an approach, patients with AS who received a dose reduction (n = 53) were matched using propensity score to similar patients in the registry but who did not receive a dose reduction (n = 83). The HR (95% CI) of the reduced versus standard dosing group for relapse and any adverse event was 1.46 (0.66–3.19) and 0.56 (0.22–1.44), respectively. Mean difference (95% CI) in cost of TNFi drugs was €−4214 (€−4707 to €−3701) per year of treatment in favour of reduced dosing strategy (44) . It will be important to merge the differential impact on disease activity and side-effects into an overall health measure (QALY) and understand the impact on all costs in order to estimate an iCUR from a societal perspective.

None of the studies calculated a budget impact of the drug or the strategy for their region or country.

Future perspectives of cost-effectiveness analyses

All published cost-effectiveness analyses have addressed AS. The main question remaining is what is the cost-effectiveness of diagnosing and treating nr-axSpA? Insight into the cost-effectiveness of the new diagnostic criteria, the role of rheumatologists (as opposed to the GP) in managing axSpA, and different drug strategies to treat the disease are lacking. An increasing number of cohorts now have data available and should be able to model the cost-effectiveness of the new criteria. As there is some concern that the criteria still lack specificity and as it is observed than the effectiveness of TNFi may be somewhat less than for AS, the advances in modelling can actually help to understand the source of uncertainty (expected value of perfect information) and even to identify groups for which the new technology is not cost-effective (expected value of individualized care). This could help research planning going forward and provide information on where to spend money in order to improve health QALY of patients at acceptable extra costs. One of the interesting questions could be whether research into a biomarker for the disease or for non-response could contribute to cost-effective management of axSpA.

Preferably, such models should be supported by the clinical research community and have open access. Such open-access models can have different 'parts' or 'modules', such as, for example, a module 'pure AS'. A universal model would improve collaborations of researchers in a large consortium so that they may perform true cost-effective translational research. A simpler version of the open-access model could be to model the cost-effectiveness of the new biologics in axSpA and of remission induction strategies followed by dose reduction or stop-strategies.

Transferability and inequality or inequity

Several economists argue against the possibility of having a universal open-access model, as there is concern that the course of disease and healthcare provision across countries would be too diverse. However, there is no evidence of strong difference in severity of axSpA across world regions. Also, the close collaboration among clinical researchers who also aim for consensus of treatment strategies has improved uniform implementation of recommendations (47) in most regions of the world. Therefore transferability of economic evaluations mainly depends on health utility valuation, costs, resources, and productivity, which can be easily adjusted for (48).

The issue of international transferability of economic evaluations brings us to another gap in the current literature. All evaluations in AS have been done in high-income countries. As pricing of new medications is protected by a patent, prices in national currency of innovative medications are quite similar across countries but not when adjusted for purchasing power parities. When realizing that healthcare resources and especially loss of productivity have a much lower cost/price in low-income countries, it is unlikely that new drugs can provide sufficient monetary returns for biologics to reach favourable cost-effectiveness. While European recommendations account for cost-effectiveness considerations when developing guidelines, they do not account for the huge differences in economic wealth between countries. Although reimbursement criteria for biologics in AS are quite homogeneous across countries, it would be relevant to explore access to recommended healthcare in real life (49).

Conclusion

The economic implications of axSpA, in particular since the advent of TNFi, have generated great interest. Interventions for axSpA will compete for funding with interventions in other diseases. Overall, use of biologics after failing NSAIDs in patients with active disease is cost-effective. As new technologies emerge, the role of cost-effectiveness analyses to evaluate the efficiency of treatments will become even more important. The issue of diagnosing and treating axSpA early is especially challenging. Economic evaluations will increasingly be used to inform decision making on which interventions will be used, and help guide further research, so that better decisions can be made later. It is likely that future clinical research will have to pay more attention to the economic considerations of interventions, through more pragmatic trials, and collection of economic endpoints.

References

1. Fries JF, Spitz P, Kraines RG, Holman HR. Measurement of patient outcome in arthritis. Arthritis Rheum 1980;23:137–45.
2. Fries JF, Spitz PW, Young DY. The dimensions of health outcomes: the health assessment questionnaire, disability and pain scales. J Rheumatol 1982;9:789–93.
3. Saslaw MS, Vieta A, Myerburg RJ. Cost of rheumatic fever and of iets prevention. J Public Health Nations Health 1965;55:429–34.
4. Thompson MS, Read JL, Hutchings HC, Paterson M, Harris ED Jr. The cost-effectiveness of auranofin: results of a randomized clinical trial. J Rheumatol 1988;15:35–42.
5. Organisation for Economic Co-operation and Development. http://www.oecd.org/health/.
6. O'Donnell JC, Pham SV, Pashos CL, Miller DW, Smith MD. Health technology assessment: lessons learned from around the world—an overview. Value Health 2009;12(Suppl 2):S1–5.
7. Committee on Quality of Health Care in America; Institute of Medicine. Crossing the Quality Chasm: A New Health System for the 21st Century. Washington, DC, National Academy of Sciences, 2001.
8. Drummond MF, Sculpher MJ, Torrance GW, O'Brien BJ, Stoddart GL. Methods for the Economic Evaluation of Health Care, 3rd edn. Oxford, Oxford University Press, 2005.
9. Kobelt G (2013) Health Economics: An Introduction to Economic Evaluation, 3rd edn. London, Office of Health Economics, 2013.
10. Koopmanschap MA, Rutten FF. A practical guide for calculating indirect costs of disease. Pharmacoeconomics 1996;10:460–6.
11. Franke LC, Ament AJ, van de Laar MA, Boonen A, Severens JL. Cost-of-illness of rheumatoid arthritis and ankylosing spondylitis. Clin Exp Rheumatol 2009;27(4 Suppl 55):S118–23.
12. Boonen A, van den Heuvel R, van Tubergen A, et al. Large differences in cost of illness and wellbeing between patients with fibromyalgia, chronic low back pain, or ankylosing spondylitis. Ann Rheum Dis 2005;64(3):396–402.
13. Boonen A, van der Heijde D, Landewé R, et al. Costs of ankylosing spondylitis in three European countries: the patient's perspective. Ann Rheum Dis 2003;62:741–7.
14. Moltó A, Etcheto A, van der Heijde D, Landewé R, van den Bosch F, Dougados M. Prevalence of comorbidities and evaluation of their screening in spondyloarthritis: results of the international cross-sectional ASAS-COMOSPA study. Ann Rheum Dis 2015;74(Suppl 2):743.
15. Kvamme MK, Lie E, Kvien TK, Kristiansen IS. Two-year direct and indirect costs for patients with inflammatory rheumatic joint diseases: data from real-life follow-up of patients in the NOR-DMARD registry. Rheumatology (Oxford) 2012;51(9):1618–27.
16. Cooksey R, Husain MJ, Brophy S, The cost of ankylosing spondylitis in the UK using linked routine and patient-reported survey data. PLoS One 2015;17;10(7):e0126105.
17. Rafia R, Ara R, Packham J, Haywood KL, Healey E. Healthcare costs and productivity losses directly attributable to ankylosing spondylitis. Clin Exp Rheumatol 2012;30:246–53.
18. Akkoç N, Direskeneli H, Erdem H, et al. Direct and indirect costs associated with ankylosing spondylitis and related disease activity scores in Turkey. Rheumatol Int 2015;35(9):1473–8.
19. Tsifetaki N, Migkos MP, Papagoras C, Voulgari PV, Athanasakis K, Drosos AA. Counting costs under severe financial constraints: a cost-of-illness analysis of spondyloarthropathies in a tertiary hospital in Greece. J Rheumatol 2015;42:963–7.
20. Malhan S, Pay S, Ataman S, et al. The cost of care of rheumatoid arthritis and ankylosing spondylitis patients in tertiary care rheumatology units in Turkey. Clin Exp Rheumatol 2012;30:202–7.
21. Moots RJ, Ostor AJ, Loft AG, et al. Reduction of direct and indirect costs in patients with AS receiving etanercept: results from an open-label 36-week extension of the ASCEND study in four European countries. Rheumatology (Oxford) 2012;51:393–6.
22. Petříková A, Doležal T, Klimeš J, Vocelka M, Sedová L, Kolář J. The economic burden of the ankylosing spondylitis in the Czech Republic: comparison between 2005 and 2008. Rheumatol Int 2013;33:1813–19.
23. van der Burg LR, Ter Wee MM, Boonen A. Effect of biological therapy on work participation in patients with ankylosing spondylitis: a systematic review. Ann Rheum Dis 2012;71:1924–33.
24. Kristensen LE, Petersson IF, Geborek P, et al. Sick leave in patients with ankylosing spondylitis before and after anti-TNF therapy: a population-based cohort study. Rheumatology (Oxford) 2012;51:243–9.
25. Marra CA, Marion SA, Guh DP, et al. Not all 'quality-adjusted life years' are equal. J Clin Epidemiol 2007;60:616–24.
26. Joore M, Brunenberg D, Nelemans P, et al. The impact of differences in EQ-5D and SF-6D utility scores on the acceptability of cost-utility ratios: results across five trial-based cost-utility studies. Value Health 2010;13:222–9.
27. Herdman M, Gudex C, Lloyd A, et al. Development and preliminary testing of the new five-level version of EQ-5D (EQ-5D-5L). Qual Life Res 2011;20(10):1727–36.
28. Kiltz U, van der Heijde D, Boonen A, et al. Development of a health index in patients with ankylosing spondylitis (ASAS HI): final result of a global initiative based on the ICF guided by ASAS. Ann Rheum Dis 2015;74:830–5.
29. Bansback N, Harrison M, Brazier J, et al. Health state utility values: a description of their development and applicationfor rheumatic diseases. Arthritis Rheum 2008:15;59:1018–26.
30. Van Tubergen A, Boonen A, Landewé R, et al. Cost effectiveness of combined spa-exercise therapy in ankylosing spondylitis: a randomized controlled trial.Arthritis Rheum 2002;47:459–67.
31. Boonen A, Patel V, Traina S, Chiou CF, Maetzel A, Tsuji W. Rapid and sustained improvement in health-related quality of life and utility for 72 weeks in patients with ankylosing spondylitis receiving etanercept. J Rheumatol 2008;35:662–7.
32. Gooch K, Feeny D, Wong RL, et al. Is the Health Utilities Index 3 valid for patients with ankylosing spondylitis? Value Health 2011;14:160–5.
33. Wailoo A, Hernández M, Philips C, Brophy S, Siebert S. Modeling health state utility values in ankylosing spondylitis: comparisons of direct and indirect methods. Value Health 2015;18:425–31.
34. Kimel M, Revicki D, Rao S, et al. Norms-based assessment of patient-reported outcomes associated with adalimumab monotherapy in patients with ankylosing spondylitis. Clin Exp Rheumatol 2011;29:624–32.
35. Boonen A, van der Heijde D, Landewé R, et al. How do the EQ-5D, SF-6D and the well-being rating scale compare in patients with ankylosing spondylitis? Ann Rheum Dis 2007;66:771–7.
36. Husereau D, Drummond M, Petrou S, et al. Consolidated Health Economic Evaluation Reporting Standards (CHEERS) statement. Med Econ 2013;16:713–19.
37. Bansback N, Maetzel A, Drummond M, et al. Considerations and preliminary proposals for defining a reference case for economic evaluations in ankylosing spondylitis. J Rheumatol 2007;34:1178–83.

38. Tran-Duy A, Boonen A, van de Laar MA, Severens JL. Impact on total population health and societal cost, and the implication on the actual cost-effectiveness of including tumour necrosis factor-α antagonists in management of ankylosing spondylitis: a dynamic population modelling study. Cost Eff Resour Alloc 2015;13:18.
39. Gaujoux-Viala C, Fautrel B. Cost effectiveness of therapeutic interventions in ankylosing spondylitis: a critical and systematic review. Pharmacoeconomics 2012;30:1145–56.
40. Bakker C, Hidding A, van der Linden S, van Doorslaer E . Cost effectiveness of group physical therapy compared to individualized therapy for ankylosing spondylitis. A randomized controlled trial. J Rheumatol 1994 Feb;21(2):264–8.
41. Tran-Duy A, Boonen A, van de Laar MA, Franke AC, Severens JL. A discrete event modelling framework for simulation of long-term outcomes of sequential treatment strategies for ankylosing spondylitis. Ann Rheum Dis 2011;70:2111–18.
42. Armstrong N, Joore M, van Asselt T, et al. Golimumab for the treatment of ankylosing spondylitis: a NICE single technology appraisal. Pharmacoeconomics 2013;31:415–25.
43. Borrás-Blasco J, Gracia-Pérez A, Rosique-Robles JD, Casterá ME, Abad FJ. Clinical and economic impact of the use of etanercept 25 mg once weekly in rheumatoid arthritis, psoriatic arthropathy and ankylosing spondylitis patients. Expert Opin Biol Ther 2014;14:145–50.
44. Závada J, Uher M, Sisol K, et al. A tailored approach to reduce dose of anti-TNF drugs may be equally effective, but substantially less costly than standard dosing in patients with ankylosing spondylitis over 1 year: a propensity score-matched cohort study. Ann Rheum Dis 2016;75(1):96–102.
45. van der Velde G, Pham B, Machado M,et al. Cost-effectiveness of biologic response modifiers compared to disease-modifying antirheumatic drugs for rheumatoid arthritis: a systematic review. Arthritis Care Res (Hoboken) 2011;63:65–78.
46. Fautrel B, Benhamou M, Breban M, et al. Cost effectiveness of two therapeutic regimens of infliximab in ankylosing spondylitis: economic evaluation within a randomised controlled trial. Ann Rheum Dis 2010;69:424–7.
47. van den Berg R, Stanislawska-Biernat E, van der Heijde DM. Comparison of recommendations for the use of anti-tumour necrosis factor therapy in ankylosing spondylitis in 23 countries worldwide. Rheumatology (Oxford) 2011;50:2270–7.
48. Drummond M, Barbieri M, Cook J, et al. Transferability of economic evaluations across jurisdictions: ISPOR Good Research Practices Task Force report. Value Health 2009;12:409–18.
49. Ottersen OP, Dasgupta J, Blouin C, et al. The political origins of health inequity: prospects for change. Lancet 2014;383(9917):630–67.

CHAPTER 26

Physical functioning and work ability

Michael M. Ward

Introduction to physical functioning and work ability

Similar to most musculoskeletal diseases, AS has the potential to impact physical functioning and work ability. Physical functioning refers to the ability to move to accomplish a task, and includes activities such as self-care, mobility, and doing chores. Physical functioning provides the foundation for the ability to work. Both of these activities can be impacted by specific aspects of AS, as well as by barriers in the environment (1, 2). Although patients with AS tend to have fewer functional limitations than patients with other rheumatic diseases, most patients are affected to some degree on occasion, and some patients can be profoundly and persistently affected (3).

Physical functioning

Assessment of physical functioning

Physical functioning can refer to performance on tasks actually undertaken (for example, ascending two flights of stairs) or the capacity to perform tasks (for example, ascending a 2000-m mountain). Measures of performance are generally preferred because these capture a person's typical experience. Functional ability can be assessed by direct observation, either naturalistically or in a designed test, such as timed chair stands. More often, self report of functional limitations is used, because this method allows assessment of a broad range of functions quickly. In addition, self-reports provide the patient's perspective of his or her experiences, which can be important for planning treatment. However, self-reports capture limitations beyond the specific tasks assessed, and should be viewed as general measures of overall frailty (4, 5).

The scope of items included in self-report measures of physical functioning depends implicitly on what level of functioning is considered normal. Most questionnaires include everyday tasks. Therefore, most physical function questionnaires have a ceiling effect, wherein they do not distinguish well among patients at the fit end of the scale. Some new measures, such as those of the Patient-Reported Outcome Measurement Information System (PROMIS), include distinctions between whether one can or cannot run 2 miles, and therefore redefine what is considered normal functioning (6). The PROMIS measure and the SF-36 physical functioning scales are also normalized to provide comparisons with the general population (7).

The measures most commonly used in AS are the BASFI, HAQ-S, and Dougados Functional Index (DFI) (8-10). These measures emphasize tasks involving axial movement. Scores are not referenced to the general population. Although termed 'disease-specific', these measures capture limitations regardless of the cause, and can be influenced by conditions other than AS. The BASFI is a 10-item questionnaire that uses a visual analogue or numerical rating scale format (possible range 0–10, with higher scores indicating more limitations) (see Box 26.1) (8).

The HAQ-S includes five questions on difficulty working at a desk and difficulty driving, in addition to the standard HAQ (9). The DFI is a 20-item questionnaire that asks about difficulty with dressing, mobility, bending, sleeping, and deep breathing (10).

Although each measure has been shown to have good psychometric properties, the BASFI has been preferred because of its focus on axial functions and because it is somewhat more sensitive to change than the other measures (11). In a recent study, the HAQ-S captured limitations due to peripheral arthritis better than the BASFI, and yet captured limitations in axial functions equally

Box 26.1 Items of the BASFI. Respondents are asked to rate difficulty doing each task over the past week

1. Putting on your socks or tights without help or aids (e.g. sock aid).
2. Bending forward from the waist to pick up a pen from the floor without an aid.
3. Reaching up to a high shelf without help or aids (e.g. helping hand).
4. Getting up out of an armless dining-room chair without using your hands or any other help.
5. Getting up off the floor without help from lying on your back.
6. Standing unsupported for 10 minutes without discomfort.
7. Climbing 12–15 steps without using a handrail or walking aid. One foot on each step.
8. Looking over your shoulder without turning your body.
9. Doing physically demanding activities (e.g. physiotherapy exercises, gardening, or sports).
10. Doing a full day's activities, whether it be at home or at work.

Table 26.1 Levels of the BASFI in large registry and cohort studies

Reference	Country	*n*	Source of sample	Mean age (years)	Mean duration of AS (years)	Mean BASFI (SD)
Taylor, 1998 (14)	UK	2965	Specialty rheumatology clinic and patient support group	44	19	4.0
Dagfinrud, 2004 (15)	Norway	314	University rheumatology clinic	44	13	3.1 (2.5)
Wei, 2007 (16)	Taiwan	329	University rheumatology clinic	39	7	1.9 (2.1)
Kobelt, 2008 (17)	Spain	601	Rheumatology clinics	48	19	3.8 (2.9)
Boonen, 2009 (18)	Belgium	619	Rheumatology clinics	44	17	5.2 (2.4)
Bakland, 2011 (19)	Norway	360	Regional registry	45	–	3.5
Bodur, 2012 (20)	Turkey	1381	University rheumatology clinics	40	12	3.3 (2.6)
Ward, 2013 (21)	USA	801	University rheumatology clinics	46	20	3.0†

†Median.

well (12). Difficulty in performing individual tasks of the BASFI and HAQ-S correlated well with the degree of impairment in corresponding physical movements (for example, difficulty looking behind oneself and restricted cervical rotation), but the BASFI had more non-specific associations.

Prevalence and severity of limitations in physical functioning

Mobility is the function most impacted by AS. One-third of patients report some difficulty with mobility, and 15% rated these limitations as very important, in contrast to only 25% who reported any difficulty in household tasks and 20% with any difficulty in self-care (13).

In studies of AS registries or large unselected cohorts, most patients had mild limitations in physical functioning (14–21). The BASFI averaged between 3 and 4 (out of 10) among patients with a mean age in the fifth decade and mean duration of AS of between 7 and 20 years (see Table 26.1).

Physical limitations typically increase with age and the duration of AS. In a large British study primarily of members of a patient support group, the median BASFI among men ranged from 2.5 at onset to 4 at 40 years of AS; among women, the median ranged from 3 at onset to 4.2 at 40 years (14). Among 801 US patients, 19% had a BASFI of 1 or lower, and 50% had a BASFI less than 3 (21). Functional limitations were more common among those with longer durations of AS, but 50% of those with AS for longer than 30 years had a BASFI less than 3.5. For comparison, among 223 healthy persons, the median BASFI was 0.2 (range 0–4.7), with higher scores among women, older persons, less well-educated individuals, and the obese (22).

In three studies that used the SF-36 physical functioning scale, mean scores were consistently 67 among men, compared to 87 in the general population (score of 100 indicates no limitations) (13, 15, 23). Scores were slightly worse among women. Scores were 1 SD lower than the general population, indicating appreciable difficulties by this measure (15). It is important to recognize that these studies included patients attending rheumatology clinics, and therefore likely represent a more severely affected subset. Physical functioning in patients with AS is generally better than in patients with RA (3, 23).

Causes of functional limitations

Measures of functional limitations describe the status of the patient, but do not indicate what is causing the limitation. Limitations can result from either acute temporary disturbances in mechanics or physiology, or more permanent impairments (24). This principle applies to virtually all measures of functioning. For example, renal function can be decreased by acute tubular necrosis or by chronic scarring of the kidney, and from a single measurement of serum creatinine one cannot distinguish between these two potential causes. Similarly, in AS, limitations in physical functioning can result from either acute limitations due to disease activity, or chronic changes related to structural damage, or from a combination of the two (see Fig. 26.1) (25).

For example, inability to look behind oneself while driving can be the result of pain due to spinal inflammation with acute muscle spasm, or from cervical spine fusion. When assessing functional limitations clinically, it is important to distinguish how much of the limitation may be due to disease activity and potentially reversible with treatment.

The most common disease activity-related causes of functional limitations in AS are spinal pain, stiffness, fatigue, and peripheral

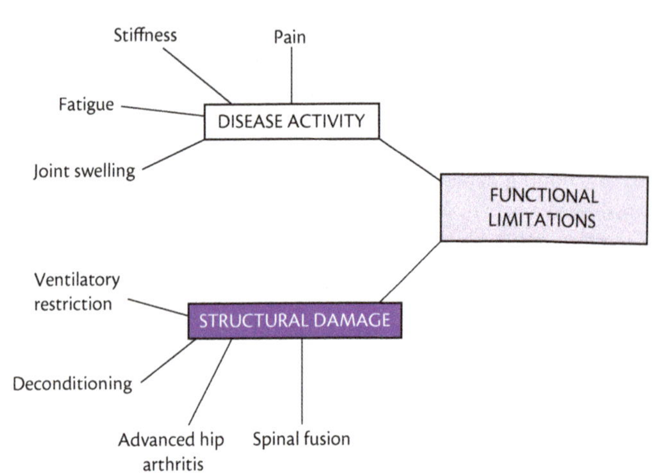

Fig. 26.1 Causes of functional limitations in AS.

joint pain and swelling (26). Each of these inflammatory manifestations can cause temporary limitations by interfering with normal body movement, strength, or endurance. Enthesitis can also have a major impact on physical functioning, but this association may partly represent an overlap between widespread enthesial tenderness and fibromyalgia (12). The most common structural damage-related causes of functional limitations are spinal fusion and advanced hip arthritis (18, 21). Extreme kyphosis, including patients who lack horizontal gaze, and advanced hip arthritis frequently result in the most severe functional limitations. Deconditioning may play a larger role than appreciated because it is rarely assessed. Ventilatory compromise due to a fixed rib cage and restrictive lung disease may also contribute (27). These manifestations are generally slowly progressive and not amenable to short-term treatment.

The impact of spinal fusion on functional ability varies with the duration of AS (21). Lumbar spine fusion has a greater influence on physical functioning in early AS, when it is often the predominant site of involvement, and has less strong associations after 20 years of AS, when cervical spine fusion comes to have the largest impact. Hip arthritis has the largest impact after 30 years of AS. Associations between the extent of spinal damage and functional limitations are stronger in early AS than in later AS, suggesting that patients with long-standing spinal fusion accommodate to this impairment to some degree.

Risk factors

The risk factors for functional limitations in AS are those that influence the two main mediators of disease activity and structural damage. As noted in the section 'Prevalence and severity of limitations in physical functioning', functional limitations tend to increase with age and duration of AS (14, 16, 21, 28–30). It is unclear if functional limitations differ by gender, although women report more limitations than men at the same degree of spinal fusion (13, 28 31). Patients of lower socioeconomic status have more limitations than others (13, 30, 32). Those with symptom onset before age 16 may have more limitations than those with onset at an older age (30).

Smokers have been consistently found to have more functional limitations than non-smokers, and limitations progress faster among smokers (28, 29, 32, 33). These associations may be mediated by both higher disease activity and more structural damage among smokers. Occupational physical activity is also a risk factor for functional limitations in AS (29). BASFI scores were on average 0.9 points higher (on a 0–10 scale) among those whose lifetime jobs required moderate physical activity than among those who only had sedentary occupations. Among individual occupational activities, dynamic flexibility, defined as repeated bending, twisting, and stretching, had the strongest association with functional limitations (34). This activity is common among masonry workers, roofers, construction laborers, timber cutters, and automobile repairmen, among others. Those whose past jobs required frequent dynamic flexibility had BASFI scores that averaged 1.1 points higher than those without such jobs. Although stretching is thought to improve AS symptoms, occupational activities are not discretionary, and may be required for longer periods and at times when the patient cannot move comfortably. Repeated stress of an inflamed back may underlie the association between occupational physical activity and long-term limitations.

Prevention and treatment

Interventions to prevent functional limitations in AS are limited to smoking cessation or avoidance, and occupational retraining for those with physically demanding jobs. Jobs that do not require excessive bending and twisting and that permit freedom of movement throughout the day should be encouraged as part of vocational counselling.

Recreational exercise and daily back stretching are beneficial for overall fitness and flexibility. However, evidence that these activities can prevent functional limitations or improve physical functioning in AS over the long term is limited. Extended follow-up of patients is needed to detect an effect, yet frequent changes in exercise habits over time can attenuate associations. High recreational activity during adolescence and young adulthood, as recalled by patients, was not associated with the degree of functional limitations in middle-aged patients with AS (29). In a prospective study, patients who did back exercises frequently had improvement in physical functioning compared to those who did not (33). Benefit was seen only among those who did back exercises at least 5 days per week (35). In this study, recreational exercise was not associated with improved physical functioning even though it was associated with less pain and stiffness.

Short-term physical therapy is effective in improving physical functioning in patients with AS, compared to no therapy (36). However, benefits are often not sustained after therapy. Improvements in physical functioning did not differ between group therapy or intensive spa therapy and individual physical therapy, even though the former interventions were more effective in improving pain (36). For patients with ventilatory limitations due to chest wall immobility, inspiratory muscle training may improve respiratory capacity and physical functioning (37).

For patients with advanced hip arthritis, total hip arthroplasty is a very effective treatment to decrease pain and increase mobility, with durable results (38, 39). Spinal osteotomy may be used to correct extreme cervical or thoracic kyphosis and improve functioning, but this surgery entails risks of spinal cord injury or mortality in 4–8% of patients (40, 41).

Medications that improve inflammatory symptoms, such as NSAIDs and TNFα inhibitors, also improve functional limitations that are due to disease activity. At present, no medications are known to improve physical functioning through mechanisms other than improvement in disease activity.

Work ability

Work is one of the central activities of adulthood. In addition to providing economic benefits, work provides psychological benefits by validating one's self-worth and providing opportunities for personal growth and social interactions. Therefore, when a chronic illness threatens one's ability to work, the consequences can extend beyond the loss of income. Because AS usually begins during young adulthood, it has the potential to impact the work ability of most patients. Permanent work disability is the main concern, but AS can also cause decreased work productivity or lead to changes in one's type of job.

Permanent work disability

Prevalence

Permanent work disability, or permanent withdrawal from the labour force due to illness, is the most consequential social outcome of AS (42, 43). In studies published since 2000, the prevalence of permanent work disability in cohorts of patients with AS ranged from 13% to 43% (see Table 26.2) (19, 44–56).

These cross-sectional studies each examined cohorts with a wide range of ages and durations of AS. Most studies examined patients attending university rheumatology clinics, and therefore likely included a greater proportion of patients with more severe AS than patients in the community at large. Consequently, the frequency of work disability in these studies is likely higher than would be observed in a population-based study of patients with AS (57). Studies also differed in the criteria used to define work disability. Some studies based the definition on receipt of a government or insurance disability pension, while others used patients' reports of inability to work due to illness. Variation among countries in

Table 26.2 Employment and work disability in persons with AS

Study (reference)	Country	n	Source of sample	Percentage male	Mean age (years)	Mean duration of AS (years)	Percentage employed	Work disability criterion	Percentage work disabled
Zink, 2000 (44)	Germany	8776	University and private rheumatology clinics	69	44	15	71	–	–
Ward, 2001 (45)	USA	234	University rheumatology clinic and community	70	48	21	87	Patient report	13
Boonen, 2001 (46)	Netherlands	529	Nationwide rheumatology practices	76	44	11.7	71	Pension	23
Barlow, 2001 (47)	UK	133	Specialty rheumatology clinic and patient support group	73	49	28	80	Patient report	20
Boonen, 2002 (48)	Europe	209	University rheumatology clinics	70	43	11	54	Pension	29
Zhu, 2008 (49)	China	145	University rheumatology clinic	79	40	10	67	Patient report	17
Forejtová, 2008 (50)	Czech Republic	989	Patient support group	62	50	23	–	Pension	27
Marengo, 2008 (51)	Argentina	64	Tertiary rheumatology clinic	90	43	–	74	Pension	9
Ariza-Ariza, 2009 (52)	Spain	699	University rheumatology clinics	77	48	14	–	Pension	25
Healey, 2011 (53)	UK	521	Specialty rheumatology clinics	72	51	17	60	Patient report	26
Ramos-Remus, 2011 (54)	Mexico	185	Rheumatology clinics	66	42	12	71	Pension	29
Bakland, 2011 (19)	Norway	360	University rheumatology clinic	73	45	22	–	Pension	43
Abdul-Sattar, 2014 (55)	Egypt	90	University rheumatology clinic	94	38	12	–	Patient report	40
Tu, 2014 (56)	China	257	University rheumatology clinic	83	28	6	64	Patient report	10

how liberal or strict the regulations are regarding disability pensions, and the ability of patients to navigate administrative regulations, can contribute to differences in the prevalence of work disability using this definition. The socioeconomic composition of the sample also influences the prevalence of work disability, with higher prevalences among cohorts with more blue-collar or manual workers (45, 46, 58, 59). Few studies reported the occupations of participants.

In most cohorts, 70% or more of working-age patients were employed. The proportion employed provides a different perspective on work ability than the proportion work disabled, as it represents individuals who have successfully adapted to their work circumstances. However, it is a less specific indicator of work disability because it is influenced by many factors other than illness, including age-related retirement, being a homemaker or student, and economic recessions. AS may also prompt premature retirement. While patients may elect early retirement in part due to symptoms or functional difficulty, this is not captured as work disability, but contributes to lower prevalences of employment.

Work disability is a cumulative process that increases with the duration of AS. Estimates of the overall proportion of individuals with work disability are difficult to interpret because not all patients will have had AS long enough to know if they will develop work disability. A more accurate representation comes from studies that report life-table analysis, which standardize follow-up among patients. Boonen et al. reported that 21% of Dutch patients were work disabled at 10 years of AS, and 31% were work disabled at 20 years of AS (46). In a Norwegian study, 30% of men and 40% of women were work disabled at 20 years of AS, increasing to 55% and 70%, respectively, at 30 years (19). Work disability accrued at a constant rate, without acceleration in late AS. In a small Argentinian study, 5% of patients were work disabled at age 40, but this proportion increased to 25% at age 50 (51). Work disability may also occur early. In one study, 15% of patients with SpA for less than 5 years were work disabled (60).

Comparisons with the general population

Persons with AS are two to three times more likely to be work disabled than persons in the general population of the same age and sex (46, 61). These elevated ratios are due in part to the low frequency of disability in young adults in the general population, and reflect the experience of patients with AS attending rheumatology clinics. Among college graduates with AS, the frequency of work disability was similar to the general population (61). In studies from the USA and Germany, employment among women with AS was similar to the general population, while men with AS were 6–39% less likely to be employed (61, 62). Among men, high relative unemployment was limited to those with long-standing AS or low education levels.

Trends in work disability

New work disability pensions for men with AS in Germany decreased from 32 per million in 2001 to 14 per million in 2011; among women with AS, the rate decreased from 11 per million in 2001 to 5 per million in 2011 (63). These impressive improvements paralleled those observed for patients with RA, and suggest that recent treatment advances have helped decrease the likelihood of work disability in AS at the population level.

Risk factors for work disability

As noted in the section 'Risk factors', the risk factors for work disability identified most consistently have been older age and lower levels of formal education (or lower socioeconomic status). Persons with university-level educations are 1.4–4 times more likely to remain employed than persons with less formal education (19, 44–47). This association is presumably related to the greater likelihood of heavy occupational physical activity among those with less formal education. Heavy physical activity at work increases the risk of work disability (45, 46, 58, 59). This may be due to the strain that physical activity places on inflamed joints, by the physical flexibility required in some jobs, added fatigue, or by less opportunity to regulate the pace of work.

Other risk factors are less well established, partly because studies often examine different risk factors (64). Although work disability is cumulative, it is unclear if the duration of AS has an effect on work disability independent of age. Studies differ on whether gender is associated with work disability (19, 44–48, 52, 53, 62). Peripheral arthritis, total hip arthroplasty, more extensive spinal fusion, more comorbid conditions, and functional limitations have also been identified as independent predictors of work disability in some studies (19, 45, 46, 52, 53). These results indicate that work disability is largely due to the extent and severity of musculoskeletal impairment. Aspects of the work environment that contribute to work disability have been less well studied, but the lack of workplace accommodations and poor employer support have been associated with higher risks of unemployment in persons with AS (65).

Work instability and the prevention of work disability

Withdrawal from work due to disability occurs after a period of increasing difficulty managing at work. This period of threatened work loss has been termed 'work instability'. Up to 40% of patients with AS attending rheumatology clinics may have work instability (66, 67). Identification of these patients can help to target interventions to prevent loss of work. Unfortunately, little research has been done on the effectiveness of vocational interventions to prevent work loss in AS (68). Results of one small clinical trial have suggested that treatment with TNFα inhibitors may decrease work instability in patients with AS, but larger studies are needed (69, 70).

Absenteeism

Sick leave, temporary disability, and reduced work hours all represent aspects of absenteeism. Like permanent work disability, absenteeism is a function of the worker's health status (due to possibly only a temporary exacerbation of symptoms), the type of work, and the worker's social circumstances. Risks differ between those with physically demanding and sedentary jobs, between those who are family breadwinners and those who can depend on others for support, and between those whose employers have supportive and those with restrictive policies regarding temporary absences (65).

Sick leaves are prevalent among workers with AS, occurring in 16–44% of patients annually (45, 49, 53, 54, 56, 71–74). However, the average number of sick days per year was generally low, ranging from 8 to 12 days. Extended sick leaves were uncommon, with 3% of workers reporting sick leave of 10 days or more in one study, and 10% reporting a sick leave of at least 30 days in another study (45, 53). Most sick days were due to AS rather than other causes. In Sweden, 52% of workers with AS had a sick leave of longer than 14 days at some time during a 7-year follow-up, compared to 36% of unaffected workers (75). Again, these studies were based largely on patients attending rheumatology clinics, and therefore likely show higher rates than those occurring in the population of workers with AS. Sick leave accounted for only 1.6–13% of indirect costs (costs due to lost productivity) of AS (43, 49, 56). Sick leave was more common among older workers and smokers, and those with more active AS, functional limitations, learned helplessness, depression, and those who valued work less (45, 53, 72–74).

Twenty percent to 30% of workers with AS work part-time or reduce their hours (45, 76). Part-time employment is more common among women, and reduced work hours is most associated with active symptoms (45, 62).

Presenteeism

Presenteeism refers to reduced work productivity among persons who come to work despite being ill. Presenteeism represents a decrease in the quantity or quality of work, due to physical, cognitive, or emotional limitations, or problems focusing, meeting deadlines, or interacting with coworkers. Nationally, presenteeism costs employers billions of dollars in expenses (77). Presenteeism can be manifested by a worker doing tasks more slowly, needing assistance from coworkers, or isolating himself or herself. Presenteeism was estimated to result in 20% lower productivity in workers with AS than in unaffected workers (range 6–49%) (43, 53, 56, 71, 73, 74). One to two additional hours of work per week were needed to compensate for presenteeism (71, 73). Higher disease activity was the most consistent predictor of presenteeism (53, 56, 71, 73, 74).

Choice of occupation

Because the type of occupation is closely related to the risk of work loss in AS, it is important that vocational counselling be part of the treatment plan for adolescents and young adults with AS. They should be discouraged from occupations that require heavy physical activity, particularly those involving dynamic flexibility and exposure to whole-body vibration (34). Jobs that allow for freedom of movement and control of the pace of work are more suited to maintenance of employment in the long term.

For those already in the workforce, changes in job type are uncommon. Among patients attending rheumatology clinics, 8–17% reported a change in their type of work over the course of AS, more often to a less physically demanding job (45, 46, 74). Job changes may not be motivated by illness in all cases. Women and those with more AS symptoms and physically demanding jobs were more likely to change their type of work (45).

The low frequency of changes in type of job contrast with the relatively high rates of permanent work disability, suggesting room for improvement in interventions to retrain patients for different types of work so they can remain in the workforce. Workplace accommodations can help prevent work loss. The effectiveness of specific vocational rehabilitation interventions is unclear, however (68). A Dutch study suggested that work disability could be prevented in 25% of patients with AS by job training, and in 73% by accommodations (76). Vocational rehabilitation may be more effective early in the work instability process, and monitoring of work instability may signal those who would be good candidates for intervention.

Conclusion

Most patients with AS have few limitations in physical functioning, with notable exceptions of temporary limitations due to active symptoms, advanced hip arthritis, and extreme kyphosis. Treatment to control symptoms and exercise are effective in maintaining functional ability. Many patients accommodate to spinal inflexibility. Work ability is most impacted by the job's physical demands, particularly those requiring dynamic flexibility. Maintenance of work ability is higher with less physically demanding jobs.

Acknowledgement

This work was funded by the Intramural Research Program, National Institute of Arthritis and Musculoskeletal and Skin Diseases, National Institutes of Health.

References

1. World Health Organization. Towards a Common Language for Functioning, Disability and Health: ICF. Geneva, WHO, 2002. http://www.who.int/classifications/icf/training/icfbeginnersguide.pdf.
2. Boonen A, van Berkel M, Cieza A, Stucki G, van der Heijde D. Which aspects of functioning are relevant for patients with ankylosing spondylitis: results of focus group interviews. J Rheumatol 2009;36:2501–11.
3. Louie GH, Reveille JD, Ward MM. Challenges comparing functional limitations in rheumatoid arthritis and ankylosing spondylitis. Clin Exp Rheumatol 2009;27:S83–91.
4. Louie GH, Ward MM. Association of measured physical performance and demographic and health characteristics with self-reported physical function: implications for the interpretation of self-reported limitations. Health Qual Life Outcomes 2010;8:84.
5. van Weely SF, van Denderen JC, Steultjens MP, et al. Moving instead of asking? Performance-based tests and BASFI-questionnaire measure different aspects of physical function in ankylosing spondylitis. Arthritis Res Ther 2012; 14:R52.
6. Fries JF, Cella D, Rose M, Krishnan E, Bruce B. Progress in assessing physical function in arthritis: PROMIS short forms and computerized adaptive testing. J Rheumatol 2009; 36:2061–6.
7. Ware JR Jr, Kosinski M, Dewey JE. How to score version 2 of the SF-36 health survey. Lincoln, Rhode Island, QualityMetric Incorporated, 2000.
8. Calin A, Garrett S, Whitelock H, et al. A new approach to defining functional ability in ankylosing spondylitis: the development of the Bath Ankylosing Spondylitis Functional Index. J Rheumatol 1994; 21:2281–5.
9. Daltroy LH, Larson MG, Roberts WN, Liang MH. A modification of the Health Assessment Questionnaire for the spondyloarthropathies. J Rheumatol 1990;17:946–50.
10. Dougados M, Gueguen A, Nakache JP, Nguyen M, Amor B. Evaluation of a functional index for patients with ankylosing spondylitis. J Rheumatol 1990; 17:1254–5.
11. Zochling J. Measures of symptoms and disease status in ankylosing spondylitis: Ankylosing Spondylitis Disease Activity Score (ASDAS), Ankylosing Spondylitis Quality of Life Scale (ASQoL), Bath Ankylosing Spondylitis Disease Activity Index (BASDAI), Bath Ankylosing Spondylitis Functional Index (BASFI), Bath Ankylosing Spondylitis Global Score (BAS-G), Bath Ankylosing Spondylitis Metrology Index (BASMI), Dougados Functional Index (DFI), and Health Assessment Questionnaire for the Spondylarthropathies (HAQ-S). Arthritis Care Res 2011;63(Suppl 11):S47–58.
12. Bethi S, Dasgupta A, Weisman MH, et al. Functional limitations due to axial and peripheral joint impairments in patients with ankylosing spondylitis: are focused measures more informative? Arthritis Care Res 2013;65:607–14.
13. Ward MM. Health-related quality of life in ankylosing spondylitis: a survey of 175 patients. Arthritis Care Res 1999;12:247–55.
14. Taylor AL, Balakrishnan C, Calin A. Reference centile charts for measures of disease activity, functional impairment, and metrology in ankylosing spondylitis. Arthritis Rheum 1998;41:1119–25.
15. Dagfinrud H, Mengshoel AM, Hagen KB, et al. Health status of patients with ankylosing spondylitis: a comparison with the general population. Ann Rheum Dis 2004;63:1605–10.

16. Wei JC-C, Wong R-H, Huang J-H, et al. Evaluation of internal consistency and re-test reliability of Bath ankylosing spondylitis indices in a large cohort of adult and juvenile spondylitis patients in Taiwan. Clin Rheumatol 2007;26:1685–91.
17. Kobelt G, Sobocki P, Mulero J, et al. The burden of ankylosing spondylitis in Spain. Value Health 2008;11:408–15.
18. Boonen A, van der Cruyssen B, de Vlam K, et al. Spinal radiographic changes in ankylosing spondylitis: association with clinical characteristics and functional outcome. J Rheumatol 2009;36:1249–55.
19. Bakland G, Gran JT, Becker-Merok A, Nordvåg BY, Nossent JC. Work disability in patients with ankylosing spondylitis in Norway. J Rheumatol 2011;38:479–84.
20. Bodur H, Ataman S, Bugdayci DS, et al. Description of the registry of patients with ankylosing spondylitis in Turkey: TRASD-IP. Rheumatol Int 2012;32:169–76.
21. Ward MM, Learch TJ, Gensler LS, et al. Regional radiographic damage and functional limitations in patients with ankylosing spondylitis: differences in early and late disease. Arthritis Care Res 2013;65:257–65.
22. Wariaghli G, Allali F, Berrada K, et al. Normative values for the Bath Ankylosing Spondylitis Functional Index in the general population compared with ankylosing spondylitis patients in Morocco. BMC Musculoskelet Disord 2012;13:40.
23. Chorus AMJ, Miedema HS, Boonen A, et al. Quality of life and work in patients with rheumatoid arthritis and ankylosing spondylitis of working age. Ann Rheum Dis 2003;62:1178–84.
24. Aletaha D, Smolen J, Ward MM. Measuring function in rheumatoid arthritis. Identifying reversible and irreversible components. Arthritis Rheum 2006;54:2784–92.
25. Landewé R, Dougados M, Mielants H, et al. Physical function in ankylosing spondylitis is independently determined by both disease activity and radiographic damage of the spine. Ann Rheum Dis 2009;68:863–7.
26. Spoorenberg A, van Tubergen A, Landewé R, et al. Measuring disease activity in ankylosing spondylitis: patient and physician have different perspectives. Rheumatology 2005;44:789–95.
27. Berdal G, Halvorsen S, van der Heijde D, Mowe M, Dagfinrud H. Restrictive pulmonary function is more prevalent in patients with ankylosing spondylitis than in matched population controls and is associated with impaired spinal mobility: a comparative study. Arthritis Res Ther 2012;14(1):R19.
28. Doran MF, Brophy S, MacKay K, et al. Predictors of longterm outcome in ankylosing spondylitis. J Rheumatol 2003;30:316–20.
29. Ward MM, Weisman MH, Davis JC Jr, Reveille JD. Risk factors for functional limitations in patients with long-standing ankylosing spondylitis. Arthritis Rheum 2015;53:710–17.
30. Stone M, Warren RW, Bruckel J, et al. Juvenile-onset ankylosing spondylitis is associated with worse functional outcomes than adult-onset ankylosing spondylitis. J Rheumatol 2005;53:445–51.
31. Lee W, Reveille JD, Davis JC Jr, et al. Are there gender differences in severity of ankylosing spondylitis? Results from the PSOAS cohort. Ann Rheum Dis 2007;66:633–8.
32. Mattey DL, Dawson SR, Healey EL, Packham JC. Relationship between smoking and patient-reported measures of disease outcome in ankylosing spondylitis. J Rheumatol 2011;38:2608–15.
33. Ward MM. Predictors of the progression of functional disability in patients with ankylosing spondylitis. J Rheumatol 2002;29:1420–5.
34. Ward MM, Reveille JD, Learch TJ, Davis JC Jr, Weisman MH. Occupational physical activities and long-term functional and radiographic outcomes in patients with ankylosing spondylitis. Arthritis Rheum 2008;59:822–32.
35. Uhrin Z, Kuzis S, Ward MM. Exercise and changes in health status in patients with ankylosing spondylitis. Arch Intern Med 2000;160:2969–75.
36. Dagfinrud H, Kvien TK, Hagen KB. Physiotherapy interventions for ankylosing spondylitis. Cochrane Database Syst Rev 2008;(1):CD002822.
37. Drăgoi RG, Amaricai E, Drăgoi M, Popoviciu H, Avram C. Inspiratory muscle training improves aerobic capacity and pulmonary function in patients with ankylosing spondylitis: a randomized controlled study. Clin Rehabil 2015 Mar 25;pii:0269215515578292.
38. Sweeney S, Gupta R, Taylor G, Calin A. Total hip arthroplasty in ankylosing spondylitis: outcome in 340 patients. J Rheumatol 2001;28:1862–6.
39. Joshi AB, Markovic L, Hardinge K, Murphy JC. Total hip arthroplasty in ankylosing spondylitis: an analysis of 181 hips. J Arthroplasty 2002;17:427–33.
40. Etame AB, Than KD, Wang AC, La MF, Park P. Surgical management of symptomatic cervical or cervicothoracic kyphosis due to ankylosing spondylitis. Spine 2008;33:E559–64.
41. Van Royen BJ, De Gast A. Lumbar osteotomy for correction of thoracolumbar kyphotic deformity in ankylosing spondylitis. A structured review of three methods of treatment. Ann Rheum Dis 1999;58:399–406.
42. Ward MM. Functional disability predicts total costs in patients with ankylosing spondylitis. Arthritis Rheum 2002;46:223–31.
43. Rafia R, Ara R, Packham J, Haywood KL, Healey E. Healthcare costs and productivity losses directly attributable to ankylosing spondylitis. Clin Exp Rheumatol 2012;30:246–52.
44. Zink A, Braun J, Listing J, Wollenhaupt J. Disability and handicap in rheumatoid arthritis and ankylosing spondylitis—results from the German Rheumatological Database. J Rheumatol 2000;27:613–22.
45. Ward MM, Kuzis S. Risk factors for work disability in patients with ankylosing spondylitis. J Rheumatol 2001;28:315–21.
46. Boonen A, Chorus A, Miedema H, et al. Withdrawal from labour force due to work disability in patients with ankylosing spondylitis. Ann Rheum Dis 2001;60:1033–9.
47. Barlow JH, Wright CC, Williams B, Keat A. Work disability among people with ankylosing spondylitis. Arthritis Care Res 2001;45:424–9.
48. Boonen A, van der Heijde D, Landewe R, et al. Work status and productivity costs due to ankylosing spondylitis: comparison of three European countries. Ann Rheum Dis 2002;61:429–37.
49. Zhu TY, Tam L-S, Lee VW-Y, et al. Costs and quality of life of patients with ankylosing spondylitis in Hong Kong. Rheumatology (Oxford) 2008;47:1422–5.
50. Forejtová Š, Mann H, Stolfa J, et al. Factors influencing health status and disability of patients with ankylosing spondylitis in the Czech Republic. Clin Rheumatol 2008;27:1005–13.
51. Marengo MF, Schneeberger EE, Citera G, Maldonado Coco JA. Work status among patients with ankylosing spondylitis. J Clin Rheumatol 2008;14:273–7.
52. Ariza-Ariza R, Hernández-Cruz B, Collantes E, et al. Work disability in patients with ankylosing spondylitis. J Rheumatol 2009;36:2512–16.
53. Healey EL, Haywood KL, Jordan KP, Garrett A, Packham JC. Impact of ankylosing spondylitis on work in patients across the UK. Scand J Rheumatol 2011;40:34–40.
54. Ramos-Remus C, Hernandez-Rios G, Duran-Barragan S, et al. Fifteen-year trends of long-term disability and sick leaves in ankylosing spondylitis. Clin Rheumatol 2011;30:361–7.
55. Abdul-Sattar A, Abou El Magd S. Prevalence and associated risk factors for work disability in Egyptian patients with ankylosing spondylitis from one center. Int J Rheum Dis 2014 Feb 15;doi 10.1111/1756-185X.12306.
56. Tu L, Rai JC, Cao S, et al. Costs and work limitation of patients with ankylosing spondylitis in China. Clin Exp Rheumatol 2014;32:661–6.
57. Gran JT, Husby G. Ankylosing spondylitis: a comparative study of patients in an epidemiological survey, and those admitted to a Department of Rheumatology. J Rheumatol 1984;11:788–93.
58. Roussou E, Kennedy LG, Garrett S, Calin A. Socioeconomic status in ankylosing spondylitis: relationship between occupation and disease activity. J Rheumatol 1997;24:908–11.
59. Boonen A, Chorus A, Landewe R, et al. Manual jobs increase the risk of patients with ankylosing spondylitis withdrawing from the labour force, also when adjusted for job related withdrawal in the general population. Ann Rheum Dis 2002;61:658.

60. van der Weijden MAC, Boonen A, van der Horst-Bruinsma IE. Problems in work participation and resource use should not be underestimated in patients with early spondyloarthritis. J Rheumatol 2014;41:2413–20.
61. Ward MM, Reveille JD, Learch TJ, Davis JC Jr, Weisman MH. Impact of ankylosing spondylitis on work and family life: comparisons with the US population. Arthritis Rheum 2008;59:497–503.
62. Mau W, Listing J, Huscher D, Zeidler H, Zink A, German Collaborative Arthritis Centers. Employment across chronic inflammatory rheumatic diseases and comparison with the general population. J Rheumatol 2005;32:721–8.
63. Mau W, Thiele K, Lamprecht J. Trends in work force participation of patients with rheumatic diseases. Results from German social insurance data and the national database of the German collaborative arthritis centers. Z Rheumatol 2014;73:11–19.
64. Boonen A, de Vet H, van der Heijde D, van der Linden S. Work status and its determinants among patients with ankylosing spondylitis. A systematic literature review. J Rheumatol 2001;28:1056–62.
65. Stolwijk C, Castillo-Ortiz J-D, Gignac M, Luime J, Boonen A, OMERACT Worker Productivity Group. Importance of contextual factors when measuring work outcome in ankylosing spondylitis: a systematic review by the OMERACT Worker Productivity Group. Arthritis Care Res (Hoboken) 2015 Mar 2;doi 10.1002/acr.22573 .
66. Gilworth G, Emery P, Barkham N, Smyth MG, Helliwell P, Tennant A. Reducing work disability in ankylosing spondylitis—development of a work instability scale for AS. BMC Musculoskelet Disord 2009;10:68.
67. Fabreguet I, Koumakis E, Burki V, et al. Assessment of work instability in spondyloarthritis: a cross-sectional study using the Ankylosing Spondylitis Work Instability scale. Rheumatology (Oxford) 2012;51:333–7.
68. Hoving JL, Lacaille D, Urquhart DM, et al. Non-pharmacological interventions for preventing job loss in workers with inflammatory arthritis. Cochrane Database Syst Rev 2014;11:CD010208.
69. Barkham N, Coates LC, Keen H, et al. Double-blind placebo-controlled trial of etanercept in the prevention of work disability in ankylosing spondylitis. Ann Rheum Dis 2010;69:1926–8.
70. van der Berg LRA, ter Wee MM, Boonen A. Effect of biological therapy on work participation in patients with ankylosing spondylitis: a systematic review. Ann Rheum Dis 2012;71:1924–33.
71. Boonen A, Chorus A, Miedema H, et al. Employment, work disability, and work days lost in patients with ankylosing spondylitis: a cross-sectional study of Dutch patients. Ann Rheum Dis 2000;60:353–8.
72. Boonen A, Brinkhuizen T, Landewe R, van der Heijde D, Severens JL. Impact of ankylosing spondylitis on sick leave, presenteeism, and unpaid productivity, and estimation of the societal cost. Ann Rheum Dis 2010;69:1123–8.
73. Gordeev VS, Maksymowych WP, Schachna L, Boonen A. Understanding presenteeism in patients with ankylosing spondylitis: contributing factors and association with sick leave. Arthritis Care Res 2014;66:916–24.
74. Boonen A, Boone C, Albert A, Mielants H. Understanding limitations in at-work productivity in patients with active ankylosing spondylitis: the role of work-related contextual factors. J Rheumatol 2015;42:93–100.
75. Strömbeck B, Jacobsson LT, Bremander A, et al. Patients with ankylosing spondylitis have increased sick leave—a registry-based case-control study over 7 yrs. Rheumatology (Oxford) 2009;48: 289–92.
76. Chorus AMJ, Boonen A, Miedema HS, van der Linden S. Employment perspectives of patients with ankylosing spondylitis. Ann Rheum Dis 2002;61:693–9.
77. Mitchell RJ, Bates P. Measuring health-related productivity costs. Popul Health Manag 2011;14:93–8.

CHAPTER 27

Patient support and advocacy

Seoirse Smith and Laurie M. Savage

Introduction to patient support and advocacy

Patient advocacy groups grew out of a need to provide support to and education for patients and to fuel research to better understand diseases, their diagnosis, and treatment options for patients. These organizations, while first viewed with skepticism by many, have become integral partners with the medical community in developing healthcare policy, patient education, and scientific research (1). Such organizations typically focus on a specific disease, conduct fundraising and public awareness, participate in scientific research, and publish and disseminate educational materials and services. These patient advocacy organizations serve as an important means for the public at large to learn about a specific disease, share stories about their experiences, participate in scientific research, and, more importantly, change their health behaviour (2).

In its current form, patient advocacy traces its roots to the early days of modern cancer research and treatment. In the 1950s, Dr Sidney Farber, a Harvard Medical School cancer researcher, coined the phrase 'total care' to describe all the services that children suffering from leukaemia and their families should receive, including clinical care, nutrition, social work, and emotional and psychological support (3). Everyone involved in the care of a child with leukaemia, thus, should be involved in and advocate for the child's treatment planning and aftercare activities. A manifestation of 'total care' is now practiced at many healthcare institutions. Educated patient advocacy organizations provide a unique perspective that few others share. To be effective, these organizations must be patient-centred (and often patient-led) and blend the ability and knowledge to participate in a range of activities to improve community health and enhance health policy initiatives (4).

Ankylosing Spondylitis International Federation

Vision

The vision of the Ankylosing Spondylitis International Federation (ASIF) is '*to be the global voice of those living with Ankylosing Spondylitis*'. The clear use of the phrase '*those living with Ankylosing Spondylitis*', rather than '*patient*', is completely intentional, as the impact of a person diagnosed with a chronic condition generally affects more people than that one person who has been diagnosed. With this in mind, ASIF is trying to be more inclusive and to involve all of the stakeholders that are impacted by or have an interest in the condition beyond the diagnosed person, as well as the diagnosed person him- or herself—be they family, friends, work colleagues, or healthcare professionals.

Mission

The ASIF Mission that is charged with supporting that vision of being the global voice of AS is as follows: '*To increase awareness of Ankylosing Spondylitis (AS) and disseminate knowledge of the disease around the world to all key stakeholders—be they people living with AS, health professionals, researchers, pharmaceutical organizations, policy makers or the general public.*'

Once again, the more inclusive and hopefully collaborative involvement of all of the stakeholders that are impacted by, have an interest in, or are involved somehow in managing the condition and its outcomes is reflected in the Mission Statement.

With improving awareness and education for the person diagnosed, the rise of the knowledgeable diagnosed person (sometimes referred to as the 'competent patient') as someone who becomes actively involved in collaborating in, and contributing to, the management of his or her condition is more a reality than ever before.

Objectives

In order to deliver on this mission, ASIF has five objectives. Each is simple in its desired outcome, but all are set out to deliver on the mission stated in the section 'Mission', with one primary underlying principle—support for all of those who need that support.

- To exchange information and experiences among the member societies.
- To support the development of newly formed societies.
- To cooperate in international research projects.
- To encourage the exchange of articles for publication in the journals of member societies.
- To contact Ankylosing Spondylitis stakeholders (primarily people living with AS and health professionals involved in managing the condition), in countries where an AS society does not yet exist.

Over the years of its operation, the Vision, Mission, and Objectives have developed, and will develop further, as the environment in which the member organizations operate continues to change. The specific goals that ASIF has developed to meet these objectives are the following:

- To have an AS support organization in every country. ASIF encourages the formation of support groups in all countries and is happy to provide advice and encouragement to enable this. The website currently has some information on how to set up a new organization, information that has been gathered over years of experience.

- To facilitate the exchange of information and cooperation among AS patients, scientists, rheumatologists, healthcare professionals, physicians, and physiotherapists.
- To provide an active voice for patients input into understanding and management of their condition by doctors and allied healthcare professionals.
- To work with media to get coverage of patient issues and promote awareness of AS and its implications for those living with the condition.

History

The idea for ASIF arose from discussions that started in 1984 amongst a number of patient support groups focused on AS (or Morbus Bechterew as it is known in some European countries) that already existed within Europe. Some of these organizations are still very active and have been a key part of ASIF's development and progress since then; for example, (1) the National Ankylosing Spondylitis Society (NASS) in the UK, which was founded in 1976; (2) Deutsche Vereinigung Morbus Bechterew (DVMB) in Germany, which was founded in 1980; and (3) Gigtforeningen for Morbus Bechterew in Denmark, which was founded in 1973.

These discussions and efforts to help support one another given their similar aims and intentions led the participants to organize a federation of patient support and advocacy groups focused on AS and culminating in an inaugural meeting in April 1988 in Bath, England. The current membership of ASIF stands at 39 organizations in 35 countries, as some countries have more than one representative organization. The most recent additions to the membership have been organizations from China, Cyprus, Russia, and Lithuania.

In keeping with the vision to be the global voice for those living with AS, ASIF seeks to reach out and encourage the formation of patient organizations and membership in more countries. All those living with AS need to know that they are not alone and deserve representation through patient organizations and membership in a worldwide community.

Since its foundation, ASIF has existed to support AS organizations around the world through sharing information, experiences, and knowledge. It exists to promote international cooperation on mutually beneficial projects. It exists to help develop support groups where none currently exists. There are some fundamental principles that all organizations in ASIF have. How these principles are met, what the priorities are, and what the outcomes are may differ across the organizations, across their geographies, and even across their timelines. However, the basic principles remain the same: to deliver holistic support to people living with AS, as effectively as possible, using all possible means at our disposal, and thereby empowering them to manage their condition.

The national organizations for AS wish to empower people living with AS

- by informing them on their condition and its management;
- by informing their medical team on their condition and its management;
- by educating all related stakeholders and the general public;
- by removing barriers and obstacles associated with living with this chronic illness.

The latter includes social, regulatory, financial, and employment barriers, where possible. While this last point is important for any disease advocacy organization, there is perhaps some added importance that we see within the AS community. This is principally due to the age of onset and the profile of the people that are diagnosed with AS—frequently they are in their late teens or early 20s, just at the beginning of their active participation in society as adults, with significant new elements to their lives being undertaken with careers, financial commitments, life partners, and family.

ASIF-promoted projects

There have been significant advances in AS through ASIF promoting and supporting a number of international projects. Aside from the published outcomes of these projects, there is another more specific value that ASIF seeks to promote amongst stakeholders, and that is to engage geographically dispersed patient groupings with varying experiences and also larger cohorts of people to contribute to the studies.

On top of this, it has been extremely valuable to endorse the principle of the more 'mature', usually larger, organizations being able to provide support, assistance, and guidance in participating in research projects to the less mature organizations, along with the 'develop once and use many times' approach of creating project elements once, to be reused by many others on a repeatable basis.

There are a number of examples of these principles and approaches by ASIF-supported projects over the years since its inception. Amongst the many significant studies are the following:

Pregnancy and AS—1998 (5)

A questionnaire was developed by Prof. Dr Monika Østensen, Department of Rheumatology, University Hospital, Trondheim in Norway. This was then published in newsletters of AS societies or sent to female members in Canada, the USA, and 11 European countries. After analysis there then followed a publication of the results in the *Journal of Rheumatology*, with patient-adapted publications appearing in newsletters of contributing AS societies.

Car Driving with AS—1998 (6)

Car safety has increased in recent decades and it continues to improve. However, safety systems are designed primarily with regard to healthy people. Those suffering from AS with moderate to marked severity present special problems in driving a car. ASIF and its member organizations saw it as their task to provide members with some guidelines on safe car driving. This booklet was the result.

Comparison of HLA-B27—2003 (7)

Prof. Dr Ernst Feldtkeller (Munich, Germany), who was then the vice-president of ASIF, in cooperation with Prof. Dr M. Asim Khan (Cleveland, Ohio, USA), Prof. Dr Désirée van der Heijde and Prof. Dr Sjef van der Linden (University of Maastricht, Netherlands), and Prof. Dr Jürgen Braun (Herne, Germany) undertook this study. A questionnaire was developed and published in the June 2000 newsletters of the AS societies in Germany (DVMB) and Austria (Österreichische Vereinigung Morbus Bechterew, OVMB). After analysis there then followed a publication of the study in *Rheumatology International*, with patient-adapted publications appearing in newsletters of contributing AS societies.

Survey of Vertebral Fractures—2005, 2005 & 2006 (8)

Questions on vertebral fractures were included in the questionnaire published in the June 2000 newsletters of the AS societies in Germany and Austria (see above). A second questionnaire with detailed questions on vertebral fractures to be answered only by patients with a history of a vertebral fracture was printed in the membership journals of the AS societies in Germany and Denmark in June 2001. X-rays of some of the fractures were available to be inspected. Prof. Dr Ernst Feldtkeller (Munich, Germany) and Debby Vosse MD (University of Maastricht, Netherlands), in cooperation with Jon Erlendsson MD (consulting rheumatologist of AS society in Denmark), Piet Geusens MD (Professor of Rheumatology, Limburg University Center, Diepenbeek, Belgium, and University of Maastricht, Netherlands), and Sjef van der Linden MD (Professor of Rheumatology, University of Maastricht, Netherlands) completed this work.

The results were published in two steps: step 1—Prevalence and Annual Incidence of Vertebral Fractures in Patients with Ankylosing Spondylitis. *Rheumatology International*; and step 2—Clinical Vertebral Fractures in Patients with Ankylosing Spondylitis. *Journal of Rheumatology* (9).

A patient-adapted publication of the result of both steps appeared in the March 2005 issue of *Morbus-Bechterew-Journal*, the journal of the AS society in Germany, with translations published in the newsletters of other AS societies around the world.

NSAID Therapy of AS—2006 (10)

Questions on the efficacy and side-effects of NSAID treatment were included in the questionnaire published in the June 2000 newsletters of the AS societies in Germany and Austria. The study was completed by Jane Zochling (Herne) in cooperation with Martin Bohl-Bühler (Brandenburg and Berlin), Prof. Dr Ernst Feldtkeller (then vice-president of ASIF, Munich), and Prof. Dr Jürgen Braun (Herne, Germany). The results were published in *Clinical Rheumatology*, with patient-adapted publications appearing in newsletters of contributing AS societies.

Disease Triggers of AS—2006 (11)

Questions on possible triggers of the disease were included in the questionnaire published in the June 2000 newsletters of the AS societies in Germany and Austria. The study was conducted by Jane Zochling (Herne) in cooperation with Martin Bohl-Bühler (Brandenburg and Berlin), Prof. Dr Ernst Feldtkeller (then vice-president of ASIF, Munich), and Prof. Dr Jürgen Braun (Herne, Germany). The scientific results were published in *Clinical Rheumatology*.

Disease Duration of AS—2008 (12, 13)

Answers were developed by the ASIF vice-president (Prof. Dr Ernst Feldtkeller) and president (Jon Erlendsson MD) on a publication in which the duration since diagnosis was regarded as a possible definition of the term 'disease duration' for AS. This piece covered the definition of disease duration in AS as a comment on the article by Davis et al. published as an 'electronic letter' in *Annals of Rheumatic Diseases*.

Common Infections in AS—2006 (14)

Questions on common infections were included in the questionnaire published in the June 2000 newsletters of the AS societies in Germany and Austria. The study was completed by Jane Zochling (Herne) in cooperation with Martin Bohl-Bühler (Brandenburg and Berlin), Prof. Dr Ernst Feldtkeller (vice-president of ASIF, München), and Prof. Dr Jürgen Braun (Herne, Germany). The results of the study were published in *Clinical Rheumatology*, with a patient-adapted publication of the results appearing in the June 2006 issue of *Morbus-Bechterew-Journal*, the journal of the AS society in Germany—this was then made available for other AS organizations to reproduce.

Behaviour and Environmental Adaptations in AS—2013 (15)

This was a project for the development of a core set of recommendations to be given to patients by their rheumatologists, preferably in connection with the diagnosis of AS. This was achieved by literature search of the scientific and patient-oriented literature, evaluation of raw recommendations by participants of the ASIF Council meeting in 2011, followed by the selection of final recommendations by extensive discussion later. The resulting recommendations were documented in *Rheumatology International*.

Don't Turn Your Back on It—2014 (16)

With Prof. Joachim Sieper, the ASIF president co-chaired a task force on this European IBP awareness initiative. This initiative was undertaken to increase awareness of IBP and to encourage people to move towards a solution for the frequent delay in diagnosis. Being proactive and visiting a healthcare professional to get a correct diagnosis can lead to appropriate and timely care. A key element of the initiative was to develop the core assets, materials, and approach centrally, before making them available for adoption by each of the countries taking up this initiative. A critically important aspect of the initiative was the collaborative nature of the plan, involving relevant stakeholders from a pharmaceutical company (in this case AbbVie), healthcare professionals, rheumatologists, and patient advocates/representatives.

Initially, the awareness programme was launched in France, Germany, Italy, Spain, and the UK. This was then followed by Australia, Japan, New Zealand, Portugal, Ireland, and Norway. There are plans for a further ten countries to use the awareness programme in 2015.

What has changed since the foundation of ASIF?

Increased number of stakeholders

In the years that ASIF and its member organizations have been in existence, there has been an increase in the number of stakeholders involved in managing AS. The stakeholder group now includes more healthcare professionals and for more sustained periods of time than before. In the early days, referral to a specialist rheumatologist and possibly, but not always, to a physiotherapist appeared to be the limit of the healthcare team involved in managing the condition. Now, the physiotherapist is definitely part of managing the condition over the longer term, and the diagnosis may be made by the specialist rheumatologist, but now also contributed to by the GP, and possibly the nurse specialist or occupational therapist. There is also a more recognizable role for researchers, scientists, and pharmaceutical companies. Lastly, the realization that the person diagnosed should have a role alongside an expanded team of healthcare professionals is particularly noticeable.

The rise of the 'competent patient'

One of the major changes in the period since ASIF was founded is the increasing knowledge of those diagnosed, what has been called the 'competent patient', and the increasing knowledge of those that assist and support those with AS. A great deal of that increase in knowledge is attributable to the organizations that now exist, many on a voluntary basis, to provide help, assistance, support, and information. An excellent example of this is the SAA, as discussed in the section 'Spondylitis Association of America', in addition to the other member organizations of ASIF. The role of the diagnosed person, alongside healthcare professionals, in proactively participating in the management of his or her own condition and not as a passive spectator is a big step forward and a noticeable change.

Greater collaboration across those stakeholders

Along with the expanded team of stakeholders involved in managing the chronic condition that is AS is a realization that greater collaboration among all of those concerned can lead to more effective treatment regimes, better management, greater adherence to the treatment plan, including exercise, lifestyle, and pharmaceutical therapies, and ultimately better outcomes for the diagnosed person.

Changing engagement models for patients

A key development over the time period is the changed focus on patient journeys. The ability to 'map' the journey from symptom to diagnosis to treatment to ultimately living with the condition for better outcomes has resulted in changed engagement models for patients. These changed engagement models and the move away from being diagnosed meaning the patient is a spectator in the management of his or her condition is having a positive effect on prognosis and outcomes, particularly when viewed in quality of life terms.

Where does ASIF go from here?

ASIF has completed some good work and there is more on the way; however, there is a need to continue to change and adapt ASIF's work to the current environment, at all levels, including:

- financial and commercial;
- political and social;
- medical and technical.

The challenge is how to do that—while continuing to support member organizations to fulfil their basic operational commitments to support people living with AS.

The areas that have been identified so far as offering the best path forward are as follows:

Greater collaboration with similar organizations

Greater connection and collaboration with organizations that are similar to ASIF but possibly from different or related disease areas; for example, the International Federation of Psoriasis Associations (IFPA), the European Federation of Crohn's and Ulcerative Colitis Associations (EFCCA), and the Platform of Organizations of People with Rheumatic Diseases in Southern Europe (AGORA).

Greater engagement with international law makers and political representatives

An increased role and engagement at EULAR/People with Arthritis and Rheumatism (PARE) will help strengthen our collective voice and hopefully lead to a greater impact at the political and social level. The opportunities for ASIF and AS patient groups to address this chronic condition with the WHO must be organized—one way of doing this is to connect with similar organizations to approach WHO jointly.

More collaborative efforts in a number of areas

- Engaging with the healthcare professional organizations to jointly develop the desire for collaborative management of the condition for better outcomes, promoting the knowledgeable patient as a key stakeholder in the management of the condition.
- Building on the relationships already developed with the pharmaceutical industry will help develop a better conversation about treatment programmes that deliver for the diagnosed person more effectively.
- Further improvements on initiatives to 'develop/build once and use many ...', allowing smaller, less mature patient groups to benefit from the more mature, larger organizations.

Branding and inclusion of nr-axSpA

AS is a chronic condition that suffers from poor awareness and understanding. Part of that is attributable to the fact that the disease is not well recognized and in the past has been called a number of different names (not least Morbus Bechterew and AS). There is a need to 'rebrand' AS. There is a need for it to be understood in the same way that CF (cystic fibrosis), MS (multiple sclerosis), and ALS (amyotrophic lateral sclerosis) are known by the public. These days, one rarely hears the full name of any of those three conditions, yet it is generally understood what is meant by just their initials. Also, there is a public awareness challenge regarding nr-axSpA, as well as AS, recognizing that these are related and deserving of the same attention, support, advice, and information. This is a question that needs to be answered by any efforts to 'rebrand' and increase awareness of the condition.

The Spondylitis Association of America

As the only non-profit organization in the USA dedicated to advocacy on behalf of individuals affected by SpA, the SAA seeks to promote education, research, and optimal care for all SpA patients. Among its advocacy priorities are promoting earlier diagnosis and treatment of SpA, promoting public awareness and education about the disease, improving access to appropriate quality healthcare and medications for patients, increasing federal funding for research, and influencing public policy that impacts patients' lives.

History

In 1983, two physicians and ten patients met in Los Angeles to create the country's first-ever SpA support group. A year later, the organization became a tax-exempt, non-profit corporation under the name of the Ankylosing Spondylitis Association (ASA). Jane Bruckel, a volunteer, nurse, and SpA patient, was elected the group's first president. The ASA gained national attention in 1985 when a *Los Angeles Times* article, 'Dealing with the Back Pain with a Funny Name,' (16) elicited more than 500 letters and phone calls from across the country, creating a surge in support. Bruckel retired from the ASA in 2006. As the ASA grew, it established a national Medical and Scientific Advisory Board, comprising SpA researchers and health professionals. In 1992, the organization changed its name to the Spondylitis Association of America (SAA) to reflect a broadened mission that encompassed diseases related to AS. Its board of directors changed the organization's major focus 4 years later to funding and helping to organize research efforts.

The 1990s saw steady growth for the SAA, with efforts focusing on research, public awareness, educational programming, and fundraising. By 2011, the SAA received its third consecutive Four Star Charity Navigator Award and, in 2012, was named by Charity Navigator as one of the top ten charities in the USA 'worth watching'. In 2013, the SAA teamed up with the ACR and SPARTAN to develop new axSpA treatment guidelines, which were published in September 2015. The SAA served as SPARTAN's fiscal agent from the group's inception through December 2013.

An advocacy organization for millions

Since its founding in 1983, the SAA has been the only patient advocacy organization in the USA that dedicates all of its resources to meeting the needs and improving the lives of the SpA community. Thirty-two years ago in the USA, there were no public support networks, no resources for educating physicians or the general public, no pamphlets or information guides for people living with SpA. There were few treatment options, no media coverage, and no research groups dedicated to this disease. Since then, the SAA has been at the forefront of every major milestone in SpA research, education, and advocacy in the USA, and remains what it is today: the first and largest resource for millions of Americans who are affected by SpA.

The SAA's advocacy efforts range from publications and videos, educational programming for patients, physicians, and caregivers, patient support services, and tools that help patients manage their disease.

Soon after the *Los Angeles Times* article mentioned in the section 'History', the SAA produced the first comprehensive patient self-management book, *Straight Talk on Spondylitis* (17), which received praise from medical professionals worldwide. Written specifically for SpA patients, the book contains information on therapies and treatment; a comprehensive list of medications, activities, and exercise programmes; and tips for coping with the psychological challenges of living with a chronic illness. The SAA published subsequent editions in 1992 and 2009.

In 2009, the SAA completed the development and production of the first-ever training video for emergency first responders, 'Ankylosing Spondylitis: Managing Patients in an Emergency Setting, a Primer for First Responders'. Accredited by the Continuing Education Coordinating Board for Emergency Medical Services, the programme has been incorporated into the permanent curricula of multiple emergency medical technician (EMT) training programmes in the USA. Many of the SpA member organizations of the ASIF are currently collaborating with the SAA to adapt the programme for other healthcare delivery systems and to translate it into other languages (18). In addition, the SAA produces a wide range of publications and materials with information specifically targeted to the SpA community, including educational brochures on topics ranging from childhood-onset SpA to exercise and iritis, as well as *Spondylitis Plus*, the SAA's award-winning quarterly news magazine.

Each year, SAA professional staff travel across the country to host free educational seminars in different metropolitan areas throughout the USA. All seminars include an experienced rheumatologist, who provides an overview of SpA, and other speakers who complement the programme with presentations on a host of other topics. The SAA offers multimedia resources as well—free online webinars on a variety of issues, monthly podcasts on topics of interest to the SpA community, and video highlights of its many educational seminars. In addition, the SAA sponsors scientific symposia to create cross-discipline dialogues among researchers and clinicians in both SpA and conditions that are related to the disease.

The SAA offers several different ways for patients and their families to connect with others in the SpA community. Through the National Educational Support Group Network, the SAA sponsors more than 30 support groups across the USA, focusing on education and support while providing a safe and friendly environment for people to discuss the day-to-day practical challenges of living with SpA. Through the Internet, message boards, and other social media platforms (19–23), the SAA has an online community that provides an opportunity for SpA patients and their loved ones to contribute to discussions related to managing SpA. The SAA's website had more than 422 000 visits (including nearly 324 000 unique visitors) in the fourth quarter of fiscal year (FY) 2013 (1 April–30 June 2014). The organization received 7692 likes on its Facebook page and has 3157 Twitter followers. The SAA's forums and message boards were viewed more than 692 000 times in the last quarter of FY 2013. Two additional SAA websites—its Spondylitis Update Newsletter (*eSUN*) electronic newsletter and Spondylitis Web Info for Teens (SWIFT)—are also popular; nearly 17 000 people subscribed to *eSUN*, and SWIFT had 789 unique visitors in FY 2013's fourth quarter.

Accelerating research

Since 1996, networks of individuals affected with a specific disease or group of diseases have become partners with laboratory scientists and clinical investigators to further research the biology and treatment of disease (24). For more than 25 years the SAA has encouraged and facilitated collaborations among prominent physician-scientists as a means of accelerating advances in SpA research, diagnosis, and treatment. The SAA was instrumental in the collaborative establishment of SPARTAN, which comprises a group of North American health professionals dedicated to research, awareness, and treatment of SpA (25).

In 1998, the SAA provided the seed money to launch the AS Genetics Study (26), the first major genetic study of SpA in North America. The National Institutes of Health (NIH) followed with a multi-million-dollar grant to expand the project, enabling collaboration among ten university medical centres and SAA, to identify the genetic causes of SpA. SAA spearheaded the collection of data from 400 families with sibling pairs who have SpA. Through this important data collection, principal investigator John D. Reveille, MD, at the University of Texas Health Science Center at Houston, who was successful in obtaining NIH funding, and his colleagues made the remarkable discovery of seven genetic abnormalities that contribute to the susceptibility and cause of SpA.

In a 2005 study, Dr Tammy M. Martin and colleagues, with patient recruitment support from the SAA, sought to uncover whether a specific gene or multiple genes are involved in susceptibility to iritis, or AAU, which is a serious inflammation of the eye (27). AAU occurs in the absence of other inflammatory diseases or in the presence or SpA and related diseases. Since 40% of patients with SpA also have AAU, the study enrolled a large proportion of participants with SpA. The study identified aberrations in the 9p chromosomal region, which contains as many as 100 different genes, as the potential cause of AAU. It was the first study to employ a genome-wide scan to identify a genetic region for AAU.

A collaborative effort in 2007 by an international team of researchers in the UK, Australia, and the USA—called the Australo-Anglo-American Spondylitis Consortium (TASC) (28) and headed by Dr Reveille and Dr Matthew Brown at the University of Queensland—led to the discovery of two genes that increase susceptibility to SpA. This was the most significant breakthrough since HLA-B27, a predisposing gene that accounts for most of the genetic susceptibility to SpA, was identified in 1970. The two newly identified genes, ERAP1 and IL-23R, also play a role in susceptibility to SpA. The findings of the study, which was partially funded through the SAA, resulted from the largest and most comprehensive GWAS ever conducted at the time.

The SAA funded TASC's precursor, the North American Spondylitis Consortium (NASC), and served as NASC's Clinical Coordinator Centre. It then went on to serve as one of the Clinical Coordinator Centres of the multinational coalition TASC, and the SAA's executive director and associate executive director served as co-principal investigators in the Administrative Core of TASC. In subsequent TASC studies, Dr Reveille, Dr Brown, and colleagues discovered additional regions of the genome associated with SpA. In 2011, the researchers uncovered three variants in the RUNX3, LTBR-TNFRSF1A, and IL-12B regions of the genome, as well as additional areas that also seem to play a role in SpA. Together, these and earlier TASC genetic findings identified potential new treatment targets for the disease (29).

Additionally, the SAA has been involved in other major SpA research efforts, including the first SpA epidemiology study conducted by the Centers for Disease Control and Prevention (CDC), which used data and statistical methodology from the SAA Spondylitis Screening Tool in SpA as the foundation for the patient questionnaire developed by the CDC.

In 2013, the SAA seeded a national patient registry on SpA. By combining existing patient databases that have been used in research, the composite registry can examine thousands and potentially tens of thousands of patients and track health trends, disease severity over time, age, gender, race, and many other factors, in order to improve understanding of SpA. Without the SAA's ability and commitment to patient recruitment, much of the work accomplished today would not have been possible.

The SAA is also supporting research conducted by Dr James Rosenbaum of the Oregon Health and Science University on the role of the gut microbiome (the collective genomes of the microbial population living in the intestine) in SpA, which may be a promising future target for SpA therapy (30), and laboratory studies by Dr Joel Taurog of the University of Texas Southwestern Medical Center in Dallas on the role of HLA-B27 and other genes implicated in SpA.

In the coming years, the SAA will continue to help participate in and drive important research, as well as keep its constituents informed of the latest scientific breakthroughs.

Addressing the needs of spondyloarthritis patients

The SAA has conducted two major studies of how SpA impacts patients' quality of life. These studies examined issues ranging from time to diagnosis and pain to employment and medication.

The 2002 AS Life Impact Study (31) was conducted by Harris Interactive (known as the Harris Poll) on behalf of the SAA. Harris surveyed 2190 adults to learn more about the experiences of people with AS and the impact of the disease on their daily lives. This formed the basis of a study, led by Drs Millicent Stone and Robert Inman at the University of Toronto, which was the first-ever extensive nationwide survey of juvenile- and adult-onset AS patients. Among the key findings, which were published in the June 2005 issue of *Arthritis Care and Research* (32), were that:

- AS is difficult to diagnose and often takes up to 10 years from the time a patient first experiences symptoms to the time the patient receives a proper diagnosis. More than half of the respondents were not diagnosed with AS until at least 5 years after the onset of symptoms, and 30% endured symptoms for more than 10 years before being diagnosed.
- AS causes permanent physical damage. Two-thirds of those surveyed said that AS has forced them into a forward-stooped posture to some degree, and more than half said their spine had at least partially fused—or become rigid.
- AS is a painful disease. More than 70% of the patients said that back pain or stiffness was one of the first symptoms that caused them to seek treatment. Three out of ten said that they were incapacitated when their AS pain was at its worst and could not move.
- AS causes people to change jobs or stop working. Nearly 44% of those surveyed said they had to avoid certain careers or jobs because of AS. Seventeen percent of those under age 65 described themselves as 'not working'. Of those, six out of ten said AS was the reason for their unemployment.
- AS greatly affects patients' daily lives. More than 60% of respondents said that AS is at least somewhat limiting in terms of getting into a car, walking, or having a satisfying sex life. Eighty percent said AS limits quality sleep.
- Patients try a variety of treatments to help them cope with AS. More than 80% of patients had taken a prescription medication in the past year to manage their AS and almost half had taken an over-the-counter drug to do so.

A follow-up AS Life Impact Study (33) was launched in 2011 to poll AS patients about symptoms, diagnosis, treatment, medication, and quality of life issues. In this survey, conducted by Launch Box, LLC, 865 interviews were conducted with people who have AS and related diseases, including uSpA, JoSpA, enteropathic arthritis, and ReA.

The findings built on the first AS Life Impact Survey. More than half of the respondents had had their disease for more than 20 years. On average, it took between 1 and 5 years to be diagnosed. Uveitis was most likely to be diagnosed quickly, while uSpA, JoSpA, PsA, and general spondylitis often took five or more years to detect. More than 75% of the respondents suffered from pain in the lumbar spine, neck, and hip, while they had pain to a lesser extent in their knees, ribs, and fingers. Pain appeared to be inversely related to income, suggesting that lower-income patients may not be receiving equal treatment.

Among the survey participants, comorbidity was high. More than 34% had high blood pressure and another 23% had high cholesterol. Irritable bowels, balance issues, and sexual dysfunction affected at least one-quarter of respondents. Again, those with lower incomes showed a higher incidence of these conditions. The most common treatments prescribed by physicians included NSAIDs such as ibuprofen and acetaminophen. Of the biologics, Enbrel was taken by 19% of patients, followed by Humira (14%) and Remicade (12%). MTX was used by only 11%. Stretching, strengthening, biking, walking, and running, as well as proper posture techniques were the most common non-medical treatments used by respondents. Three out of 10 patients reported seeing one doctor, typically a rheumatologist, while another third saw two doctors, and yet another third saw three or more doctors. The remaining 10% did not see a doctor for their AS; 36% of these individuals said they were not bothered by their disease.

As part of the survey, the SAA incorporated the Evaluation of Ankylosing Spondylitis Quality of Life (EASi-QoL) (34), a self-reporting measurement tool used to evaluate patients' physical function, disease activity, emotional well-being, and social participation. Physical function had the most impact on QoL scores. Disease activity appeared to have only a moderate impact, while emotional well-being had the smallest impact.

The results of the two surveys led to major, never-before-documented findings, highlighting a need for increased awareness and earlier treatment of AS and enabling physicians and the SAA to better address the needs of the AS community.

Lobbying and legislating

In addition to the patient education, public awareness, and scientific research components of its advocacy activities, the SAA has taken a leadership role in legislative advocacy, working with the US Congress and other elected officials to raise awareness of SpA and to increase federal funding for basic research and clinical trials. The SAA is a member of the NIH's National Institute of Arthritis and Musculoskeletal and Skin Diseases (NIAMS) Coalition. Composed of nearly 60 voluntary and professional associations, the NIAMS Coalition annually visits congressional offices in Washington, DC, to showcase broad support for NIAMS initiatives and to instruct Congress about research opportunities and findings related to musculoskeletal and skin diseases. As a member of the Coalition, the SAA's Executive Director served a 2-year term as Co-Chair of the NIAMS Coalition in 2008 and 2009. In 2008, the SAA contributed to the lobbying effort that resulted in the passage of the Genetic Information Non-Discrimination Act (GINA), a federal law that protects Americans from being treated unfairly by health insurers and employers 'because of differences in their DNA that may affect their health' (35).

More recently, the SAA has joined a powerful coalition of organizations (including the ACR, the Arthritis Foundation, and the National Psoriasis Foundation) to support passage of the Patient's Access to Treatment Act of 2013 (HR406), which would 'enable patients with chronic, disabling, and life-threatening conditions to access the treatment they need'.

Conclusion

As healthcare reform continues apace, the SAA will focus its future efforts on, among other initiatives, economic considerations and access-to-care issues related to SpA. The rising cost of healthcare has hit the middle-class particularly hard. The cost of employer-sponsored health insurance plans rose 119% from 1999 to 2008, far outpacing median household income, which increased only 29% over that time (36). Patients in the USA with chronic conditions such as SpA have been hit particularly hard. They report spending considerably more (41% spend more than $1000) on their disease than their counterparts in either Canada or the UK, difficulty complying with taking prescription medications, and poor access to healthcare services (37). The cost of providing care to these individuals eats up nearly 75% of all national healthcare expenditures (38). As the largest SpA advocate in the USA, the SAA is uniquely positioned to help patients with SpA deal with rising healthcare costs, access issues, and disease-related concerns. Among the initiatives the SAA may propose is continued development of Treatment Guidelines to standardize and improve patient outcomes.

The SAA's extensive network of supportive programmes, educational offerings, and research initiatives ensure that those affected by SpA do not have to face this disease alone. They will, in the words of the SAA's mission, 'empower those affected to live life to its fullest'.

References

1. Nijsten T, Bergstresser P. Patient advocacy groups: let's stick together. J Invest Dermatol 2010;130:1757.
2. Davison KP, Pennebaker JW, Dickerson SS. Who talks?: the social psychology of illness support groups. Am Psychol 2000;55(2):205.
3. Dana-Farber Cancer Institute. History of Dana-Farber Cancer Institute. http://www.dana-farber.org/About-Us/History-and-Milestones.aspx .
4. National Breast Cancer Coalition. The Breast Cancer Deadline 2020. http://www.breastcancerdeadline2020.org/homepage.html.
5. Østensen M, Østensen H. Ankylosing spondylitis—the female aspect. J Rheumatol 1998;25:120–4.
6. Erlendsson J. Consultant Rheumatologist. Car Driving with Ankylosing Spondylitis. ASIF, 1998, http://www.asif.info/en/.
7. Feldtkeller E, Khan MA, van der Heijde D, van der Linden S, Braun J. Age at disease onset and diagnosis delay in HLA-B27 negative vs. positive patients with ankylosing spondylitis. Rheumatol Int 2003;23:61–6.
8. Feldtkeller E, Vosse D, Geusens P, van der Linden S. Prevalence and annual incidence of vertebral fractures in patients with ankylosing spondylitis. Rheumatol Int 2006;26(3):234–9.
9. Vosse D, Geusens P, Erlendsson J, Feldtkeller E, van der Linden S. Clinical vertebral fractures in patients with ankylosing spondylitis. J Rheumatol 2004;31;1981–5.
10. Zochling J, Bohl-Bühler MH, Baraliakos X, Feldtkeller E, Braun J. Non-steroidal anti-inflammatory drug use in ankylosing spondylitis—a population-based survey. Clin Rheumatol 2006;25:794–800.
11. Zochling J, Bohl-Bühler MH, Baraliakos X, Feldtkeller E, Braun J. Infection and work stress are potential triggers of ankylosing spondylitis. Clin Rheumatol 2006;25:660–6.
12. Feldtkeller E, Erlendsson J. The definition of disease duration in ankylosing spondylitis: comment on the article by Davis et al. published as 'electronic letter' in Annals of Rheumatic Diseases. 12 July 2006.

13. Feldtkeller E, Erlendsson J. Definition of disease duration in ankylosing spondylitis. Rheumatol Int 2008;28:693–6.
14. Zochling J, Bohl-Bühler MH, Baraliakos X, Feldtkeller E, Braun J. The high prevalence of infections and allergic symptoms in patients with ankylosing spondylitis is associated with clinical symptoms. Clin Rheumatol 2006;25:648–58, with corrections in Clin Rheumatol 2006;25:659.
15. Feldtkeller E, Lind-Albrecht G, Rudwaleit M. Core set of recommendations for patients with ankylosing spondylitis concerning behaviour and environmental adaptations. Rheumatol Int 2013;33(9):2343–9.
16. Anderson PB. Dealing with the back pain with the funny name. *Los Angeles Times*, 28 May 1985.
17. Savage LM. Straight Talk on Spondylitis. Sherman Oaks, California, SAA, 2009.
18. SAA. Ankylosing spondylitis: managing patients in an emergency setting, a primer for first responders. *Spondylitis Plus*, Summer 2009.
19. SAA. http://www.spondylitis.org.
20. SAA. Facebook page. http://tinyurl.com/bzwmw9.
21. SAA. Twitter page. https://twitter.com/spondylitis.
22. SAA. eSUN—Our Free Monthly Newsletter. http://www.spondylitis.org/eSUN.
23. SWIFT. http://www.teen.spondylitis.org.
24. Landy DC, Brinich MA, Colten ME, et al. How disease advocacy organizations participate in clinical research: a survey of genetic organizations. Genet Med 2012;14(2):223.
25. SPARTAN. http://www.spartangroup.org.
26. SAA. Ankylosing spondylarthrits research: celebrating a major research milestone. *Spondylitis Plus*, Sept/Oct 2005.
27. Savage LM. Acute anterior uveitis: researchers uncover genetic region involved with a potential loss of vision in people with AS. *Spondylitis Plus*, Mar/Apr 2005.
28. Edwards SP. New genes provide additional targets for spondylitis treatment. *Spondylitis Plus*, Winter 2008.
29. SAA. A new genetic discovery brings ankylosing spondylitis further into focus. *Spondylitis Plus*, Fall 2011.
30. Rosenbaum J. Does the microbiome cause ankylosing spondylitis? *Spondylitis Plus*, Winter 2011.
31. SAA. First, national AS Life Impact Study of ankylosing spondylitis identifies need for patient, physician awareness. *Spondylitis Plus*, June 2005.
32. Stone M, Warren RW, Bruckel J, et al. Juvenile-onset ankylosing spondylitis is associated with worse functional outcomes than adult-onset ankylosing spondylitis. Arthritis Care Res 2005;53(2):445.
33. SAA. About us. http://www.spondylitis.org/About-Us .
34. Haywood KL, Garret AM, Jordan KP, et al. Evaluation of ankylosing spondylitis quality of life (EASi-QoL): reliability and validity of a new patient-reported outcome measure. J Rheumatol 2010, 37(10): 2100-9.
35. NIH. Genetic Information Nondiscrimination Act of 2008. http://www.genome.gov/10002328.
36. Schoen C, Nicholson JL, Rustgi SD. Paying the Price: How Health Insurance Premiums Are Eating up Middle-Class Incomes. Commonwealth Fund, 2009, http://www.commonwealthfund.org/publications/data-briefs/2009/aug/paying-the-price-how-health-insurance-premiums-are-eating-up-middle-class-incomes.
37. Reveille JD, Ximenes A, Ward MM. Economic considerations of the treatment of ankylosing spondylitis. Am J Med Sci 2012;343(5):371.
38. CDC. The Power of Prevention: Chronic Disease … the Public Health Challenge of the 21st Century. CDC, 2009, http://www.cdc.gov/chronicdisease/pdf/2009-Power-of-Prevention.pdf.

CHAPTER 28

Axial spondyloarthritis in Asia

Huji Xu, Feng Huang, Chan-Bum Choi, and Tae-Hwan Kim

Axial spondyloarthritis in China

Clinical aspects

Epidemiology

AxSpA is a common rheumatic disease in China, which has a population of 1.3 billion, accounting for nearly 20% of the world's population, and is associated with considerable burden regarding local and global public health. Therefore, epidemiological studies of axSpA in China are pivotal. Rheumatology is a relatively new discipline of clinical medicine in China. The first rheumatology department in mainland China was established in the early 1980s. Since then, Chinese physicians specializing in rheumatology have conducted several epidemiological studies of rheumatic diseases nationally (1).

To date, nearly 30 local and nationwide epidemiological studies have reported on the prevalence of SpA in China, which was found to vary from 0.38 to 1.61% among the Han Chinese (1–3). Recently, local epidemiological surveys of SpA have been performed independently in Beijing and Shandong province, and the estimated prevalence in these areas is 0.58% and 0.42%, respectively (4).

The prevalence of AS was reported in early 1994 to be approximately 0.26%, without significant geographic differences between northern (Beijing) and southern (Shantou) China (5). Based upon epidemiological studies of SpA conducted from 1980 to 2006 in China, the prevalence of AS was found to be 0.2–0.54% among the ethnic Han Chinese, which was relatively higher than that observed among other ethnic populations (mainly Muslim and Manchu) (1). The prevalence of PsA ranged from 0.01% to 0.1%, which was generally similar to most other countries, whereas this figure was much lower in Japan. However, only 1–9% of Asian patients with psoriasis were reported to have PsA, which was much lower than this proportion in Caucasians (6–42%) (6). More recent data have revealed that the prevalence of PsA is 0.02% according to a report on eight common rheumatic diseases in suburban Beijing (7). The prevalence of ReA was found to be 0.02%, and that of uSpA was 0.64–1.2% (1). Regarding the prevalence of uSpA, the Han Chinese population comprises a larger proportion of people affected by SpA than those with AS, which calls for physicians to improve their skills in detecting uSpA.

Aetiology and pathogenesis

As in European Caucasians, SpA in Chinese subjects has a strong genetic component. Genetic factors, particularly HLA-B27, play pivotal roles in the pathogenesis of SpA. As in other ethnic populations, more than 80% of Chinese AS patients are HLA-B27 positive, with the predominant subtype being HLA-B*2704. The incidence of HLA-B27 positivity in the Chinese population ranges from 4% to 8%, which is lower than that in Caucasians but much higher than that in the Japanese population (1%). Furthermore, a study of 2144 Chinese AS patients revealed that HLA-B27 was highly associated with distinct clinical features. The HLA-B27-positive AS group had a higher percentages of males, more frequently a family history of AS, and more axial joint involvement compared to the HLA-B27-negative AS group (8).

The pathogenesis of axSpA is not completely understood but almost certainly involves immune-mediated inflammation and disrupted bone homeostasis. Although the exact role of cytokines in the pathogenesis of AS cannot be pinpointed, the serum levels of TNF-α (9), IL-17, and IL-23 (10) were significantly higher in Chinese patients with AS than in the normal control subjects. The frequencies and ratios of lymphocyte subsets were also changed in the peripheral blood of patients with SpA. Furthermore, the surface receptors of lymphocytes, such as TLRs and B-cell activation factor (BAFF), appeared to be abnormal in Chinese patients with AS (4).

Clinical features

There is no predominant difference in the clinical features between the Chinese population and other ethnic populations. The age at onset in Chinese patients with AS has been reported to be mainly between 20 and 25 years. HLA-B27 positivity may correlate with an earlier onset. The diagnostic delay from the onset of disease has been reported to be 5–7 years in China (1). As in other populations, Chinese patients with AS are likely to develop early limited mobility, and radiographic progression seems to vary among individuals. However, Chinese AS patients have higher frequencies of peripheral arthritis and hip joint involvement (11, 12). Regarding EAMs, AAU has been reported in 25–40% of Chinese AS patients, which seems to be HLA-B27-related (13). Cardiovascular disorders and metabolic syndromes are commonly found; the occurrence of cardiac arrhythmia is noteworthy (14). Notably, apical lung fibrosis due to either the disease itself or latent tuberculosis infection has a relatively high incidence in Chinese AS patients (12, 15).

Chinese AS patients have higher frequencies of JoSpA, which ranges from 20% to 36% (11); in Caucasians, this prevalence varies from 9% to 21% (16, 17). A total of 190 cases of JoSpA were enrolled in a clinical study in China. Among these patients, 90% were HLA-B27 positive. The male:female ratio was 6:1. More than 90% of the patients reported their disease onset after 8 years of age, and most were 12–15 years old. Notably, the prevalence of axial arthritis, including lower back pain (10%) and heel pain (5%), was much lower than that of peripheral arthritis (80%), which included the hip and shoulder joints. Sacroiliitis was present in 76% of the studied patients, while enthesitis was present in 35%, and 10% exhibited dactylitis. AAU was observed in 5% of those studied (11).

Differences exist between the populations of southern and northern China regarding clinical manifestations and therapeutic interventions. Disease duration between the age of onset and age of diagnosis was significantly longer in southern AS patients. Hip joint involvement and peripheral arthritis at disease onset were more prevalent in northern AS patients than in their southern counterparts (18).

Current research

Genetic studies

The distribution of HLA-B27 subtypes reveals substantial demographic and geographic diversity (19). The main subtype is HLA-B*2704 in Chinese populations, whereas HLA-B*2705 is the next most common HLA-B27 subtype of the remaining individuals. Although HLA-B*2704 is a major subtype in Chinese individuals, it has been reported that the prevalence of HLA-B*2704(+) in AS patients was increased from northern to southern China, whereas HLA-B*2705 positivity was the reverse (4). Moreover, several minor subtypes seem to be derived from HLA-B*2704 in the Chinese population. For example, HLA-B*2715 only has a single amino acid altered at position 163 compared to HLA-B*2704. It has been repeatedly demonstrated that HLA-B*2704 is more commonly associated with AS than HLA-B*2705 in both Taiwan and the mainland Chinese Han population (20, 21).

HLA-B*2706 is more likely to appear in Malay descendants than Chinese descendants. It has been suggested that HLA-B*2706 has a relatively weak association with AS compared to the HLA-B*2704 subtype in Southeast Asia (22–24). However, a study reported carriers of HLA-B*2706 in Han Chinese descendants in Taiwan, revealing the complicated effect of the HLA-B*2706 subtype (25).

Although the basis for the association of HLA-B27 and AS remains unknown, Chinese researchers have been studying approaches to unravelling the promoters of HLA-B27. Using high-throughput techniques to screen chemical libraries, Zhao et al. discovered eight chemicals with pharmaceutical potential that might trigger or inhibit the activity of the HLA-B27 promoter (26). Two suppressors were derived from a traditional Chinese herbal medicine (*Tripterygium wilfordii* Hook f., known as lei gong teng and thunder-god vine). Six activators belonged to the flavonoid compounds, which are found in common dietary products (26). In an HLA-B27-transfected U937 cell line, cytokines, including TNF-α, IFNα, IFNβ, and IFNγ, triggered the expression of HLA-B27. The in vitro stimulation by IFNγ, which was the strongest activating factor among these cytokines, elevated the expression levels of CHOP, glucose-regulated protein 78 kDa (GRP78), and X-box binding protein 1 (XBP-1) in the peripheral blood and synovial fluid of HLA-B27-positive patients with AS. These phenomena were less significant in HLA-B27-negative patients and healthy controls. These findings present novel ideas for unravelling the mechanism of HLA-B27 in the pathogenesis of SpA (4, 27).

In China, HLA-B27 is responsible for no more than one-third of the genetic risk in modifying disease penetrance, with AS resulting in only 1–5% of HLA-B27 carriers. It has been long suspected that genetic factors in other MHC and non-MHC regions may contribute to disease susceptibility. To date, several genetic variants associated with AS in the Chinese population have been identified, including HLA-B60, major histocompatibility complex class I chain-related gene A (MICA), STAT3, tumour necrosis factor receptor superfamily member 1A (TNFRSF1A), and ERAP1 (28, 29). Regarding the IL-23R gene, the associated allele exhibits diversity among different ethnic groups, although, in most cases, it is the same, which is consistent with a shared ancestor origin of the disease-associated SNP(s). rs11209026, a non-synonymous SNP in IL-23R, is a key polymorphism associated with AS in Caucasians and was reported to not be polymorphic in Chinese subjects (28). A rare variant in IL-23R has been reported to potentially attenuate the protective effects of IL-23R against AS in Han Chinese (30). A recent multi-ethnic GWAS provided a new perspective on the similarities and differences in AS susceptibility between Asians and Caucasians. A total of 13 loci had at least nominal levels of association in East Asians (Chinese, Koreans, Taiwanese), whereas 23 achieved genome-wide significance in white Europeans (31).

A GWAS in Han Chinese identified two novel susceptibility SNP loci (rs4552569 and rs17095830) in non-MHC regions, loci at chromosomes 5q14 and 12q12(32). Limited evidence of an association of these two loci has been observed in large-scale independent replication studies in East Asians and Caucasians (31).

It has been confirmed in the Chinese population that genes in both MHC and non-MHC regions are associated with PsA, including HLA-B27 and IL-12B (33). A GWAS of psoriasis was conducted in Han Chinese and identified a novel locus (rs4085613) at chromosome 1q21 within the late cornified envelope (LCE) gene (34). Subsequent association analyses have further identified six new psoriasis susceptibility loci in the Chinese population (35). These outcomes indicated an obvious discrepancy across different populations. However, further GWAS of PsA to unveil the interrelationship between psoriasis and spondylitis are ongoing.

The similarities and differences in the genetic features of SpA between Chinese and other ethnic populations have demonstrated the utility of gene mapping in probing the genetic diversity among different ethnic groups. The heterogeneity among various ethnic groups may help discriminate valid associations from false positives. Moreover, the identification of new genetic risks in the Chinese population may provide additional details for defining the genetic basis of axSpA. Thus further genetic studies in Han Chinese are expected.

Immunopathogenesis

In addition to genetic studies, a number of centres in China have been investigating the immunopathogenesis of SpA. Several intracellular cytokines have been studied in Chinese patients with SpA. Increased levels of IL-6 were detected in both the synovial fluid and peripheral blood of SpA patients, which correlated with elevated inflammatory biomarkers, such as ESR and CRP level (12). IFNγ and IL-4 in the peripheral blood suppressed the activity of type 1 cytotoxic T (Tc1) cells and type 1 T helper (Th1) cells in active AS patients with elevated ESR and CRP level (19). A positive correlation between the level of serum MMP-3 and disease activity in AS has also been confirmed in Chinese patients (36). Serum levels of TNF-like weak inducer of apoptosis (TWEAK) in patients with PsA were significantly elevated in parallel with disease activity (37). In addition to an imbalance of cytokines and chemokines, lymphocyte profiles are altered in patients with SpA. Zhang et al. reported that the differentiation of

CD8-positive Treg cells, which can produce IL-4 in the peripheral blood, was changed in AS patients and in healthy HLA-B27-positive controls (38). The generation of IL-4+CD8+ T cells implicated a role it might play in the pathogenesis of SpA (38). Lin et al. observed higher levels of CD3+CD154+ T cells in the peripheral blood of patients with active axSpA (39). The percentage of CD3+CD154+ T cells, which appeared to be a potential biomarker, decreased in patients receiving treatment with TNFi treatment. Moreover, elevated levels of IgA generated against infections of enterobacteria have been observed in Chinese patents with AS (40, 41). However, the mechanisms underlying these phenomena remain unknown.

Challenges to diagnosis

Diagnostic criteria

An early diagnosis is essential to interventions that may relieve symptoms, control disease activity, and minimize spinal deformity. The diagnostic criteria of SpA in China are mainly adopted from the mNY criteria, the ESSG, Amor criteria for adult SpA, and the new ASAS criteria. The reliability and validity of many of these criteria have been evaluated in the Chinese population. Although more evidence is required to validate the new criteria in the Chinese population, the ASAS criteria have already been applied in clinical trials in China, which include detection of early SI involvement by MRI. The ability of the ASAS criteria to clinically define axSpA was demonstrated to surpass that of the ESSG and Amor criteria in China (41). In a cohort of Chinese patients with SpA, the ASAS criteria demonstrated the highest sensitivity (98.4%) compared to the mNY criteria (71.9%) and the ESSG (83.6%) criteria. It has been reported in a Chinese cohort study that uSpA patients defined by the ASAS or ESSG criteria had an earlier onset and less long-term functional impairment than AS patients diagnosed according to the mNY criteria (42). In discriminating axial PsA from peripheral PsA, spinal mobility measurements, especially lumber side flexion and the Schober test, were valid and practical (43). In classifying axial uSpA patients in China, HLA-B27 may be more useful than MRI in examining the SI joint (44).

Laboratory and radiographic findings

Without a specific diagnostic laboratory test, SpA is identified mainly by the clinical manifestations and radiographic findings. HLA-B27 is widely used as a screening test for patients with lower back pain in clinical settings due to its strong association with AS. There are several methods for HLA-B27 testing, including a microlymphocytotoxicity test, flow cytometry (FC), and a PCR assay. The standard PCR assay is a time-consuming method of detecting HLA-B27, with a contamination risk. Duplex real-time TaqMan PCR may be a high-throughput approach with a specificity and accuracy comparable to those of the sequence-based PCR typing for HLA-B27 detection in Han Chinese (45). Chou et al. reported a fast screening method for HLA-B27 detection that uses immunomagnetic separation and enzyme-linked immunosorbent assay (IMS-ELISA) (46). The study demonstrated that an IMS-ELISA is an effective method with equivalent accuracy to FC for HLA-B27 testing. Additionally, by sieving a phage-display random peptide library, Wang et al. discovered a peptide (LALPPLAPNHHH) in the serum of patients with AS, which might be a promising biomarker (47). However, the sensitivity and specificity of the peptide for AS requires validation in future studies (47). BMPs have been associated with axial involvement and AS progression. In AS patients with spinal fusion, serum levels of BMP-2, BMP-4, and BMP-7 were higher than those of either patients without spinal fusion or healthy control subjects; additionally, elevated serum levels of BMP-4 and BMP-7 were correlated with hip joint involvement in AS patients (48).

Imaging plays an important role in the diagnosis of SpA, including X-ray, CT, and MRI. MRI is regarded as a method with high specificity in the diagnosis of early sacroiliitis. However, high costs and insufficient sensitivity of MRI limits its widespread application in detecting early sacroiliitis. Gong et al. revealed that needle biopsy could detect sacroiliitis earlier than MRI (49). Early diagnosis and early treatment may be important to achieve a better prognosis. US has been proposed as an alternative, convenient, and safe approach to detect oedema of soft tissue or cartilage, entheseal perfusion, and spinal vascularization due to sacroiliitis (50, 51).

To achieve better management of SpA, the development of early diagnostic techniques remains a major challenge for future studies of SpA.

Challenges in treatment

Guidelines

Treatments for axSpA in China and other parts of the world are similar, with minor differences. The therapeutic targets of SpA are to ameliorate the symptoms of the patients as well as to prevent subsequent clinical deformity. SpA is a group of disorders with diverse clinical features that require individualized evaluation and treatment. The therapeutic strategies in SpA consist of two complementary approaches: non-pharmacological and pharmacological treatments. The cornerstone of non-pharmacological treatment of patients with SpA is patient education and regular exercise. The pharmacological treatment mostly comprises NSAIDs, DMARDs, and biologic agents. Management of SpA requires a combination of these two parts coordinated by rheumatologists (52).

In addition to diagnosis and treatment, disease monitoring is vital in managing SpA. Disease monitoring helps physicians assess and follow the efficacy and safety of therapies with effective instruments. The ASDAS, BASDAI, BASFI, BASMI, ESR, and CRP level have good reference values for assessing a patient's condition. A Chinese cohort study of AS compared the validity and reliability of BASDAI and ASDAS. Both of these have been validated as highly discriminatory measurements of assessing disease activity in AS, and ASDAS performed better in a subgroup with raised levels of CRP (53). In China, BASDAI and BASFI have been validated to have good reliability in the evaluation of a patient's condition and TNFi treatment response. Application of these validated instruments has contributed to better management of SpA.

Non-pharmacological therapy and traditional medication

Non-pharmacological therapy consists of education, exercise, and physical therapy. Patient education is central in the management of SpA to help the patient alter daily behaviour and improve quality of life. However, few well-organized educational programmes for patients are accessible in China due to the lack of consultation time and lack of facilities for education. Physical exercise has been recommended as an important treatment to maintain mobility and relieve pain in AS, but the high cost of and lack of well-trained physical therapists restrict the use of supervised exercise in China (52).

NSAIDs are a first-line option for pain relief, the inhibition of inflammation, and, possibly, decrease in new bone formation. A large-scale controlled trial showed good efficacy and tolerability of celecoxib in the pain management of Chinese patients with AS (54). Local corticosteroid injection was recommended only for patients with severe peripheral arthritis and enthesitis. SSZ was usually given for peripheral arthritis and early-stage spinal disease. However, head-to-head clinical trials on the efficacy and safety of SSZ and that of ETN indicated the inferiority of SSZ. In China, short-term MTX administration in early AS has been studied (52). Thalidomide exhibited a beneficial effect and fair tolerability in the treatment of Chinese SpA patients. It has been reported that thalidomide potentially reduces serum levels of macrophage colony stimulating factor (M-CSF) and TGF-β1 (12). Further large-scale, double-blind, placebo-controlled trials are required to evaluate the efficacy and safety of such treatments for axSpA.

In China, traditional Chinese medicine (TCM), comprised mainly of herbal medicine, acupuncture, and moxibustion, and therapeutic massages provide more options to patients as alternative therapeutic modalities. Therapeutic massages, acupuncture, and moxibustion are considered to be non-pharmacological treatments to diminish pain and improve function. Although the feedback of patients and data from a few local studies provide evidence for benefits of acupuncture and moxibustion in the treatment of SpA, well-designed trials are required to validate the efficacy of these treatments (52). Herbal medicine and herbal extracts (*T. wilfordii* polyglycosidium, total glucosides of peony, etc.) are commonly used in the treatment of SpA in China. However, few studies of high quality are available to assess the efficacy and tolerability of herbal medicine in the treatment of SpA.

Biologics

TNFi agents are a major successful therapeutic advance in the treatment of active SpA. The efficacy and safety of these agents has been demonstrated in Chinese patients with AS (55–57). TNFi therapies are effective in targeting not only axial involvement but also peripheral arthritis, enthesitis, and EAMs. With the rapid economic growth in China, increasing numbers of SpA patients have received TNFi therapies, including ETN, infliximab, adalimumab, and golimumab (52).

In China, a number of clinical studies of TNFi therapies in AS have been reported. The efficacy and safety profiles of TNFi in the treatment of Chinese patients with AS and uSpA have been assessed and confirmed in several clinical trials. At the end point of a 12-week period, significantly more patients with AS and uSpA who were treated with ETN reached disease remission than the placebo group (56, 58). A short-term open-label study of infliximab reported that 84% of active AS patients achieved ASAS 20 in a 10-week period (59). It has been reported that infliximab performed better than ETN in the treatment of SpA with EAMs, including IBD and uveitis. However, more supportive evidence in the Chinese population is necessary for further confirmation.

Adalimumab was demonstrated to be effective in the treatment of Chinese patients with active AS in a 12-week RCT. A significantly greater percentage of individuals in the adalimumab group were ASAS 20 responders (42.8%) than in the placebo group (6.1%) at week 2 of treatment. The well-tolerated profile of adalimumab has been confirmed in this population (55). A 1-year, placebo-controlled, phase III study demonstrated good efficacy and adequate safety of golimumab in the treatment of AS in China. In another study, golimumab-treated patients had a significantly higher percentage of ASAS 20 responders than the placebo group (50.0% vs 22.9%). Moreover, golimumab treatment significantly improved HRQoL and quality of sleep in the study at week 52 (57).

Although these TNFi are highly effective in the treatment of SpA, rheumatologists encounter several limitations of their application in Asian populations. First and foremost, the costs of biologic therapies are prohibitively high. Currently, most Asian countries are still developing. The limited incomes of patients and poor health insurance coverage for biologics make biologic therapies unaffordable for many Asian patients. Physicians in Asia have been trying to establish cost-effective treatment strategies. In China, thalidomide has been demonstrated to be an effective maintenance regimen for AS patients who discontinued TNFi therapy after reaching remission (60). Local injections of ETN into the involved joints have been reported to be effective and safe in the treatment of SpA (61). A second concern regarding TNFi therapy relates to infections, which appear to be the most frequent adverse effects of such therapies. A high prevalence of hepatitis B virus (HBV) and latent tuberculosis in China poses a risk to patients who receive TNFi. To minimize the potential reactivation of such infections, screening tests for HBV and tuberculosis remain necessary before the initiation of TNFi therapy. Finally, studies to date in China suggest that TNFi fail to prevent new bone formation in SpA (52).

Patient considerations

AxSpA severely impairs HRQoL and the socioeconomic well-being of patients in China. Chinese physicians have been giving increased recognition to patient-oriented outcomes. Chan et al. reported that SpA patients in China were more likely to develop depressive and anxiety disorders, as measured by the Hospital Anxiety and Depression Scale (10.6% and 15.6%, respectively) (62). Furthermore, it has been shown that patients with axial PsA incur twice as much in indirect costs as patients with peripheral PsA in Hong Kong (63). Indirect costs and burden of disease issues caused by SpA implicitly yet profoundly affect patients individually and society at large. These important aspects of SpA need to be further recognized and addressed in China.

Conclusion

Rheumatologists and scientists in China have been putting forth their best efforts to achieve optimal therapeutic outcomes and to elucidate the still-elusive mechanisms underlying SpA. Studies on SpA have highlighted the shared and distinct factors and features of various clinical subsets of SpA. Differences in SpA among different ethnic groups have also been investigated. Genetic and immunological studies among Han Chinese are required to explain the clinical heterogeneity observed. With its rapid economic development, China has witnessed major advances in research and the clinical management of SpA. Well-accepted classification criteria and sensitive detection methods are contributing to earlier diagnosis of axSpA. Currently, most SpA patients in China are still treated with traditional medications, mainly NSAIDs. Fortunately, an increasing number of patients in China have access to anti-TNFi therapy. However, there is still a long way to go for both the healthcare system and physicians in China to develop better policies and strategies for axSpA management.

Axial spondyloarthritis in Korea

Introduction

The ancient history of Korea dates back over 5000 years and a number of dynasties have enriched the art, culture, and science of Korea over the centuries. In modern history, the Republic of

Korea, established in 1948, has achieved enormous development in economy, science, and technology in a relatively short period. This presents some interesting parallels with the development of rheumatology in general and AS in particular: despite their short history compared to other diseases, they have seen immense advances in recent years.

It is only since the 1980s that rheumatology was recognized as a specialty in Korea. Before the emergence of rheumatology, AS was managed mainly by orthopaedic surgeons. The first report of AS in Korea, which came from an ophthalmologist, described uveitis in a patient with AS (64). The patient was a 35-year-old male who had enthesitis of the heel and arthritis of the knee for 12 years and IBP for 8 years. He had been treated by an orthopaedic surgeon with aspirin and dexamethasone. He had been experiencing alternating visual loss 3 to 4 times a year since the first onset of enthesitis, but vision improved with the use of intermittent dexamethasone. Only later was it determined that he had AS with vertebral body ankylosis secondary to syndesmophytes formation. The reports on AS in the early 1980s mainly concerned uveitis in these patients. Many such cases probably reflected the clinical picture of undiagnosed AS.

The first research article on AS, which was by a rheumatologist, was published in 1982 and it examined the diagnostic utility and significance of quantitative SI joint scintigraphy in the assessment of sacroiliitis (65). The first publication on AS from Korea in a Science Citation Index (SCI) journal was in 1997. This was a case report of aneurysmal dilatation of ascending aorta and aortic insufficiency in a patient with JoSpA (66). More than 250 domestic and 190 SCI journal articles on SpA by Korean investigators have been published since.

Korea now has rheumatologists with dedicated research and patient-care interests in SpA, and there has been enormous progress in the diagnosis and management of SpA. There is now a research society for SpA within the Korean College of Rheumatology where SpA researchers hold regular symposia to share ideas, present research, and collaborate on nationwide studies on SpA.

The following section provides an introduction to SpA research as well as epidemiologic features and current treatment for SpA in Korea.

Clinical aspects

Epidemiology

The prevalence of axSpA in Korea has not been systematically investigated yet. It is presumed that axSpA is still underdiagnosed in Korea. Patients are often seen with IBP for several years who fulfill the ASAS classification criteria for axSpA but who have not been properly diagnosed. The prevalence of RA is known to be about 27 per 10 000 population (67) in Korea and the mean prevalence of AS in East Asian countries is estimated as 25.5 per 10 000. Studies have generally shown the prevalence in Asia to be lower than that in Europe and North America (68). The prevalence of axSpA is expected to approximate that of RA and to be not much different from that in neighbouring countries.

According to the reports of hospital-based cohorts of Korean AS patients, the male:female ratio is over 8:1 (69). AS was previously reported as male-predominant in studies of Caucasian patients in the past, but in western countries AS is now estimated to have a male:female ratio of about 3:1. There is no good evidence to date whether this is also the case for Koreans. A study of uSpA fulfilling the ESSG criteria has shown a lower male:female ratio of 1.2:1 (70) and in the study of nr-axSpA it was 3:1, while it was 8:1 for AS patients in the same study (71).

The mean age of onset is 20.9 years for AS, and 19.6% of patients have a family history of axSpA (69). The age of onset is older for uSpA (27.4 years) (70) and nr-axSpA (29.5 years) (72). While there is no difference between men and women (20.6 vs 23.3 years, $p = 0.05$), there is a trend of men having the earlier onset. Women have a significantly higher rate of having a family history of SpA (29.3% vs 18.3%, $p = 0.01$) and uveitis (40.8% vs 28.2%, $p = 0.03$) (69).

The mNY criteria for AS are commonly used in Korea for the diagnosis of AS and endorsed by the Korean Ministry of Health and Welfare as the eligibility criteria to receive special consideration and a reduction in insurance copayment. Although not adopted by other specialties, the ASAS classification criteria are also widely accepted by Korean rheumatologists, who are the physicians mainly making the diagnosis of axSpA. The diagnosis is frequently delayed. One study has shown that the average delay in diagnosis is 8 years for axSpA and 4 years for peripheral SpA (72).

Clinical features

Inflammatory lower back pain is the most common initial symptom (47.1%), followed by hip joint pain (15.8%), knee joint pain (13.7%), Achilles tendinitis (7.2%), ankle joint pain (4.2%), plantar fasciitis (2.3%), tarsal joint pain (1.7%), and shoulder pain (1.4%).

Peripheral and hip joint involvement are higher in Korean patients with AS than in AS patients of other ethnicities. Hip joints are involved in 73.9% of patients and peripheral joints in 47.1% (69). Peripheral joint involvement was even higher in a study of uSpA. Over 91% showed peripheral joint arthritis in the knee (72%), ankle (46%), elbow (27%), wrist (21%), and hand (23%) (70). However, peripheral involvement was low in a study of nr-axSpA, with only 39.4% showing peripheral joint involvement, among which 57.4% had only the lower limb involvement, 13.1% upper limb involvement, and 29.5% involvement of both limbs (72).

Enthesitis is also common and more frequent among Koreans than among other ethnicities. Eighty-two percent of the patients manifest enthesitis in uSpA (70), 42.7% exhibited enthesitis in AS (69), and 19.4% did so in nr-axSpA (72).

Uveitis is the most common EAM, with a prevalence similar to that reported for other ethnicities. It is 29.7% in AS, 13% in uSpA, and 23.9% in nr-axSpA (69–71). It is unilateral in 63.6% of cases, but 11.8% are bilateral and the alternating involvement of both eyes occurs in 24.6%. Only 33.5% of the cases have one episode of uveitis and 20.9% experienced five or more episodes. The mean frequency of uveitis episodes per year is 3.7 (69). Other extra-articular involvement included renal involvement (3.9%) and cardiac involvement (1.6%).

Research

Genetic studies

HLA-B27 positivity in the general Korean population has not been studied extensively. Some studies have reported the prevalence to be from 2.3% to 7%, which is lower than that of Caucasians. On the other hand, HLA-B27 positivity in patients with AS is high and is reported to be from 94.8% to 96.3% (69, 73). B*2705 is the predominant subtype in Koreans (73, 74), which is similar to Caucasians but different from other Asians, among whom B*2704 is predominant.

ERAP1, which is known to be associated with AS in Caucasians and Chinese, is associated with AS in Koreans as well. SNPs rs27044 and rs30187 of ERAP1 show significant association with AS in Koreans (75). In another study, ERAP1 SNPs rs27037 and rs27434, as well as rs10865331 at 2p15, also show an association with AS (76).

Programmed cell death protein 1 (PD-1) were reported to be associated with susceptibility to AS (77) and BMP-6 SNPs rs270378 and rs1235192 were associated with radiographic severity (78). However, other studies have shown no association with IL-23R (79), IL-1 (80, 81), caspase recruitment domain-containing protein 15 (CARD15) (82), and NF-κB (81) polymorphisms and AS.

A genome-wide copy number variant (CNV) association study has been performed in 309 patients with AS and 309 controls. The results showed that 227 CNV regions were associated with AS. In two replication sets of 625 AS patients and 891 controls, 1q32.2 (HHAT), 2q31.2 (PRKRA), 6p21.32 (HLA-DPB1), and 16p13.3 were replicated in both sets, while 1q32.2, 1p34.2 (BMP-8A), 2q31.2, 6p21.32, 11q22.1 (CNTN5), 13q13.1 (EEF1DP3), 14q24.2 (RGS6), 16p13.3, and 22q11.1 (IL-17RA) were replicated only in one set (83).

Clinical studies

Korea is a country with an intermediate tuberculosis (TB) burden, with an incidence rate of 78.9 per 100 000 person years (PY) in 2011, and the introduction of TNFi has raised concerns about reactivation of latent TB. Both interferon-gamma release assays (IGRAs) and tuberculin skin test are recommended for screening latent TB in patients initiating TNFi. However, the concordance of these two tests was low (84). Positive conversion of IGRA was investigated in patients with AS and 7.9% of the patients had positive conversion (85), although its clinical significance is still unclear and there are no related recommendations as yet.

There have been several studies of the incidence rate of TB in patients with rheumatic diseases treated with TNFi. Compared to the TB incidence rate of 73 per 100 000 PY in the general population, patients with AS had higher incidence rates, ranging from 123 to 308 per 100 000 PY (86, 87). AS patients treated with TNFi showed higher incidence of TB, with 561–715 per 100 000 PY (86–88), which was lower compared to RA (772–1143 per 100 000 PY) (86, 88) and IBD (3710 per 100 000 PY) (88). Non-tuberculous mycobacteria (NTM) was also increased in patients with rheumatic diseases treated with TNFi, with incidence rates of 231–238 per 100 000 PY (89, 90).

Patients with a history of TB may be at increased risk of TB, but the incidence rate of TB after initiation of TNFi in patients with either CD, RA, or AS who had a history of TB was calculated as 336 per 100 000 PY (91), which was comparable to those without previous TB.

Re-administration of TNFi in patients who previously discontinued TNFi after developing active TB during the treatment is controversial. One study found no recurrence of TB in eight patients in whom TNFi was re-administered (92). Another study with six patients re-administered with TNFi also showed no relapse during mean follow-up of 30.6 months (93).

Investigation of eight inactive HBsAg carrier patients with RA or AS treated with TNFi showed one hepatitis B reactivation (94). Of 49 patients with RA or AS receiving TNFi, 20 received antiviral prophylaxis with either lamivudine or entecavir and 29 received no antiviral agents; 6.9% of the patients not receiving antiviral prophylaxis showed reactivation within 1 year, and one of the patients who received antiviral prophylaxis developed viral activation after 64 weeks (95).

The COI and quality of life was assessed in the study of 192 AS patients, which showed that the yearly COI was $10 200 and EQ-5D was 0.62 (96).

Radiologic studies

Radiologic studies of AS using plain-film radiography and MRI have proved to be a productive line of research in Korea. Important risk factors for spinal ankylosis are disease duration and elevation of inflammatory markers. Analysis of Korean patients with AS shows that progress in ankylosis is slower when peripheral arthritis accompanies AS (97). Neck pain in AS patients is usually associated with ankylosis, or inflammation of the cervical vertebral body and cervical facet joints. However, atlantoaxial subluxation (AAS) and atlantoaxial ankylosis (AAA) should be taken into consideration as differential diagnosis (98). Patients with atlantoaxial distance greater than 3 mm made up approximately 14.1% of AAS patients, and those with greater than 4 mm made up approximately 5%. AAS was directly associated with CRP and a history of peripheral arthritis. AAA was associated with the disease duration.

As a measurement tool for spinal ankylosis, mSASSS is most commonly used. The change in vertebral bodies is semiquantitatively measured, but facet joints, which are commonly affected, are not included in the scoring. Squaring is important as a component of mSASSS. However, since it is difficult to distinguish squaring even in normals, it has been suggested that only the 3rd and 4th cervical vertebrae should be considered in calculation (99).

Patients with AS may complain of intermittent lower abdominal pain. Prostatitis may be contributory, but symphysis pubis inflammation should also be considered as a possible cause. Osteitis pubis is relatively common in AS compared with the general population or patients with other rheumatic diseases. Patients with high mSASSS and longer disease duration have more inflammation of the symphysis pubis (100). Radiologic studies in AS hold great potential to shed light on bony ankylosis research through MRI-defined fat quantification, osteoblastic activity research, etc. Radiologic imaging studies such as MRI, positron emission tomography (PET)-CT, and PET-MRI are currently being used to investigate pathologic findings and disease progression.

Guidelines for treatment

In Korea, population data on axSpA are scarce and the Health Insurance Review and Assessment Service (HIRA) is developing treatment guidelines for AS (101). All patients should have adequate therapeutic trials of at least two NSAIDs. All patients should have NSAIDs for at least 3 months at the maximum tolerated dose, unless contraindicated. DMARD therapy is not mandated for patients with primarily axial manifestations, whereas patients with predominantly symptomatic peripheral arthritis should have appropriate trials of NSAIDs, low-dose steroids, and DMARDs. If symptomatic control is not achieved, then TNFi should be instituted. This standard approach is in agreement with the ASAS-EULAR treatment recommendations. Approximately 30% of AS patients are treated with TNFi agents. Biologics other than TNFi are not covered by insurance and many are currently being studied in AS.

When patients with SpA complain of hip or back pain secondary to sacroiliitis, the degree of the pain often varies greatly. In some cases, mild and intermittent pain may disappear without treatment or after NSAID administration. However, if the pain is severe and continuous despite NSAID administration, it is important to find other treatment options. Because Korean health insurance does not cover the administration of TNFi in this case, clinicians are using fluoroscopy-guided corticosteroid injections into the SI joint as an alternative. Fluoroscopy-guided intra-articular injections were performed in 53 patients with AS who visited the outpatient clinic over the past 2 years. Patients were followed up for 13.6 months after injection, on average (range 0–32 months). For 37 out of 53 patients, pain was relieved and obviated the need for additional intra-articular injections or the initiation of TNFi. However, 4 out of 53 patients (7.5%) needed a second injection and 12 patients started TNFi because of the high disease activity and lack of response to local injections. These results have led to the recommendation that fluoroscopy-guided corticosteroid injection should be considered at an early stage for axSpA patients who do not suffer from extensive spinal involvement.

Conclusion

Both basic and clinical researchers in the field of AS are scarce, even though there is a significant number of patients with AS in Korea. Social circumstances and medical training programmes have tended to emphasize treatment of patients rather than research. Expansion of web-based networking and international cooperation has enabled Korean rheumatologists to treat AS patients with current best practices comparable to that in western countries. There is great potential to expand research in AS. All contemporary treatments for AS are available in Korea, but access remains a problem for many patients because of insurance issues.

AS patients in western cohorts usually suffer from IBP, and thus the treatment focuses on back pain. More than half of Korean patients exhibit significant peripheral arthritis (69). Although most of the AS patients with peripheral arthritis respond to conventional treatment, some patients will need more aggressive treatments. However, insurance coverage for TNFi is limited to treatment of spinal symptoms. Thus one domestic research imperative is to collect more data in order to change insurance policy.

Ongoing collaborative research projects are being conducted with orthopaedic surgeons using osteoblasts and osteoclasts harvested from surgical procedures on spine and joints. Currently, these studies are focusing on facet joints rather than the vertebral body, which is done in collaboration with radiologists. Development of new image modalities which can quantitate inflammation is an active area of research as well.

Acknowledgement

Drs Xu and Huang thank Dr Geng Wang for his assistance in preparing this manuscript.

References

1. Zeng QY, Chen R, Darmawan J, et al. Rheumatic diseases in China. Arthritis Res Ther 2008;10(1):R17.
2. Ng SC, Liao Z, Yu DT, Chan ES, Zhao L, Gu J. Epidemiology of spondyloarthritis in the People's Republic of China: review of the literature and commentary. Semin Arthritis Rheum 2007;37(1):39–47.
3. Liao ZT, Pan YF, Huang JL, et al. An epidemiological survey of low back pain and axial spondyloarthritis in a Chinese Han population. Scand J Rheumatol 2009;38(6):455–9.
4. Rong J, Jieruo G. Spondyloarthritis in China. Curr Opin Rheumatol 2013;25(4):460–7.
5. Wigley RD, Zhang NZ, Zeng QY, et al. Rheumatic diseases in China: ILAR-China study comparing the prevalence of rheumatic symptoms in northern and southern rural populations. J Rheumatol 1994;21(8):1484–90.
6. Tam LS, Leung YY, Li EK. Psoriatic arthritis in Asia. Rheumatology 2009;48(12):1473–7.
7. Li R, Sun J, Ren LM, et al. Epidemiology of eight common rheumatic diseases in China: a large-scale cross-sectional survey in Beijing. Rheumatology 2012;51(4):721–9.
8. Yang M, Xu M, Pan X, et al. Epidemiological comparison of clinical manifestations according to HLA-B*27 carrier status of Chinese ankylosing spondylitis patients. Tissue Antigens 2013;82(5):338–43.
9. Xueyi L, Lina C, Zhenbiao W, Qing H, Qiang L, Zhu P. Levels of circulating Th17 cells and regulatory T cells in ankylosing spondylitis patients with an inadequate response to anti-TNF-alpha therapy. J Clin Immunol 2013;33(1):151–61.
10. Mei Y, Pan F, Gao J, et al. Increased serum IL-17 and IL-23 in the patient with ankylosing spondylitis. Clin Rheumatol 2011;30(2):269–73.
11. Huang F, Zhang J, Zhu J, Guo J, Yang C. Juvenile spondyloarthropathies: the Chinese experience. Rheum Dis Clinic North Am J 2003;29(3):531–47.
12. Ho HH, Chen JY. Ankylosing spondylitis: Chinese perspective, clinical phenotypes, and associated extra-articular systemic features. Curr Rheumatol 2013;15(8):344.
13. Chou CT. Spondyloarthritis in Asian countries—an overview. Curr Rheumatol 2008;4:81–6.
14. Ho HH, Yeh SJ, Tsai WP, Wang CM, Chen JY. Paroxysmal supraventricular tachycardia and Wolff-Parkinson-White syndrome in ankylosing spondylitis: a large cohort observation study and literature review. Semin Arthritis Rheum 2012;42(3):246–53.
15. Ho HH, Lin MC, Yu KH, Wang CM, Wu YJ, Chen JY. Pulmonary tuberculosis and disease-related pulmonary apical fibrosis in ankylosing spondylitis. J Rheumatol 2009;36(2):355–60.
16. O'Shea FD, Boyle E, Riarh R, Tse SM, Laxer RM, Inman RD. Comparison of clinical and radiographic severity of juvenile-onset versus adult-onset ankylosing spondylitis. Ann Rheumatic Dis 2009;68(9):1407–12.
17. Zhang S, Li Y, Deng X, Huang F. Similarities and differences between spondyloarthritis in Asia and other parts of the world. Curr Opin Rheumatol 2011;23(4):334–8.
18. Ma HJ, Yin QF, Hu FP, et al. Different clinical features in patients with ankylosing spondylitis from southern and northern China. Int J Rheum Dis 2012;15(2):154–62.
19. Feltkamp TE, Mardjuadi A, Huang F, Chou CT. Spondyloarthropathies in eastern Asia. Curr Opin Rheumatol 2001;13(4);285–90.
20. Liu Y, Jiang L, Cai Q, et al. Predominant association of HLA-B*2704 with ankylosing spondylitis in Chinese Han patients. Tissue Antigens 2010;75(1):61–4.
21. Yang KL, Chen IH, Hsiao CK, et al. Polymorphism of HLA-B27 in Taiwanese Chinese. Tissue Antigens 2004;63(5):476–9.
22. Ren EC, Koh WH, Sim D, Boey ML, Wee GB, Chan SH. Possible protective role of HLA-B*2706 for ankylosing spondylitis. Tissue Antigens 1997;49(1):67–9.
23. Lopez-Larrea C, Sujirachato K, Mehra NK, et al. HLA-B27 subtypes in Asian patients with ankylosing spondylitis. Evidence for new associations. Tissue Antigens 1995;45(3):169–76.
24. Gonzalez-Roces S, Alvarez MV, Gonzalez S, et al. HLA-B27 polymorphism and worldwide susceptibility to ankylosing spondylitis. Tissue Antigens 1997;49(2):116–23.
25. Hou TY, Chen HC, Chen CH, Chang DM, Liu FC, Lai JH. Usefulness of human leucocyte antigen-B27 subtypes in predicting ankylosing spondylitis: Taiwan experience. Intern Med J 2007;37(11):749–52.
26. Zhao L, Liu CH, Yu D. High-throughput screening of chemical libraries for modulators of gene promoter activity of

HLA-B2705: environmental pathogenesis and therapeutics of ankylosing spondylitis. J Rheumatol 2011;38(6):1061–5.
27. Feng Y, Ding J, Fan CM, Zhu P. Interferon-gamma contributes to HLA-B27-associated unfolded protein response in spondyloarthropathies. J Rheumatol 2012;39(3):574–82.
28. Davidson SI, Wu X, Liu Y, et al. Association of ERAP1, but not IL23R, with ankylosing spondylitis in a Han Chinese population. Arthritis Rheum 2009;60(11):3263–8.
29. Davidson SI, Liu Y, Danoy PA, et al. Association of STAT3 and TNFRSF1A with ankylosing spondylitis in Han Chinese. Ann Rheum Dis 2011;70(2):289–92.
30. Davidson SI, Jiang L, Cortes A, et al. Brief report: high-throughput sequencing of IL23R reveals a low-frequency, nonsynonymous single-nucleotide polymorphism that is associated with ankylosing spondylitis in a Han Chinese population. Arthritis Rheum 2013;65(7):1747–52.
31. International Genetics of Ankylosing Spondylitis Consortium, Cortes A, Hadler J, et al. Identification of multiple risk variants for ankylosing spondylitis through high-density genotyping of immune-related loci. Nat Genet 2013;45(7):730–8.
32. Lin Z, Bei JX, Shen M, et al. A genome-wide association study in Han Chinese identifies new susceptibility loci for ankylosing spondylitis. Nat Genet 2012;44(1):73–7.
33. Leung YY, Tam LS, Li EK. The perspective on psoriatic arthritis in Asia. Curr Rheumatol Rep 2011;13(4):369–75.
34. Zhang XJ, Huang W, Yang S, et al. Psoriasis genome-wide association study identifies susceptibility variants within LCE gene cluster at 1q21. Nat Genet 2009;41(2):205–10.
35. Sun LD, Cheng H, Wang ZX, et al. Association analyses identify six new psoriasis susceptibility loci in the Chinese population. Nat Genet 2010;42(11):1005–9.
36. Chen CH, Lin KC, Yu DT, et al. Serum matrix metalloproteinases and tissue inhibitors of metalloproteinases in ankylosing spondylitis: MMP-3 is a reproducibly sensitive and specific biomarker of disease activity. Rheumatology 2006;45(4):414–20.
37. Xia L, Shen H, Xiao W, Lu J. Increased serum TWEAK levels in psoriatic arthritis: relationship with disease activity and matrix metalloproteinase-3 serum levels. Cytokine 2011;53(3):289–91.
38. Zhang L, Jarvis LB, Baek HJ, Gaston JS. Regulatory IL4+CD8+ T cells in patients with ankylosing spondylitis and healthy controls. Ann Rheum Dis 2009;68(8):1345–51.
39. Lin Z, Liao Z, Huang J, et al. Evaluation of Assessment of Spondyloarthritis international Society classification criteria for axial spondyloarthritis in Chinese patients with chronic back pain: results of a 2-year follow-up study. Int J Rheum Dis 2014;17(7):782–9.
40. Chou CT, Uksila J, Toivanen P. Enterobacterial antibodies in Chinese patients with rheumatoid arthritis and ankylosing spondylitis. Clin Exp Rheumatol 1998;16(2):161–4.
41. Howe HS, Zhao L, Song YW, et al. Seronegative spondyloarthropathy—studies from the Asia Pacific region. Ann Acad Med, Singapore 2007;36(2):135–41.
42. Chung HY, Lau CS, Wu KP, Wong WS, Mok MY. Comparison of performance of the Assessment of SpondyloArthritis international Society, the European Spondyloarthropathy Study Group and the modified New York criteria in a cohort of Chinese patients with spondyloarthritis. Clin Rheumatol 2011;30(7):947–53.
43. Leung YY, Ho KW, Tam LS, et al. Evaluation of spinal mobility measurements in predicting axial psoriatic arthritis. Clin Rheumatol 2011;30(9):1157–62.
44. Liao Z, Lin Z, Xu M, et al. Clinical features of axial undifferentiated spondyloarthritis (USpA) in China: HLA-B27 is more useful for classification than MRI of the sacroiliac joint. Scand J Rheumatol 2011;40(6):439–43.
45. Fan W, Huang L, Zhou Z, et al. Rapid and reliable genotyping of HLA-B*27 in the Chinese Han population using a duplex real-time TaqMan PCR assay. Clin Biochem 2012;45(1–2):106–11.
46. Chou CT, Tsai YF, Liu J, et al. The detection of the HLA-B27 antigen by immunomagnetic separation and enzyme-linked immunosorbent assay-comparison with a flow cytometric procedure. J Immunol Meth 2001;255(1–2):15–22.
47. Wang M, Li X, Chen J, et al. Screening and evaluating the mimic peptides as a useful serum biomarker of ankylosing spondylitis using a phage display technique. Rheumatol Int 2011;31(8):1009–16.
48. Chen HA, Chen CH, Lin YJ, et al. Association of bone morphogenetic proteins with spinal fusion in ankylosing spondylitis. J Rheumatol 2010;37(10):2126–32.
49. Gong Y, Zheng N, Chen SB, et al. Ten years' experience with needle biopsy in the early diagnosis of sacroiliitis. Arthritis Rheum 2012;64(5):1399–406.
50. Arslan H, Sakarya ME, Adak B, Unal O, Sayarlioglu M. Duplex and color Doppler sonographic findings in active sacroiliitis. Am J Roentgenol 1999;173(3):677–80.
51. Unlu E, Pamuk ON, Cakir N. Color and duplex Doppler sonography to detect sacroiliitis and spinal inflammation in ankylosing spondylitis. Can this method reveal response to anti-tumor necrosis factor therapy? J Rheumatol 2007;34(1):110–16.
52. Huang Z, Huang F. Update on the management of spondyloarthritis in Asian countries. Curr Rheumatol Rev 2012;8(1):39–44.
53. Au YL, Wong WS, Mok MY, Chung HY, Chan E, Lau CS. Disease activity assessment in ankylosing spondylitis in a Chinese cohort: BASDAI or ASDAS? Clin Rheumatol 2014;33(8):1127–34.
54. Huang F, Gu J, Liu Y, et al. Efficacy and safety of celecoxib in chinese patients with ankylosing spondylitis: a 6-week randomized, double-blinded study with 6-week open-label extension treatment. Curr Therap Res Clin Exp 2014;76:126–33.
55. Huang F, Gu J, Zhu P, et al. Efficacy and safety of adalimumab in Chinese adults with active ankylosing spondylitis: results of a randomised, controlled trial. Ann Rheum Dis 2014;73(3):587–94.
56. Lee TY, Huang F. Anti tumor necrosis factor alpha (TNFα) therapy in ankylosing spondylitis—Asian perspective. Curr Rheumatol Rev 2009;5(3):158–64.
57. Bao C, Huang F, Khan MA, et al. Safety and efficacy of golimumab in Chinese patients with active ankylosing spondylitis: 1-year results of a multicentre, randomized, double-blind, placebo-controlled phase III trial. Rheumatology 2014;53(9):1654–63.
58. Huang F, Zhang J, Huang JL, et al. [A multicenter, double-blind, placebo-controlled, randomized, phase III clinical study of etanercept in treatment of ankylosing spondylitis.] Zhonghua Nei Ke Za Zhi 2010;49(9):741–5.
59. Huang F, Zhang LY, Zhang JL, et al. [A short-term efficacy and safety study of infliximab in active ankylosing spondylitis.] Zhonghua Nei Ke Za Zhi 2006;45(2):122–6.
60. Deng X, Zhang J, Zhang J, Huang F. Thalidomide reduces recurrence of ankylosing spondylitis in patients following discontinuation of etanercept. Rheumatol Int 2013;33(6):1409–13.
61. Cui Y, Xiao Z, Shuxia W, et al. Computed tomography guided intra-articular injection of etanercept in the sacroiliac joint is an effective mode of treatment of ankylosing spondylitis. Scand J Rheumatol 2010;39(3):229–32.
62. Chan CY, Tsang HH, Lau CS, Chung HY. Prevalence of depressive and anxiety disorders and validation of the Hospital Anxiety and Depression Scale as a screening tool in axial spondyloarthritis patients. Int J Rheum Dis 2014 Oct 7; doi 10.1111/1756-185X.12456.
63. Zhu TY, Tam LS, Leung YY, et al. Socioeconomic burden of psoriatic arthritis in Hong Kong: direct and indirect costs and the influence of disease pattern. J Rheumatol 2010;37(6):1214–20.
64. Kim HB, Oh JH, Choi O. Anterior uveitis and ankylosing spondylitis. J Korean Ophth Soc 1976;17(2):235–9.
65. Lee YY, Park S, Lee MC, et al. Sacroiliac joint/sacrum uptake ratio measured by quantitatibe sacroiliac joint scintigraphy. Korean J Nucl Med 1982;16(2):63–70.
66. Kim TH, Jung SS, Sohn SJ, Park MH, Kim SY. Aneurysmal dilatation of ascending aorta and aortic insufficiency in juvenile spondyloarthropathy. Scand J Rheumatol 1997;26(3):218–21.
67. Sung YK, Cho SK, Choi CB, Bae SC. Prevalence and incidence of rheumatoid arthritis in South Korea. Rheumatol Int 2013;33(6):1525–32.

68. Dean LE, Jones GT, MacDonald AG, Downham C, Sturrock RD, Macfarlane GJ. Global prevalence of ankylosing spondylitis. Rheumatology (Oxford) 2014;53(4):650–7.
69. Kim TJ, Kim TH. Clinical spectrum of ankylosing spondylitis in Korea. Joint Bone Spine 2010;77(3):235–40.
70. Kim TH, Lee HS, Ji JD, et al. Undifferentiated spondyloarthropathy in Korea: focusing on peripheral arthritis. J Korean Med Sci 2002;17(1):71–4.
71. Jeong H, Yoon JY, Park EJ, et al. Clinical characteristics of nonradiographic axial spondyloarthritis in Korea: a comparison with ankylosing spondylitis. Int J Rheum Dis 2015;18(6):661–8.
72. Seo MR, Baek HL, Yoon HH, et al. Delayed diagnosis is linked to worse outcomes and unfavourable treatment responses in patients with axial spondyloarthritis. Clin Rheumatol 2015;34(8):1397–405.
73. Park KS, Kang SY, Lee WI. [HLA-B27 subtypes in Korean patients with ankylosing spondylitis.] Korean J Lab Med 2008;28(1):46–52.
74. Park SH, Kim J, Kim SG, Kim SK, Chung WT, Choe JY. Human leucocyte antigen-B27 subtypes in Korean patients with ankylosing spondylitis: higher B*2705 in the patient group. Int J Rheum Dis 2009;12(1):34–8.
75. Choi CB, Kim TH, Jun JB, et al. ARTS1 polymorphisms are associated with ankylosing spondylitis in Koreans. Ann Rheum Dis 2010;69(3):582–4.
76. Bang SY, Kim TH, Lee B, et al. Genetic studies of ankylosing spondylitis in Koreans confirm associations with ERAP1 and 2p15 reported in white patients. J Rheumatol 2011;38(2):322–4.
77. Lee SH, Lee YA, Woo DH, et al. Association of the programmed cell death 1 (PDCD1) gene polymorphism with ankylosing spondylitis in the Korean population. Arthritis Res Ther 2006;8(6):R163.
78. Joo YB, Bang SY, Kim TH, et al. Bone morphogenetic protein 6 polymorphisms are associated with radiographic progression in ankylosing spondylitis. PLoS One 2014;9(8):e104966.
79. Sung IH, Kim TH, Bang SY, et al. IL-23R polymorphisms in patients with ankylosing spondylitis in Korea. J Rheumatol 2009;36(5):1003–5.
80. Kim TJ, Kim TH, Lee HJ, et al. Interleukin 1 polymorphisms in patients with ankylosing spondylitis in Korea. J Rheumatol 2008;35(8):1603–8.
81. Kim TH, Stone MA, Rahman P, et al. Interleukin 1 and nuclear factor-kappaB polymorphisms in ankylosing spondylitis in Canada and Korea. J Rheumatol 2005;32(10):1907–10.
82. Kim TH, Rahman P, Jun JB, et al. Analysis of CARD15 polymorphisms in Korean patients with ankylosing spondylitis reveals absence of common variants seen in western populations. J Rheumatol 2004;31(10):1959–61.
83. Jung SH, Yim SH, Hu HJ, et al. Genome-wide copy number variation analysis identifies deletion variants associated with ankylosing spondylitis. Arthritis Rheumatol 2014;66(8):2103–12.
84. Kim JH, Cho SK, Han M, et al. Factors influencing discrepancies between the QuantiFERON-TB gold in tube test and the tuberculin skin test in Korean patients with rheumatic diseases. Semin Arthritis Rheum 2013;42(4):424–32.
85. Son CN, Jun JB, Kim JH, Sung IH, Yoo DH, Kim TH. Follow-up testing of interferon-gamma release assays are useful in ankylosing spondylitis patients receiving anti-tumor necrosis factor alpha for latent tuberculosis infection. J Korean Med Sci 2014;29(8):1090–3.
86. Kim HW, Park JK, Yang JA, et al. Comparison of tuberculosis incidence in ankylosing spondylitis and rheumatoid arthritis during tumor necrosis factor inhibitor treatment in an intermediate burden area. Clin Rheumatol 2014;33(9):1307–12.
87. Kim EM, Uhm WS, Bae SC, Yoo DH, Kim TH. Incidence of tuberculosis among korean patients with ankylosing spondylitis who are taking tumor necrosis factor blockers. J Rheumatol 2011;38(10):2218–23.
88. Jung SM, Ju JH, Park MS, et al. Risk of tuberculosis in patients treated with anti-tumor necrosis factor therapy: a nationwide study in South Korea, a country with an intermediate tuberculosis burden. Int J Rheum Dis 2015;18(3):323–30.
89. Yoo JW, Jo KW, Kang BH, et al. Mycobacterial diseases developed during anti-tumour necrosis factor-alpha therapy. Eur Respir J 2014;44(5):1289–95.
90. Lee SK, Kim SY, Kim EY, et al. Mycobacterial infections in patients treated with tumor necrosis factor antagonists in South Korea. Lung 2013;191(5):565–71.
91. Jo KW, Hong Y, Jung YJ, et al. Incidence of tuberculosis among anti-tumor necrosis factor users in patients with a previous history of tuberculosis. Respir Med 2013;107(11):1797–802.
92. Suh YS, Kwok SK, Ju JH, Park KS, Park SH, Yoon CH. Safe re administration of tumor necrosis factor-alpha (TNFα) inhibitors in patients with rheumatoid arthritis or ankylosing spondylitis who developed active tuberculosis on previous anti-TNFα therapy. J Korean Med Sci 2014;29(1):38–42.
93. Kim YJ, Kim YG, Shim TS, et al. Safety of resuming tumour necrosis factor inhibitors in patients who developed tuberculosis as a complication of previous TNF inhibitors. Rheumatology (Oxford) 2014;53(8):1477–81.
94. Chung SJ, Kim JK, Park MC, Park YB, Lee SK. Reactivation of hepatitis B viral infection in inactive HBsAg carriers following anti-tumor necrosis factor-alpha therapy. J Rheumatol 2009;36(11):2416–20.
95. Ryu HH, Lee EY, Shin K, et al. Hepatitis B virus reactivation in rheumatoid arthritis and ankylosing spondylitis patients treated with anti-TNFα agents: a retrospective analysis of 49 cases. Clin Rheumatol 2012;31(6):931–6.
96. Lee TJ, Park BH, Kim JW, Shin K, Lee EB, Song YW. Cost-of-illness and quality of life in patients with ankylosing spondylitis at a tertiary hospital in Korea. J Korean Med Sci 2014;29(2):190–7.
97. Kim TJ, Lee S, Joo KB, et al. The presence of peripheral arthritis delays spinal radiographic progression in ankylosing spondylitis: Observation Study of the Korean Spondyloarthropathy Registry. Rheumatology (Oxford) 2014;53(8):1404–8.
98. Lee JS, Lee S, Bang SY, et al. Prevalence and risk factors of anterior atlantoaxial subluxation in ankylosing spondylitis. J Rheumatol 2012;39(12):2321–6.
99. Kim TJ, Kim HS, Joo KB, Kim S, Kim TH. Do we really need to evaluate entire cervical spines for squaring score in modified stoke ankylosing spondylitis spinal score? J Rheumatol 2008;35(3):477–9.
100. Koo BS, Song Y, Joo KB, et al. Radiologic changes in the symphysis pubis of male patients with ankylosing spondylitis. J Rheumatol 2015 Dec 15;pii: jrheum.150711.
101. J Braun, J Davis, M Dougados, et al. First update of the international ASAS consensus statement for the use of anti-TNF agents in patients with ankylosing spondylitis. Ann Rheum Dis 2006;65(3):316–20.

CHAPTER 29

Axial spondyloarthritis in Latin America

Percival Sampaio-Barros and Rafael Valle-Oñate

Introduction to axial spondyloarthritis in Latin America

The modern concept of axSpA, proposed by ASAS in 2009 (1), encompasses the characteristic group of patients with AS, as well as the group with axSpA without radiologic sacroiliitis, but presenting characteristic BME on MRI (2). In 2011, the concept of SpA was even enlarged with the publication of the classification criteria for peripheral SpA (3). Two Latin American countries contributed with patients for these studies.

These concepts are especially important for the patients with SpA in Latin America, as they quite frequently present axial and peripheral symptoms in the course of their disease. This pattern is more frequently presented by the populations in which there was a significant miscegenation among Amerindians, whites, and blacks, as opposed to the more homogeneous white populations in the extreme south of South America (4).

This chapter focuses on axSpA in Latin America, as well as the peripheral and EAMs that are common in those Latin American patients with axSpA.

Brief description of Latin America

Latin America is a subregion of the Americas that comprises 20 countries where Spanish and Portuguese are spoken. It covers an area that stretches from the southern border of the USA to the extreme south of South America, including the Caribbean (Fig. 29.1). Latin America has an area of approximately 19 200 000 km^2 and a population of around 604 million inhabitants (estimated 2013).

Latin America also presents one of the most diverse ethnic variabilities in the world. The specific ethnic composition varies from country to country. Some are dominated by inhabitants of European ancestry (ex. Argentina). Others are dominated by Amerindian populations (ex. Peru). The predominance of European-Amerindians, more commonly referred as Mestizos, is characteristic of countries like Mexico. The mixture of Europeans and black populations is common in Brazil, where around 50% of the population is considered Mulattos (mixture of white and blacks). The only nation with a majority of blacks is the Dominican Republic. The ethnic distribution in the Latin American countries is shown in Table 29.1.

Presentation of axial spondyloarthritis in Latin America

The RESPONDIA cohort

Latin American cohorts of SpA present different demographic characteristics when compared with European cohorts. The first cohort that analysed clinical, demographic, and therapeutic parameters in Latin American countries was the Ibero-American Registry of Spondyloarthropathies (RESPONDIA), which was an association of 85 centres in 11 countries (Argentina, Brazil, Chile, Costa Rica, Ecuador, Mexico, Peru, Uruguay, and Venezuela, and also Portugal and Spain) which used a common protocol of investigation for SpA, originating from the Spanish Registry of Spondyloarthropathies of the Spanish Society of Rheumatology (REGISPONSER). As patients were analysed previously according to the new ASAS classification criteria for SpA, the RESPONDIA protocol used the ESSG classification criteria (5). Despite the difficulties in the standardization of the different parameters to be applied to the SpA patients in such a heterogeneous group of 85 centres, RESPONDIA was very important for the spread of knowledge about SpA in Latin America.

A study comparing a cohort of 1083 Latin American SpA patients from RESPONDIA with a European cohort of 2356 patients from the Spanish and Belgian registries of SpA found that the Latin American patients presented with a significantly higher frequency of peripheral arthritis (57% vs 42%) and enthesitis (54% vs 38%), while the European patients had a greater frequency of HLA-B27 positivity (83% vs 71%). Regarding treatment, Latin American patients were frequently more often prescribed NSAIDs (89% vs 75%), corticosteroids (19% vs 8%), MTX (34% vs 10%), and SSZ (32% vs 19%), while there was no difference in the prescription of anti-TNF therapy (15% in Europe vs 14% in Latin America) (6). The higher prescription of corticosteroids, MTX, and SSZ in the Latin American SpA patients can be associated with the higher frequency of peripheral joint symptoms in these patients. Another publication focused on hip disease in Latin Americans, comparing 466 patients from RESPONDIA with 2252 patients from Spain and Belgium, and found a higher prevalence of hip involvement in the Latin American group (36% vs 24%). Functional status, measured by BASFI, was significantly worse in patients with hip involvement. The necessity of hip replacement surgery was associated with early-onset, entheseal, and axial disease (7).

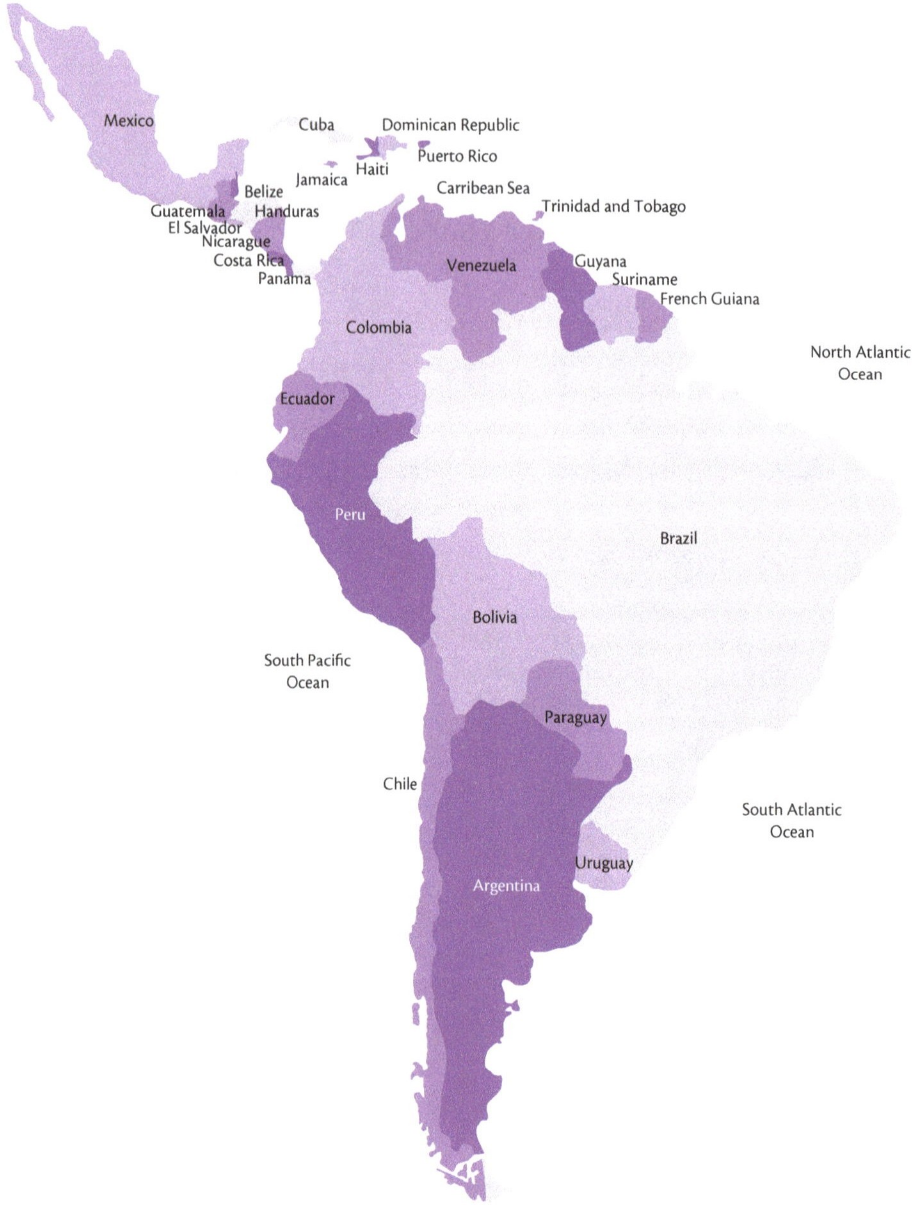

Fig. 29.1 (See colour plate section). Map of Latin America.

Two other studies analysed the importance of EAMs for the characterization of Latin American SpA patients. The first study analysed 1072 patients with primary AS, 147 patients with PsA, and 45 patients with enteropathic axSpA. Although functional capacity, disease activity, and quality of life were similar among the different groups, primary AS was associated with younger age at onset, male gender, IBP, and SI pain, whereas psoriatic spondylitis was associated with dactylitis, enthesitis, and peripheral arthritis (8). These data confirmed that late-onset SpA in Latin American patients is frequently associated with psoriasis and IBD. The other study investigated anterior uveitis in a group of 2012 SpA patients. Anterior uveitis was present in 372 patients (18.5%), and was associated predominantly with IBP, radiographic sacroiliitis, enthesopathies, hip involvement, and HLA-B27 positivity. Logistic regression analysis showed that AS and HLA-B27 positivity (trend) were significantly associated with anterior uveitis, whereas EAMs (predominantly psoriasis) were negatively associated (9).

National cohorts

The presentation of axSpA in Latin America is associated with diverse clinical and demographic factors, such as ethnicity, gender, and age at onset. We will analyse these different factors individually.

Ethnicity

The diverse ethnic background observed in Latin America (as shown in Table 29.1) is extremely important for the characterization of axSpA in the different countries of the continent.

In a prospective and multicentric Argentinian study with 402 SpA patients, there were 70.8% of whites and 22.8% of white-natives, originated from the miscegenation among whites and

Table 29.1 Ethnic distribution in the most important Latin American countries

Country	Population/ethnic distribution
Argentina	40 million inhabitants Whites—86%; non-whites—14%
Bolivia	10 million inhabitants Amerindians—55%; Mestizos—30%; whites—15%
Brazil	202 million inhabitants Whites—49%; Mulattos—43%; blacks—7%
Chile	17 million inhabitants Whites—59%; Mestizos—25%; Indians—8%
Colombia	47 million inhabitants Amerindians—45%; whites—37%; blacks—11%
Costa Rica	4 million inhabitants Whites—80%; Mestizos—15%; blacks—4%
Cuba	11 million inhabitants Whites—65%; Mulattos—30%; blacks—5%
Dominican Republic	9 million inhabitants Blacks—70%; Mulattos—24%; whites—4%
Ecuador	14 million inhabitants Mestizos—71%; Amerindians—14%; whites—6%
El Salvador	7 million inhabitants Mestizos—90%; whites—9%
Guatemala	15 million inhabitants Mestizos—60%; Indians—40%
Mexico	106 million inhabitants Mestizos—70%; Amerindians—20%; whites—10%
Nicaragua	5 million inhabitants Mestizos—69%; whites—17%; blacks—9%
Panama	3 million inhabitants Mestizos—68%; whites—15%; blacks—10%
Peru	29 million inhabitants Amerindians—45%; white-Indians—37%; whites—15%
Uruguay	3 million inhabitants Whites—88%; Mestizos—8%; blacks—4%
Venezuela	28 million inhabitants White-Indians—45%; whites—21%; African-Indians—10%

The ethnic distributions were adapted from the last demographic census in the mentioned countries. Countries without ethnic data in the last national census were not mentioned.

native Amerindians. As many participating centres were focused preferentially on PsA, the cohort had a predominance of patients with PsA (40.2%), followed by AS (21.4%) and uSpA (8.2%). A family history of SpA was present in 16.8% of the patients, and 18.3% of patients were unemployed, with a significant number of AS patients (10).

A Brazilian study focusing on ethnicity in a cohort of 1318 patients from the Brazilian Registry of Spondyloarthritis (Registro Brasileiro de Espondiloartrites (RBE)) confirmed an expected association of white ethnicity with psoriasis and positive HLA-B27. Nevertheless, the African-Brazilian patients (predominantly miscegenated) showed an association with hip involvement, axial inflammatory pain, and radiographic sacroiliitis. It is important to note that most African-Brazilian patients in the study were biracial, products of miscegenation between whites and blacks, and only a few were considered to be black only (11).

A Chilean study with 102 SpA patients, in a setting of predominantly white-indigenous ethnicity (81.4%), found AS in 58.7%, PsA in 25.6%, and uSpA in 7.3% of the patients (12).

A Colombian prospective study analysing 218 patients without a definite diagnosis of SpA found 71 patients (32.5%) with uSpA. IBP was a common complaint, but radiographic evidence of sacroiliitis was detected in only 55% of the patients (predominantly unilateral and/or asymmetric), and HLA-B27 was positive in only 39% of the patients. Only 7% of the patients evolved to a definite diagnosis of SpA in a short-term follow-up (13). Another Colombian study, focusing on HLA-B27 subtypes in a cohort of 59 patients with AS in the two more prevalent ethnic groups of the country (Mulattos and Mestizos), found a high prevalence of HLA-B*2705 (84.7%), with no difference between the two ethnic groups (14).

A recent epidemiologic study has estimated the prevalence of SpA in Mexico at 0.6%, with a prevalence of AS of 0.1% (15). Overall, the initial combination of axial and peripheral symptoms in the JoSpA patient, followed by axial disease, and then peripheral arthritis and enthesitis in the adult patient is the classical clinical pattern most frequently observed in the highly miscegenated Mexican population (16).

Gender

SpA cohorts in Latin America show a male predominance; female gender is frequently associated with a more peripheral disease pattern.

An Argentinian study analysing 402 patients with SpA showed a male predominance (59% vs 41% compared with female gender), although diseases with a peripheral involvement (PsA 60.2%; uSpA 8.2%, and ReA 6.2%) were frequent in the cohort (10).

A recent study from the RBE, analysing gender in a cohort of 1505 SpA patients, found a predominance of male gender (72.4%). Importantly, female gender was associated with peripheral SpA, upper limb arthritis, higher number of painful and swollen joints, dactylitis, psoriasis, nail involvement, and a family history of SpA. Patients' global assessment scores, as well as disease activity (BASDAI), functionality (BASFI), enthesitis score (MASES), and quality of life (ASQoL) were also higher in female SpA patients (17). Although these indexes (BASDAI, BASFI, MASES, and ASQoL) were designed for measuring predominantly axial disease, their higher scores in the female gender can be associated with higher frequency of peripheral involvement in female SpA patients.

A male predominance was observed in the RESPONDIA cohort of SpA patients from Chile (58.4%) (12), Costa Rica (57.6%) (18), Mexico (59.3%) (19), Peru (65%) (20), Uruguay (66%) (21), and Venezuela (62.3%) (22).

In Colombia, multiple studies have found a male predominance, between 56.9 and 63.4% (23–25). Of interest, in a study of enteropathic SpA, the female gender was more frequent (66.7%) (26).

Interestingly, a recent publication describing 183 SpA patients from Guatemala revealed a female predominance (60%); axial and peripheral components were observed frequently, and the most common diseases in the group were ReA (67%) and uSpA (26%) (27). It is important to note that Guatemala has an ethnic distribution of 60% Mestizos and 40% Indians, with an extremely low percentage of white people (see Table 29.1).

Age at onset

In the new classification criteria of axSpA, age at onset of less than 45 years is mandatory, emphasizing that SpA constitutes a group of diseases that rarely start after 45 years old (1). In a Brazilian cohort of 1424 SpA patients, in 151 (10.6%) the disease started after 45 years; these later onset SpA patients were predominantly females with peripheral arthritis, dactylitis, nail involvement, and psoriasis (28).

In the national cohorts participating in RESPONDIA, the mean age at onset was 38.4 years in Argentina (29), 35.3 years in Chile (12), 34.5 years in Costa Rica (18), 30.6 years in Peru (20), 31 years in Uruguay (21), and 29.4 years in Venezuela (22). Similarly, the mean age at onset in Colombian studies was 36.6 years (23–26).

Regarding JoSpA, it is important to consider that its initial manifestation is not IBP but peripheral arthritis and/or enthesitis (30). An interesting aspect related to JoSpA is associated with its long-term follow-up. A follow-up study showed that 75% of the Mexican JoSpA cases fulfilled the mNY criteria for AS 5–10 years after onset. Similarly, 42% of the uSpA patients developed AS within 3 years. Radiographic sacroiliitis, grade 2 bilateral or grade 3 unilateral, and previous uveitis were the most important prognostic factors influencing this transition. Although patients with peripheral arthritis, particularly JoSpA, may receive an early diagnosis because of early referral to a rheumatologist, those with axial disease may be diagnosed late in the course of the disease (31).

A recent publication of the RBE found that in 235 (16.5%) of 1424 SpA patients there was disease onset at less than 16 years; these JoSpA patients were associated with male gender, HLA-B27 positive, lower limb arthritis, enthesitis, anterior uveitis, and lower scores of BASDAI and BASFI (32).

JoSpA is discussed in detail in Chapter 15.

Peripheral involvement

As mentioned in the section 'The RESPONDIA cohort', peripheral involvement is significantly more common in the Latin American RESPONDIA cohort than in the Spanish and Belgian SpA cohorts (6). Although genetic factors may be associated with this increased frequency of peripheral involvement, it is important to consider that Amerindian and black populations have lower socioeconomic status than white populations. Poverty and less access to healthcare and education are variables to be considered in this characterization.

An analysis of the national cohorts participating in the RESPONDIA cohort has shown that peripheral involvement was significantly frequent in the SpA patients (33). Associated peripheral involvement was referred by 66% of the Argentinian (29), 59% of the Chilean (12), 79.2% of the Mexican (19), 43.3% of the Peruvian (20), 42% of the Uruguayan (21), and 50.7% of the Venezuelan (22) patients.

Peripheral involvement is a common clinical characteristic in Brazilian SpA patients. When analysing 1505 SpA patients from the five Brazilian geographic regions, it was observed that combined axial and peripheral involvement, as well as higher mean ESR and CRP values, were more common in areas with a strong component of miscegenation (northeast and north), while purely axial involvement and the occurrence of anterior uveitis were significantly more frequent in the south (with a predominant white population) (4).

In another highly miscegenated country, Guatemala, the percentage of patients with peripheral involvement (associated or not with axial involvement) is high, and the most frequent diseases in the SpA spectrum are ReA and uSpA (27).

In a Colombian study analysing 144 patients with SpA, 77.1% had axial involvement and 50.7% had peripheral arthritis (26). In another study with patients from the northwest region of the country, axial (84.5%) and peripheral (64.7%) involvement were higher than in the previous study (24).

Enthesitis

Enthesitis, predominantly affecting the Achilles tendon and plantar fascia, is a common complaint of SpA patients in Latin America. In the RESPONDIA cohort, clinical enthesitis was referred by 32.8% of patients in Argentina (29), 52.3% in Chile (12), 57.6% in Costa Rica (18), 79.7% in Mexico (19), 52.8% in Uruguay (21), and 34.8% in Venezuela (22).

High frequencies of enthesitis were found in Colombian studies, ranging between 41.7% (26) and 67% (24). A single study applying MASES found a mean score of 4 (24). A study assessing MASES scores in 1505 Brazilian SpA patients found that 54% of the patients reported at least one enthesitic site. The presence of enthesitis was significantly associated with axial (buttock, cervical, and hip pain) and peripheral symptoms (lower limb arthritis, number of painful and swollen joints), as well as higher mean BASDAI, BASFI, and ASQoL scores. Multivariate logistic regression showed that Achilles tendinitis, as well as higher scores of BASFI and ASQoL, were associated with work incapacity (34).

Genetics: HLA-B27

There are no specific studies analysing the incidence and prevalence of HLA-B27 in Latin American populations. Probably due to its ethnic heterogeneity, Latin American SpA cohorts generally present a lower frequency of HLA-B27 when compared with European populations (6).

As details on HLA-B27 are not commonly available in the national health systems in Latin American countries, just a few countries have published data about this topic. The early studies of HLA-B27 in Brazilian populations of AS found a positivity of 75–86% (35). In a study analysing 147 AS patients from a single centre, HLA-B27 was positive in 78.2% of the cases (36). The main HLA-B27 allele observed in the AS Brazilian population was HLA-B*2705 (37), which was also the most frequent allele in uSpA (38), PsA (39), and ReA (40). The HLA-B*2705 allele was also associated with recurrence of anterior uveitis in a single-centre study (41).

HLA-B27 subtypes in Colombia are similar to those found in the Brazilian population. In a study of 59 patients with AS, HLA-B*2705 was found in 87.1% of Mulattos and 80% of Mestizos, whereas HLA-B*2702 was found in 12.8% of Mulattos and 20% of Mestizos (14). The frequency of HLA class II alleles in SpA patients was also studied. A total of 56 patients from the Colombian northwest region were analysed; HLA-DRB4*01 (35.7%) and HLA-DQB1*0501 (28.6%) were the most frequent alleles. Dactylitis was associated with HLA-DRB4*01 in 64.3% of patients, while enthesitis was associated with HLA-DQB1*0501 in 37.9% of patients.

Axial and peripheral involvement were almost equally associated with HLA-DRB4*01 (37% and 36.1%, respectively) (25).

In a Mexican study with 172 patients with SpA (83 with uSpA, 64 with AS, and 25 with ReA) and 99 healthy controls, HLA-B27 was associated with younger age at onset and increased disease severity, and HLA-DR1 with older age at onset. The strength of HLA-B15, HLA-B27, and HLA-DR1 associations varied in different forms of SpA in Mexicans, and are independent from HLA-B27 (42).

In a cohort of 48 AS patients and 55 healthy controls from Zulia, Venezuela, the alleles HLA-B*2705 (68.8%) and HLA-B*2702 (31.2%) were found in the AS population, while in the control group HLA-B*2708 was the most frequent allele (43).

Two Brazilian studies analysed the long-term follow-up of patients with uSpA. The first study analysed 111 patients fulfilling ESSG and Amor criteria for SpA in a long-term (2, 5, 7, and 10 years) follow-up. Patients were predominantly male (81.1%), white (78.4%), and HLA-B27 positive (61.3%). Twenty-seven patients (24.3%) had a final diagnosis of AS and three patients (2.7%) were considered PsA, whereas 25 patients (22.5%) went into remission during the follow-up. Multivariate logistic regression analysis showed that progression to AS was associated with HLA-B27 positivity (OR 6.720) and buttock pain (OR 6.211) (44). Another study analysing the 8-year follow-up of 40 patients with a diagnosis of uSpA, also fulfilling ESSG criteria, showed a predominance of female gender (58%), African-Brazilian ethnicity (60%), and HLA-B27 negativity (55%). Ten patients (27.8%) had AS progression during the 8-year follow-up; buttock pain (OR 10.55) and low-grade radiographic sacroiliitis (OR 11.50) at baseline were associated with definite SpA (45).

HLA-B27 is positive in 90% of the juvenile-onset AS patients, and the HLA-B*2705 allele is present in more than 95% of the AS patients (16). A Mexican study analysing the long-term follow-up of JoSpA patients demonstrated that 75% of these patients fulfilled the mNY criteria for AS 5–10 years after onset. In a similar way, 42% of the patients with uSpA developed AS within 3 years. Radiographic sacroiliitis, grade 2 bilateral or grade 3 unilateral (OR 11.18), and previous uveitis (OR 19.25) were the most important prognostic factors (31).

A recent study also analysed disease progression in a cohort of 139 consecutive Colombian patients with SpA (according to ESSG criteria). Mean age at onset was 26.8 years, mean disease duration was 8.5 years, HLA-B27 was positive in 60% of the tested patients, and 18% reported a family history of SpA. Follow-up in 51 patients revealed that 22% (11 patients, with ReA initially diagnosed in six and uSpA in five) developed AS (13).

Other biomarkers

In a Mexican study with a cohort of SpA patients (AS, uSpA, and ReA) and a group of ethnically matched healthy individuals, the authors found that, besides HLA-B27, low molecular weight protein 2 (LMP2) genotypes (46) and heath shock protein 70 polymorphisms (47) were also involved in the genetic susceptibility to develop AS.

A Colombian study analysed different serum biomarkers (TNFα, IL-1α, IL-6, IL-17, IL-23, and ultrasensitive CRP) and factors associated with clinical activity and poor prognosis in 62 SpA patients (19 with AS, 13 with ReA, and 30 with uSpA); there was predominance of males (69.4%), with IBP in 67.7%, arthritis in 71.0%, enthesitis in 54.8%, and positive HLA-B27 in 41.9%. Patients with SpA had significantly higher levels of IL-17, IL-23, TNFα, IL-6, IL-1α, and ultrasensitive CRP compared with controls. An increase in serum levels of ultrasensitive CRP, IL-6, IL-1α, and lipopolysaccharide binding protein (LBP) was associated with HLA-B27, IBP, and arthritis, and was correlated with poor prognosis in SpA (48). Another potential biomarker, serum monocyte chemoattractant protein-1 (MCP-1), was studied in order to distinguish AS from low back pain; a sensitivity of 96% and a specificity of 83.3% were found (49).

Treatment

The percentage of patients using NSAIDs, corticosteroids (CS), MTX, SSZ, and anti-TNF drugs in the different Latin American cohorts of RESPONDIA are described in Table 29.2. These data reflect the national preferences for the treatment of different forms of SpA in the period 2006–2009.

An Argentinian study focusing on adherence to treatment in a cohort of 59 patients with AS (male predominance (72.9%), with a mean age of 47 years and mean disease duration of 120 months) and 53 patients with RA (female predominance (69.8%), with a mean age of 56 years and mean disease duration of 156 months) found a better adherence in RA patients, although the AS adherence was not bad (50).

In 2013, the second update of the Guidelines for the Diagnosis and Treatment of Ankylosing Spondylitis of the Brazilian Society of Rheumatology were published. These guidelines follow the Brazilian Medical Association's strict rules for evidence-based medicine (51).

In Mexico, patients rarely receive standard treatment for SpA from their general physicians or orthopaedic surgeons. However, once they are referred to a rheumatologist, their SpA is more likely to be treated appropriately and in agreement with ASAS and EULAR recommendations for the treatment of AS (16).

Table 29.2 Drugs used in the treatment of SpA in different Latin American countries participating in the RESPONDIA cohort (2006–2009)

Country	NSAID(%)	CS(%)	MTX(%)	SSZ(%)	Anti-TNF(%)
Argentina (*n* = 405)	77.5	29.0	49.0	12.0	10.4
Brazil (*n* = 1036)	77.0	7.5	26.2	21.3	5.4
Chile (*n* = 109)	83.4	40.3	44.0	27.5	0.0
Costa Rica (*n* = 33)	97.0	39.4	33.3	45.5	12.1
Mexico (*n* = 172)	94.0	11.0	30.0	35.0	12.1
Peru (*n* = 60)	–	15.3	23.3	56.7	1.7
Uruguay (*n* = 53)	98.0	9.0	36.0	28.0	0.0
Venezuela (*n* = 69)	97.1	46.4	53.6	40.6	27.0

In Colombia, a study from the northwest region showed that DMARDs were the most frequently used drugs (68%), followed by NSAIDs (52%) and anti-TNF drugs (42%); among these, infliximab was prescribed in 20% of patients, followed by adalimumab (16%) and ETN (6%) (24). A study on the use of anti-TNF in four major cities in Colombia found that 21.2% of all prescribed anti-TNFs were for SpA treatment (AS: 17.1%, PsA: 2.5%, CD: 1.6%) (52). A Colombian study was designed to distinguish responders from non-responders to three standard pulses of infliximab at week 6 in a series of 47 AS patients. Although 22 different cytokines were measured as potential biomarkers, only higher levels of serum IL-1 helped distinguish the responders, with a sensitivity of 84.9% and a specificity of 23.8% (53).

References

1. Rudwaleit M, van der Heijde D, Landewé R, et al. The development of Assessment of SpondyloArthritis international Society classification criteria for axial spondyloarthritis (part II): validation and final selection. Ann Rheum Dis 2009;68:777–83.
2. Rudwaleit M, Jurik AG, Hermann KG, et al. Defining active sacroiliitis on magnetic resonance imaging (MRI) for classification of axial spondyloarthritis: a consensual approach for the ASAS/OMERACT MRI group. Ann Rheum Dis 2009;68:1520–7.
3. Rudwaleit M, van der Heijde D, Landewé R, et al. The Assessment of SpondyloArthritis international Society classification criteria for peripheral spondyloarthritis and for spondyloarthritis in general. Ann Rheum Dis 2011;70:25–31.
4. Saad CG, Gonçalves CR, Sampaio-Barros PD. Seronegative arthritis in Latin America: a current review. Curr Rheumatol Rep 2014;16(9):438.
5. Dougados M, van der Linden S, Juhlin R, et al. The European Spondylarthropathy Study Group preliminary criteria for the classification of spondylarthropathy. Arthritis Rheum 1991;34:1218–27.
6. Benegas M, Muñoz-Gomariz E, Font P, et al. Comparison of the clinical expression of patients with ankylosing spondylitis from Europe and Latin America. J Rheumatol 2012;39:2315–20.
7. Vander Cruyssen B, Muñoz-Gomariz E, Font P, et al. Hip involvement in ankylosing spondylitis: epidemiology and risk factors associated with hip replacement surgery. Rheumatology (Oxford) 2010;49:73–81.
8. Pérez Alamino R, Maldonado Cocco JA, Citera G, et al. Differential features between primary ankylosing spondylitis and spondylitis associated with psoriasis and inflammatory disease. J Rheumatol 2011;38:1656–60.
9. Sampaio-Barros PD, Pereira IA, Hernández-Cuevas C, et al. An analysis of 372 patients with anterior uveitis in a large Ibero-American cohort of spondyloarthritis: the RESPONDIA group. Clin Exp Rheumatol 2013;31:484–9.
10. Buschiazzo E, Maldonado-Cocco JA, Arturi P, et al. Epidemiology of spondyloarthritis in Argentina. Am J Med Sci 2011;341:289–92.
11. Skare TL, Bortoluzzo AB, Gonçalves CR, et al. Ethnic influence in clinical and functional measures of Brazilian patients with spondyloarthritis. J Rheumatol 2012;39:141–7.
12. Gutierrez MA, Pérez C, Saavedra J, et al. Registro Iberoamericano de Espondiloartritis: Chile. Reumatol Clin 2008;4(Suppl 4):S41–7.
13. Valle-Oñate R, Candia L, Romero-Sánchez C, et al. Epidemiology of spondyloarthritis in Colombia. Am J Med Sci 2011;341:293–4.
14. Martínez B, Caraballo L, Hernández M, Valle R, Avila M, Iglesias Gamarra I. HLA-B27 subtypes in patients with ankylosing spondylitis (AS) in Colombia. Rev Invest Clin 1999;51:221–6.
15. Peláez-Ballestas I, Navarro-Zarza JE, Julian J, et al. A community-based study on the prevalence of spondyloarthritis and inflammatory back pain in Mexicans. J Clin Rheumatol 2013;19:57–61.
16. Burgos-Vargas R, Peláez-Ballestas I. Epidemiology of spondyloarthritis in Mexico. Am J Med Sci 2011;341:298–300.
17. Carvalho HM, Bortoluzzo AB, Gonçalves CR, et al. Gender characterization in a large series of Brazilian patients with spondyloarthritis. Clin Rheumatol 2012;31:687–95.
18. Saenz-Castro R. Registro Iberoamericano de Espondiloartritis: Costa Rica. Reumatol Clin 2008;4(Suppl 4):S36–40.
19. Casasola-Vargas JC, Flores-Alvarado DE, Huerta-Gil G, et al. Registro Iberoamericano de Espondiliartritis (RESPONDIA): México. Reumatol Clin 2008;4(Suppl 4):S56–62.
20. Chavez-Corrales JE, Jauregui MM, Linares MA, et al. Registro Iberoamericano de Espondiloartritis: Peru. Reumatol Clin 2008;4(Suppl 4):S63–7.
21. Palleiro D, Spangenberg E. Registro Iberoamericano de Espondiloartritis (RESPONDIA): Uruguay. Reumatol Clin 2008;4(Suppl 4):S73–8.
22. Chacón R, Granados Y, Esteva MH, et al. Registro Iberoamericano de Espondiloartritis (RESPONDIA): Venezuela. Reumatol Clin 2008;4(Suppl 4):S79–86.
23. Londoño JD, González LA, Ramírez LA, et al. Caracterización de las espondiloartropatías y determinación de factores de mal pronóstico en una población de pacientes colombianos. Rev Colomb Reumatol 2005;12:195–207.
24. Márquez J, Pinto LF, Candia DL, et al. Espondiloartritis em el Hospital Pablo Tobón Uribe. Descripción de una cohorte. Rev Colomb Reumatol 2010;17:80–5.
25. Velásquez EP, Quintero JC, Aristizábal BH, et al. Frecuencia de alelos de HLA de clase I y II en uma cohorte de pacientes con espondiloartritis provenientes del noroccidente colombiano. Biomedica 2012;32:43–51.
26. Pérez-Fernández OM, Mantilla RD, Cruz-Tapias P, Rodriguez-Rodriguez A, Rojas-Villarraga A, Anaya JM. Spondyloarthropathies in autoimmune diseases and vice versa. Autoimmune Dis 2012;736384.
27. Garcia-Kutzbach A, Montenegro A, Iraheta I, Bará C, Saenz R. Epidemiology of spondyloarthropathies in Central America. Am J Med Sci 2011;341:295–7.
28. Skare TL, Leite N, Bortoluzzo AB, et al. Effect of age at disease onset in the clinical profile of spondyloarthritis: a study of 1424 Brazilian patients. Clin Exp Rheumatol 2012;30:351–7.
29. Bellomio V, Berman A, Sueldo RR, et al. Registro Iberoamericano de Espondiloartrites (RESPONDIA): Argentina. Reumatol Clín 2008;4(Suppl 4):S23–9.
30. Burgos-Vargas R. The Assessment of the Spondyloarthritis international Society concept and criteria for the classification of axial spondyloarthritis and peripheral spondyloarthritis: a critical appraisal for the pediatric rheumatologist. Pediatr Rheumatol Online J 2012;10:14.
31. Huerta-Sil G, Casasola-Vargas JC, Londoño JD, et al. Low-grade radiographic sacroiliitis as prognostic factor in patients with undifferentiated spondyloarthritis fulfilling diagnostic criteria for ankylosing spondylitis throughout follow up. Ann Rheum Dis 2003;65:642–6.
32. Duarte AP, Marques CD, Bortoluzzo AB, et al. Epidemiologic profile of juvenile-onset spondyloarthritis compared with adult-onset spondyloarthritis in a large Brazilian cohort. Braz J Rheumatol 2014;54:424–30.
33. Gallinaro AL, Ventura C, Sampaio Barros PD, Gonçalves CR. Spondyloarthritis: analysis of a Brazilian series compared with a large Ibero-American registry (RESPONDIA group). Braz J Rheumatol 2010;50:581–9.
34. Carneiro S, Bortoluzzo AB, Gonçalves CR, et al. Effect of enthesitis on 1505 Brazilian patients with spondyloarthritis. J Rheumatol 2013;40:1719–25.
35. Sampaio-Barros PD, Gonçalves CR, Silva JAB, et al. Registro Iberoamericano de Espondiloartritis (RESPONDIA): Brasil. Reumatol Clin 2008;4(Suppl 4):S30–5.
36. Sampaio-Barros PD, Bertolo MB, Kraemer MHS, Marques Neto JF, Samara AM. Primary ankylosing spondylitis: patterns of disease in a Brazilian population of 147 patients. J Rheumatol 2001;28:560–5.
37. Conde RA, Sampaio-Barros PD, Donadi EA, et al. Frequency of the HLA-B27 alleles in Brazilian patients with ankylosing spondylitis. J Rheumatol 2003;30:2511–12.
38. Sampaio-Barros PD, Conde RA, Donadi EA, et al. Undifferentiated spondyloarthropathies in Brazilians: importance of HLA-B27 and

the B7-CREG alleles in characterization and disease progression. J Rheumatol 2003;30:2632–7.
39. Bonfiglioli R, Conde RA, Sampaio-Barros PD, Louzada-Junior P, Donadi EA, Bertolo MB. Frequency of HLA-B27 alleles in Brazilian patients with psoriatic arthritis. Clin Rheumatol 2008;27:709–12.
40. Sampaio-Barros PD, Conde RA, Donadi EA, et al. Frequency of HLA-B27 and its alleles in patients with Reiter syndrome: comparison with the frequency in other spondyloartrhropathies and a healthy control population. Rheumatol Int 2008;28:483–6.
41. Sampaio-Barros PD, Conde RA, Bonfiglioli R, Bértolo MB, Samara AM. Characterization and outcome of uveitis in 350 patients with spondyloarthropathies. Rheumatol Int 2006;26:1143–46.
42. Vargas-Alarcón G, Londoño J, Hernandez-Pacheco G, et al. Effect of HLA-B and HLA-DR genes on susceptibility and severity of spondyloarthropathies in Mexican patients. Ann Rheum Dis 2002;61:714–17.
43. Cipriani A, Rivera S, Hassanhi M, et al. HLA-B27 subtypes determination in patients with ankylsoing spondylitis from Zulia, Venezuela. Human Immunol 2003;64:745–9.
44. Sampaio-Barros PD, Bortoluzzo AB, Conde RA, Costallat LT, Samara AM, Bertolo MB. Undifferentiated spondyloarthritis: a long-term followup. J Rheumatol 2010;37:1195–9.
45. Lage RC, Bomtempo CAS, Kakehasi AM, de Carvalho MA. Undifferentiated spondyloarthritis in a heterogeneous Brazilian population: an eight-year follow-up study. Rheumatol Int 2014;34:1019–23.
46. Vargas-Alarcón G, Gamboa R, Zuñiga J, et al. Association study of LMP gene polymorphisms in Mexican patients with spondyloarthritis. Human Immunol 2004;65:1437–42.
47. Vargas-Alarcón G, Londoño J, Hernandez-Pacheco G, et al. Heath shock protein gene polymorphisms in Mexican patients with spondyloarthropathies. Ann Rheum Dis 2002;61:48–51.
48. Londoño J, Romero-Sanchez MC, Torres VG, et al. The association between serum levels of potential biomarkers with the presence of factors related to the clinical activity and poor prognosis in spondyloarthritis. Braz J Rheumatol 2012;52:536–44.
49. Romero-Sánchez C, Tsou HK, Jan MS, et al. Serum monocyte chemotactic protein-1 concentrations distinguish patients with ankylosing spondylitis from patients with mechanical low back pain. J Spinal Disord Tech 2011;24:202–7.
50. Arturi P, Schneeberger EE, Sommerfleck F, et al. Adherence to treatment in patients with ankylosing spondylitis. Clin Rheumatol 2013;32:1007–15.
51. Sampaio-Barros PD, Keiserman M, Meirelles ES, et al. Recommendations for the management and treatment of ankylosing spondylitis. Braz J Rheumatol 2013;53:242–57.
52. Machado J, Moncada JC, Pineda R. Perfil de utilización de los anti-factor de necrosis tumoral en pacientes de Colombia. Biomedica 2011;31:250–7.
53. Romero-Sánchez C, Robinson WH, Tomooka BH, et al. Identification of acute phase reactants and cytokines useful for monitoring infliximab therapy in ankylosing spondylitis. Clin Rheumatol 2008;27:1429–35.

CHAPTER 30

Axial spondyloarthritis in India

Anand Malaviya and Ashok Kumar

Introduction to axial spondyloarthritis in India

SpA is among the commonest rheumatological conditions in India, second only to RA (1). This is consistent with the fact that the prevalence of SpA is linked to the prevalence of HLA-B27 in that population (2). Its prevalence in different regions of India has been reported to be approximately 6% of the general population (3). That would put the country prominently on the SpA map of the world, reflected in the large number of publications from the late 1970s onwards, dispelling any earlier misconceptions that it is largely a 'white man's disease'. This chapter summarizes the various aspects of SpA as reported from India.

Early reports (late 1970s–1980s)

The earliest publications on SpA from India were by our group from New Delhi in 1979 (4, 5). These papers included a broader group of patients with 'seronegative spondarthritis', as defined by Moll and colleagues (6). In these early papers the emphasis was on the prevalence of HLA-B27 among patients with SpA. Included in this report were 19 patients with AS, but their clinical details were not provided. AS was diagnosed according to Calin's clinical criteria (7). Twelve of the cases were predominantly axial and the other seven had prominent extra-axial features.

In 1983, our group reported a hitherto poorly described entity that we called 'unclassifiable' SpA (8). Patients classifiable as AS using Rome criteria (9) were excluded. There were 29 patients who could not be classified under any of the described subtypes of SpA (PsA, IBD-related, ReA). In retrospect, this could have been the first report of nr-axSpA as only 4 of 29 patients had possible sacroiliitis on standard radiograph. Several years later this subgroup of SpA was named 'undifferentiated' SpA, along with the description of its classification criteria (10, 11). It is noted that these studies did not cite our earlier publication (6).

In 1986, investigators in Mumbai (on the west coast of India) reported 86 males and 122 females between 16 and 40 years of age, with arthritis of more than 6 weeks' duration, studied over a period of 3 years (12). Fifty-two percent (45) of the male patients were reported to have clinical features of SpA. This was in contrast to only 9.8% (12) of the female patients. Among patients with features of SpA, these workers reported 12.8% patients who could not be classified as AS, but the classification criteria used were not specified. The authors commented that these 'unclassifiable' patients had similarities to the incomplete form of Reiter's disease, where some of the typical features of the disease were not present. This study compared this subgroup with our earlier report on uSpA (8).

The first Indian study exclusively on AS was in 1984 from New Delhi (13). In 1984, using Rome classification criteria for AS (9), we described 51 patients (Table 30.1). In 1989, workers from Mumbai reported on 82 patients with AS classifiable with mNY criteria (14), in which the differences between male and female patients with AS were described (15) (Table 30.1).

HLA status in earlier studies

The earliest report on HLA-B27 in AS occurring in India was from Chandigarh in northern India (16). These investigators reported an HLA-B27 frequency of 94% and 3% among 17 AS patients and 60 controls, respectively. Two years later, we from New Delhi reported the frequency of HLA-B27 among patients with a broad spectrum of conditions included under the SpA family (4, 5). We used the acronym SSA (seronegative spondarthritis) for this group of related diseases, which became popular among Indian rheumatologists and remained so until the end of the last century. By that time, the acronym SpA had become widely accepted by rheumatologists around the world and replaced 'SSA' among Indian rheumatologists as well. Two reports from 1979 included AS but also several other conditions within the broad SpA family, including persons having chronic back pain generally diagnosed as lumbar sprain, intervertebral disc disease, and non-specific back pain (4, 5). The frequency of HLA-B27 in AS was 74% in one study (4) and 87.5% in another (5). Soon after, another study described that patients with uSpA (8) had an 84% frequency of HLA-B27, as against 6% in normal controls.

These publications established two important points: HLA-B27 frequency in the SpA group was highest among patients with AS (approximately 95%), but decreased to approximately 50% if PsA and other members of the SpA family were included. This was similar to Khan's 2002 report that HLA-B27 frequency is highest in AS and declines among other members of the SpA family of diseases (2). The second point was that frequency of HLA-B27 among normal controls around Delhi (in northern India) was approximately 6%, which is similar to that of the western European population (2). If the projections from Khan are applied to the northern Indian population, then approximately 0.2% of the general population and approximately 2% of those with HLA-B27 would have SpA-related conditions in northern India (2). In the 1989 report from Mumbai mentioned in the section 'Early reports (late 1970s–1980s)' (15), 78% of males and 89% of females were HLA-B27 positive. In 1996, workers from Chennai (earlier called Madras, in the southern part of India) reported results on 177 patients with AS and found 153 (86%) to be positive for HLA-B27 (17). In summary, these early reports established the fact that in AS among Indians, HLA-B27 positivity is high (between 80% and 90%.)

Table 30.1 AS/axSpA reports from India: demographic, clinical, imaging, and genetic characteristics and acute-phase reactants

Variables studied	Delhi (northern India), 1984, n = 51 (13), using Rome criteria	Mumbai (western India), 1989, n = 82 (15), using mNY criteria (14)	Chennai (southern India), 1990, n = 102 (18), using mNY criteria (14)	Delhi, 2009, n = 70 (24, 25), using mNY criteria (14)	Delhi, 2014 (26–28), n = 347 using ASAS 2009 criteria (23)	Remarks
Age of onset (years)	21.2	M 20.56, F 25.4	26	M 23.6, F 32.5	24.8 (SD 8.91); M 23 (SD 8.6), F 24.7 (SD 0.8)	Similar to textbook figures and major reviews (19)
Disease duration (years) prior to diagnosis	8.7	–	–	9.3 (± 6.5)	7.23 (SD ± 6.2); M 7.34 (SD 6.32), F 6.8 (SD 7.4)	See Table 30.3 for details
Delay in diagnosis (years)	–	M 6.3, F 5.71	–	6.9 (± 5.2); M 6.5, F 8.6*	7.5 (SD ± 6, range 0.04–50, IQR 7) M/F	Similar to accepted figures of 5–6 years (2, 133)
Male: female ratio	16:1	7.2:1	16:1	5:1	3.75:1	
Symptoms at onset (%)						
◆ IBP, neck pain	41	42 (51.2); M 34 (47.2), F (80); cervical spine 2 (2.4%)	57.8	–	78.3; M 80, F 72.6*	Much higher than in earlier reports, no definite reason could be attributed
◆ Peripheral arthritis	47 (knee 11 (21.5), hip 15 (29.9), ankle, shoulder, and elbow 1 each (1.96))	38 (46.3); M 49.97; F 20	37.25	–	22; M 20, F 30*	Much lower than earlier reports; no definite reason could be attributed
◆ Root joint involvement	–	–	–	–	2; M 1.5, F 4*	–
◆ AAU	10	1 (1.2)	10.8	25.7	<1*	Much less than that reported in 2009; no definite reason could be attributed
◆ Enthesitis	2 (heel pain)	NA	17.6 (heel pain)	–	5; M 6.2, F 0, statistically significant (p = 0.028)	–
Clinical features (%)						
◆ Inflammatory spinal–sacroiliac symptoms (back pain)	100	82 (100 by selection criteria)	NA	87.1#	100 (by selection criteria)	By selection criteria, 100
◆ Peripheral arthritis—mainly knee, ankle, hip, oligo, prominent asymmetry	61	Overall figure 39	48	65.7	49.4; M 43, F 63.7*	Higher than textbook figures of 30 (19, 20)
Extra-articular features (%)						
◆ Enthesitis	Heel pain 24	NA	Heel pain 34.3, costochondral 10.8	Achilles tendonitis 24.3, costochondral 30, Achilles tendon 24.3, planter fasciitis 20, tibial tuberosity 14.3	34 (chest and scapular region 20.2, heel, planter fascia, iliac crest, ischium, feet 13.6)*	Similar to generally acceptable textbook figures of 30–50 (19)

(*continued*)

Table 30.1 Continued

Variables studied	Delhi (northern India), 1984, *n* = 51 (13), using Rome criteria	Mumbai (western India), 1989, *n* = 82 (15), using mNY criteria (14)	Chennai (southern India), 1990, *n* = 102 (18), using mNY criteria (14)	Delhi, 2009, *n* = 70 (24, 25), using mNY criteria (14)	Delhi, 2014 (26–28), *n* = 347 using ASAS 2009 criteria (23)	Remarks
◆ Anterior uveitis/ iridocyclitis	22	1.12	13.7	25.7	11.3; M 11, F 12.3*	Similar to generally acceptable textbook figures of 30–40 (19)
◆ Urethritis/ mucositis	18	NA	NA	NA	2.6; M 3, F 1.4*	–
◆ Dactylitis	NA	NA	NA	NA	0.3; M 0.4, F 0*	–
◆ Tendinitis	NA	NA	NA	NA	0.3; M 0.44, F 0*	–
◆ Apical pulmonary fibrosis	4	NA	4.9	NA	NA	–
◆ Aortic incompetence	4	NA	7.8	NA	NA	–
HLA-B27 (%)	94	79.4, M 78, F 89	86.7	92.9	92.6*	Similar to 90% mentioned by Khan (2)
History of smoking (%)	NA	NA	NA	NA	17.34 current smokers (M 58 (16.76), F 2 (0.58)), difference highly significant (*p* < 0.001); 5 (1.44) ex-smokers	Much lower than reports from developed countries (see Table 30.3)
Family history	NA	34	NA	52.9	68; M 67, F 71*	Higher than earlier reports; could be because of increasing awareness
Overweight/obesity (%)	NA	NA	NA	NA	75; overweight 20, obese 55*	Similar to that reported by Durcan et al. (134) (see Table 30.3)
Radiographic sacroiliitis (%)	51 (100 by selection criteria)	100 (by selection criteria)	78.4#	87.1#	64.8; M:F 71.2 vs 48.3, significant difference (*p* = 0.016)	
ESR (%)	–	–	–	51.45 ± 28.9	High 61.8; M 59.3, F 70.2*	Similar to textbook figures of 60 (19)
CRP (%)	NA	NA	NA	NA	65.7; M 64.8, F 69.2*	Similar to textbook figures of 60 (19)

#These figures could be inaccurate because in these studies mNY criteria were used for patient selection, according to which 100% of the selected patients should have had radiographic sacroiliitis.

*Statistically no difference between genders.

NA, Not available; IQR, interquartile range.

Reports in the 1990s

In 1990, workers from Chennai reported 102 patients with AS classified with mNY criteria (18). Age at onset, gender distribution, clinical features at disease onset, clinical characteristics of the disease—including subjective and objective manifestations of axial involvement, peripheral disease, and EAMs—HLA-B27 status, and radiographic sacroiliitis are summarized in Table 30.1. Most of the observed features were similar to the common characteristics of AS in general, except for the high male:female ratio of 16:1 as against the commonly cited figure of 2:1 (19) and a high proportion of patients with typical predominantly asymmetrical lower limb peripheral arthritis (48% as against 30–35%) (19, 20). Radiographic sacroiliitis was reported only in 78% of the patients.

The same group of workers reported on another 177 AS patients classified with mNY criteria in 1994, with comparable results (21). In this paper, the mean age was 26.4 years, with a male:female ratio that was even higher (18.7:1) than the previous report of 16:1. Moreover, 12.4% of patients were juveniles. Reported clinical features included IBP in 45%, peripheral arthritis of SpA pattern (lower extremity asymmetrical affecting large joints) in 42%, positive Schober's test in 80.2%, SI joint tenderness in 69%, heel enthesitis in 23%, anterior uveitis in 21%, and positive HLA-B27 in 86.7% of patients.

In 1995, a study from our group included only HLA-B27-positive uSpA patients and compared the clinical and radiographic features in 39 males and 25 females (22). The study could be of relevance because 92% of females and 74% of males were reported to have IBP. Radiographic sacroiliitis was present in 56% of females and 74% of males. In retrospect, such males and females may have had true AS, according to mNY criteria. This study also reported longer delay in diagnosis among females (8 years vs 2 years in males) that was statistically significant. Peripheral arthritis was present in approximately 70%, with no significant difference between genders. Family history was reported in 48% of males, as against 15% of females, which was, however, statistically not significant.

Recent reports: before and after publication of 2009 ASAS classification criteria

In 2009, our group restudied the clinical features of AS and reasons for the delay in diagnosis (24, 25). mNY classification criteria were used in these two studies. The salient findings are summarized in Table 30.1. In the absence of any report on axSpA using 2009 ASAS criteria, in 2014 we restudied 288 patients classifiable as axSpA using ASAS criteria (23). The results were presented recently (26–28) and are also summarized in Table 30.1.

Among these 288 patients, 187 had AS (mNY criteria). Another 101 patients not classifiable with mNY criteria were classified as having nr-axSpA, using ASAS criteria. Thus a larger number of patients were included in the axSpA category. Also, the male:female ratio was only 3.75:1, which was much less than the earlier reports using mNY criteria. Baseline disease activity, functional status, and spinal damage among patients were as follows: BASDAI, ASDAS, BASFI, and BASMI were 3.5, 2.86, 2.63, and 2, respectively. Enthesitis as a presenting symptom was seen in 5% of patients, exclusively among males. However, overall history of enthesitis was present in 34%, which is similar to commonly cited figures (19). An important observation of this study was the chest enthesitis that was seen in 20% of patients. In the past, this often led to unnecessary investigations to decipher the cause of chest pain. In a small number of patients, the initial symptoms were with root joints, extra-articular involvement, or non-specific symptoms.

Another important observation in the Indian studies was the much higher peripheral joint involvement (Tables 30.1 and 30.2). AAU is reported to be the most frequent extra-articular feature, seen in 25–30% of patients (29), not dissimilar to the usual figures of 30–40% (19). As can be seen in Table 30.1, two series from India have reported similar figures, but three others, including our 2014 series, have reported much lower figures, the reason for which is not obvious. High ESR and CRP were seen in 62% and 66% of patients, respectively, which is within the internationally cited range of 50–70% (19, 29). Table 30.2 gives the salient features of Indian studies until 2009 (using Rome or mNY criteria) and the 2014 study of axSpA using ASAS classification criteria of 2009. Additional features are also summarized in Tables 30.1 and 30.2.

Comparison of patients with ankylosing spondylitis (mNY criteria) and non-radiographic axial spondyloarthritis (ASAS criteria)

Two recent publications from our group in New Delhi compared patients with AS (mNY criteria) and nr-axSpA (ASAS criteria) (30, 31). In these studies several differences were noted between these two groups of patients. These included significantly longer disease duration, onset more often with axial and SI joint symptoms, more males, predominantly axial involvement, higher BASMI scores, and more syndesmophytes among the AS patients. In other parameters including age of onset, delay in diagnosis, and BASDAI, BASFI, ASDAS, MASES, ESR, CRP, and HLA-B27 status, there was no statistically significant difference between these two groups. These results showed that AS patients (mNY criteria) reveal several features that are distinct from nr-axSpa (ASAS criteria). This issue has been discussed recently and needs resolution (32).

Uncommon complications of axial spondyloarthritis

In a paper published in 2007 from a northern Indian city, 7% of AS patients with disease duration longer than 5 years were found to have subclinical amyloidosis by abdominal subcutaneous fat-pad aspiration (33). Renal involvement in SpA has also been reported by our group from India (34). The study included 23 patients with AS, 16 with Reiter's disease, ten with uSpA, and one with features of SpA overlapping with RA. All patients were HLA-B27 positive. Nine (4.5%) had significant persistent proteinuria. Renal biopsy in seven of them revealed proliferative glomerulonephritis. Immunofluorescence studies revealed immune-complex deposition in only three of them, but circulating immune complexes were present in five of seven patients with proteinuria. However, serum complement levels (C3 and C4) were normal in these patients, and antinuclear antibody was negative by immunofluorescence.

Other diseases of the spondyloarthritis family

Psoriatic arthritis

PsA is a common form of arthritis seen in rheumatology clinics in India. In a prospective study on 18,924 patients seen in a dermatology department in Delhi, 530 (2.8%) were diagnosed with psoriasis, of whom 290 (55%) had joint symptoms: arthralgia only in 48 (9%), seven (1.3%) had a deforming variety of arthritis, and one (0.2%) had bilateral sacroiliitis (35). The first publication on PsA from India was by our group in 1984 (36). The paper described 20 patients with PsA, their clinical features, and HLA-B27 status. Since then, additional studies from India have been published. The results are summarized in Table 30.3. Generally, the clinical profile conformed to what is reported in the literature.

In 2003, Rajendran et al. from Chennai described radiographic findings among 116 patients with PsA (37). Thirteen (11.2%) had bilateral involvement. In the lumbar spine, non-marginal syndesmophytes were noted in six patients (5.2%) and squaring of the vertebrae in one patient (0.86%). Of the six patients with joint

Table 30.2 Notable differences in AS/axSpA reported from India compared to the usually acceptable standard textbook features

Variables studied	Observation	Comments
Gender ratio—M:F	Fell from a high of 16:1 and 18:1 (18, 21) to 7:1 (15), 5.1:1 in (24), and 3.75:1 in 2014 (26)	Cause could be increasing awareness of relatively subtle and atypical clinical features and less severe disease among females (135). An older paper also mentions M:F ratio of 10:1 that fell to 5:1 over time (136). Presently, the accepted textbook figure on M:F ratio is 2:1 (19)
Delay in diagnosis with delayed presentation to rheumatologist	6.9 (± 5.2) years in 2009 (24), 5.9 (± 5.9) in 2014 (26)	Similar to accepted figures of 5–6 years (2, 137). Incorrect diagnosis (e.g. non-specific back pain (35.1%), degenerative disc disease (25.9%), RA (20.37%), and TB of spine (16.6%) in that order) was the main cause. Absence of EAMs and juvenile age add to the delay that resulted in significantly worse BASDAI, BASFI, and BASMI at presentation. Incorrect diagnoses were made by non-rheumatologists who are the primary caregivers to patients with back pain in India (86% by orthopaedicians; 14% by general physicians, physicians of other specialties, and practitioners of alternative systems of medicine) (96). Improvement over time has been discussed in several earlier studies (133, 138–140)
Peripheral arthritis	Reported in 39–65% of patients in different series from India	Much higher than 22% in a recent study (141) and the textbook figure of 30% (19). It is possible that environmental factors could be playing a role; many of our patients could have had trivial post-infectious ReA that was forgotten over time. In this context it is interesting to note that a study from Korea reported a frequency of 70% AS patients having peripheral joint involvement (19)
Smokers and tobacco users	17.34% current smokers (58 males (16.76%) and 2 females (0.58%); the difference was highly significant ($p < 0.001$); 5 (1.44%) ex-smokers	Smoking is much less prevalent among Indian SpA patients compared to a European country (57% in Turkey) (142). It is the single most important risk factor for developing more severe disease that worsens damage and increases cardiovascular disease risk (143–145). This could be one of the reasons for the milder form of disease among females (19, 135, 136)
Overweight and obesity	Obesity was estimated using body mass index with cut-off values for overweight and obesity as recommended for Indians (146). No difference was observed between genders. More than 65% of axSpA patients were overweight or obese (20% and 55.4%, respectively)	These findings were similar to that reported by Durcan et al., who observed increased disease burden and poor perceptions regarding benefits of exercise among overweight or obese patients (134). This could also be true among Indian patients and could be the main hurdle against doing regular exercise and efforts to lose weight
Sacroiliitis on imaging	Radiographic in 64.8% of patients on MRI, 35.2% (nr); 71.2% in males, 48.3% in females ($p = 0.016$)	Similar to reports in the literature that radiographic sacroiliitis is seen significantly more among males than females (147). Yet the inflammatory burden of disease (ASDAS, BASDAI) was comparable (147). This finding has therapeutic implications; patients not classifiable with mNY criteria but only with ASAS criteria would still be entitled to similar appropriate treatment (including biologics)

Details of the different studies from India are given in Table 30.1.

Studies until 2009 used Rome or mNY criteria. The 2014 study used ASAS classification criteria for axSpA.

EAM = extra-articular manifestations.

erosions (5.2%), five had erosions in the PIP/DIP of their hands and one in the MTP of the foot. In four patients, Achilles tendon calcification (3.5%) was observed. One patient had 'pencil-in-cup' deformity (0.86%). The mean duration for the peripheral joint erosions to occur in their patients was 34.2 months.

A study on PsA from Mumbai reported ESR of >20 in 60/85 (70.5%) and >100 in 9/85 (10.5%), Hb <10 in 10/96 (10.4%), serum uric acid >6.5 in 6/42 (14.2%), and rheumatoid factor (RF) in 6/41 (14.6%) (38). Radiography was not reported. Roussou et al. reported on PsA in three ethnic groups living in northeast London, including South Asians (39). They found elevated ESR (average 20.5 ± 17.6) among Asian females (23.9%), which was not significantly different from other races. In their series of 116 patients with PsA, Rajendran et al. (37) reported elevated ESR and CRP in 51.7% and 43.9% (>0.6 mg/dL) of patients, respectively. RF was positive in 3.4% and antinuclear antibody (ANA) was present in 5.4% (3/56) of patients. In another study from southern India on 141 patients with PsA classified according to CASPAR criteria (40), SpA was present in 29 (20.6%) (41). This is in contrast to earlier reports of 12.1% and 11.2% with SpA described above (36, 37, 42). However, it is to be noted that while the earlier papers used Moll and Wright criteria for PsA (6), the paper by Mithun et al. (41) used CASPAR criteria (40).

Reiter's disease

In 1983, our group published findings on 36 patients with Reiter's syndrome (43). Male:female ratio was 4:1. The mean duration at presentation in males and females was 5.5 and 6.5 years, respectively. The mean age of onset was 24 and 28 years in males and females, respectively. Clinical manifestations included IBP in 69%, mono- or oligoarthritis mainly affecting large joints in lower extremities with significant asymmetry in 83%, non-specific urethritis in 53%, heel enthesitis in 44%, radiographic sacroiliitis in 42%, conjunctivitis in 39%, dysentery in 33%, mucosal ulcerations in 17%, renal disease in 14%, anterior uveitis in 19%, and keratoderma blenorrhagicum in 8%.

IBD-associated arthritis

Studies available on IBD-associated arthritis are few and poorly detailed. The Indian Society of Gastroenterology (ISG) Task Force

Table 30.3 Demography, clinical characteristics, and HLA-B27 status in PsA

Variables studied	Delhi, 1984, *n* = 20 (36)	Mumbai, 1995, *n* = 102 (38)	Chennai, 2003, *n* = 116 (37)	Faridabad, 1995, *n* = 55 (35)
Male:female ratio	1.85:1	1.83:1	2:1	2.4:1
Mean age of onset of psoriasis (years)	NA	M 33, F 28	NA	NA, 95% < 50
Mean age of onset of arthritis (years)	NA, range 16–60	38	41 (range 10–65)	NA
Median interval between onset of psoriasis and arthritis (years)	NA	2.5	2.8	NA
Psoriasis onset antedated arthritis	12 (60%)	64 (63.8%)	58 (50.8%)	NA
Psoriasis and arthritis onset concomitantly	NA	20 (19.7%)	43 (37.1%)	NA
Arthritis antedated psoriasis	40%	5.8%	12.1%	NA
Psoriasis not observed	NA	12 (11.6%)	–	0%
Polyarticular arthritis	6 (30%; 1 was seropositive RA overlap)	26 (25.4%)	48.3%	54 (98%)
Mono-/oligoarticular enthesopathic spondyloarthritis	5 (25%); HLA-B27 positive in 3 (60%)	51 (50%); HLA status not reported	48.3%	1 (1.8%)
Mutilans variety	1 (5%); HLA-B27 positive	1 (0.98%); HLA status not reported	0.86%	7 (12.7%)
DIP only	2 (40%)	1 (0.98%)	2.6%	1 (1.8%)
Joints affected	Limited details available	Limited details available	NA	Limited details available
Spine–sacroiliac	5 (25%)	26 (25.5%)	NA	1 (1.8%)
Knee	NA	Among the commonest	66.4%	NA
Ankle	NA	Among the commonest	50%	NA
Hip	NA	NA	5.2%	NA
Foot	NA	NA	Toes 33.6%, MTP 19.8%	NA
Shoulder	NA	NA	25.9%	NA
Elbow	NA	NA	30.2%	NA
Finger joints	NA	Among the commonest	MCP 52.6%, PIP 34.5%	NA
Wrist	NA	NA	35.3%	NA
DIPs only	2 (10%)	1 (0.98%)	32.8%	1 (1.8%)
Mutilans variety	3 (15%)	2 (1.96%)	0.86%	7 (12.7%)
Sausage digits	NA	30 (29.4%)	16%	Nil

NA, Not available; PIP, proximal interphalangeal joint; DIP, distal interphalangeal joint; MTP, metatarsophalangeal joint.

reported on the clinical spectrum of IBD recently (44). The survey comprised data on 745 (64.3%) patients with ulcerative colitis (UC), 409 (35.3%) with Crohn's disease (CD), and five with indeterminate colitis. Arthralgia/arthritis was reported in 33% of UC and 26% of CD patients. Back pain was present in 31% and 36% of UC and CD patients, respectively. Kochhar et al. from Chandigarh in northern India reported a series of 150 patients with UC (79 males, 71 females, age 13–78 years) (45). Peripheral arthritis was seen in 16 (10.7%) patients and sacroiliitis was seen in 21 (14%). There was no relationship between the severity of sacroiliitis and extent of colitis. Rheumatic symptoms were more common in males (15:6). In this series, 12 (8%) patients had ocular complaints—anterior uveitis (five patients), conjunctivitis (four patients), and episcleritis (three patients). Uveitis occurred mostly in female patients (4/5) and was coincident with exacerbations of colitis in all instances. Mucocutaneous manifestations occurred in four patients—pyoderma gangrenosum in two and oral aphthous ulcers in two. Extraintestinal features of UC were, in general, similar to those reported from the west. Pokharna et al. from Bikaner (northwestern India) reported on 46 patients with UC (46). They found peripheral arthritis in one patient and anterior uveitis in two patients. No patient had sacroiliitis, vascular, mucocutaneous, or hepatobiliary manifestations.

Danda et al. from Vellore (southern India) looked for biopsy-proven CD and its predictors in suspected cases of enteropathic arthritis (47). All 29 patients underwent ileocolonoscopy and colonic biopsies. Fourteen out of the 29 patients on whom studies were done had histologically confirmed CD. Those with CD were younger (34.7 vs 41.6 years, $p = 0.057$), had history of weight loss more often (12 vs 1), fever (11 vs 0), perianal fistula (4 vs 0), abdominal pain (8 vs 2), history of dysentery (4 vs 0), and uveitis

(6 vs 1). However, logistic regression analysis showed loss of weight as the only independent predictor of CD in this subset of patients.

Solitary rectal ulcer syndrome

Tandon et al., from New Delhi, prospectively studied 22 patients with solitary rectal ulcer (48). In 15 of these patients, a single rectal ulcer was found, whereas seven patients had two ulcers each. Nineteen of these 29 ulcers were located on the anterior or anterolateral wall of the rectum. Histological features of the solitary rectal ulcer comprised fibrous obliteration of the lamina propria with disorientation of the muscularis mucosa and extension of muscle fibres into the lamina propria. Evident rectal prolapse was present in only three patients. Four patients had recurrent oral ulcerations and one had erythema nodosum. Radiographic sacroiliitis was present in six of 19 (31%) patients and HLA-B27 occurred in four of the 20 (20%) tested for HLA class I antigens. All four HLA-B27-positive patients had associated sacroiliitis and showed good response to sulfasalazine (SSZ). These associations raise the possibility that solitary rectal ulcers may be a part of a systemic disease or of several diseases with varied aetiology.

Acute anterior uveitis

In AS/SpA-associated uveitis in Asian Indian patients, the most frequent HLA phenotype was A9-B27, unlike the A2-B27 observed among American whites and blacks (49). A more recent study on AS/SpA-related uveitis in Asian Indians reported increased frequency of B*27:04-positive AS patients compared with B*27:05-positive patients, while B*27:02 was rare and observed only in AAU (50, 51). Another paper reported on 89 patients with uveitis (80 with AAU), out of which 56.3% were HLA-B27 positive (52). This figure was much less than the 64.3% reported earlier from Chandigarh (53).

Epidemiology of spondyloarthritis in India

AxSpA/AS

There are only a handful of epidemiological reports on SpA and AS from India. There are two reports on the prevalence of AS from India, both from the western region (Maharashtra), describing the prevalence of AS as approximately 7 and 9 per 10 000 population, respectively (54, 55). A large hospital-based study from southern India reported 0.6% patients having AS; 87% were HLA-B27 positive (21). Some of the hospital-based studies from India have reported uSpA to be the commonest subset (5, 17). Such patients could be a forme-fruste of ReA triggered by a wide array of gut and genitourinary infections (56). However, these studies were carried out prior to the publication of ASAS classification criteria for axial and peripheral SpA (23, 57). Therefore these conclusions may not reflect the actual status in the community.

Juvenile spondyloarthritis and enthesitis-related arthritis

Literature on JoSpA and ERA from India is scant. There are two publications that deal with the aetiopathogenesis, clinical features, and articular damage related to this disease (58, 59), but none on epidemiology. Despite the lack of epidemiological studies on JIA, most paediatric rheumatologists from India have noted the fact that within the broad category of JIA, ERA is the commonest among Indian patients, which is in contrast to reports from the West, where oligoarthritis is the commonest subset of JIA (60). In India, both at the community level from the state of Maharashtra (west India), as reported by Kunjir et al., and from a hospital setting in Delhi, ERA is the commonest category, representing 36–40% of all JIA patients (58, 61). Earlier reports from India classified patients with juvenile arthritis as per the American Rheumatism Association (ARA) criteria, which did not distinguish SpA subtypes. In the previous systems, most ERA patients were classified as 'pauciarticular type II', which was reported to be 30–47% (62, 63).

Immunological and immunopathological studies

In our early studies, only a few simple immunological parameters were reported (64). Thus high IgG levels were observed among SpA patients and high IgA levels were seen among patients with ReA. Serum complement C3 and autoantibodies were normal or not detected among SpA patients, but high levels of circulating immune complexes were found. An unusual SpA case with undetectable IgM and IgA was also reported (65). More recent studies from India have shown presence of lipoproteins related to *Escherichia coli*, *Klebsiella*, and *Salmonella typhi* among AS and ReA patients (66). In another study using PCR technique, *Salmonella*-genus-specific DNA was detected in synovial fluid of three acute post-dysenteric ReA patients (67). In another study, nine novel peptides having similarities with outer membrane proteins from arthritogenic bacteria were identified that bound to HLA-B*27.05 (68).

Studies on ERA have reported antigen-specific lymphoproliferative responses against enteric bacteria (69). The same group also showed innate immune-gene dysregulation involvement in antigen presentation, scavenger function, and chemotaxis (70.). It has been postulated that endogenous ligands may activate TLRs, causing persistence of the disease even in the absence of infection. Rahman et al. (71) from the same institution studied ERA patients for a calcium-binding protein complex of myeloid-related proteins (MRPs) 8 (S100A8) and 14 (S100A9), expressed by several cells involved in inflammation (granulocytes, monocytes, activated macrophages). These are endogenous ligands for TLR4. Their study showed an increase of these proteins in the plasma of ERA patients that was even higher in those with active disease. The same workers also showed that there were no specific polymorphisms in TLR2 and TLR4 among these patients (72). Upregulation of TLRs and their adaptors (probably in response to microbial inducers) has been reported by the same group, which could lead to uncontrolled inflammation and tissue injury (73). The same group also described stimulation of TLRs on binding with their ligands, leading to increased release in proinflammatory cytokines and MMPs by fibroblast-like synoviocytes derived from the synovial fluid of children with ERA (74). They have also reported that in patients with ERA, peripheral blood Th1, Th2, Th17, and Treg cells were unchanged, but Th1 and Th17 cells were increased and Th2 cells were reduced in synovial fluid compared with blood (75).

Recent studies on HLA-B27

Genetic studies in SpA

As discussed in the section 'HLA status in earlier studies', the first paper from India describing the frequency of HLA-B27 in AS patients was published from Chandigarh in 1977 (16), and reported the frequency of HLA-B27 to be 94% and 3%, respectively, in patients and controls. Two years later, our group reported on HLA-B27 in patients with SpA and found 90% positivity (4). In another paper, our group from Delhi reported on HLA-B27 in 29 patients consisting of different subsets of SpA and 118 normal controls (8). HLA-B27 was positive in 84% of patients but only 5.9% of controls. In 1984, our group studied HLA-B27 in 51 AS patients and 118 normal controls (13). Ninety-four percent of patients compared to 6% controls were HLA-B27 positive.

Disease associations with HLA-B27 subtypes

Studies carried out in India have reported a strong association of AS/SpA with HLA-B27 subtypes (4, 8, 16). As mentioned in the section 'Early reports (late 1970s–1980s)', in 1983 we reported HLA-B27 in 84% of uSpA patients and also a higher RR of some other antigens, including A11, Aw30, A28, Bw63, Bw41, B37, and Bw35 (8). Initial studies on SpA also revealed an association of B*27:05 and B*27:04 with AS, while B*27:07 was observed in northern Indian AS patients with a frequency similar to that in healthy controls (50). On the other hand, B*27:02 was rare and observed only in patients with AAU (50). These observations were further confirmed in a larger disease cohort, suggesting an association of B*27:05 with uSpA and of B*27:04 primarily with AS (51). Studies conducted in Mumbai (western India) reported an association of B*27:05, B*2704, B*27:14, B*27:07, and B*27:02 with AS, while B*27:08 was observed more frequently among patients with haemophilia with chronic synovitis (76, 77). Among southern Indian AS patients, predominant association was observed with B*27:05 and B*27:04, and no other subtypes were observed in this cohort (78). Another study on AS patients living in the Mumbai region has confirmed a strong association of B*27:05 with AS, along with other subtypes including B*27:04, B*27:07, and B*27:02 (79). Thus, in summary, the most AS-associated B27 subtypes in Asian Indians are B*27:05, B*27:02, B*27:04, and B*27:07.

These findings may be compared with HLA-B27 association with AS/SpA in other populations. Thus the most commonly observed association is with B*27:05, B*27:02, B*27:04, and B*27:07. Additionally, several other subtypes that include B*27:01, B*27:03, B*27:08, B*27:10, B*27:13, B*27:14, B*27:15, B*27:19, B*27:23, B*27:24, B*27:25, and B*27:49 have been reported to occur among patients, even if one case only (80, 81).

MHC loci other than HLA-B27

Our studies revealed that MHC loci other than HLA-B27 also govern susceptibility to AS. For example, while HLA-A2 and HLA-B27 together were elevated in AS and uSpA, those with Reiter's syndrome showed a decreased frequency of B35 and B27 (82). Another study evaluating MHC haplotypes including human MHC class I chain related (MIC) genes and TNF polymorphisms in AS patients (Indians, Caucasians, and Africans) revealed that B27 alone rather than B27-related class I haplotypes contributed to AS susceptibility. Further interesting observations were seen when MICA was evaluated together with the B27 gene as MIC-B27 haplotypes, for example MICA-A4 with B*2705,02,03 and 08; MICA-A5 with B*2704 and B*2707; and MICA-A.5.1 with B*2706 (83). Among SpA patients from southern India, significant association has been reported with an extended six locus haplotype B*2705-Cw*02-STR-MICA (A4)-C1_4_1 (213 bp)-C1_2_5 (178 bp)-MIB (340 bp) (78). In this study, a significant association of HLA-B27 and Cw*02 with SpA was also reported, but B*44 revealed a negative association. Studies on B7 CREG alleles in patients from the Mumbai region reported significantly increased frequencies of HLA-B7 and HLA-B-40 alleles in HLA-B27-negative patients when compared to the HLA-B27-positive group (84).

AS/SpA-associated uveitis

In AS/SpA-associated uveitis in Asian Indian patients, the most frequent HLA phenotype was A9-B27, unlike the A2-B27 observed among American whites and blacks (49). A more recent study on AS-related uveitis in Asian Indians reported an increased frequency of B*27:04-positive AS patients than B*27:05-positive patients, while B*27:02 was rare and observed only in AAU (50, 51). Another paper reported on 89 patients with endogenous uveitis (80 with AAU), of whom 56.3% were HLA-B27 positive (52). This figure was much less than the 64.3% reported earlier from Chandigarh (53).

Genetic studies in PsA

Prevalence of HLA-B27 in PsA has been reported to be 11.3% in Indians (41). This was lower than 19–30% reported from other regions of the world (85–88). Prevalence was much less than that in AS (> 90%) (89). Studies from other countries have reported an association between palmoplantar pustulosis and HLA-B27 positivity (90, 91). However, Mithun et al. found no such association (41). Extra-articular features were less prevalent (41). Apart from HLA-B27, which has a significantly higher prevalence in PsA, association with HLA-B38, B-8, and C-6 was observed by Canadian workers (85).

Genetic studies in uSpA

One of the earliest studies from India reported HLA-B27 in 84% of cases of uSpA, and the RR of some other antigens, including A11, Aw30, A28, Bw63, Bw41, B37, and Bw35, was also higher (8).

Disease associations with HLA-B27 subtypes

Prevalence of HLA-B27 in PsA has been reported as 11.3% in Indians as against 30% in Caucasians (53). Apart from HLA-B27, which has a significantly higher prevalence in PsA, association with HLA-B38, B-8, and C-6 has been observed in other populations (85). In a paper on JoSpA from Varanasi (northern India), urinary tract infection, diarrhoea, and constipation were more common in HLA-B27-positive cases (92). In a report from Mumbai, HLA-B27 alleles were characterized in a sample population of 51 persons (93). B*2704, B*2705, B*2707, B*2708, and B*2714 alleles were detected, and two novel B27 alleles, B*2708 and B*2714, were found in this Indian population. In addition, B*2714 was observed in a patient with AS. This association was not previously reported in ethnic groups from India. In another study, workers from northern India looked for additional genetic factors in AS, because HLA-B27's contribution to disease susceptibility is only 15% (94). They studied IL-1R antagonist polymorphism in Indian patients with AS. This large study concluded that the IL-1RN*2 allele is a susceptibility marker for AS in the Indian population, but it does not influence disease phenotype.

Management of axSpA

Management of axSpA in India is unsatisfactory and the main reason would appear to be that, by-and-large, rheumatology has been a neglected subject in medical school curricula (95, 96). The issues related to delayed diagnosis by primary care providers, delayed referral to specialists, incorrect past diagnoses, and inappropriate prior drug use have been highlighted in our 2009 and 2014 studies. The consequences of this neglect are discussed in the next section.

Primary care providers, specialist referrals, and delayed diagnoses

Traditionally, patients with musculoskeletal aches and pain in India seek help from orthopaedists or practitioners of alternative medicine, and often from several of them. 'Doctor shopping' for musculoskeletal ailments is widespread. This is mainly due to little awareness about rheumatology in the community (95, 96). Thus the patients in our 2014 study had been under the care of orthopaedists (86.2%), ayurvedic practitioners (27.2%), homeopaths (24.3%), internists (20.8%), neurologists (11.2%), yogasana therapists (8.65%), GPs (8%), physiotherapists (1.9%), gastroenterologists, dermatologists, and practitioners of Unani medicine (all approximately 0.5%), and others (e.g. home remedies, reiki, massage, and bone setters/manipulators called *pehalwans*) (14%). More recently, rheumatologists had also been consulted by one-third of the patients.

These figures show that the majority of orthopaedists do not refer SpA patients to rheumatologists. They also revealed a range of prior diagnoses these patients received, which were as follows: non-specific back pain or 'some arthritis' 50%; prolapsed intervertebral disc 7%; TB of spine 5% (in our 2009 report this figure was even higher, at 8.5% (25); others (RA, gout, rheumatic fever, JIA, septic discitis, back sprain) 10%; while a large group remained without any diagnostic label. Some 50% of these patients after prolonged delay were ultimately diagnosed as having SpA.

The treatment received by these patients prior to the diagnosis of SpA also reflected the knowledge deficit among primary caregivers. In the absence of a proper referral system for patients to specialists and little awareness of rheumatology as a speciality, the patients reached a rheumatologist through a variety of channels, which included patients, friends, or relatives who knew a rheumatologist (24.4%); referral by an orthopaedician (13.8%) or doctors other than orthopaedicians (41.21%); internet search and self-referral (12.4%); and other means (conferences and newspapers, television programmes, clinical laboratories, allied health professionals, medical representatives, etc.) (approximately 3%). These factors appear to be the main cause of delay in diagnosis and institution of appropriate treatment among axSpA patients. In one recent publication by our group, the delay was more than 6 years (25). These observations indicated that the diagnosis of SpA was being missed by non-rheumatologists. Moreover, in the absence of an organized referral system for patients to reach specialists, they get treated by a variety of non-rheumatologists, as well as practitioners of alternative systems of care. Commonly, such patients seek orthopaedic consultation. However, unfortunately, orthopaedists (and other non-rheumatologist physicians) seem to miss the diagnosis, as a result of which such patients receive irrelevant, incorrect, or substandard treatment. DMARDs and NSAIDs, if used, are commonly prescribed in suboptimal doses.

Patient-centric and logistic issues

Patients in India with musculoskeletal problems are generally unsure of the type of caregiver they should consult. These patients end up referring to either orthopaedists or non-rheumatologists, simply because rheumatology is a new speciality and there are not enough trained rheumatologists. Also, there are widespread misconceptions and misbeliefs among patients with rheumatological conditions; for example, 'English medicines' (a term used for modern scientific medicines) have 'side-effects' and they do not 'cure' the ailment. Implied in that view is that ayurvedic medicines, homeopathy, and other alternative systems are free of side-effects and also they 'cure the disease permanently'!

In addition to this, there are difficulties of logistics. Since rheumatology services are available only in metropolitan centres and larger cities, most patients living in smaller towns and rural areas have to travel long distances to reach such centres or clinics. For poorer patients, travelling in the country is an ordeal because buses and trains are extremely crowded and there are absolutely no provisions and facilities for differently abled persons.

Financial issues

Affordability of modern medicines is a major issue in India. The reasons are easy to understand. India's per capita income is $1219 (i.e. $101 per month) (97). Approximately 25% of the nation's population earns less than the government-specified poverty threshold of $0.40 per day, and 27.5% of the population was living below the poverty line in 2004–2005 (98). The World Bank further estimated that 33% of the global poor population resides in India (2012). The Global Hunger Index (GHI) of the Food and Agriculture Organization of the United Nations stated that out of 842 million hungry people in 2011–2013, 210 million were in India (99). Less than 5% of the population has health insurance. The projection is that by 2015, this figure may go up to 5.5%, and this increase would be almost entirely among urban Indians (100). The third-party payer system is almost non-existent in India. It is obvious that the cost of drugs for the treatment of axSpA is a major constraint in disease management. These statistics clearly explain the reason why a majority of axSpA patients in India cannot be prescribed biologics. Patients simply cannot bear the cost, as there is hardly any arrangement for payment from government or private insurance.

Drug treatment

The drug treatment taken by axSpA patients prior to presentation has been studied by us (28). Patients had received various medications at different times. These included simple analgesics (76%); NSAIDs (16%) (the majority used them 'on demand' as pain killers; only 0.6% received continuous NSAIDs); and others (ayurvedic medicines, homeopathic medicines, vitamins, calcium, glucosamine-chondroitin, iron, nutraceuticals, acupressure, acupuncture, etc.) (49%). They had also received uric acid-lowering drugs (2.25%); anti-TB drugs (6.3%); antibiotics (7.5%); and procedures/interventions (joint drainage, arthroscopy, plastering) (1.5%). In a small number (less than 0.5%), back pain was considered to be due to osteoporosis and treated with anti-osteoporosis agents. Glucocorticoids (GCs) were taken orally off and on by 23%; intra-articular steroid preparations were received by 0.3%; GC was given parentally to 2%; and unsupervised self-medication with GC was taken by 0.3% patients. After receiving the diagnosis of SpA (by orthopaedists or other non-rheumatologists), these patients had received DMARDs that included SSZ (37.2%), MTX (22.4%), hydroxychloroquine (8%), LFN (2.56%), and biologics (0.32%); 38.1% of them had not received any DMARDs. When prescribed DMARDs, they received optimal doses in only 35% of cases.

Beyond this report, there is little reliable published information on how axSpA is treated in India. The Indian Rheumatology Association (IRA) appointed a nine-member committee to draft a consensus statement on the diagnosis and treatment of axSpA (101). In the absence of any credible data from India, the final statement was based upon EULAR and other recommendations and publications (102–104)), as well as on the experience of Indian rheumatologists and prevalent practices in the country. Since publication of the IRA consensus statement in 2010, the newer recommendations (105, 106) have been presented and discussed during several rheumatology continuing medical education (CME) courses and regional and national rheumatology meetings in different parts of the country, ensuring a regular update for Indian rheumatologists. This has ensured that rheumatologists in India follow standard recommended management procedures for SpA patients in the country as far as possible.

General measures

Physical therapy is a standard recommendation for SpA (104); it is recommended by most caregivers in India. However, there are problems in the optimal implementation of this therapeutic modality. First, there are only a few centres with a separate physiatry department. Also, there are only a few practising rheumatologists and rheumatology clinics with attached physiotherapists/occupational therapists to provide expert help and guidance to patients. More importantly, counsellors are not available in rheumatology set-ups to counsel patients about the importance of physiotherapy, exercise, and overall lifestyle changes (including smoking, obesity, and avoidance of metabolic syndrome, which is so prevalent in India). Rheumatology specialist nurses do help to some extent, but they are overburdened with providing information about the disease, explaining medicines, administering different therapies, and so on. Moreover, rheumatology specialist nurses are available only in a few centres in India.

There are additional problems, as most of the patients are young adults; they are busy in their studies or careers. Therefore, noncompliance with physical therapy and exercises is quite common. Most rheumatologists in India feel that the physical therapy aspect of the management of axSpA is not optimal.

Use of non-biologic agents

According to the recommendations by IRA consensus statement in 2010 discussed in the section 'Drug treatment', NSAIDs are recommended to be used as the cornerstone for the treatment of axSpA in India. 'Continuous' use of NSAIDs/coxibs (such as a disease-modifying drug) as against 'on-demand' use (like a pain killer), has been shown to not only suppress inflammation but also act in some circumstances as an anti-osteoproliferative measure (107, 108). Therefore ASAS/EULAR has recommended continuous treatment with NSAIDs/coxibs for patients with persistently active, symptomatic disease, taking into account cardiovascular, gastrointestinal, and renal risks (105).

Based upon this evidence and these recommendations, many rheumatologists, including one of the authors (ANM), prescribe NSAIDs to be taken continuously for at least 2 years and not as pain killers 'on demand'. As the majority of patients with axSpA are young adults with no background renal disease, the risk factors mentioned in the previous paragraph are generally non-issues. Such patients tolerate continuous NSAIDs/coxibs without problems. Regular monitoring for adverse effects is carried out in such patients. Most rheumatologists use an empirical approach for choosing these drugs, incorporating patient preference. However, etoricoxib has been shown to be highly effective in an RCT (109). Therefore this has become the drug of choice by most rheumatologists, unless the patient expresses a personal choice. Among patients with cardiovascular disease (CVD) issues (including family history of premature CVD) and for those relatively older, the cardio-neutral drug naproxen is preferred. Besides these, diclofenac, indomethacin, and a large number of other NSAIDs and coxibs available in the country are also used. As the original study on continuous use of etoricoxib was only for 2 years (107), the usual practice is to change the prescription to 'on-demand' use of NSAIDs/coxibs after 2 years. Also, most Indian rheumatologists would use at least two NSAIDs/coxibs sequentially before labelling the patient unresponsive to this class of drugs. It needs to be mentioned that there are probably an equal number of Indian rheumatologists, including one of the authors (AK), who would not be willing to take the risk of causing the adverse effects of NSAIDs/coxibs on kidney, cardiovascular, gastrointestinal, and other organs by continuous use of these drugs. They prefer prescribing this class of drugs only for 'on-demand' use.

There are several adjunct therapies widely used by rheumatologists for axSpA patients in India. Intra-articular depo-GCs (usually depot-triamcinolone acetonide) are very popular. With increasing use of musculoskeletal US, difficult joints (e.g. hip and SI joints) are now being injected quite regularly. Simple analgesics (e.g. paracetamol, tramadol) are also quite popular for pain control. Amitriptyline in small doses is often used as a muscle relaxant and for improved quality of sleep. Vitamin D supplementation and calcium are prescribed to most patients. Lifestyle modifications, including weight and blood-lipid control, smoking cessation, and regular exercise are being advised by most rheumatologists. Recommended vaccination coverage among SpA patients is also increasing gradually.

Disease-modifying antirheumatic drugs

Rheumatologists in India are generally aware of the recommendations for DMARD use only in peripheral SpA (102–105). Trials of commonly used DMARDs, including SSZ, low-dose methotrexate (LD-MTX), and leflunomide (LFN) in SpA have often been topics of discussion in the various rheumatology forums (110–114). Despite weak evidence, a large majority of axSpA patients in India are being prescribed SSZ, irrespective of whether they do or do not have peripheral arthritis. One of the authors (AK) is a strong believer that SSZ is effective in axSpA among Indian patients. In a recent in-depth evaluation of SSZ in SpA, Fagrli et al. have stated that it might have some role in its treatment (110). Original enthusiasm for LD-MTX in SpA (115, 116) has waned due to contradictory reports (117, 118). However, it is often used in difficult-to-treat peripheral disease. There is ongoing debate on the use of MTX with biologics to minimize the formation of anti-drug antibodies. LFN is often used in difficult peripheral arthritis and enthesitis, frequently in combination with LD-MTX.

Biologics

Indian rheumatologists generally follow the international recommendations for the use of biologics in axSpA (103, 106). Accordingly, patients who can be classified with mNY criteria or ASAS criteria for axSpA with active disease, usually with a BASDAI of ≥ 4, despite trial of full dose of at least two NSAIDs/coxibs given sequentially, are recommended anti-TNFα inhibitors. Infliximab, ETN, and 2 ETN-biosimilars are available in India. Golimumab was launched only in October 2014 but only for use in RA. Unfortunately, the high cost of these agents is a major stumbling block. As discussed in the section 'Financial issues', only a minority of patients have medical insurance or financial resources to afford these drugs; the majority have to pay from their own resources. In our own database, 182/347 (52.3%) patients were considered for biologics, but only 43 out of 347 (12.3%) could afford them, and that too only for a few doses; 139 (40%) could not take them due to financial constraints. Infliximab was preferred by 60% of those who took it. The additional issue is of flare-up of TB that was seen soon after biologics were introduced in India in 2000. Therefore a strategy for stringent screening for latent TB infection (LTBI) was worked out (119). A modified approach for LTBI screening has been followed since 2004 (120). Such screening has almost completely eliminated the problem of TB flare-ups among patients receiving TNFi.

Alternative management strategy for patients unable to afford biologics

Analysis of our own patients has revealed that approximately 50% of the patients merited treatment with biologics but could not afford them (see section 'Biologics'). Under the circumstances, some alternative to biologics had to be offered to such patients. This issue was also discussed by Braun and Seiper in 2002 (121). In this context, there were reports on the safety and efficacy of LD-MTX in axSpA (115, 116). Of course there were also some contradictory reports as well (117). Similarly, there were a few earlier reports on the safety and efficacy of SSZ in axSpA (122). Interestingly, there was a report from Japan that combination of LD-MTX and SSZ was superior to monotherapy (124). Also, there were several earlier reports on the efficacy of high-dose intravenous methylprednisolone (MP) pulse therapy in AS (125–129). Lastly, Maksymowych and colleagues have published reports of the efficacy of pamidronate in the treatment of refractory AS (130, 131).

Based upon this evidence, the author's (ANM's) group used a combination of these four therapeutic modalities in patients with inadequate response to NSAIDs/coxibs (132). The study included 46 patients with mNY criteria classifiable AS. Some 63% of the patients had high disease activity, with BASDAI ≥ 4 and ESR > 30 mm after the first hour. Besides the standard dose of MTX and 1 g BID SSZ, they were administered 'pulses' of 500 mg MP synchronized with 60 mg pamidronate. The first cycle consisted of 500 mg MP given intravenously on three consecutive days. The next 5-monthly cycles consisted only of 500 mg MP on two consecutive days synchronized with pamidronate 60 mg. These cycles were given for a total of 6 months. The results were very encouraging: 39 of the 46 patients achieved ASAS 20 and BASDAI-50 improvement (85%; 95% CI, range 71–94%). Seven (15.2%) patients did not achieve ASAS 20 or BASDAI-50 response. The total expense of 6 months' treatment was INR 40 000. The comparative expense in giving 6 months of infliximab to a person weighing 70 kg would be INR 408 000, which is approximately a ten-fold higher cost. With these encouraging early results, most patients who are unable to afford biologics are being treated with this regimen, with further modifications currently being evaluated.

Conclusion

The SpA group of conditions are among the most common inflammatory rheumatological disorders in India, and have been extensively reported over since the 1970s. Epidemiological studies have shown the prevalence of SpA to be 7–9 per 10 000 persons. The main observation related to management was minimal use of biologic agents due to the high cost. Sparse medical insurance coverage of the population and overall poverty are the main reasons. With the lack of access to biologics, alternative strategies with other agents are being evaluated. However, the situation may change soon because of a spurt in the availability of biosimilars from late 2014 onwards. This development has brought down the cost and may lead to an increased access to biologics in SpA.

References

1. Malaviya AN, Singh RR, Kapoor SK, Sharma A, Kumar A, Singh YN. Prevalence of rheumatic diseases in India: results of a population survey. J Ind Rheumatol Assoc 1994;2:13–17.
2. Khan MA. Update on spondyloarthropathies. Ann Intern Med 2002;136:896–907.
3. Malaviya AN, Sawhney S, Mehra NK, Kanga U. Seronegative arthritis in South Asia: an up-to-date review. Curr Rheum Rep 2014;16:413–26.
4. Malaviya AN, Mehra NK, Adhar GC, et al. HLA B27 in patients with seronegative spondarthritis. J Rheumatol 1979;6:413–16.
5. Malaviya AN, Mehra NK, Adhar GC, et al. The clinical spectrum of HLA-B27 related rheumatic diseases in India. J Assoc Physicians India 1979;27:487–92.
6. Moll JM, Haslock I, Macrae IF, Wright V. Associations between ankylosing spondylitis, psoriatic arthritis, Reiter's disease, the intestinal arthropathies, and Behcet's syndrome. Medicine (Baltimore) 1974;53:343–64.
7. Calin A, Porta J, Fries JF, Schurman DJ. Clinical history as a screening test for ankylosing spondylitis. JAMA 1977:237:2613–14.
8. Prakash S, Mehra NK, Bhargava S, Malaviya AN. HLA B27 related 'unclassifiable' seronegative spondyloarthropathies. Ann Rheum Dis 1983;42:640–3.
9. Kellgren JH, Jeffrey MR, Ball J. The Epidemiology of Chronic Rheumatism. Oxford, Blackwell, 1963, Vol 1, p. 326.
10. Amor B, Dougados M, Mijiyawa M. Criteres de classification des spondylarthropathies. Rev Rhum 1990;57:85–9.
11. Dougados M, van Der LS, Juhlin R, et al. The European Spondylarthropathy Study Group preliminary criteria for the classification of spondylarthropathy. Arthritis Rheum 1991;34:1218–27.
12. Borges NE, Desai HR, Joshi AD, Siqueira RD, Mangat G, Joshi VR. Unclassifiable seronegative spondyloarthritides. J Assoc Physicians India 1986;34:387 .
13. Prakash S, Mehra NK, Bhargava S, Vaidya MC, Malaviya AN. Ankylosing spondylitis in India. Ann Rheum Dis 1984;43:381–5.
14. Van der Linden SM, Valkenburg HA, Cats A. Evaluation of the diagnostic criteria for ankylosing spondylitis: a proposal for modification of the New York criteria. Arthritis Rheum 1984;27:361–8.
15. Mathew CM, Bhandarkar P, Siqueria RD, Boerges NE, Joshi VR. Ankylosing spondylitis in females—similarities and differences from male spondylitis. J Assoc Physicians India 1989;37: 334–6.
16. Sengupta S, Sehgal S, Aikat BK, Deodhar SD. HLA B27 in ankylosing spondylitis in India. Lancet 1977;309:1209–10.
17. Madhavan R, Chandrasekaran AN, Parthiban M, Achutan K, Porkodi R, Rajendran CP. HLA profile of seronegative spondyloarthropathies

in a referral hospital in South India. J Indian Rheumatol Assoc 1996;4-3:91–5.
18. Achuthan K, Porkodi R, Ramakrishnan S, et al. Pattern of rheumatic diseases in south India. V. Ankylosing spondylitis. A clinical and radiological study. J Assoc Physicians India 1990;38:774–6.
19. Sieper J. Ankylosing spondylitis. In: Watts RA, Conaghen PG, Denton C, Foster H, Isaacs J, Ladner UA (eds), Oxford Textbook of Rheumatology, 4th edn. Oxford, Oxford University Press, 2013, pp 879–89.
20. Paramarta JE, Baeten D. Spondyloarthritis: from unifying concepts to improved treatment. Rheumatology (Oxford) 2014;53(9):1547–59.
21. Chandrasekaran AN, Porkodi R, Achutan K, Madhavan R, Parthiban M. Spectrum of clinical and immunological features of systemic rheumatic disorders in a referral hospital in south India: primary ankylosing spondylitis. J Indian Rheumatol Assoc 1994;2-4:149–52.
22. Uppal SS, Pande I, Singh G, et al. Profile of HLA B27 related unclassifiable seronegative spondyloarthropathy in females and its comparison with the profile in males. Br J Rheumatol 1995;34:137–40.
23. Rudwaleit M, van der Heijde D, Landew R, et al. The development of Assessment of SpondyloArthritis international Society classification criteria for axial spondyloarthritis (part II): validation and final selection. Ann Rheum Dis 2009;68:777–83.
24. Aggarwal R, Malaviya AN. Clinical characteristics of patients with ankylosing spondylitis in India. Clin Rheumatol 2009;28:1199–205.
25. Aggarwal R, Malaviya AN. Diagnosis delay in patients with ankylosing spondylitis: factors and outcomes—an Indian perspective. Clin Rheumatol 2009;28:327–31.
26. Malaviya AN Rawat R, Gogia SB, Arya V. Axial-spondyloarthritis (ax-SpA) from single rheumatology clinic in New Delhi—I: demography, HLA B27 status, spinal indices, delay in diagnosis and classification. Indian J Rheumatol 2014;9(Suppl 1),S47–8.
27 Kalyani A, Malaviya A, Aggarwal V, Rawat R, Gogia S, Sharma P. Axial-spondyloarthritis (ax-SpA) from single rheumatology clinic in New Delhi—II: symptoms at onset, articular and extra-articular features, family history and acute phase reactants. Indian J Rheumatol 2014;9(Suppl 1),S49.
28. Malaviya A, Aggarwal V, Rawat R, Gogia S. Axial-spondyloarthritis (ax-SpA) from single rheumatology clinic in New Delhi—III: how did they find a rheumatologist (with whose reference), who were the prior care-givers, what was the diagnosis and what treatments were given. Indian J Rheumatol 2014;9(Suppl 1),S47.
29. Sieper J, Braun J, Rudwaleit M, Boonen A, Zink A. Ankylosing spondylitis: an overview. Ann Rheum Dis 2002;61(Suppl 3):iii8–18.
30. Malaviya AN, Kalyani A, Rawat R. Is radiographic axial SpA a distinct subset with more severe axial involvement? Comment on the article by Deodhar et al. Arthritis Rheumatol 2015;67:856.
31. Malaviya AN, Kalyani A, Rawat R, Gogia SB. Comparison of patients with ankylosing spondylitis (AS) and non-radiographic axial spondyloarthritis (nr-axSpA) from a single rheumatology clinic in New Delhi. Int J Rheum Dis 2015; 18(7):736–41.
32. Deodhar A, Reveille JD, van den Bosch F, et al. The concept of axial spondyloarthritis: joint statement of the Spondyloarthritis Research and Treatment Network and the Assessment of SpondyloArthritis international Society in response to the US Food and Drug Administration's comments and concerns. Arthritis Rheumatol 2014;66: 2649–56.
33. Singh G, Kumari N, Aggarwal A, Krishnani N, Misra R. Prevalence of subclinical amyloidosis in ankylosing spondylitis. J Rheumatol 2007;34:371–3.
34. Mittal VK, Malhotra KK, Bhuyan UN, Malaviya AN. Kidney involvement in seronegative spondarthritides. Indian J Med Res 1983;78:670–5.
35. Bedi TR. Clinical profile of psoriasis in north India. Indian J Dermatol Venereol Leprol 1995;61:202–5.
36. Malaviya AN, Dasgupta B, Tiwari SC, Khan KM, Pasricha JS, Mehra NK. Psoriatic arthritis: a clinical and immunological study in 20 cases from India. J Assoc Physicians India 1984;32:403–5.
37. Rajendran CP, Ledge SG, Rani KP, RadhaMadhavan R. Psoriatic arthritis. J Assoc Physicians India 2003;51:1065–8.
38. Shah NM, Mangat G, Balakrishnan C, Joshi VR. Psoriatic arthritis—a study of 102 patients. J Indian Rheumatol Assoc 1995;3:133–6.
39. Roussou E, Chopra S, Ngandu DL. Phenotypic and clinical differences between Caucasian and South Asian patients with psoriatic arthritis living in north east London. Clin Rheumatol 2013;32:591–9.
40. Helliwell PS, Porter G, Taylor WJ, CASPAR Study Group. Polyarticular psoriatic arthritis is more like oligoarticular psoriatic arthritis, than rheumatoid arthritis. Ann Rheum Dis 2007;66:113–17.
41. Mithun CB, Antony PT, Mariaselvam CM, Negi VS. Clinical and immunogenetic characteristics of psoriatic arthritis: a single-center experience from South India. J Rheumatol Clin Immunol 2013;1(1).
42. Singh YN, Verma KK, Kumar A, Malaviya AN. Methotrexate in psoriatic arthritis. J Assoc Physicians India 1994;42:860–2.
43. Prakash S, Mehra N, Bhargava S, Malaviya A. Reiter's disease in north India: a clinical and immunogenetic study. Rheumatol Int 1983;3:101–4.
44. Makharia GK, Balakrishnan S, Abraham R, et al. Survey of inflammatory bowel diseases in India. Indian J Gastroenterol 2012;31:299–306.
45. Kochhar R, Mehta SK, Nagi B, Bhatia V, Goenka MK, Malik AK. Extraintestinal manifestations of idiopathic ulcerative colitis. Indian J Gastroenterol 1991;10:88–9.
46. Pokharna RK, Kabra PK, Sharma R, Kochar DK. Extraintestinal manifestations of idiopathic ulcerative colitis in northwestern India. Indian J Gastroenterol 2004;23:89–90.
47. Danda D, Kurian G, Chacko A, et al. Crohn's disease in rheumatology clinic—an Indian experience. J Postgrad Med 2005;51:269–72.
48. Tandon RK, Atmakuri SP, Mehra NK, Malaviya AN, Tandon HD, Chopra P. Is solitary rectal ulcer a manifestation of a systemic disorder? J Clin Gastroenterol 1990;12:286–90.
49. Mehra NK, Khan MA, Vaidya MC, Malaviya AN, Batta RK. HLA antigens in acute anterior uveitis and spondylarthropathies in Asian Indians and their comparision to American whites and blacks. J Rheumatol 1983;10:981–4.
50. López-Larrea C, Sujirachato K, Mehra NK, et al. HLA-B27 subtypes in Asian patients with ankylosing spondylitis. Evidence for new associations. Tissue Antigens 1995;45:169–76.
51. Kanga U, Mehra NK, Larrea CL, Lardy NM, Kumar A, Feltkamp TE. Seronegative spondyloarthropathies and HLA-B27 subtypes: a study in Asian Indians. Clin Rheumatol 1996;15(Suppl 1):13–18.
52. Mishra MN, Bharucha KM. HLA-B27 Association with uveitis in an Asian Indian Population. Iran J Immunol 2011;8:85–9.
53. Sen Gupta S, Jain IS, Jain GC, Deodhar SD. HLA antigens in acute anterior uveitis in North Indians. Indian J Ophthalmol 1978;26:26–9.
54. Chopra A, Patil J, Billempelly V, et al. Prevalence of rheumatic diseases in a rural population in western India: a WHO-ILAR COPCORD study. J Assoc Physicians India 2001;49:240–6.
55. Joshi VL, Chopra A. Is there an urban-rural divide? Population surveys of rheumatic musculoskeletal disorders in the Pune region of India using the COPCORD Bhigwan model. J Rheumatol 2009;36:614–22.
56. Aggarwal A, Misra R, Chandrasekara S, Prasad KN, Dayal R, Ayyagiri A. Is undifferentiated seronegative spondyloarthropathy a forme frusta of reactive arthritis? Br J Rheumatol 1997;36:1001–4.
57. Rudwaleit M, van der Heijde D, Landew R, et al. The Assessment of SpondyloArthritis international Society classification criteria for peripheral spondyloarthritis and for spondyloarthritis in general. Ann Rheum Dis 2011;70:25–31.
58. Sawhney S. Spectrum of Juvenile idiopathic arthritis in a tertiary level centre in India. Indian J Rheumatol 2006;14:3–6.
59. Agarwal M, JariwalaM, Prakash R, Sawhney S. 110 Patients with enthesitis related arthritis: a demographic and clinical study from a tertiary level pediatric rheumatology centre In India. Ann Rheum Dis 2012;71(Suppl 3):264.
60. Espinosa M, Gottlieb BS. Juvenile idiopathic arthritis. Pediatr Rev 2012;33:303–13.

61. Kunjir V, Venugopalan A, Chopra A. Profile of Indian patients with juvenile onset chronic inflammatory joint disease using the ILAR classification criteria for JIA: a community-based cohort study. J Rheumatol 2010;37:1756–62.
62. Seth V, Kabra SK, Semwal OP, Jain Y. Clinico-immunological profile in juvenile rheumatoid arthritis—an Indian experience. Indian J Pediatr 1996;63:293–300.
63. Singh S, Salaria M, Kumar L, Minz R, Datta U, Sehgal S. Clinicoimmunological profile of juvenile rheumatoid arthritis at Chandigarh. Indian Pediatr 1999;36: 449–54.
64. Prakash S, Bansal R, Rajagopalan P, Mehra NK, Malaviya AN. Immunological studies in seronegative spondyloarthropathies. Br J Rheumatol 1983;26:146–50.
65. Prakash S, Mehra NK, Malaviya AN. Immunoglobulin A and M deficiency in 'unclassified' HLA B27-related arthropathy. Arthritis Rheum 1983;26:1175–6.
66. Madhavan R, Porkodi R, Rajendran CP, Chandrasekaran AN, Umadevi KR, Alamelu R. IgM, IgG, and IgA response to enterobacteria in patients with ankylosing spondylitis in southern India. Ann N Y Acad Sci 2002;958:408–11.
67. Rodrigues JJ, Joshi VR. Bacterial DNA detection in spondyloarthropathies. Proceedings of International Symposium on Recent Advances in Molecular Biology, Allergy and Immunology, 3–5 September 2000, Baroda, India.
68. Singh AK, Aggarwal A, Chaurasia S, Misra R. Identification of immunogenic HLA-B*27:05 binding peptides of salmonella outer membrane protein in patients with reactive arthritis and undifferentiated spondyloarthropathy. J Rheumatol 2013;40:173–85.
69. Saxena N, Aggarwal A, Misra RN. Is the enthesitis-related arthritis subtype of juvenile idiopathic arthritis a form of chronic reactive arthritis? Rheumatology (Oxford) 2006;45:1129–32.
70. Myles A, Tuteja A, Aggarwal A. Synovial fluid mononuclear cell gene expression profiling suggests dysregulation of innate immune genes in enthesitis-related arthritis patients. Rheumatology (Oxford) 2012;51:1785–9.
71. Rahman MT, Myles A, Gaur P, Misra R, Aggarwal A. TLR4 endogenous ligand MRP8/14 level in enthesitis-related arthritis and its association with disease activity and TLR4 expression. Rheumatology (Oxford) 2014;53:270–4.
72. Myles A, Aggarwal A. Lack of association of single nucleotide polymorphisms in toll-like receptors 2 and 4 with enthesitis related arthritis category of juvenile idiopathic arthritis in Indian population. Rheumatol Int 2013;33:417–21.
73. Myles A, Rahman MT, Aggarwal A. Membrane-bound toll-like receptors are overexpressed in peripheral blood and synovial fluid mononuclear cells of enthesitis-related arthritis category of juvenile idiopathic arthritis (JIA–ERA) patients and lead to secretion of inflammatory mediators. J Clin Immunol 2012;32:488–96.
74. Agarwal S, Misra R, Aggarwal A. TLR ligands induce metalloproteinases expression in human fibroblast like synoviocytes from patients with juvenile idiopathic arthritis. Indian J Med Res 2010;131:771–9.
75. Mahendra A, Misra RN, Aggarwal A. Th1 and th17 predominance in the enthesitis-related arthritis form of juvenile idiopathic arthritis. J Rheumatol 2009;36:1730–6.
76. Chavan H, Samant R, Deshpande A, Mankeshwar R. Correlation of HLA B27 subtypes with clinical features of ankylosing spondylitis. Int J Rheum Dis 2011;14:369–74.
77. Ghosh K, Shankarkumar U, Shetty S, Mohanty D. Chronic synovitis and HLA-B27 in patients with severe haemophilia. Lancet 2003;361:933–4.
78. Thomas R, Philip J, Banerjee M. Association of an extended haplotype of HLA class I alleles and their flanking microsatellites with spondyloarthropathies in South Indian patients. Hum Immunol 2006;67:318–23.
79. Chhaya SU. HLA-B27 polymorphism in Mumbai, western India. Tissue Antigens 2005;66:48–50.
80. Akkoc N, Khan MA. HLA B27 and ankylosing spondylitis. APLAR J Rheumatol 2005;8:146–53.
81. Khan MA. Polymorphism of HLA-B27: 105 subtypes currently known. Curr Rheumatol Rep 2013;15:362.
82. Mehra NK, Taneja V, Jhingan B,Malaviya AN. Evidence to show MHC-linked factors other than HLA-B27 governing susceptibility to spondyloarthropathies in Asian Indians. Asian Pac J Allergy Immunol 1985;3:143–6.
83. Martinez-Borra J, Gonzalez S, López-Vazquez A, et al. HLA-B27 alone rather than B27-related class I haplotypes contributes to ankylosing spondylitis susceptibility. Hum Immunol 2000;61:131–9.
84. Dhurandhar PS, Shankarkumar U. HLA association in seronegative spondyloarthritis patients from Mumbai, India. Int J Hum Genet 2007;7:235–9.
85. Eder L, Chandran V, Pellet F, et al. Human leucocyte antigen risk alleles for psoriatic arthritis among patients with psoriasis. Ann Rheum Dis 2012;71:50–5.
86. Queiro R, Torre JC, González S, López-Larrea C, Tinturé T, López-Lagunas I. HLA- antigens may influence the age of onset of psoriasis and psoriatic arthritis. J Rheumatol 2003;30:505–7.
87. Dalbeth N, Dockerty JL,Williamson L. Influence of HLA-B27 on the clinical presentation of psoriatic arthritis. J Rheumatol 2003;30:2511–12.
88. Liao HT, Lin KC, Chang YT, et al. Human leukocyte antigen and clinical and demographic characteristics in psoriatic arthritis and psoriasis in Chinese patients. J Rheumatol 2008;35:891–5.
89. Brown MA. Genetics of ankylosing spondylitis. Curr Opin Rheumatol 2010;22:126–32.
90. Sheehan NJ. The ramifications of HLA-B27. J R Soc Med 2004 Jan;97(1):10–14.
91. Zachariae H, Overgaard Peterson H, Kissmeyer Nielson F, Lamm L. HLA-antigens in pustular psoriasis. Dermatologica 1977;154:73–7.
92. Sonkar GK, Usha, Singh S. Is HLA-B27 a useful test in the diagnosis of juvenile spondyloarthropathies? Singapore Med J 2008;49:795–9.
93. Shankarkumar U, Ghosh K, MohantyD. HLA B27 polymorphism in western India. Tissue Antigens 2002;60:98–101.
94. Agrawal S, Srivastava R, Sharma B, Pandya S, Misra R, Aggarwal A. IL1RN*2 allele of IL-1 receptor antagonist VNTR polymorphism is associated with susceptibility to ankylosing spondylitis in Indian patients. Clin Rheumatol 2008;27:573–6.
95. Handa R. Rheumatology in postgraduate curriculum. Indian J Rheumatol 2014;9:127–30.
96. Handa R. Rheumatology in India—quo vadis? Nat Rev Rheumatol 2015:11:183–8.
97. International Monetary Fund. Report for Selected Countries and Subjects. 2006. https://www.imf.org/external/pubs/ft/scr/2006/cr06170.pdf.
98. Poverty estimates for 2004–05. Planning Commission, Government of India, 2007. http://planningcommission.nic.in/news/prmar07.pdf.
99. Varma S. India home to a quarter of the world's hungry: Global Hunger Index Report. The Times of India, 14 October 2013. http://timesofindia.indiatimes.com/india/India-home-to-a-quarter-of-the-worlds-hungry-Global-Hunger-Index-report/articleshow/24171694.cms.
100. Saraswathi M. Over 630 million Indians to have health insurance coverage by 2015. Business Standard, 11 October 2012. http://www.business-standard.com/article/pf/over-630-mn-indians-to-have-health-insurance-coverage-by-2015-112101100272_1.html.
101. Malaviya AN, Shankar S, Arya V, et al. Indian Rheumatology Association consensus statement on the diagnosis and treatment of axial spondyloarthropathies. Ind J Rheumatol 2010:5:16–34.
102. Toussirot E, Wendling D. Current guidelines for the drug treatment of ankylosing spondylitis. Drugs 1998:56:225–40.
103. Keat A, Barkham N, Bhalla A, et al. BSR guidelines for prescribing TNF-alpha blockers in adults with ankylosing spondylitis. Rheumatology (Oxford) 2005;44:939–47.
104. Zochling J, van der Heijde D, Burgos-Vargas R, et al. ASAS/EULAR recommendations for the management of ankylosing spondylitis. Ann Rheum Dis 2006:654:442–52.
105. Braun J, van den BR, Baraliakos X, et al. 2010 update of the ASAS/EULAR recommendations for the management of ankylosing spondylitis. Ann Rheum Dis 2011:70:896–904.

106. van Der Heijde D, Sieper J, Maksymowych WP, et al. 2010 Update of the international ASAS recommendations for the use of anti-TNF agents in patients with axial spondyloarthritis. Ann Rheum Dis 2011:70:905–8.
107. Wanders A, Heijde D, Landewe R, et al. Nonsteroidal anti-inflammatory drugs reduce radiographic progression in patients with ankylosing spondylitis: a randomized clinical trial. Arthritis Rheum 2005:52:1756–65.
108. Poddubnyy D, Rudwaleit M, Haibel H, et al. Effect of non-steroidal anti-inflammatory drugs on radiographic spinal progression in patients with axial spondyloarthritis: results from the German Spondyloarthritis Inception Cohort. Ann Rheum Dis 2012:71:1616–22.
109. van Der Heijde D, Baraf HS, Ramos-Remus C, et al. Evaluation of the efficacy of etoricoxib in ankylosing spondylitis: results of a fifty-two-week, randomized, controlled study. Arthritis Rheum 2005:52:1205–15.
110. Fagerli KM, van Der Heijde D, Heiberg MS, et al. Is there a role for sulphasalazine in axial spondyloarthritis in the era of TNF inhibition? Data from the NOR-DMARD longitudinal observational study. Rheumatology (Oxford) 2014:53:1087–94.
111. Ward MM. Sulfasalazine for the treatment of ankylosing spondylitis: relic or niche medication? Arthritis Rheum 2011:63:1472–4.
112. Braun J, van der Horst-Bruinsma I, Huang F, et al. Clinical efficacy and safety of etanercept versus sulfasalazine in patients with ankylosing spondylitis: a randomized, double-blind trial. Arthritis Rheum 2011:63:1543–51.
113. Altan L, Bingol U, Karakoc Y, Aydiner S, Yurtkuran M. Clinical investigation of methotrexate in the treatment of ankylosing spondylitis. Scand J Rheumatol 2001:30:255–9.
114. van Denderen JC, van der Paardt M, Nurmohamed MT, de Ryck YM, Dijkmans BA, van der Horst-Bruinsma IE. Double blind, randomised, placebo controlled study of leflunomide in the treatment of active ankylosing spondylitis. Ann Rheum Dis 2005;64:1761–4.
115. Gonzalez-Lopez L, Garcia-Gonzalez A, Vazquez-Del-Mercado M, Munoz-Valle JF, Gamez-Nava JI. Efficacy of methotrexate in ankylosing spondylitis: a randomized, double blind, placebo controlled trial. J Rheumatol 2004:31:1568–74.
116. Creemers MC, Franssen MJ, van de Putte LB, Gribnau FW, van Riel PL. Methotrexate in severe ankylosing spondylitis: an open study. J Rheumatol 1995:22:1104–7.
117. Anandarajah A, Ritchlin CT. Treatment update on spondyloarthropathy. Curr Opin Rheumatol 2005:17:247–56.
118. Boulos P, Dougados M, Macleod SM, Hunsche E. Pharmacological treatment of ankylosing spondylitis: a systematic review. Drugs 2005:65:2111–27.
119. Malaviya AN, Kapoor S, Garg S, et al. Preventing tuberculosis flare in patients with inflammatory rheumatic diseases receiving tumor necrosis factor-alpha inhibitors in India—an audit report. J Rheumatol 2009;36:1414–20.
120. Malaviya AN, Kapoor S, Garg S, Rawat R. Recommended screening strategy for preventing tuberculosis flare in patients with inflammatory rheumatic diseases receiving tumor necrosis factor-alpha inhibitors in India—follow-up report. J Rheumatol 2010;37:209.
121. Braun J, Sieper J. Therapy of ankylosing spondylitis and other spondyloarthritides: established medical treatment, anti-TNF-alpha therapy and other novel approaches. Arthritis Res 2002;4:307–21.
122. Amor B, Kahan A, Dougados M, Delrieu F. Sulfasalazine and ankylosing spondylitis. Ann Intern Med 1984;101:878.
123. Ferraz MB, Tugwell P, Goldsmith CH, Atra E. Meta-analysis of sulfasalazine in ankylosing spondylitis. J Rheumatol 1990;17:1482–6.
124. Calguneri M, Cobankara V, Ozturk MA, Ertenli I, Kiraz S, Apras S. Combination therapies in spondyloarthropathies. Kobe J Med Sci 2004;50:31–7.
125. Mintz G, Enriquez RD, Mercado U, Robles EJ, Jimenez FJ, Gutierrez G. Intravenous methylprednisolone pulse therapy in severe ankylosing spondylitis. Arthritis Rheum 1981;24:734–6.
126. Richter MB, Woo P, Panayi GS, Trull A, Unger A, Shepherd P. The effects of intravenous pulse methylprednisolone on immunological and inflammatory processes in ankylosing spondylitis. Clin Exp Immunol 1983;53:51–9.
127. Peters ND, Ejstrup L. Intravenous methylprednisolone pulse therapy in ankylosing spondylitis. Scand J Rheumatol 1992;21:134–8.
128. Yoshida S, Motai Y, Hattori H, Yoshida H, Torikai K. A case of HLA-B27 negative ankylosing spondylitis treated with methylprednisolone pulse therapy. J Rheumatol 1993;20:1805–6.
129. Mercado U. The use of methylprednisolone pulse therapy in a severe case of HLA-B27 negative ankylosing spondylitis. J Rheumatol 1994;21:1582–3.
130. Maksymowych WP, Jhangri GS, Leclercq S, Skeith K, Yan A, Russell AS. An open study of pamidronate in the treatment of refractory ankylosing spondylitis. J Rheumatol 1998;25:714–17.
131. Maksymowych WP, Lambert R, Jhangri GS, et al. Clinical and radiological amelioration of refractory peripheral spondyloarthritis by pulse intravenous pamidronate therapy. J Rheumatol 2001;28:144–55.
132. Malaviya AN, Kapoor S, Garg S, Ahmad I, Raja RR. A new strategy of drug treatment in NSAID-unresponsive ankylosing spondylitis: combination of pamidronate and methylprednisolone monthly intravenous infusions on the background of a combination of disease modifying drugs sulfasalazine and methotrexate. J Assoc Physicians Ind 2007;55:193–7.
133. Jones A, Harrison N, Jones T, Rees JD, Bennett AN. Time to diagnosis of axial spondylarthritis in clinical practice: signs of improving awareness? Rheumatology (Oxford) 2014;53:2126–7.
134. Durcan L, Wilson F, Conway R, Cunnane G, O'Shea FD. Increased body mass index in ankylosing spondylitis is associated with greater burden of symptoms and poor perceptions of the benefits of exercise. J Rheumatol 2012;39:2310–14.
135. Busquets-Pérez N, Marzo-Ortega H. How important is early diagnosis of ankylosing spondylitis for therapy in clinical practice? Int J Clin Rheumatol 2012;7:575–8.
136. Heart FD, Robinson KC. Ankylosing spondylitis in women. Ann Rheum Dis 1959;18:15–23.
137. Jones A, Harrison N, Jones T, Rees JD, Bennett AN. Time to diagnosis of axial spondylarthritis in clinical practice: signs of improving awareness? Rheumatology (Oxford) 2014;53:2126–7.
138. Calin A, Elswood J, Rigg S, Skevington SM. Ankylosing spondylitis—an analytical review of 1500 patients: the changing pattern of disease. J Rheumatol 1988;15:1234–8.
139. Feldtkeller E, Khan MA, van Der HD, van Der LS, Braun J. Age at disease onset and diagnosis delay in HLA-B27 negative vs. positive patients with ankylosing spondylitis. Rheumatol Int 2003;23:61–6.
140. Clegg DO. Treatment of ankylosing spondylitis. J Rheumatol Suppl 2006;78:24–31.
141. Rudwaleit M, Claudepierre P, Kron M, Kary S, Wong R, Kupper H. Effectiveness of adalimumab in treating patients with ankylosing spondylitis associated with enthesitis and peripheral arthritis. Arthritis Res Ther 2010;12:R43.
142. Pehlivan Ö, Yalçınkaya Y, Hüseyinsinoğlu N, et al. Spondyloarthropathies (including psoriatic arthritis)—effects of smoking in patients with ankylosing spondylitis and nonradiographic axial spondyloarthritis receiving TNF inhibitors. Rheumatology (Oxford) 2014;53(Suppl 1):i1451.
143. Peters MJ, van der Horst-Bruinsma IE, Dijkmans BA, Nurmohamed NM. Cardiovascular risk profile of patients with spondylarthropathies, particularly ankylosing spondylitis and psoriatic arthritis. Semin Arthritis Rheum 2004;34:585–92.
144. Braun J, Sieper J, Zink A. The risks of smoking in patients with spondyloarthritides. Ann Rheum Dis 2012;71:791–2.
145. Wendling D, Prati C. Spondyloarthritis and smoking: towards a new insight into the disease. Expert Rev Clin Immunol 2013;9: 511–16.
146. Misra A, Shrivastava U. Obesity and dyslipidemia in South Asians. Nutrients 2013;5:2708–33.
147. Wallis D, Haroon N, Ayearst R, Carty A, Inman RD. Ankylosing spondylitis and nonradiographic axial spondyloarthritis: part of a common spectrum or distinct diseases? J Rheumatol 2013;40:2038–41.

Index

Page numbers followed by *b*, *f* or *t* refer to boxes, figures or tables respectively. Alphabetical order is letter-by-letter.

A
abatacept 66–7, 161, 207
abdominal pain 272
absenteeism 107, 255–6
aceclofenac 190*b*
acupuncture 183, 270
acute anterior uveitis (AAU) *see* uveitis
acute phase reactants 22, 103, 106–7, 192, 289
adalimumab
  axSpA/AS 203–4, 270
  IBD 158
  peripheral SpA 33
adaptive immune system 63–7, 155–6
advocacy organizations 259
  ASIF 259–62
  SAA 262–5
aetiology
  genetics 37–42
  infections 71, 75–6, 138
  patient questionnaire on 261
  of uveitis 146
Africa 4, 38
age at onset 37, 93, 137, 267, 271, 280
alternative medicine 182–4, 270, 293
aminopeptidases 38–40, 49, 55, 66, 133, 271–2
Amor criteria 14*t*, 24, 32*t*
anakinra 66, 207
analgesics 189–91
Andersson's lesions 213, 216, 225, 226*f*
animal models of disease *see* HLA-B27 tg rat model; SKG mouse model; TNFΔ^{ARE} mouse model
animals with SpA 1–2
ankylosing spondylitis (AS), definition 19, 91
Ankylosing Spondylitis International Federation (ASIF) 259–62
ankylosing tarsitis 134, 135*f*, 137*f*, 139
anterior chest wall stretch exercise 179*f*
anteroposterior pelvic compression test 96*b*
antibiotics 33–4, 74
antidrug antibodies 204
anti-IL-17 biologics 160–1, 172, 206–7
anti-IL-23/IL-12 biologics 42, 160, 172, 205–6
anti-integrins 158–60
aortitis 7, 94
apremilast 207
ARAD registry (Australia) 235
archaeology 2–4
Argentina 278–9, 281
arthritogenic peptide hypothesis 45, 46–7, 53–5, 74, 76, 156
arthroplasty of the hip 134, 213, 253
ARTIS registry (Sweden) 230–1, 234–5
AS (ankylosing spondylitis), definition 19, 91
ASAS Berlin diagnostic algorithm 25–7
ASAS classification criteria for axSpA 14*t*, 24–5, 118, 269
ASAS classification criteria for peripheral SpA 32–3
ASAS/EULAR recommendations for management of AS 175, 199, 204*f*
ASAS Health Index 104
ASAS outcome measures 102–8, 176*t*, 182, 269
ASAS response/remission criteria 108
ASCEND study 199
ASDAS (Ankylosing Spondylitis Disease Activity Score) 102, 103, 108
Asia
  China 14, 17*t*, 267–70
  epidemiology 14, 16, 267, 271, 291
  HLA-B27 14, 267, 268, 271, 285, 290*t*, 291–2
  India 285–95
  Korea 230, 270–3
ASIF (Ankylosing Spondylitis International Federation) 259–62
ASQoL (Ankylosing Spondylitis Quality of Life Questionnaire) 104
ATG16L1 (autophagy-related protein 16–1) 55, 155
ATTRA registry (Czech) 232, 234
autoantibodies 64–5
autoimmune disease 53
autoinflammatory disease 53
autophagy 55, 155
axis of vision measurement 214, 215*f*

B
back pain
  assessment 103
  in axSpA 16, 19–20, 21, 83, 93, 264
  CAM treatments 183–4
  IBP awareness programmes 261
  indication for surgery 213
  and NSAIDs 21, 189–90
  postoperative 218, 221
  prevalence of IBP 14
bacteria *see* infections; microbiome, gastrointestinal
Bacteroides infections 76
ball exercises 179*f*
balneotherapy 10, 177, 180, 246
bamboo spine 82, 123, 125*f*
  surgery 217, 218, 219
BASDAI (Bath Ankylosing Spondylitis Disease Activity Index) 102, 103
  BASDAI 50 response 108
BASFI (Bath Ankylosing Spondylitis Functional Index) 102, 251–2, 251*b*
BASMI (Bath Ankylosing Spondylitis Metrology Index) 104, 105
B cells 64–5
  depletion with rituximab 161, 207
Bechterew, Wladimir Michailowitsch 5, 6, 10
Behçet's disease 38
BEI (Berlin Enthesitis Index) 106*t*
Berlin diagnostic algorithm 25–7
beta 2-microglobulin (β_2m) 46
BIOBADABRASIL registry (Brazil) 234
BIOBADASER registry (Spain) 231, 233–4, 234
biologics 159*t*, 203*t*
  abatacept 66–7, 161, 207
  antibodies to 204
  anti-IL1 66, 207
  anti-IL6 66, 207
  anti-IL12 42, 160, 172, 203*t*, 205–6
  anti-IL17 160–1, 172, 206–7
  anti-IL23 160, 172, 205–6
  anti-integrins 158–60
  in axSpA/AS 66–7, 203–4, 206, 207, 232–5, 270, 282, 295
  economics 242, 246–7, 295
  in IBD 158–61
  JAK3 inhibitors 160
  in JoSpA 139
  patient registries 230–1, 232–5
  in psoriasis/PsA 160–1, 172, 204, 205, 206, 207
  in reactive arthritis 74
  rituximab 161, 207
  in uveitis 206
  see also tumour necrosis factor inhibitors
biomarkers 281
  acute phase reactants 22, 103, 106–7, 192, 289
  of bone pathology 86, 87, 269
bird-dog exercise 178*f*
bisphosphonates 87, 201, 295
BMD (bone mineral density) 86
BME *see* bone marrow oedema
BMPs (bone morphogenetic proteins) 83, 86, 269

bone
biomarkers 86, 87, 269
degenerative changes 113, 119, 123, 124*f*, 129
normal modelling and remodelling 81, 82*f*
osteoporosis 82, 86–7, 94, 120, 129–30
osteoproliferation 81–6, 87, 135
bone marrow oedema (BME)
on MRI 23, 23*f*, 32, 116, 117, 118
and NSAIDs 190
scoring methods 120
bone mineral density (BMD) 86
bone morphogenetic proteins (BMPs) 83, 86, 269
Brazil 234, 279, 280, 281
bridge exercise 177*f*
brodalumab 203*t*, 207
Brodie, Benjamin Collins 5, 71
Bruckel, Jane 263
BSRBR registry (UK) 231, 232, 233, 234
buttock pain 21

C
calcium pyrophosphate deposition disease (CPPD) 1
Campylobacter infections 30, 71, 138
Canada
epidemiology 15–16, 17*t*
patient registries 230
CARD9 41, 64, 155
cardiovascular disease 7, 94
and NSAIDs 192–3
cardiovascular training 178
car driving 252, 260
cauda equina syndrome 8, 95, 130, 221, 227
MRI 129*f*, 217*f*
CD4+ T cells (T helper cells) 50, 63, 64, 65–6, 205
in IBD 151, 155
CD8+ T cells (cytotoxic) 45, 46, 47, 53, 65, 66, 269
CD163 32, 58–9, 156
CD (Crohn's disease) *see* inflammatory bowel disease
celecoxib 190*b*, 192
certolizumab, in axSpA 203*t*, 204
cervical spine pathology 93, 95, 272
assessment of mobility 105, 214
fractures 94, 95, 222, 223*f*
surgery 216, 216*f*, 218, 220
cervicitis 73
Charlson comorbidity index 107
CHEERS taskforce 244
chest expansion, limitation of 93, 95, 104, 126
chest pain 94
children *see* juvenile-onset spondyloarthritis (JoSpA)
child's pose exercise 178*f*
Chile 279
China 14, 17*t*, 267–70
Chinese medicine 183, 270
chiropractic treatment 183
Chlamydia infections
ankylosing spondylitis 75
reactive arthritis (CiReA) 31, 64, 71, 72–4, 75, 138
CHOP protein 55
circinate balanitis 72, 73
classification
axSpA 13, 14*t*, 23–5, 91, 112, 118
JoSpA 133
peripheral SpA 32–3
psoriasis 167
sacroiliitis grade 19*t*, 112, 118
clazikizumab 203*t*
climate, and rehabilitation 180
clinical features 21–2, 91–6
age at onset 37, 93, 137, 267, 271, 280
in Chinese patients 267–8
extra-articular 22, 94–5, 267, 278, 288
first description of 6
in Indian patients 287–8*t*
JoSpA 94, 134–6, 135*f*, 136*f*, 137*f*, 267–8
JoSpA variant forms 137–9
in Korean patients 271, 272
in Latin American patients 277–8
musculoskeletal manifestations 93–5, 134–6
peripheral SpA 29, 30–1, 31*f*
posture 6*f*, 7*f*, 91*f*, 215*f*
psoriasis 22, 168–9, 168*f*
psoriatic arthritis 138–9, 170–1, 288–9
reactive arthritis 71–2, 73, 138, 289
see also imaging
clinical outcomes/assessment 101–8
ability to work 107–8, 253–6
ASAS/OMERACT core set 102–7, 176*t*, 182, 269
ASDAS score 102, 103, 108
BASDAI 102, 103, 108
comorbidity measures 107
imaging assessment 107, 120–1, 125–7
physical functioning 102, 251–2
psoriasis/PsA 169, 171
QALYs 104–5, 242–3
response and remission criteria 108
spinal mobility/posture 22, 104–5, 213–16
theory 101–2
clinical trials 25, 229–30, 235–6
cohort studies 229
Colombia 279, 280, 281, 282
comorbidities 94–5, 107, 265
'competent patients' 262
complementary medicine 182–4, 270, 293
computed tomography (CT) 113, 113*f*, 217
conjunctivitis 73
Connor, Bernard 4
corticosteroids 273, 294
peripheral SpA 33
uveitis 147–8
cost-effectiveness studies 246–7
cost-of-illness (COI) studies 240–2
costosternal/costovertebral joints 93, 94, 126, 128*f*
costs of healthcare 239–48
India 293, 295
USA 265
cost-utility studies 234, 242–3
counselling *see* patient education
COX-2 inhibitors 190, 192, 193, 246, 294
COX (cyclooxygenase) enzymes 189
cranio-cervical junction 213, 216, 216*f*, 218, 220, 223*f*
C-reactive protein (CRP) 22, 103, 106–7, 192, 289
Crohn's disease (CD) *see* inflammatory bowel disease
CT (computed tomography) 113, 113*f*, 217
CTLA4 antigen 66–7, 161, 207
curdlan 57
see also SKG mouse model
cyclosporin 172
cytokines *see* IL-1; IL-6; IL-10; IL-17; IL-22; IL-23; IL-36; interferon; tumour necrosis factor
cytotoxic T cells (CD8+) 45, 46, 47, 53, 65, 66, 269

D
dactylitis 22, 31, 33*t*, 135*f*
DANBIO registry (Denmark) 231, 232, 233
death rates 96, 222
dectin-1 41, 64, 155
degenerative bone disease
sacroiliac joints 113, 119
spine 123, 124*f*, 129
dendritic cells (DCs) 56–7, 63, 66, 153, 170
Denmark 231
dermatology 72, 73, 135*f*, 169
see also psoriasis
DESIR study 229
developing countries, drug costs 247, 293, 295
DFI (Dougados Functional Index) 251
diagnosis
axSpA 19–27, 91–2, 95–6, 128
Berlin algorithm 25–7
in China 269
delayed/underdiagnosis 13–14, 16, 91–3, 222, 264, 271, 289*t*, 293
differentials 1, 30, 113, 119–20, 129–30, 134, 216
imaging of the SI joints 19, 20*f*, 22–3, 23*f*, 24, 91–2, 111–14, 117–19, 269
imaging of the spine 7, 22, 23, 27, 123–4, 124*f*, 128, 216–17
inflammatory back pain 21, 93
JoSpA 134
in Korea 271
laboratory tests 22, 269
peripheral SpA 30–2
physical examination 21–2, 30, 95
psoriasis 169, 170*f*
red flags 96*b*
spinal fractures 129–30, 216, 222–3
uveitis 22, 145–6, 146*f*
see also classification
diarrhoea 3
diclofenac 189, 190*b*, 191, 192
diffuse idiopathic skeletal hyperostosis (DISH) 128*f*, 129
in the pharaohs 3–4
difluprednate 148
dinosaurs with SpA 2
disease activity measurement 102–3, 108
disease-modifying antirheumatic drugs
biological *see* biologics
synthetic *see* DMARDS
DKK1 (dickkopf-1) 84, 86
DLQI (Dermatology Life Quality Index) 169
DMARDs (disease-modifying antirheumatic drugs) (synthetic)
axSpA/AS 199–201, 270, 294, 295
in combination with TNFi 234–5
JoSpA 139
peripheral SpA 33
psoriatic arthritis 172
reactive arthritis 74
uveitis 147
see also biologics
Doppler ultrasound 114
dorsal lordosating spondylodesis 218–19
driving ability 252, 260
duodenal ulcers 193–4

E
EAMs (extra-articular manifestations) 22, 94–5, 267, 278, 288
see also inflammatory bowel disease; psoriasis; uveitis
early disease see non-radiographic axSpA
E-cadherin 153
economic analysis 239–48
cost-effectiveness studies 246–7
cost-of-illness studies 240–2
cost-utility studies 234, 242–3
methodologies 243–6
treatment costs in India 293, 295
treatment costs in the USA 265
education see patient education
Egypt, ancient 3–4, 8–9
electrophysical agent therapies 181
Elixhauser et al. comorbidity measure 107
emergency medicine 222–3, 227, 263
employment (dis)ability 107–8, 234, 253–6, 264
economic evaluations 240b, 241, 242
employment-related risk factors 231, 253, 255, 256
endoplasmic reticulum stress hypothesis 47–9, 55
ENRADAS trial 191
enteral nutrition 152
enteric infections 71, 72, 75, 76, 138
enthesitis
assessment 105–6
axSpA/AS 22, 94, 96
JoSpA 134
in Latin America 280
peripheral SpA 27, 31–2, 33t
reactive arthritis 72, 73
enthesitis-related arthritis (ERA) 133, 137
see also juvenile-onset spondyloarthritis (JoSpA)
epidemiology
Asia 14, 16, 267, 271, 291
axial SpA/AS 13–17, 92–3, 267, 271, 278–80, 291
gender 16–17, 37, 92–3, 271, 279–80, 289t
HLA-B27 14–15, 37, 38, 267
IBD 30, 151
IBP 14
JoSpA 133, 291
Latin America 278–80
peripheral SpA 30
psoriatic arthritis 170, 267
reactive arthritis 30, 71
registry studies 231–2
spinal fractures 222
uveitis 145
work disability 253–5
EQ-5D (EuroQol Five Dimensions questionnaire) 104, 242–3
ERAP1/ERAP1 (endoplasmic reticulum aminopeptidase 1) 38–40, 49, 55, 66, 133, 156, 271–2
ERAP2/ERAP2 (endoplasmic reticulum aminopeptidase 2) 40, 55, 133
ERASURE trial 206
erythema nodosum 72
erythrocyte sedimentation rate (ESR) 103, 106–7, 289
erythroderma 167, 168f
ESSG criteria (European Spondylarthropathy Study Group) 14t, 24, 32t
ESTHER trial 199–200
etanercept (ETN)
in AxSpA/AS 203–4, 270
in combination with rehabilitation therapy 180–1
compared with SSZ 199–200
cost-effectiveness studies 246–7
in IBD 158
in peripheral SpA 33
in uveitis 147
ethnicity 14–15, 37, 267
in Latin America 277, 278–9, 280
etoricoxib 190–1, 246, 294
Europe
costs 241–2
epidemiology 14, 16, 17t
patient registries 230–1
exercise 176–9, 184, 246, 253
extension in lying exercise 177f
extra-articular manifestations (EAMs) 22, 94–5, 267, 278, 288
see also inflammatory bowel disease; psoriasis; uveitis
eye disease see uveitis

F
FABERE test 96b
facet joint involvement 124, 125f, 126, 128f
faecal microbial transplantation 152
Fagge, Charles Hilton 5
family history 21, 37
fatigue 94, 103
fat metaplasia in SI joints 117, 117f, 118, 121
females
clinical features 93, 279
epidemiology 16–17, 37, 92–3, 271, 279–80, 289t
fibromyalgia 30
fingers, swollen (dactylitis) 22, 31, 33t
Finland 17t, 232
FIXTURE trial 206
flagellins 156
foot
enthesitis 22, 31–2, 94, 134
JoSpA 134, 135f, 137f, 139
peripheral SpA 31f
foot orthotics 139
Forestier's disease (DISH) 128f, 129
in the pharaohs 3–4
fossil record 1–2, 3f
fractures see spinal fractures
Fraenkel, Eugen 7

G
gadolinium-enhanced MRI 23, 114, 118–19, 125
Gaenslen's test 96b
gastrointestinal tract
enteric infections causing ReA/SpA 71, 72, 75, 76, 138
IBD see inflammatory bowel disease
microbiome 50, 55, 75, 76, 152–3, 156, 157, 264
risks of NSAID use 193–4
gender
clinical features 93, 279
epidemiology 16–17, 37, 92–3, 271, 279–80, 289t
genetics 37–42
China 268
ERAP1/ERAP2 38–40, 49, 66, 271–2
family history 21, 37
IBD/SpA overlap 41, 153–6
IL-1 56
IL-23 pathway 40–2, 56, 268
JoSpA 133
Korea 271–2
MHC antigens/HLA-B27 37–8, 45, 167–8, 171–2, 268, 271, 280–1, 292
psoriasis 37, 38, 41–2, 167–8, 170
psoriatic arthritis 37, 38, 171–2, 268
registry studies 232
research sponsored by the SAA 263–4
TNF 56
uveitis 264
geographic prevalence 14–15
GESPIC study 229
glaucoma 145
Glisson, Francis 9
global assessment of disease activity 103
global posture re-education (GPR) therapy 179
golimumab, in AxSpA/AS 203–4, 247, 270
group-based exercises 177, 179
Guatemala 279–80, 280
guselkumab 206
guttate psoriasis 167, 168f

H
H_2 receptor antagonists 193
haemangioma, spinal 129
hamstring stretch exercise 177f
HAQ-S (Health Assessment Questionnaire) 251
Hawthorne effect 229
heart disease 7, 94
and NSAIDs 192–3
heat, therapeutic 180, 181
hedgehog signalling 84
heel enthesitis 22, 31–2, 94, 134
Helicobacter pylori infection 194
hepatitis B (HBV) 270, 272
hepatotoxicity of NSAIDs 194
herbal medicines 183–4, 270
herpes simplex uveitis 146–7
hidradenitis suppurativa (HS) 29t, 30
hip
compensation for kyphosis 213
functional assessment 105
JoSpA 134
pathology 93–4, 134, 253, 271, 277
replacement 134, 213, 253
Hippocratic luxation table 9f
histopathology
bowel inflammation 151, 151f
JoSpA 133–4
peripheral SpA 32, 58–9
psoriasis 169, 170f
SI joints 58, 85f
history, at presentation 21, 30
history, of the disease 1–10, 71
HLA-B27
arthritogenic peptide hypothesis 45, 46–7, 53–5, 74, 76, 156
and AS 38, 45, 49–50, 260–1
in China 14, 267, 268
diagnostic tests for 22, 147, 269
epidemiology 14–15, 37, 38, 267
ERAP1 interaction 38–40, 49, 156
homodimers 47, 55, 66, 156
and IBD 155–6
in India 285, 290t, 291–2
and JoSpA 133
in Korea 271

HLA-B27 (*Cont.*)
in Latin America 280–1
microbial interactions 55, 65, 76, 156
misfolding 47–9, 55, 66, 156, 158
pathogenesis 45–50, 53–5, 63–4, 156
and PsA 38, 50, 171, 292
and ReA 38, 72
structure 47*f*
subtypes 38, 49, 268, 280–1, 292
suppressors and promoters 268
and uveitis 146–7, 147, 291, 292
HLA-B27 tg rat model 47, 55, 63, 152, 157–8
HLA-B60 38
HLA-B alleles in PsA 171–2
HLA-C*06 167–8, 171
HNF4A (hepatocyte nuclear factor 4 alpha) 153
home-based exercises 177, 178, 253
hyperthermy therapy 181

I

IBD *see* inflammatory bowel disease
IBP *see* inflammatory back pain
ibuprofen 190*b*, 192
IFN (interferon) 42, 63, 268
IgA (immunoglobulin A) 153
IL-1 (interleukin-1) 55–6, 66, 207
IL-6 (interleukin-6) 66, 207, 268
IL-10 (interleukin-10) 72, 155
IL-17 (interleukin-17) 56, 57, 59, 65–6, 87, 205
anti-IL-17 treatment 160–1, 172, 206–7
in psoriasis/PsA 160–1, 170, 172, 206–7
IL-22 (interleukin-22) 57, 64
IL-23 (interleukin-23) and IL-23/IL-17 pathway 56–8, 59, 64, 155
anti-IL-23/IL-12 treatment 42, 160, 172, 205–6
and ER stress 48, 55
genetics 40–2, 56, 268
and IBD 155
and JoSpA 133
and psoriasis/PsA 204–5
IL-36 (interleukin-36) 170
ILCs (innate lymphoid cells) 58*t*, 157
NK cells 47, 55
imaging
Andersson's lesions 226*f*
assessment of disease activity 19*t*, 107, 120–1, 125–7
cauda equina syndrome 129*f*, 217*f*
classification criteria 24, 112, 118
differential diagnoses 113, 119–20, 129–30
drawing (17th century) 4*f*
JoSpA 112–13, 113*f*, 119, 135*f*, 136–7, 136*f*, 138*f*
in Korea 272
peripheral SpA 32
SI joints 111–21, 289*t*
SI joints: advanced features 116–17, 116*f*, 117*f*, 135*f*
SI joints: diagnostic 19, 20*f*, 22–3, 23*f*, 24, 91–2, 111–14, 117–19, 269
SI joints: early features 111, 111*f*, 114–16, 116*f*
SI joints: JoSpA 112–13, 113*f*, 119, 135*f*, 136*f*
SI joints: normal 112*f*, 114, 115*f*
SI joints: osteoarthritis/OCI 119, 120*f*
spine *see* spinal imaging
whole-body 125, 138*f*
immune system 268–9, 291
adaptive immunity 63–7, 155–6
aminopeptidases 38–40, 49, 55, 66, 133, 271–2
B cells 64–5
cytokines *see* IL-1; IL-6; IL-10; IL-17; IL-22; IL-23; IL-36; interferon; tumour necrosis factor
dendritic cells 56–7, 63, 66, 153, 170
and IBD/SpA overlap 151, 153–7
immune-mediated inflammatory diseases 53, 54*f*
innate immune system 53–9, 153–5, 156–7
macrophages 32, 56–7, 58–9, 156
T cells *see* T cells
tolerance to the GI microbiome 153
see also HLA-B27
incidence 13
axSpA 16
JoSpA 133
psoriatic arthritis 170
reactive arthritis 30, 71
incremental cost-effectiveness ratio (iCER) 246–7
India 285–95
axSpA/AS 285–8, 291
HLA-B27 285, 290*t*, 291–2
IBD 289–91
JoSpA 291
psoriatic arthritis 288–9, 292
Reiter syndrome 289
treatment 292–5
uveitis 291, 292
indomethacin 190*b*
INFAST trial 189–90
infections
axSpA/AS 74–6
bacterial spondylodiscitis 129
in India 291
JoSpA 75, 133, 138
patient questionnaires 261
psoriasis 169
reactive arthritis 30, 31, 64, 71–4, 138
surgical-site 221
and TNFi treatment 75, 270, 272, 295
uveitis 146–7
see also microbiome, gastrointestinal
inflammatory back pain (IBP)
assessment 103
awareness programmes 261
clinical features 21, 93
NSAIDs 21, 189–90
prevalence 14
inflammatory bowel disease (IBD) 151–61
animal models 157–8
in children 139
epidemiology 30, 151
genetics 41, 153–6
and the GI microbiome 75, 152, 156, 157
histopathology 151, 151*f*
and the immune system 151, 153–7
in India 289–91
pathogenesis 151–7
treatment 152, 158–61
and uveitis 147
infliximab 203*t*
in axSpA/AS 140*f*, 189–90, 203–4, 270
cost of the drug in India 295
cost-effectiveness studies 247
in uveitis 147
information provision 182
by advocacy organizations 260–1, 263
innate immune system 53–9
cytokines *see* IL-1; IL-6; IL-10; IL-17; IL-22; IL-23; IL-36; interferon; tumour necrosis factor
and IBD 153–5, 156–7
macrophages 32, 56–7, 58–9, 156
see also HLA-B27
innate lymphoid cells (ILCs) 58*t*, 157
NK cells 47, 55
inpatient rehabilitation programmes 179–80
insomnia 94
integrins (and anti-integrins) 158–60
interferon (IFN) 42, 63, 268
interleukin-1 (IL-1) 55–6, 66, 207
interleukin-6 (IL-6) 66, 207, 268
interleukin-10 (IL-10) 72, 155
interleukin-17 (IL-17) 56, 57, 59, 65–6, 87, 205
anti-IL-17 treatment 160–1, 172, 206–7
in psoriasis/PsA 160–1, 170, 172, 206–7
interleukin-22 (IL-22) 57, 64
interleukin-23 (IL-23) and IL-23/IL-17 pathway 56–8, 59, 64, 155
anti-IL-23/IL-12 treatment 42, 160, 172, 205–6
and ER stress 48, 55
genetics 40–2, 56, 268
and IBD 155
and JoSpA 133
and psoriasis/PsA 204–5
interleukin-36 (IL-36) 170
intermalleolar distance (IMD) 105
internal rotation of the hip (IHR) 105
International Classification of Disease (ICD) (9th/10th eds) 13
international patient advocacy organizations (ASIF) 259–62
internet as information source 182, 263
inverse psoriasis 167, 168*f*, 169
IRAP (aminopeptidase) 40
iritis 146*f*
see also uveitis
Italy 17*t*, 30
ixekizumab 203*t*, 207

J

JAK3 inhibitors 160
Japan 17*t*
juvenile idiopathic arthritis (JIA) 29, 133, 147
juvenile-onset ankylosing spondylitis 137–8, 147, 231
juvenile-onset psoriatic arthritis (JoPsA) 138–9
juvenile-onset spondyloarthritis (JoSpA) 133–41
in China 267–8
clinical features 94, 134–5, 135*f*, 136*f*, 137*f*, 267–8
epidemiology 133, 291
histopathology 133–4
imaging 112–13, 113*f*, 119, 135*f*, 136–7, 136*f*, 138*f*
in India 291
in Latin America 280
pathogenesis 75, 133
progression 135–6, 280, 281
QoL 136, 141
treatment 139–41
and uveitis 147
variant forms 137–9

K

keratoderma blennorrhagica 73, 135*f*
ketoprofen 190*b*
kidney disease 95, 288
and NSAIDs 194

KIRs (killer-cell immunoglobulin-like receptors) 47, 55, 66
Klebsiella pneumoniae 65, 75–6, 152
knees to chest exercise 176*f*
Koebner phenomenon 168–9
Korea 230, 270–3
kyphosis 7*f*, 91, 91*f*, 93
  assessment of 104–5, 213–16
  corrective surgery 213, 214*f*, 215*f*, 217–21, 227

L
lateral pelvic compression test 96*b*
lateral spinal flexion test 22, 105
Latin America 277–82
  epidemiology 278–80
  HLA-B27 280–1
  patient registries 230, 277–8
  peripheral SpA 277, 280
  treatment 234, 277, 281–2
leflunomide (LFN) 172, 200, 294
LEI (Leeds Enthesitis Index) 106*t*
liver failure, and NSAIDs 194
lobbying 262, 265
longitudinal observational studies 229
  patient registries 229–36
lower limb
  enthesitis 22, 31–2, 94, 134
  JoSpA 134, 135*f*, 137*f*, 139
  peripheral SpA 31*f*
  see also hip
lumbar surgery 218, 220
lung
  comorbidities 94–5
  postoperative embolism 221
lymecycline 74
lymphocytes *see* B cells; T cells

M
macrophages 32, 56–7, 58–9, 156
magnetic resonance imaging (MRI)
  cauda equina syndrome 129*f*, 217*f*
  contrast-enhanced 23, 114, 118–19, 125
  diagnostic 22–3, 24, 117–19, 128
  differential diagnoses 119, 129–30, 216
  JoSpA 119, 136*f*, 137, 138*f*
  peripheral SpA 32
  preoperative 216
  SI joints 114–21
  SI joints: advanced features 116–17, 116*f*, 117*f*
  SI joints: early features 22–3, 24, 114–16, 116*f*
  SI joints: normal 114, 115*f*
  SI joints: scoring of disease 120–1, 121*f*
  spine 124–30
  technical variations 23, 114, 118–19, 124–5
  whole-body imaging 125, 138*f*
major histocompatibility complex (MHC) 37–8, 292
  psoriasis/PsA 167–8, 171–2
  see also HLA-B27
males 16–17, 37, 92–3, 271, 279–80, 289*t*
mammals with SpA 1–2
Marie, Pierre 5–6
MASES (Maastricht Ankylosing Spondylitis Enthesitis Score) 106*t*
massage therapy 183, 270
mast cells 58*t*, 59
MEI (Mander Enthesitis Index) 105, 106*t*
meloxicam 190
men *see* males
mesalazine 200
methotrexate (MTX) 139, 172, 200, 294, 295
Mexico 279, 281
microbiome, gastrointestinal 50, 55, 75, 76, 152–3, 264
  and IBD 75, 152, 156, 157
Middle Eastern archaeology 3–4
minimally invasive dorso-ventral osteotomy and reconstruction 219–20, 219*f*
misoprostol 193–4
mNY (modified New York) criteria 14*t*, 23–4, 112
modified Schober test 22, 104
'Morbus Bechterew' 6–7
mortality rates 96, 222
moxibustion 270
MRI *see* magnetic resonance imaging
mSASSS (modified Stoke Ankylosing Spondylitis Spinal Score) 107, 272
multidisciplinary teams 261–2

N
nails 22, 168, 168*f*
naproxen 190*b*, 192
natalizumab 158–9
natural health products 183–4, 270
natural history *see* progression of disease
natural killer (NK) cells 47, 55
natural killer T (NKT) cells 157
Near Eastern archaeology 3–4
neck pathology 93, 95, 272
  assessment of mobility 105, 213
  fractures 94, 95, 222, 223*f*
  surgery 216, 216*f*, 218, 220
neurological complications
  cauda equina syndrome 8, 95, 129*f*, 130, 217*f*, 221, 227
  due to spinal fractures 82, 95, 222
  postoperative 218, 220
neutrophils 58*t*, 59
NIAMS Coalition (National Institute of Arthritis and Musculoskeletal and Skin Diseases) 265
NK (natural killer) cells 47, 55
NKT (natural killer T) cells 157
NOD2 (nucleotide oligomerization domain 2) 153–5
noggin 84, 84*f*
nomenclature 19
  historical 6, 7, 8
  JoSpA 137
  peripheral SpA 29, 31
  reactive arthritis 71
  uveitis 145
non-pharmacological treatment 175–84
  in children 139
  in China 269, 270
  complementary and alternative medicine 182–4, 270, 293
  cost-effectiveness studies 246
  historical 8–10
  in India 293, 294
  physiotherapy/exercise 10, 139, 175–81, 184, 253, 269, 294
  self-management 181–2, 184
non-radiographic axSpA (nr-axSpA)
  classification/diagnosis 19, 24, 91
  cost-effectiveness studies 247
  epidemiology 16, 17
  imaging 111, 111*f*, 114–16, 116*f*
  in India 288
  public awareness of 262
  treatment 176, 203*t*, 204
non-steroidal anti-inflammatory drugs *see* NSAIDs
NOR-DMARD registry 199, 200, 232, 233, 234, 235
North America
  archaeological record 2–3
  epidemiology 14–16, 17*t*
  patient registries 230, 264
  SAA 262–5
Norway 17*t*
NPEPPS (puromycin-sensitive aminopeptidase) 40, 55
nr-axSpA *see* non-radiographic axSpA
NSAIDs (non-steroidal anti-inflammatory drugs)
  adverse effects 191–4
  as analgesics 189–91
  axSpA/AS 189–94, 269–70, 272, 294
  back pain 21, 189–90
  in China 269–70
  cost-effectiveness studies 246
  disease modification by 191
  drug–drug interactions 194
  in India 294
  and osteoproliferation 84
  patient questionnaires 261
  peripheral SpA 33, 190
  pharmacology 189, 190*b*
nuclear factor κB1 42
nuclear medicine 113–14

O
OASIS study 229
obesity 289*t*
occipito-cervical junction 213, 216, 216*f*, 218, 220, 223*f*
occiput-to-wall distance measurement 104, 105, 215*f*
occupational health
  work disability 107–8, 234, 253–6, 264
  work related risk factors 231, 253, 255, 256
omeprazole 194
OMERACT outcome measures 101, 102–8, 182
online information sources 182, 263
orthopaedists (in India) 293
orthotics 139
OSKAR registry (Korea) 230, 232
osteitis condensans ilii (OCI) 113, 119, 120*f*
osteoarthritis 113, 119, 120*f*
osteoblasts 81, 82*f*
osteochondrosis 129
osteoclasts 82*f*, 87
osteoporosis 82, 86–7, 94, 120, 129–30
osteoproliferation 81–6, 87, 135
osteotomy, spinal 215*f*, 216*f*, 217–21, 227, 253
outcome measures (clinical assessment) 101–8
  ability to work 107–8, 253–6
  ASAS/OMERACT core set 102–7, 176*t*, 182, 269
  comorbidity 107
  imaging assessment 107, 120–1, 125–7
  physical functioning 102, 251–2
  psoriasis/PsA 169, 171
  QALYs 104–5, 242–3
  response and remission criteria 108
  spinal mobility/posture 22, 104–5, 213–16
  theory 101–2
overweight patients 289*t*

P

paediatrics *see* juvenile-onset spondyloarthritis (JoSpA)
pain *see* back pain
pain relief 189–91
palaeontology 1–2, 3*f*
pamidronate 201, 295
paraspinal muscles 93
PASI (Psoriasis Area and Severity Index) 169
pathogenesis
  arthritogenic peptide hypothesis 45, 46–7, 53–5, 74, 76, 156
  B cells 64–5
  Chinese studies 267, 268–9
  ERAP1/ERAP2 38–40, 49, 55, 66, 133, 156
  GI microbiome 50, 55, 75, 76, 152–3
  HLA-B27 38–40, 45–50, 53–5, 63–4, 156
  homodimer hypothesis 47, 55, 66, 156
  IBD 151–7
  IL-23/IL-17 pathway 40–2, 48, 55, 56–8, 59, 64, 87
  Indian studies 291
  infections 64, 65, 72, 73, 74–6, 156
  JoSpA 75, 133
  misfolding hypothesis 47–9, 55, 66, 156, 158
  psoriasis 170
  psoriatic arthritis 171–2
  reactive arthritis 64, 152
  T cells *see* T cells
  TNF 56, 64, 158, 170
patient education
  advocacy organizations 261, 263
  role in disease management 178, 181–2, 184, 269
  vocational counselling 256
patient global assessment 103
patient history 21, 30
patient registries 229–36
  compared with RCTs 229–30, 235–6
  disease-based 230, 277–8, 280
  medication-based 230–1
  research using 231–6, 264
patient self-management 181–2, 184, 262
patient support/advocacy 259
  ASIF 259–62
  SAA 262–5
Patrick's test 96*b*
pedicle subtraction osteotomy 218
pelvic tilt exercise 177*f*
peptic ulcers 193–4
peripheral arthritis
  in axSpA 22, 94, 105, 271, 289*t*
  in JoSpA 134
peripheral spondyloarthritis (SpA) 29–34
  histopathology 32, 58–9
  in Latin America 277, 280
  treatment 33, 190, 203*t*
  see also psoriatic arthritis (PsA); reactive arthritis (ReA)
PGA (physician global assessment) 103, 169
phenylbutazone 190*b*
physical examination 21–2, 30, 95
physical functioning 251–3, 264
  assessment 102, 251–2
  in JoSpA 141
physician global assessment 103, 169
physiotherapy 10, 139, 175–81, 184, 253
  in China 269
  cost-effectiveness study 246
  in India 294
Pilates exercises 179
piroxicam 190*b*
plaque-type psoriasis *see* psoriasis
PMM1A (protein phosphatase magnesium-dependent 1A) autoantibodies 65
political engagement 262, 265
posture
  analysis of spinal deformity 104–5, 213–16
  correct 176*f*
  examples of axSpA 6*f*, 7*f*, 91*f*, 214*f*, 215*f*, 219*f*
prednisolone acetate 147–8
pregnancy 260
presenteeism 107, 256
prevalence
  axSpA 15–17, 267, 271
  definition 13
  HLA-B27 14–15, 37, 38, 267
  inflammatory back pain 14
  JoSpA 133
  peripheral SpA 30
  psoriatic arthritis 170, 267
  work disability 253–5
progression of the disease 93, 116–17, 123
  affected by NSAIDs 191
  JoSpA 135–6
PROMIS questionnaire 251
prostaglandins 41, 191
proton pump inhibitors (PPIs) 194
PsA *see* psoriatic arthritis
PSOAS registry (North America) 230, 231–2
psoriasis 167–70
  classification 167
  clinical features 22, 168–9, 168*f*
  diagnosis 169, 170*f*
  genetics 37, 38, 41–2, 167–8, 170
  histopathology 169, 170*f*
  pathogenesis 170
  treatment 205–6, 206
psoriatic arthritis (PsA) 170–2
  axial PsA compared to primary AS 171
  epidemiology 170, 267
  genetics 37, 38, 171–2, 268
  and HLA-B27 38, 50, 171, 292
  in India 288–9, 292
  juvenile-onset 138–9
  pathogenesis 171–2
  treatment 159*t*, 160–1, 172, 203*t*, 204, 206, 207
  and uveitis 147
PSUMMIT1/PSUMMIT2 trials 206
PTGER4 (prostaglandin receptor) 41, 191
publications by advocacy organizations 260–1, 263
public awareness of axSpA 262, 263
pulmonary comorbidities 94–5
pulmonary embolism (postoperative) 221
PULSAR registry (USA) 230
pustular psoriasis 168, 168*f*, 170

Q

quadriceps stretch exercise 179*f*
quality of life (QoL)
  assessment 103–4, 169, 242–3
  in axSpA/AS 243, 264–5, 270
  cost per QALY 246
  in JoSpA 136, 141
  in psoriasis 167, 169

R

RA *see* rheumatoid arthritis
radiographic axSpA (r-axSpA) *see* ankylosing spondylitis
radiography
  classification criteria 19*t*, 112
  differential diagnoses 113
  history of 7
  JoSpA 112–13, 135*f*, 136–7
  preoperative 216
  SI joints 19, 20*f*, 22, 91–2, 111–13, 111*f*, 112*f*, 135*f*
  spine 22, 107, 123–4, 124*f*, 125*f*, 272
radionuclide scans 113–14
radiotherapy 10
Ramses II, mummy of 4*f*
randomized clinical trials (RCTs) 25, 229–30, 235–6
RASSS (Radiographic Ankylosing Spondylitis Spinal Score) 107
RDCI (Rheumatic Diseases Comorbidity Index) 107
reactive arthritis (ReA) 29*t*
  clinical features 71–2, 73, 138, 289
  epidemiology 30, 71
  and HLA-B27 38, 72
  in India 289
  infections triggering 30, 31, 64, 71–4, 138
  juvenile-onset 138
  pathogenesis 64, 152
  pathophysiology 72, 73
  progression to chronic SpA 74–5
  treatment 33–4, 73–4
rectal ulcers 291
red eye 145
referral
  to ophthalmology 145
  to rheumatology 20, 293
REGISPONSER registry (Spain) 230, 231
registries *see* patient registries
rehabilitation 175, 179–80, 184
  in combination with TNFi therapy 180–1
  vocational 256
Reiter syndrome 71, 289
  see also reactive arthritis
remission criteria 108
remission in peripheral SpA 31
renal disease 95, 288
  and NSAIDs 194
reptiles with SpA 1, 2, 3*f*
RESPONDIA registry (Ibero-American) 230, 277–8, 280
response and remission criteria 108
retrodental cysts 220
rheumatoid arthritis (RA)
  compared with peripheral SpA 32, 171
  cost-of-illness studies 241
  treatment 184, 203, 234
'rheumatoid spondylitis' 8
rituximab 161, 207
ROB-FIN registry (Finland) 232
Russia 5, 17*t*

S

SAA (Spondylitis Association of America) 262–5
sacroiliac (SI) joints 111–21, 289*t*
  advanced features on imaging 116–17, 116*f*, 117*f*, 135*f*

corticosteroid injections 273
diagnostic imaging 19, 22–3, 23*f*, 24, 91–2, 111–14, 117–19, 269
early features on imaging 111, 111*f*, 114–16, 116*f*
fat metaplasia 117, 117*f*, 118, 121
JoSpA 112–13, 119, 134, 135*f*, 136*f*
MRI scoring of lesions 120–1, 121*f*
normal 112*f*, 114, 115*f*
osteoarthritis/OCI 119, 120*f*
physical examination 95, 96*b*
radiographic grading of lesions 19*t*, 20*f*, 112
reactive arthritis 73
sacrum, surgery 220–1
Salmonella infections 30, 71, 72, 138, 234
SAPHO syndrome 29*t*
sarilumab 207
scalp psoriasis 168, 168*f*
Scandinavia
epidemiology 16, 17*t*, 38
registries 230–1
Scheuermann's disease 129
Schlayer, C. R. 7
Schober test (modified) 22, 104
scintigraphy 113–14
scleritis 145, 145*f*
sclerostin 84, 86
SCQM registry (Switzerland) 232, 233
secukinumab (SEC)
in AxSpA/AS 161, 203*t*, 207
in IBD 160, 206
in psoriasis/PsA 160–1, 206–7
in uveitis 206
self-administered comorbidity questionnaire 107
self-management 181–2, 184, 262
septic arthritis 113, 119–20
'seronegative spondyloarthropathy' 8, 64
see also ankylosing spondylitis
sex *see* gender
sexually transmitted infections *see Chlamydia* infections
SF-6D (short form 6D) 242–3
SF-36 (36-item Short-Form Health Survey) 104, 252
SFI (San Francisco Enthesitis Index) 106*t*
Shigella infections 71, 72
shoulder 94
sick leave 107, 255–6
SI joints *see* sacroiliac (SI) joints/sacroiliitis
SIRAS registry (Scotland) 230
SKG mouse model 57, 64, 148, 158
skin conditions 72, 73, 135*f*, 169
see also psoriasis
sleep disturbance 94, 95
Smith-Petersen osteotomy 218
smoking 253, 289*t*
social outcomes 182
ability to work 107–8, 253–6
societal costs of healthcare 240, 242–3
South America *see* Latin America
SPACE cohort 25–6
Spain 230, 231
SPARCC Enthesitis Index 106*t*
SPARCC registry (Canada) 230, 232
SPARCC scoring of SI joint disease 120, 121, 121*f*
SPARTAN group 230, 263
spa therapy 10, 177, 180, 246
spinal cord damage
cauda equina syndrome 8, 95, 129*f*, 130, 217*f*, 221, 227
fracture-associated 82, 95, 222
surgical complications 221
spinal degenerative disease 123, 124*f*, 129
spinal fractures 82, 94, 95, 222–7
Andersson's lesions 213, 216, 225, 226*f*
diagnosis/imaging 120, 129–30, 216, 222–3, 223*f*, 224*f*
management 223–5
patient survey 261
prevention 225–7
spinal imaging 123–30
assessment of disease activity 107, 125–7, 272
diagnosis of axSpA 7, 22, 23, 27, 123–4, 124*f*, 128, 216–17
diagnosis of fractures 120, 129–30, 216, 222–3, 223*f*, 224*f*
differential diagnoses 128*f*, 129–30, 129*f*
facet joints 124, 125*f*, 126, 128*f*
JoSpA 136*f*, 138*f*
preoperative 216–17
spondylitis 125–6, 126*f*, 127*f*
syndesmophytes 123, 124*f*, 125*f*
spinal (im)mobility
assessment 22, 103, 104–5, 213–16
characteristics 82–3, 93, 253
in diagnosis of axSpA 21–2, 95
examples 6*f*, 7*f*, 91*f*, 215*f*
spinal manipulation 183
spinal osteoporosis 82, 86–7, 94, 129
spinal pain *see* back pain
spinal surgery 213–27, 253
and cauda equina syndrome 227
complications 221
to correct deformity 215*f*, 216*f*, 217–21, 219*f*, 227
to delay progression 213, 214*f*
fracture management 225
planning 213–17
Spondylitis Association of America (SAA) 262–5
spondylitis, imaging 125–6, 126*f*, 127*f*
spondylodiscitis
abacterial 95, 126
Andersson's lesions 213, 216, 225, 226*f*
bacterial 129
spondylophytes 123, 124*f*, 129
SSATG registry 232, 234
STAT3/STAT3 155, 160
steroids *see* corticosteroids
Straight Talk on Spondylitis (SAA) 263
streptococcal infections 169
Strümpell, Adolf 5
sulfasalazine (SSZ) 295
axSpA/AS 199–200, 270, 294, 295
peripheral SpA 33
reactive arthritis 74
uveitis 147
supervised exercises 177, 179
surgery 213–27, 253
and cauda equina syndrome 227
complications 221
to correct deformity 215*f*, 216*f*, 217–21, 219*f*, 227
to delay progression 213, 214*f*
fracture management 225
planning 213–17
Sweden 17*t*, 230–1
syndesmophytes 22, 123, 124*f*, 125*f*
osteoproliferation 81–6, 87, 135
synovitis 32, 33*t*

T
Tai Chi 179
tarsitis 134, 135*f*, 137*f*, 139
TASC (Australo-Anglo-American Spondylitis Consortium) 264
T cell co-stimulation blockade (abatacept) 66–7, 161, 207
T cells
and biologic therapies 66–7
CD4+/Th17 (T helper cells) 50, 63, 64, 65–6, 151, 155, 157, 205
CD8+ (cytotoxic) 45, 46, 47, 53, 65, 66, 269
γδ cells 59, 157
and HLA-B27 45, 46, 47, 66
in IBD 151, 155, 157
ILCs 58*t*, 157
NKT cells 157
in psoriasis 170
terminology 19
historical 6, 7, 8
JoSpA 137
peripheral SpA 29, 31
reactive arthritis 71
uveitis 145
thalidomide 201, 270
thermotherapy 181
thoracic expansion, limitation of 93, 95, 104, 126
thoracic kyphosis *see* kyphosis
thoracic rotation exercise 179*f*
thoracic spinal fractures 224*f*, 226*f*
TLR4 (Toll-like receptor) 155, 291
TNF (tumour necrosis factor) 56, 64, 158, 170
TNFΔ^{ARE} mouse model 64, 157, 158
TNFi *see* tumour necrosis factor inhibitors
tobacco use 253, 289*t*
tocilizumab 207
toes, swollen (dactylitis) 22, 31, 33*t*, 135*f*
tofacitinib 160
Toronto University Health Network Spondylitis Program 230
'total care' 259
traditional Chinese medicine 183, 270
tragus-to-wall distance measurement 104–5
transcutaneous electrical nerve stimulation (TENS) 181
trauma *see* spinal fractures
treatment (*see also* biologics; DMARDs; non-pharmacological treatment; NSAIDs; surgery)
in antiquity/history 8–10
ASAS/EULAR recommendations 175, 199, 204*f*
bisphosphonates 87, 201, 295
in China 269–70
corticosteroids 33, 147–8, 273, 294
costs 265, 293, 295
IBD 152, 158–61
in India 292–5
JoSpA 139–41
in Korea 272–3
in Latin America 234, 277, 281–2
osteoporosis 87
osteoproliferation 84–5, 87
peripheral SpA 33, 190, 203*t*
psoriasis/PsA 159*t*, 160–1, 172, 204, 205, 206, 207
reactive arthritis 33–4, 73–4
response criteria 108
thalidomide 201, 270

treatment (*Cont.*)
 uveitis 147–8, 206
tuberculosis 270, 272, 295
tumour necrosis factor (TNF) 56, 64, 158, 170
tumour necrosis factor inhibitors (TNFi)
 in axSpA/AS 159*t*, 203–4, 270, 282, 295
 in combination with DMARDs 234–5
 in combination with NSAIDs 189–90
 in combination with rehabilitation therapies 180–1
 compared to DMARDS 199–200, 200
 cost-effectiveness studies 246–7
 dose reduction 247
 effectiveness 232
 in IBD 158
 infections in patients treated with 75, 270, 272, 295
 in JoSpA 139
 and osteoporosis 87
 and osteoproliferation 84, 85
 outcomes in AS and RA compared 234
 in peripheral SpA 33
 prediction of response 204, 232–3
 in psoriasis/PsA 159*t*, 172, 204
 in reactive arthritis 74
 safety 204, 233–4, 235
 switching to another TNFi 233
 in uveitis 147
twin studies 37

U
UK 230, 231
ulcerative colitis *see* inflammatory bowel disease
ultrasonography 27, 114, 137
undifferentiated SpA 31, 32, 137, 267, 281, 285, 292
unfolded protein response (UPR) 48, 55, 66, 155
urethritis 71, 73
urogenital infections *see Chlamydia* infections
USA
 early terminology 8
 epidemiology 14–15, 17*t*
 healthcare costs 265
 patient registries 230, 264
 SAA 262–5
ustekinumab (UST) 42, 160, 172, 203*t*, 205–6
uveitis 8, 145–8
 appearance 146*f*
 diagnosis 22, 145–6
 genetics 264
 and HLA-B27 146–7, 147, 291, 292
 in India 291, 292
 in Korea 271
 in Latin America 278
 and other EAMs 147
 in reactive arthritis 73
 treatment 147–8, 206

V
vedolizumab 159–60
venereal infections *see Chlamydia* infections
Venezuela 281
vertebral fractures *see* spinal fractures
vision, axis of vision measurement 214, 215*f*
vitamin D 87
Vitruvian Man (da Vinci) 21*f*
vocational counselling 256

W
Wenzel, Carl 4–5, 10
whole-body imaging 125, 138*f*
Wnt proteins/signalling 83–4, 86
women *see* females
work (dis)ability 107–8, 234, 253–6, 264
 economic evaluations 240*b*, 241, 242
work instability 255
work-related risk factors 231, 253, 255, 256
wound infections, surgical 221

X
X-rays *see* radiography

Y
Yersinia infections 71, 72, 75, 138

www.ingramcontent.com/pod-product-compliance
Lightning Source LLC
Chambersburg PA
CBHW082037231224
19443CB00004B/39

9 780198 734444